An Introduction to Children with Language Disorders

Related Titles

Oral Motor Assessment and Treatment:
Ages and Stages
Diane Chapman Bahr
ISBN: 0-205-29786-2

Articulatory and Phonological Impairments:
A Clinical Focus, Second Edition
Jacqueline Bauman Waengler
ISBN: 0-205-40248-8

The Development of Language,
Fifth Edition
Jean Berko-Gleason
ISBN: 0-205-31636-0

Language and Communication Disorders
in Children, Fifth Edition
Deena K. Bernstein and Ellenmorris Tiegerman-Farber
ISBN: 0-205-33635-3

Articulation and Phonological Disorders,
Fifth Edition
John E. Bernthal and Nicholas W. Bankson
ISBN: 0-205-34790-8

Discourse Impairments: Assessment
and Intervention Applications
Lynn S. Bliss
ISBN: 0-205-33407-5

The Hispanic Child: Speech, Language,
Culture, and Education
Alejandro E. Brice
ISBN: 0-205-29530-4

Language and Reading Disabilities
Hugh W. Catts and Alan G. Kamhi
ISBN: 0-205-27088-3

Clinical Management of Communication Disorders
in Culturally Diverse Children
Thalia J. Coleman
ISBN: 0-205-26724-6

Stuttering Therapy: Rationale and Procedures
Hugo H. Gregory with chapters by June H. Campbell,
Carolyn B. Gregory, and Diane G. Hill
ISBN: 0-205-34415-1

Diagnosis and Evaluation in Speech Pathology,
Sixth Edition
William O. Haynes and Rebekah H. Pindzola
ISBN: 0-205-38669-5

Born to Talk: An Introduction to Speech
and Language Development, Third Edition
Lloyd M. Hulit and Merle R. Howard
ISBN: 0-205-34296-5

Patterns of Narrative Discourse: A Multicultural,
Life Span Approach
Allyssa McCabe and Lynn S. Bliss
ISBN: 0-205-33869-0

Supporting Children with Communication Difficulties in
Inclusive Settings: School-Based Language Intervention,
Second Edition
Linda McCormick, Diane Frome Loeb,
and Richard L. Schiefelbusch
ISBN: 0-205-37954-0

The Supervisory Process in Speech-
Language Pathology and Audiology
Elizabeth S. McCrea and Judith A. Brasseur
ISBN: 0-205-33662-0

Childhood Language Disorders in Context:
Infancy through Adolescence, Second Edition
Nickola W. Nelson
ISBN: 0-205-19787-6

Language Development: An Introduction, Fifth Edition
Robert E. Owens
ISBN: 0-205-31926-2

Language Disorders: A Functional Approach
to Assessment and Intervention, Fourth Edition
Robert E. Owens
ISBN: 0-205-38153-7

Introduction to Communication Disorders: A Life Span
Perspective, Second Edition
Robert E. Owens Jr., Dale Evan Metz, and Adelaide Haas
ISBN: 0-205-36012-2

Communication and Communication Disorders:
A Clinical Introduction, Second Edition
Elena Plante and Pelagie M. Beeson
ISBN: 0-205-38922-8

Human Communication Disorders, Sixth Edition
George H. Shames and Noma B. Anderson
ISBN: 0-205-33706-6

Clinical Phonetics, Third Edition
Lawrence D. Shriberg and Raymond D. Kent
ISBN: 0-205-36833-6

Exploring Communication Disorders: A 21st Century
Introduction through Literature and Media
Dennis C. Tanner
ISBN: 0-205-37360-7

Speech, Language, Learning, and
the African American Child
Jean E. Van Keulen, Gloria Toliver Weddington,
and Charles E. DeBose
ISBN: 0-205-15268-6

For further information on these and other related titles, contact:
College Division
ALLYN AND BACON
75 Arlington Street, Suite 300
Boston, MA 02116
www.ablongman.com

THIRD EDITION

An Introduction to Children with Language Disorders

Vicki A. Reed

The University of Sydney
and James Madison University

Boston ■ New York ■ San Francisco
Mexico City ■ Montreal ■ Toronto ■ London ■ Madrid ■ Munich ■ Paris
Hong Kong ■ Singapore ■ Tokyo ■ Cape Town ■ Sydney

Executive Editor and Publisher: *Stephen D. Dragin*
Senior Editorial Assistant: *Barbara Strickland*
Manufacturing Buyer: *Andrew Turso*
Marketing Manager: *Kris Ellis-Levy*
Cover Designer: *Joel Gendron*
Production Coordinator: *Pat Torelli Publishing Services*
Editorial-production Service: *Omegatype Typography, Inc.*
Electronic Composition: *Omegatype Typography, Inc.*

For related titles and support materials, visit our online catalog at www.ablongman.com.

Previous editions of this book were published © 1994, 1986 by Macmillan College Publishing Company, Inc.

To obtain permission(s) to use material from this work, please submit a written request to Allyn and Bacon, Permissions Department, 75 Arlington Street, Boston, MA 02116 or fax your request to 617-848-7320.

Between the time Website information is gathered and then published, it is not unusual for some sites to have closed. Also, the transcription of URLs can result in unintended typographical errors. The publisher would appreciate notification where these errors occur so that they may be corrected in subsequent editions.

Library of Congress Cataloging-in-Publication Data

Reed, Vicki.

    An introduction to children with language disorders / Vicki A. Reed.—3rd ed.
      p. cm.
    Includes bibliographical references and index.
    ISBN 0-205-42042-7
      1. Language disorders in children.   I. Title.

RJ496.L35R44 2005
618.92'855—dc22

                                             2004047834

Printed in the United States of America

10 9 8 7 6 5 4 3 2 1   08 07 06 05 04

To Bob, Mariana, and the other mentors
for their support, wisdom, guidance,
and with some, their unfailing love

CONTENTS

7   Language and Children with Autism   253
Steven H. Long

10   Children with Acquired Language Disorders   335

Steven H. Long

PREFACE

This book is about children who do not acquire language normally. The text is an introductory book intended primarily for students who are learning about children with language disorders in order to assist them. Individuals who currently work with such children will also find valuable information in the book.

Children who have problems acquiring language do not have easy access to the most powerful and important human ability—language. Language affects educational achievements, human relationships, and entire lifestyles, yet most of us rarely think about our language abilities. We take our language skills very much for granted, until they are lost to us or disrupted, until they are lost to or disrupted in our loved ones, until we see children with language disorders struggle with their learning and their friendships, or until we see the consequences of language disorders in adolescents' lives. A language disorder in a child can alter the child's relationships with caregivers, undermine academic success, disturb interpersonal relationships, limit vocational possibilities, and generally isolate the child from the mainstream of society.

In this third edition, we have continued to organize the book into three parts. Part One consists of two overview/review chapters on aspects of normal language, one on the bases of language and communication and the other on normal language development in children. For some readers, these will serve as a review; for others, these will provide an introductory background for the chapters in the two later parts of the book.

In Part Two, we retained from the second edition of the book the nine chapters that focus on the language difficulties of different populations of children. Some of the populations discussed in these chapters are defined by the age of the children, for example, preschoolers; others are defined by the "etiological" or concomitant condition of the children's language difficulties, for example, autism. We look at language associated with learning disability, intellectual disability, autism, auditory impairment, and linguistic and cultural diversity. There are also chapters on children with acquired language disorders, young children with specific language impairment, and adolescents with language impairment, as well as a chapter looking at language of other special populations of children, such as gifted children and those with cleft palate. Together, these nine chapters cover the language characteristics of a wide range of children with language problems, some of whom are often overlooked in books about children's language disorders. The chapters also include intervention implications for the various populations of children.

More detailed discussions of language intervention are presented in Part Three, which consists of three chapters. The first of these is a chapter about augmentative and alternative communication as it relates to children with language disorders and their intervention. Two chapters follow. One deals with language assessment and another covers many of the procedures used and factors considered in intervention with children with language disorders.

In revising the book we have updated the information to reflect current knowledge. Because some new knowledge leads to changes in terminology, new terminology appears in this edition. For example, *mental retardation* has been replaced by *intellectual disability,* and *bilingual-bicultural* by *linguistically-culturally diverse.* The order in which some chapters appear in the book has also changed. The chapters on language and learning disability and adolescents with language impairment follow sequentially the chapter on toddlers and preschoolers with specific language impairment. In light of what we now know about specific language impairment in young children and the characteristics of the children as they mature, we believed this sequence of chapters better reflects the "natural history" of what is potentially a debilitating, insidious, and life-long disability. We have combined information in the background or review chapters into two instead of three chapters. This made space for a new chapter on augmentative and alternative communication considerations for children with language disorders. Such a chapter in a book on child language disorders is unique. However, its inclusion reflects the shifts in thinking and knowledge that have taken place with regard to facilitating communication and language in children. In this third edition, we believe we have retained what were the unique features of the previous edition and added others.

Acknowledgments

The assistance of a number of people was invaluable in revising this book, more than can be named in the available space. In particular, however, our reviewers—Pamela R. Gardner, Marshall University; Patricia Lohman-Hawk, New Mexico State University; Dennis M. Ruscello, West Virginia University; and Janice M. Wright, Ohio University—offered suggestions and comments that helped improve this edition. Others helped maintain a balance in our lives during the revision, especially when it seemed like we might lose our balance. These are the really important people in our private lives, and we thank you.

Vicki A. Reed

1

Language and Human Communication

An Overview

VICKI A. REED   **ELISE BAKER**

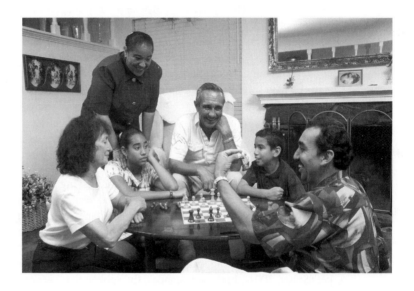

OBJECTIVES

After reading this chapter you should be able to discuss

- Communication, language, and speech, and understand the difference between them
- Extralinguistic aspects of communication, including paralinguistics, nonlinguistics, and metalinguistics
- The phonological, semantic, syntactic, morphological, and pragmatic components of oral language
- Various communication modes
- Biological, cognitive, and social bases of human communication

Have you ever stopped to think about what occurs when two people talk to each other? Usually, one person speaks while the other person listens. The speaker encodes thoughts into mental representations of words and sentences and these into a continuous stream of speech sounds or acoustic energy. The speech sounds travel through the air in the form of sound waves (acoustic energy) and reach the listener's ear. The listener then decodes the sound wave into a stream of speech sounds, and the speech sounds into the intended string of words, and the string of words miraculously into what the speaker originally thought. A breakdown in any step along the way may result in miscommunication or even a failure to communicate. Importantly, both the speaker and the listener must share the same code or symbolic system of what sounds and words represent what thoughts. Put simply, they must share the same language.

This book is concerned with the symbolic process of communication called language and the ways in which children do or do not use it. Before we can examine children's language disorders, however, we, like the speaker and the listener, must share the same language. Therefore, the purpose of this chapter is to overview for the reader the foundations of human communication and other topics that provide a platform for discussing children's language disorders. We discuss the terms *communication, language, speech,* and *extralinguistic elements of communication,* and we look at the different components of language and the relationship between understanding and using language. We also consider different communication modes. Finally, we review some of the biological, cognitive, and social bases of human communication.

Communication

Communication refers to the sending and receiving of messages, information, ideas, or feelings (Hulit & Howard, 2002). It is a broad term that not only encompasses the physical production of speech and the symbolic nature language, but any behavior or action that conveys a message. For example, a sneeze may convey a message that a person has a head cold (Crystal & Varley, 1998). A baby's cry conveys needs or discomforts that require attention, such as feeding, holding, changing a diaper, a need for a different position, or an extra blanket (Solter, 2001). In these instances, the spoken word is not essential.

Communication is not limited to humans. Other animals communicate. Unlike other animals, however, humans have the ability to communicate highly complex thoughts, feelings, and ideas through the use of language. Humans also have the capacity for speech. Extralinguistic behaviors, which will be discussed below, additionally contribute to the communicative process.

Language

Language is a code in which we make specific symbols stand for something else. Bloom (1988) defines language as "a code whereby ideas about the world are represented through a conventional system of arbitrary signals for communication" (p. 2). According to this definition, coded symbols refer to real things, concepts, or ideas, and the things that the symbols represent are the *referents.* In the English code there is no reason why an animal with four legs that is noted for tail wagging and barking is labeled a *dog.* Such an animal could as easily be coded as a *sloot*—and perhaps it is, in a code system other than English. Although the symbols are arbitrary, the symbols and their appropriate referents must be mutually agreed on by members of a community using the code if the code is to be meaningful. In this sense, language is a *convention* (Bloom, 1988).

Language is also a system in which *rules* or regularities guide what coded symbols may be combined with other symbols and in what order, and what symbols can be used in what situations. These rules or regularities are predictable and can be used to identify what are and are not acceptable uses of language. For example, in the English language the word order in the sentence, "The ball is not red," is acceptable and considered correct, whereas the word order in the sentence, "The ball not is red," violates accepted rules even though the words in the two sentences are identical.

The number of rules that delimit a language is finite. Once these finite rules are learned, however, a person can generate an infinite variety of meaningful messages by combining and recombining the symbols according to the agreed-on rules. The system of rules that results in the ability to produce an infinite number of expressions gives language its creative feature. By applying systematic rules, a language user can generate expressions never used or heard before, and another user of the same language can understand those expressions by employing the same rules. Think for a moment about a conversation you had today. Chances are, you created a sentence never spoken or written before, and you heard or read a sentence that had never been spoken or written before.

Because a language consists of regularities or sets of rules, members of a language community (including children) must learn the rules and induce the regularities in order to use the language. Among the rules that must be learned are those that determine who can say what to whom and how. Language is, therefore, a *learned* or acquired behavior.

The ability to learn language is considered an innate human ability. As Hulit and Howard (2002) point out, most human babies are "born with the *capacity* to use language in the same way that a spider is born with the ability to weave a web and a bird is born with the ability to make a nest" (p. 3). However, this does not mean that infants use language automatically. Given their innate capacity for language, they still need to *learn* the language or code of the linguistic community in which they are reared. They need to learn about the various aspects of language, including *form* (syntax, morphology, phonology), *content* (semantics), and *use* (pragmatics) (Bloom, 1988), but we will have more to say about this *linguistic code* later. Let's now turn our attention to another component of communication: speech.

Speech

Speech is the oral expression of language (Hulit & Howard, 2002). It involves the sensorimotor processes by which language users reproduce the coded symbols that are stored in their central nervous systems so that others can hear the symbols. Consequently, speech production requires the neurological control of physical movements to create sound patterns. These sound patterns are produced as a result of respiration, phonation, resonation, and articulation. *Respiration* refers to the coordinated, rapid muscular activities of the chest (which controls the lung action). Respiration provides the air in which a speech sound wave can travel. Without air, there would be no way of phonating. *Phonation* refers to the production of sound through vibration of the vocal cords (vocal folds) in the larynx (McLaughlin, 1998). Once a sound has been created, it resonates through the vocal tract (pharynx, oral cavity, and nasal cavity). According to McLaughlin (1998), resonation refers to the "modification of the vocal tone produced through changing the shape and size of the spaces in the vocal tract" (p. 440). Finally, the *articulators* (including the tongue, jaw, lips, and palate) are used to modify the sound into a vowel or a consonant. A consonant is produced by constricting the air stream, whereas a vowel is produced without significant constriction of the air stream through the mouth (Fromkin, Rodman, Collins, & Blair, 1996). Language is the code; speech is the sensorimotor production of that code.

Extralinguistic Aspects of Communication

As we saw earlier, communication can be any behavior or action that conveys a message. For example, if a speaker said, "The baby's sleeping," in a quiet whisper accompanied by a frown and an upright open-hand gesture in front of the listener, the speaker's original thought and, therefore, communicative intention may not have been to comment on the fact that the baby is asleep, but to stop the listener from speaking loudly as they enter the baby's room, in order not to wake the baby. Owens (2001) refers to behaviors such as loudness, frowning, or using gesture as *extralinguistic elements of communication.* These may enhance or even change the linguistic code. Extralinguistic elements include paralinguistics, nonlinguistics (nonverbal communication), and metalinguistics.

Paralinguistics.   Paralinguistics refers to the melodic components of speech that modify the meaning of the spoken message (McLaughlin, 1998). Melodic components include stress, pitch, and intonation. *Stress* is the relative loudness with which certain syllables in words are produced. Ladefoged (2001) defines it as "the use of extra respiratory energy during a syllable" (p. 276). For example, in the word *blackbird,* if the first syllable is said more loudly and with greater respiratory energy than the second syllable, the meaning is a specific type of bird. If there is no difference in stress between the syllables, the meaning is any bird that is black. If we take the word *pervert,* it is difficult to know whether the written word refers to a *pervert* (noun) or the act *to pervert* (verb). In spoken English, stress can communicate meaning. Stress can also be used for contrastive emphasis within utterances. For example, one speaker might say, "I like the *red* jacket," whereas a second speaker might say, "I like the *blue* jacket." In doing so, the second speaker contrasts the color *red* with the color *blue* through the use of stress.

   Pitch and intonation can also modify the meaning of a spoken message. Ladefoged (2001) describes *pitch* as the "auditory property of a sound that enables a listener to place it on a scale going from low to high" (p. 275). *Intonation,* on the other hand, refers to the pattern of pitch changes across an utterance (Ball & Lowry, 2001). Pitch and intonation both enhance a spoken message. For example, pitch can convey personal characteristics of speakers, such as their gender, age (to some extent), and emotional state (Ladefoged, 2001). Changes in pitch can also alter the meaning of a word, as is seen in tone languages, such as Mandarin Chinese, Zulu, Thai, and Vietnamese (Hwa-Froelich, Hodson, & Edwards, 2002; Ladefoged, 2001). Intonation can be used to convey syntactic information. For example, the sentence, "He went skydiving," could be said as a statement of fact, with falling intonation at the end of the utterance. The same sentence could be expressed as a question, with rising intonation at the end of the utterance. In both examples, the sequence of speech sounds remains the same, but a difference in meaning is signaled by the intonation pattern.

The combination of these melodic components of speech creates prosody. Because prosody is superimposed on the segments of an utterance (e.g., the speech sounds, words, or phrases), the melodic components are often referred to as *suprasegmental* devices (Ladefoged, 2001). These act above the level of a segment to enhance the overall meaning of an utterance to convey an emotion or an attitude. Without paralinguistics our speech would sound robotic or dull, that is, computer speech.

Nonlinguistics (Nonverbal Communication).   As indicated by the heading for this section, the nonlinguistic aspect of communication is sometimes referred to as nonverbal communication. McLaughlin (1998) writes that it consists of "nonspeech behaviors that accompany the speaker's words and transmit certain cues through facial expressions, eye contact, gestures, body language or proxemics" (p. 11). *Proxemics* refers to the ways that use of space and physical distance between speakers communicate. In the quote above, the phrase "body language" was used. Another term for body language is *kinesics,* or the way in which movements are used for communication.

In many respects, nonverbal communication can be considered a system itself. Hall (1959), in the title of his insightful and sometimes humorous book on nonverbal communication, referred to it as the "silent language." Consciously or unconsciously, we engage in nonverbal communication, sometimes to emphasize concurrent oral messages, sometimes to contradict simultaneous oral messages, and sometimes to substitute for oral messages. For example, the utterance, "That chocolate caramel fudge looks nice, thanks," could mean that the speaker thinks chocolate caramel fudge is appealing. But when spoken by a customer in a candy store, accompanied by pointing and leaning toward a piece of chocolate caramel fudge displayed in the store window, it could mean that the customer would like to purchase some fudge. Our understanding and use of nonverbal cues can largely determine the quality and effectiveness of our interpersonal relationships. In fact, some suggest that nonverbal communication carries more than half of the social meaning in interpersonal communication situations. When we are in a foreign country and unable to communicate through the use of speech and language, we often resort to using nonlinguistic cues to communicate.

It is important to note, however, that nonlinguistic behaviors are not always universal in what they communicate, and cultures differ in uses of and meanings associated with specific elements of nonverbal communication. For example, a nod of the head in the United States or Australia indicates agreement ("yes"), while the same gesture in Bengal indicates "no" (Axtell, 1991).

Inaccurate or ineffective interpretation and use of nonverbal communication may lead to problems in establishing and maintaining social relationships with others. An awareness of nonverbal communication, the nonlinguistic elements that comprise particular nonverbal systems, and the ways in which it influences relationships are important because some children struggle with language experience deficits in the ability to understand and express nonverbal cues correctly. Such difficulties can result in the development of poor self-images and self-concepts, potentially leading to even more impaired interpersonal relationships.

Metalinguistics.   The third extralinguistic element of communication is metalinguistics. The prefix *meta-* as it is used in *metalinguistics* means something like "beyond" or "higher" or "transcending," not unlike how it is used in the word *metaphysics*. As such, *metalinguistics* refers to the ability to use language to communicate or talk about and to analyze language. It involves thinking about language, seeing it as an entity separate from its function as a way of communicating, and using language to judge the correctness of language and to correct it; it is an awareness of the components of language; it is seeing language as a tool and controlling how we use language. For example, identifying and generating rhyming words involves metalinguistic ability.

Frequently, monitoring whether or not our messages are understood and consciously deciding how to clarify them involve metalinguistic skills. If we return to our example of the customer requesting a piece of chocolate caramel fudge using the utterance, "That chocolate caramel fudge looks nice, thanks," the response of the sales assistant would provide the customer with information about the success of his or her utterance. If the sales assistant nods agreeably and proceeds to pick up a piece of chocolate *almond* fudge, then the customer would recognize a need to rephrase the request emphasizing the word *caramel.* Alternatively, the sales assistant might say, "Pardon, what did you say?" from which the customer would become aware of a need to correct or clarify the utterance in order to be understood.

A Bit More about the Relationships among Speech, Language, and Communication

Communication involves the sending and receiving of messages. Although it can be as simple as a sneeze, it can also be a complex symbolic code expressed through the action of respiration, phonation, resonation, and articulation accompanied by paralinguistic and nonlinguistic cues. Figure 1.1 shows how the various terms we have addressed (speech, language, paralinguistics, nonlinguistics, metalinguistics, and communication) relate to one

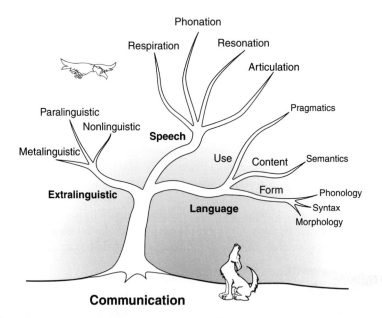

FIGURE 1.1   Components of Communication

another. Sometimes, we may communicate just using nonlinguistic behaviors, such as raising our eyebrows or frowning. We may also communicate using language without speech, as is the case with writing.

It is also important that we differentiate further between the two key terms, *speech* and *language.* As our definitions so far have indicated, language and speech are closely related but are not the same. The two sentences, "The dog is black and white," and "Is the dog black and white?," consist of the same sounds. However, the order of the sounds, and therefore the order of the words, in the two sentences are different, as is the resultant meaning of the two sentences. As another example, to produce the sentences, "I want it to *fit*" and "I want it to *sit*," a child must only alter speech movements slightly to produce the difference between "f" and "s." Yet the meaning of the two sentences is quite different based on the one speech sound variation.

It is possible for a child's code system (language) to be intact but for the same child to have difficulty with the articulation of speech sounds. For example, a child who has an interdental lisp and says "th" for "s" might say the words *thing* and *sing* the same way, but from the context we can tell that the child knows the words mean different things:

> I can "thing" Twinkle, Twinkle Little Star.
>
> I don't like that thing.

It is also possible for a child's speech production to be intact but for the child's language system to be deficient. As examples, a child who says, "I want it no to go," "The gooses are flying," or "I don't want for you to sick," with well-pronounced sounds in a highly fluent manner, is demonstrating problems with language, not speech.

As Figure 1.1 indicates, communication is a wonderfully creative human ability through which we share thoughts and feelings. Communication can be as simple as a nod of the head or as complex as the symbolic representation of language. Given the focus of this book on children's language disorders, we will now explore the components of language in greater depth.

Components of Language

Spoken languages are made up of components. Some authors call these *elements;* some call them *parameters;* others call them *aspects.* Whatever they are labeled, the intent is to break language into parts in order to discuss and describe it. Often, we consider there to be five basic components of language: (1) phonology, (2) semantics, (3) syntax, (4) morphology, and (5) pragmatics. Each is part of a system and is therefore governed by regularities and sets of rules that all speakers of a specific language must learn if they are to communicate effectively. Although we can discuss each of these components separately, they are all interrelated in language functioning, as we will see in later chapters.

Phonology

When we utter a word such as *fish,* we produce a string of speech sounds that represent the word *fish,* beginning by biting the bottom lip with the top front teeth, then producing the vowel sound, then using the tongue to produce the sound "sh." If somebody who understands English were to hear the production of this string of speech sounds, they would know that the word was *fish*. A listener who understands and speaks a language other than English would not know what was being said. This idea of using speech sounds in a particular sequence within a language to communicate meaning is the essence of phonology. Bauman-Waengler (2000) defines *phonology* as "the description of the systems and patterns of phonemes that occur in a language" (p. 49). To appreciate this definition, we need to examine the concept of speech sounds or *phonemes* more closely.

Durand (1990) defines phonemes as "sounds whose function is to distinguish words from one another" (p. 3). When we look at a string of speech sounds in words, we see that by changing just one speech sound within a word, we can differentiate one word from another. For example, in the word pair *cat/rat*, sound differences occur in the initial positions of the words. The sounds that create these meaning differences (in this case, "c" and "r") are phonemes. By replacing the "c" in "cat" with other sounds to create r̲at, m̲at, h̲at, f̲at, p̲at, t̲hat, we discover that "r," "m," "h," "f," "p," "th" are also phonemes of English because they result in words with different meanings. Phonemes can be classified as either vowels or consonants.

One problem that becomes painfully clear as we watch children attempting to learn to read is the lack of consistency between the way an English sound is said and the way it is written. For example, the letter "c" is pronounced as a "k" sound in *cat* and as an "s" sound in *center*, and the long vowel "a" is spelled *ay* in *bay*, *a* in *fade*, and *ea* in *break*. Trying to use usual alphabetic symbols to write English as it is said is very difficult. This is where the International Phonetic Alphabet (IPA) comes to the rescue. It is a system that has a correspondence between a written symbol and a sound. That is, a spoken sound is represented by one consistent printed symbol. Many of the symbols of the IPA are shown in Table 1.1. As can be seen, the symbol /s/ represents the "s" sound in *sun* and *cement*, the symbol /dʒ/ represents the "j" sound in *jump*, *badge*, and *fudge*, and the symbol /θ/ represents the "th" sound in *thumb* and *tooth*. In this text, symbols that occur between / / indicate they are IPA symbols and designate the relevant pronunciation as shown in Table 1.1. In using the IPA, a word in the language is transcribed on paper as a speaker produces it.

The exact number of phonemes in American English is difficult to determine because there are acceptable variations within the language. Some of these variations result from dialectal differences. Most estimates of the number of phonemes suggest that there are 40 to 46 (Fairbanks, 1960; Owens, 2001).

Each language has a limited set of phonemes that comprises the sound system; each language also has its own set of phonotactic rules or rules governing which phonemes can be combined with other phonemes and in what order. In English, *ksont* is not a word and never could be, even though all the individual sounds that make up the word are acceptable English phonemes. On the other hand, *skont*, which is also not an English word, potentially could be a word in the language, because the sequence of phonemes is possible. We see the application of English phonotactic rules is Lewis Carroll's opening sentence to his literary classic "Jabberwocky": "Twas brillig, and the slithy toves did gyre and gimble in the wabe: All mimsy were the borogoves, and the mome raths outgrabe." English speakers are able to read the sentence aloud and sound like they are producing acceptable English, because the nonsense words abide by the phonotactic rules. If Lewis Carroll's opening sentence began with something like "Ksee ngot, and the lsiyth ptosv did yger and rgilbe in the wabeh," we

TABLE 1.1 The International Phonetic Alphabet

Consonants				Vowels and Diphthongs			
Voiceless		Voiced					
Symbols	Key Words	Symbols	Key Words	Symbols	Key Words	Symbols	Key Words
p	pig	b	big	i	feet	u	food
t	to	d	do	ɪ	hit	ʊ	foot
k	coat, key	g	goat	e	cake	o	toll
f	fine	v	vine	ɛ	head	ɔ	fog
θ	thumb	ð	the	æ	pack	ɑ	father
s	cider, sun	z	zipper	ʌ	dug	ɒ*	law
ʃ	she	ʒ	vision, azure	ə	sofa	aɪ	time
tʃ	chair	dʒ	gem, huge	ɝ^	fur	aʊ	house
h	hello	m	me	ɚ^	mother	ɔɪ	toil
ʍ	when	n	new	ɝ*	bird	ju	fuse
		ŋ	ring	a*	mad		
		l	letter				
		r	run				
		w	we				
		j	yes				

*These vowels occur in some Eastern and/or Southern American speech patterns.

would struggle to pronounce many of the words because they fail to conform to the phonotactic rules of English. Children learning the phonological system of their language must learn to use not only the acceptable set of phonemes but also the phonotactic rules for combining these phonemes sequentially into words.

Semantics

Semantics deals with the referents for words and the meanings of utterances. At a basic level, semantics involves the vocabulary of a language, or the lexicon. Sequences of phonemes combine to form words. The words are then used to represent items, attributes, concepts, or experiences. As we know, many words can have multiple meanings depending on the situations in which they are used. *Peel* can refer to the rind of a piece of fruit or the act of stripping or tearing off. In identifying the meanings of words, we typically think of the dictionary meanings. These dictionary meanings are the *referential meanings* or denotative meanings of words. However, words may have *connotative* or *emotionally associated meanings*. These meanings can, in fact, be so strong as to actually produce physical responses to the word. To many, the word *snake* can create chills even though the denotative meaning of the word refers to one of several kinds of limbless reptiles.

A word and its referents can trigger associations with another word and its referents. In some instances, the associated words belong to the same category as the original word. For example, the word *cow* may trigger one to think of *pig, horse,* and *sheep.* In other instances, the associated word or words may be the category for the original word—*animal* or *farm animal.*

Words can be categorized and recategorized through the process of abstraction. In the process of categorizing words, we identify or abstract the similarities among the referents for the words and use the similar characteristics to form another category that is also labeled. Hayakawa (1964) used the example of Bessie the cow to demonstrate the categorization and abstraction of referents. One of the lowest levels of categorization of Bessie is that of "cow," some of the abstracted characteristics of which include animal, four legs, tail, milk giver, and *moo.* This category of abstracted qualities ignores the individual differences among all the other cows that make up the group and focuses only on the similar characteristics. The similar characteristics or attributes form the category "cow." However, cows have characteristics similar to chickens, pigs, and horses. Those abstracted similar characteristics can be categorized and labeled as "livestock." The term *livestock* becomes a superordinate category for cows, chickens, and pigs. In turn, livestock is similar to all other salable farm items, and based on these attributes a new category of "assets" is abstracted. "Livestock" is now subordinate to the superordinate category of assets. The abstracted similar attributes of all possible assets allow the formation of a new category—"wealth." Each time a new category was created, we increased our level of abstraction, and with each level of abstraction we moved farther and farther away from the concrete, or that which can be perceived by the senses. "Wealth" is an abstract concept. Its attributes cannot be perceived by the senses; therefore, its referents are said to be relatively abstract.

The use of superordinate and subordinate categories in the lexicon helps to bring order to our experiences. By categorizing and labeling our experiences, it is not necessary for us to treat each experience as a totally new one. Because we have finite memories, this skill is efficient and allows us to store cognitively more information than if it were not used. Children learning the semantic system of their language must acquire a categorization system somewhat consistent with that of others in the language community. Much of the educational system does, in fact, center on teaching children the categorization of attributes and how to move from superordinate categories to subordinate categories and vice versa—for example, units of instruction on colors, animals, and transportation.

Not only does the semantic component of language deal with the lexicon, it also involves the meanings conveyed by the relations among words. This aspect of semantics is termed *relational meaning.* In fact, some words, such as *an* or *if,* really take on meaning only as they are used with other words. Furthermore, when the individual meanings of words interrelate in a multiword statement, the statement takes on a meaning that goes beyond the separate words. This meaning is the statement's *propositional meaning* and is partly derived from the logical relationships inherent in the sequence of words. In the sentences, "The boy climbs the tree," and "The tree climbs the boy," the words are identical. The first sentence is plausible while the second is not, even though the individual words within the sentences retain their usual referents. The order in which the words are arranged imposes certain restrictions on the logical relationships among the words, and these restrictions are violated in the second sentence.

Earlier, in discussing semantics, reference was made to the multiple meanings of many individual words. In situations where a word may have several different referents, we typically determine its meaning from the contexts in which it is used and its relationship to other words uttered. We can use the word *table* to illustrate the derivation of meaning by employing cues regarding the word's logical relationship to other words in a sentence. Although *table* has several meanings, we can surmise from the sentence, "The table was too small to use six chairs," that the referent for the word is a piece of furniture; from the sentence, "As the rains continued, the table continued to rise," that the referent is probably a water level rather than a floating part of a dining set, although this could be plausible; and from the sentence, "The table contained numbers she had never seen before," that the referent for the word is an organized grouping of numerals such as those of a statistician. However, using the word in some sentences may not aid in deriving the word's meaning. For example, the sentence, "Read about the table," gives us no clue as to the meaning of *table*. This is referred to as an *ambiguous statement,* and in these instances we must depend on previous utterances or the situation in which the sentence is expressed to determine the referent of *table*. Verbal humor is frequently based on multiple meanings of words.

Two other aspects of semantics involve figurative meaning and inferential meaning. *Figurative meaning* goes beyond meaning that can be derived from literal interpretations of phrases. For example, "It's raining cats and dogs" is implausible if interpreted at its literal level. Metaphors, similes, proverbs, and idioms all involve figurative meanings. Inferential meaning refers to meaning that is derived not from what is stated explicitly, but from the logical relationships of statements. As an example, consider the following sequential statements:

> Sally went to the restaurant and ordered from the standard menu. She loved her wantons and fried rice.

The kind of restaurant is not stated explicitly. Yet, we are able to derive sufficient information through inferential meanings to increase the odds of making a correct, educated guess of a Chinese restaurant.

Syntax

All languages have systems of syntax, or sets of rules that govern how words are to be sequenced in utterances and how the words in an utterance are related. Phonemes combine to form words, and words combine to form phrases, clauses, and sentences. In the same way that phonological rules govern what phonemes can be combined in what order, syntactic rules determine what words can be combined in what order to convey meaning.

A basic English syntactic rule is the subject + verb + object sequence, which places the actor first followed by the receiver of the action. Although the words in the sentences "The boy hits the girl" and "The girl hits the boy" are identical, reversal of the word order signals a different meaning. Word combinations typically convey more specific information than any of the individual words alone do. For example, a child who utters the word *milk* may be indicating that the item is present, may simply be labeling it, may wish to have more of the item, or may not want it at all. If the child uses the utterance "more milk," additional specificity is obtained, although the child may be indicating that a larger quantity is present or that an increase in the amount is requested. But when the child says, "I want more milk," the child's meaning is specific. If the child says, "More milk I want," the listener may be able to understand the child's wish, but the utterance violates the syntactic rules for the intended meaning. In most instances, however, precise sequencing of words using correct syntactic rules is essential if the exact intended meaning of an utterance is to be conveyed. The words in the sentences, "When she was 10 years old, she reported that a dog had bitten her" and "She reported that a dog had bitten her when she was 10 years old," are identical, but the meanings of the two sentences are different, depending on the location of the clause "when she was 10 years old."

The theory that explains how children are able to learn what seem to be implicit syntactic rules is a continuing matter of considerable debate among linguists. We will not wade into the debate here. What most agree about, however, is that there is a generative element, so that once syntactic rules are learned, numerous sentences or phrases can be generated, and thus numerous ideas can be expressed. Table 1.2 shows a number of the multiple phrases and ideas that are possible with knowledge of a single syntactic rule—article + attributive + noun sequence.

Another aspect of syntax about which most theorists agree is that there is a *transformational element* involved. That is, with a set of operational rules, sentences can be changed by adding, deleting, and/or rearranging the words to derive sentences of various types. To illustrate, the sentence, "The girl is riding a horse," can, by rearranging the words, be transformed into the question, "Is the girl riding a horse?" or, by adding the word *not* in the correct place, transformed into the negative, "The girl is not riding a horse." In both transformations the meaning conveyed by the first sentence is altered. However, both transformed sentences are based on the structure of the original sentence, "The girl is riding a horse."

Chomsky's (1957, 1965, 1981) concepts of syntax and language learning have had a major influence on our thinking about how children acquire language and the syntactic components of the language in particular (e.g., government binding theory, generative transformational grammar). A discussion of his theories is not appropriate for this text. However, we can see in Table 1.3 further examples of how we can transform sentences and creatively alter meaning once we know "the rules."

TABLE 1.2   Use of a Syntactic Rule to Generate Multiple Phrases

Article	+	Attributive	+	Noun
The		Pretty		Dress
A		Big		Doll
An		Old		Apple
The		Tremendous		Crowd
An		Exhaustive		Experience

TABLE 1.3   Various Transformations and Examples

	Transformation Types	
Negation	*Question*	*Negation & Question*
The ball is not red	Is the ball red?	Isn't the ball red?
The girl does not run	Does the girl run?	Doesn't the girl run?
The flower is not blooming	Is the flower blooming?	Isn't the flower blooming?
	What color is the ball?	When isn't the girl running?
	When is the girl running?	Why isn't the flower blooming?
	Why is the flower blooming?	
	What is this?	

Morphology

Morphology deals with the rules for deriving various word forms and the rules for using grammatical markers or inflections. These derived word forms include plurals, verb tenses, adverbs, and superlatives. Table 1.4 shows how we can use morphology to change meaning.

Because morphology is concerned with sequences of phonemes, it is sometimes discussed as part of the phonological system. Sometimes it is considered part of the semantic system because of the meaning derived from the phoneme sequences, and sometimes it is classified as part of the syntactic system because of the interrelationships among varying word forms, their functions within sentences, and word order. Furthermore, morphology is sometimes considered as a separate component of language because of the unique rules affecting differing word forms.

TABLE 1.4   Examples of Morphological Derivations of Words

	Root word: *drive*	Root word: *gentle*	
drives	Third-person singular, present tense or plural noun for motor paths	*gently*	Adverb
drove	Irregular past tense	*gentleness*	Noun
driven	Past participle, functioning part of a verb form or as an adjective	*gentleman*	Noun
driving	Present participle, functioning as part of a verb form or as an adjective, as in *driving rain*	*gentlemanly*	Adverb
		ungentlemanly	Adverb

In all instances, morphology is concerned with meaning, and the smallest meaning units of a language are called *morphemes* (Berko-Gleason, 2001). In some instances, the smallest unit or form that conveys meaning is a word, such as *drive* (Table 1.4). Even though the word is composed of phonemes, none of them is meaningful by itself. Therefore, *drive* cannot be broken into smaller units and retain its meaning. *Drive* is a morpheme. In other instances, however, the smallest unit that conveys meaning is not a word. For example, *ing,* when added to a verb, denotes the progressive tense and its associated meaning. Therefore, when *ing* is added to the verb, it signals a meaning that is somewhat different from the meaning *drive* alone. While *ing* is not a word, it is still a morpheme.

There are basically two classes of morphemes: roots and affixes. *Roots* are words that cannot be divided into any smaller units, while *affixes* are morphemes that are attached to roots in order to alter meaning. In the word *driving,* the root is *drive* and the affix, in this case a suffix, is *ing.* In the word *redo,* the root is *do* and the affix, in this case a prefix, is *re.* Sometimes the affix involves deriving a grammatical form and conveying grammatical information, such as *ing* on *drive.* Other terms used for such affixes are inflections, inflectional morphemes, grammatical markers, and grammatical inflections. In other instances, the affix involves deriving an altered word meaning that conveys semantic information, such as the *re* on *do.* A term used for these affixes is *derivational morphemes.*

Another classification of morphemes uses the terms *free morphemes* and *bound morphemes* to identify the two different kinds. A free morpheme is able to occur alone in the language. In the previous example, *drive* is a free morpheme because it can occur meaningfully by itself. However, *ing* is a bound morpheme because it cannot occur by itself and be meaningful; it derives its meaning only when attached to another morpheme. Therefore, its function is bound to that of another morpheme. There is obviously a parallel between free morphemes and roots and bound morphemes and affixes. Words must be viewed in terms of the smallest units of meaning they possess to determine the number and types of morphemes they contain. The word *ungentlemanly* in Table 1.4 contains two free morphemes (*gentle* and *man*) and two bound morphemes (*un* and *ly*).

Examples of common rules for attaching bound morphemes to free morphemes include the formation of plural nouns by adding "s" (pronounced as the /s/ sound) to the root noun (*cat* to *cats*), past-tense verbs by adding "ed" (pronounced as a syllable *uhd*) to the root verb (*bait* to *baited*), superlative adjectives by adding "est" to the root adjective (*short* to *shortest*), and reflexive pronouns by adding "self" to the objective pronoun (*him* to *himself*). However, such rules do not explain the formation of plural nouns for which the "z" sound is used (*home* to *homes*), for which a syllable with "z" (pronounced as *uhz*) is used (*house* to *houses*), or for which the entire word changes (*man* to *men*). The examples do not explain past-tense verbs pronounced with a "t" or "d" at the end (*kick* to *kicked* or *comb* to *combed*), superlative adjectives that use a different word (*good* to *best*), or reflexive pronouns that use "selves" (*them* to *themselves*). The concept of allomorphs is needed to explain such variations. An *allomorph* is a variation of a morpheme that does not alter the meaning of the original morpheme. Table 1.5 lists several examples of allomorphs that are used to indicate noun plurals, verb tenses, and verb person and number.

In some cases, the use of allomorphs is determined by specific rules; for example, to form a noun plural when the root ends with a voiceless consonant, such as "p," add "s" to the root, except when the voiceless consonant is a fricative or an affricative, such as "sh" or "ch," in which case *uhz* is added to the root. However, in English many of the allomorphs to

TABLE 1.5 Examples of Allomorphs for Noun Plurals, Verb Tenses, and Verb Person and Number

Noun Plurals

book		books	/s/
robe		robes	/z/
twitch		twitches	/əz/
leaf		leaves	

Verb Tenses

kick	kicked	/t/	kicked	/t/
comb	combed	/d/	combed	/d/
eat	ate		eaten	
ring	rang		rung	
do	did		done	
bait	baited	/əd/	baited	/əd/
tear	tore		torn	

Verb Person/Number

kick	kicks	/s/
comb	combs	/z/
eat	eats	/s/
ring	rings	/z/
do	does	
have	has	

be used are irregular. That is, there are no specific rules governing their application. Why do we pluralize *child* by using *children,* and why do we use *was* as a past tense of *be?* Because no rules can be used for the irregularities, they must simply be memorized. Children, in the process of learning the morphology of their language, often overgeneralize the morphological rules and use the rules in place of the irregular allomorphs (*comed* instead of *came, deers* instead of *deer,* and *gooder* instead of *better*). Even adults may have difficulty with some of the irregular allomorphs. Context and/or syntax are often the only ways to determine the meaning of some irregular allomorphs or to know whether an allomorph has been used correctly. For example, *deer* does not change its form from singular to plural. If *deer* is the subject of a sentence, a verb may indicate whether the noun is singular or plural ("The deer is jumping" or "The deer are jumping").

Pragmatics

Language is used for specific reasons, and without these there would be no purpose for language. Language helps us achieve communicative or social functions (McLean &

Snyder-McLean, 1999). This aspect of language is referred to as pragmatics. Because the area of pragmatics is concerned with the whys, and therefore the hows of language use, some prefer to see pragmatics not as a component of language that is equal in status to the other components, such as syntax or semantics, but rather as the "super" component that drives, organizes, and encompasses the other components. Owens (2001) considers this view of pragmatics encompassing phonology, morphology, semantics, and syntax as a functionalist model of language.

When we think of people talking with each other, we visualize each taking turns during which they produce sequences of connected speech; these people are engaging in discourse. Some confusion exists in the literature about two terms often used in discussion of pragmatics—discourse and narrative. For our purposes, *discourse* will be used to refer to the connected flow of language. This frequently relates to conversations and communicative interactions between people, but different kinds of discourse may also occur in speeches or soliloquies. *Narrative* will be used to refer to one form of discourse, that of telling a story. A narrative is a frequently used logical description of a sequence of events. We employ narratives in discourse when describing a movie we have seen or giving an account of what happened when we went shopping. Stories, as in children's fairy tales or in novels, are another type of narrative.

Like the components of language we have discussed previously, the pragmatic aspect is rule-governed. Certain ways of using language vary from context to context, and what is socially and culturally acceptable in one situation violates the appropriate rules in another. For example, we might say to a 4-year-old child, "Close the door," but a more appropriate request to an adult peer would be, "Can you close the door?" Prutting (1982) even described pragmatics as social competence. Children, in the process of learning the form and content of language, must also learn how to vary these aspects to communicate effectively in a variety of situations. Pragmatics is comprised of several elements. Among these are

1. The various functions and acts that utterances serve
2. The coherence of sequential statements
3. The fluency with which messages are delivered
4. The ability to take turns during dialogues and at the same time maintain topics of conversation
5. The provision of adequate information for listeners to comprehend spoken messages without supplying redundant information
6. The responsibility to repair communication breakdowns and request additional information when messages are not understood
7. The appropriate use of nonverbal communicative cues
8. The codes or styles of communicative behavior employed in different situations, that is, our ability to code-switch

Skill in employing these elements, combined with the ability to use the phonological, semantic, syntactic, and morphological systems accurately, embodies what we refer to as *communicative competency* or *proficiency*. Becker-Bryant (2001) defines this as "the ability to use language appropriately and strategically in social contexts" (p. 241).

Two additional aspects of communication that contribute to the rich tapestry of skills that make up communicative competency include fluency and cohesion. *Fluency* in the delivery of messages refers to the number of false starts, hesitations, fillers, and revisions that take place as speakers say their utterances. While these fluency disrupters occur in most people's speech, they interfere with communication if they are too frequent or long. Sometimes we use these fluency disruptors deliberately to help convey part of our message. For example, if we wish to appear thoughtful about what we are saying, we might introduce more hesitations and false starts into our utterances than if we said the same thing with total assurance. As discussed earlier in the chapter, extralinguistic aspects of communication such as paralinguistic and nonlinguistic devices can also be used to enhance or even change the linguistic meaning of an utterance. The ability to use such devices falls within the pragmatic component of language.

In addition, effective language use requires that sequential utterances be related to each other. This aspect of pragmatics, termed *cohesion,* refers to the organization and order of utterances in a whole message so that the individual ideas of each utterance build logically on the previous ones. The following is part of an example, provided by Wiig and Semel (1984), in which cohesion problems are illustrated in the sequential utterances of a boy producing a narrative, in this case an explanation of the plot of a television show:

> So he was scared to tell John-boy that he stoled his poem, but he didn't really. He just got an idea from John-boy's poem. And then John-boy was trying to figure out what who shot this man he knows. And then the man stole the chickens and then that night he bring 'em back. (p. 288)

The adequate inclusion of temporal words and grammatical inflections indicating time references to help listeners orient themselves to the interrelationships of ideas and events, and the use of appropriate referent identification for pronouns, are parts of delivering coherent messages. Another important aspect of delivering coherent messages involves using not only coordinating conjunctions (e.g., *and, so*) but subordinating conjunctions (e.g., *because, if, when*) to produce complex sentences that contain more than one proposition. Adverbial conjuncts (e.g., *nevertheless, however*) are other devices that contribute to cohesion.

Being able to provide coherent messages also depends, in part, on determining what listeners already know about the topics under discussion. Shared knowledge between listener and speaker is not given emphasis or, in some cases, even reported. However, knowledge that only the speaker has must be stated in order for a listener to comprehend a message. This aspect of pragmatics is termed *presupposition* and refers to the provision of sufficient, but not too much, information for adequate listener comprehension. Appropriate use of presuppositions requires that a speaker gauge listeners' needs for specificity and frames of reference. We have all experienced irritation with speakers who waste valued communication time reporting what is obviously known, without proceeding to the key parts of a message. In contrast, we have attempted to engage in conversations in which we were unable to follow the speaker's sequence of ideas because adequate background information was not supplied.

In the latter situations, we would likely determine that a communication breakdown had occurred and attempt to repair it. We indicated previously that repairing communication breakdowns is one of the several elements of pragmatic language behaviors. The process of conversational repair is twofold. First, speakers are obligated to identify when listeners have not understood their messages and supply additional information or modifications of the ways in which previously given information was delivered. Second, listeners must signal their lack of understanding. These signals may be verbal, such as the statements, "I don't understand," "What did you say?," or "Would you repeat that please?" Or, listeners may use nonverbal cues, such as puzzled facial expressions, to indicate they have not understood.

During a conversation, both the speaker and the listener take turns responding to each other's utterances. One part of this rule-governed behavior is that one does not interrupt or talk over the other. However, turn taking also involves acknowledging the previous utterances but without repeating unnecessary content and expanding the content of the conversation with appropriate additional information. Such behavior facilitates topic maintenance. Topic maintenance requires that a person about to speak abide by the constraints of the topic created by a previous speaker and reply with responses appropriate to the topic. For example, an appropriate response and one that would continue the topic to the statement, "I bought a new car," would be, "What kind is it?" In contrast, the response, "It's cold outside," would be startling and disconcerting to the previous speaker and would probably discontinue the first topic, if not the interaction. However, there are times when we wish to change a topic that has already been introduced. These are referred to as *topic shifts*. Topic shifting is acceptable if it is not done so frequently that our conversational partners begin to think we are uninterested in them and if it is done smoothly rather than abruptly.

In certain situations with certain people, specific rules dictate the way we are supposed to communicate. For example, it would be very inappropriate during an interdisciplinary educational staffing on a child to relate the results of testing as "Sally sure did ace the hearing test but bombed the IQ test." In contrast, it might be acceptable to say to a friend and colleague that "Tom aced the continuing ed. course he took." Joos (1976) describes five styles of communication: intimate, casual, consultative, formal, and frozen. Effective use of language involves determining in communicative situations which styles are appropriate and wording messages accordingly.

As Halliday (1975) reminds us, language can also function as a means of establishing a human relationship. For example, if we wish to meet a person sitting next to us in an audience, we might ask what time the performance is expected to start even though we already know. The function of the utterance in this instance is not to acquire information, but rather to make contact. The same query, of course, could be made for the purpose of receiving information, and another important function of language is to acquire information (Halliday, 1975). For most adults, messages often serve more than one function at the same time, and adults usually vary their messages appropriately between direct and indirect speech acts. That is, they use alternative forms of language to accomplish similar purposes, depending on the context and the person to whom they are addressing the messages. Previously, we indicated that an imperative (a direct speech act such as "Close the door") is acceptable in some instances and a question (an indirect speech act such as "Can you close the door?") is more appropriate in others. As we can see, the form (syntax, phonology, semantics, and morphology) of a message does not always correspond to the intents or functions of the message.

Comprehension and Production

In our discussion on the pragmatic aspects of language, we saw that language use often involves at least two people interacting in a communicative situation—the sender of a message and the receiver of a message, who typically take turns in the roles of sender and receiver. This communicative process is referred to as *dyadic communication.* A basic assumption is that for the communicative act to be complete, both the sender and the receiver use the same code and know the same rules of the language. The sender takes an idea, applies the appropriate language rules to put the idea into code, and then transmits the code through speech production. The listener hears the sound transmission, applies the same language rules to match the code with the one already neurologically stored, and then, one hopes, comprehends the message. In other words, the sender *encodes* the message and the receiver *decodes* the message. Terms often used interchangably with *encoding* are *expression* and *production,* while *reception, understanding, interpretation,* and *comprehension* are terms often considered synonymous with *decoding.*

It is generally agreed that for adults in most situations, comprehension skills are greater than production abilities. For example, for most of us, our understanding vocabularies are superior to our expressive vocabularies (the words we use to convey our thoughts to others). There has also been a general belief that this superiority of comprehension over production applies to children in their acquisition. This belief appears reasonable when one considers the superiority of receptive to expressive skills in adults and when one observes that very young children often appear to understand much more language than they produce.

The research on the acquisition of comprehension and production skills in children has, however, yielded some conflicting results. It appears that in some situations children's comprehension of language does precede their production. This certainly is true in the early stages of language learning. However, in other situations, production abilities appear superior. Factors such as the definition of comprehension being used, the degree of comprehension being measured (e.g., depth and/or breath of comprehension of the word *snake*), and the amount of contextual support attached to the comprehension tasks likely affect how we interpret the relationship between production and comprehension. It may be that the relationship between comprehension and production changes with age (Bloom & Lahey, 1978; Owens, 2001). It may also be that comprehension and production are related but distinct skills. As Miller and Paul (1995) write, "One thing we have learned is that language comprehension and production, while following predictable patterns of acquisition in most children, do not always correspond perfectly to each other, even in an individual child" (p. 1).

Communication Modes

In our discussion of comprehension and production, hearing was used as the input modality for comprehension, and speaking was used as the output modality for production. These are the input–output modalities that comprise the auditory–oral system for language. The auditory–oral system is the most common way of using language and the one that most children acquire first. However, other combinations of input–output modalities that people may use include the visual–graphic (reading and writing), and the visual–gestural systems, as shown in Figure 1.2.

Auditory–Oral System: Hearing and Speech

The functional components of the auditory–oral system are hearing and speaking. Phylogenetically, humans heard and comprehended before they read, and they spoke before they

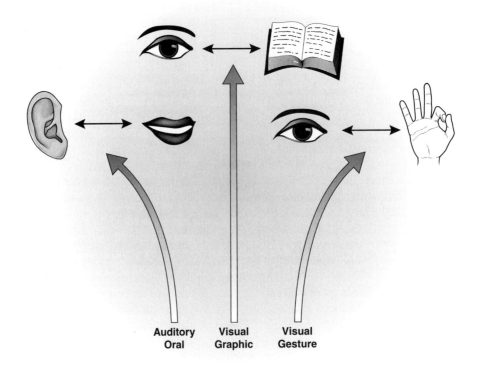

Auditory   Visual   Visual
Oral   Graphic   Gesture

FIGURE 1.2   Modes of Communication

acquired the ability to write. In the history of the human species, we have been hearing and talking for a very long time and our bodies have had lots of time to evolve to support these functions well. By comparison, we have only been reading and writing for a short time and our bodies have not had quite the same amount of time to evolve to support these functions as well. In many ways, the auditory–oral mode for language is also more flexible than the visual–graphic mode. Vision is a unidirectional sense, whereas hearing is multidirectional. We can only see in one direction at a time, but we can hear sounds originating from many directions despite the positions of our heads. Furthermore, we can talk when our hands are busy, but we cannot write. Speaking needs no special instruments, whereas writing requires the use of a pencil, pen, or these days a computer.

Children typically learn to use the auditory–oral system before they learn to use the visual–graphic system. That is, they can listen and speak before they know how to read and write. Developmentally, maturation of the physiological bases for audition and speech occurs before those used for reading and writing. Yet developmental maturation is not the only reason for children's earlier proficiencies with the auditory–oral system. For most Western languages, writing evolved as a system of visual symbols used to represent auditory symbols. The auditory–oral system is generally the basis of the visual–graphic system.

Visual–Graphic System: Reading and Writing

In the visual–graphic system, reading is employed as the input mode and writing is used as the output mode. As indicated above, reading and writing are relatively newly acquired human skills, so the neurophysiological bases of these functions have not had as much time to establish themselves in humans as the neurophysiological bases of listening and speaking. Nevertheless, the functions of reading and writing are closely related to the auditory–oral system. In many respects, the visual–graphic system is a code for another code—the auditory–oral system. As a code, language symbolizes experiences and thoughts. This code can then be represented by a system of sounds combined to form words and sentences. However, these sounds (which are themselves a code) can be recoded and rerepresented as visual, rather than auditory, symbols. That is, reading and writing are codes for hearing and speaking, which themselves are codes for the actual experiences or ideas. In the process of learning the visual–graphic language system, children learn a new coding system based on a previously learned code system.

Given the complex reciprocal relationships between the auditory–oral and visual–graphic systems, it is no surprise that children who have problems with the auditory–oral system often have difficulties learning to read and write. Most professionals emphasize the importance of an adequate auditory–oral system in learning to read and the relationship between oral language skills and reading achievement. As Wiig and Semel (1984) state, "Beginning reading depends upon accurate, deliberate, analytical decoding of letters and upon conscious translation of these letters into their auditory-vocal equivalents, which the child has already learned" (p. 33). This description is consistent with a theory of reading known as the *bottom-up theory*. A child learning to read must be able to segment printed words, decode letters in them, match them to some stored auditory model (phonetic and phonemic segmentation), and then retrieve a corresponding word (lexical retrieval). However, reading also involves using already known semantic–syntactic information, world knowledge, and narrative structure information to predict and organize what is being seen on the printed page. This is consistent with the *top-down theory* of reading, in which higher-order linguistic and cognitive skills play an important role in reading. Skills associated with both the bottom-up and top-down theories (phonological and syllabic segmentation, rapid lexical retrieval, semantic–syntactic abilities, narrative skills, general knowledge level) have been found to be factors in learning to read. It may be, however, that these different skills play more dominant roles in the process at different stages in learning to read and in different children at different times (Menyuk, Chesnick, et al., 1991; Owens, 2001; Snyder & Downey, 1991). This perspective is consistent with the *parallel, or interactive, theory* of learning to read.

There are several analogies between the visual–graphic and auditory–oral systems. The auditory and visual modalities are the receptive aspects of the two systems, whereas the oral and graphic modalities are the expressive aspects. The auditory component is based on a set of sounds that combine to form spoken words; the visual component is based on a set of letters that combine to form written words. Just as oral production for speech is a sensorimotor process, the same is true for graphic production for writing. Reception for the auditory–oral system involves transduction (conversion of waves into neural impulses) and auditory perception and processing of sound waves. Similarly, reception for the visual–graphic system involves transduction and visual perception and processing of light waves. Rules govern the use of both systems.

Although there are several analogies between the auditory–oral and visual–graphic systems, there are also differences. One difference is the sequence in which the two systems are acquired. Furthermore, although rules govern both systems and although some rules are similar, there are also different rules. One obvious difference deals with punctuation. Another relates to spelling. These are not factors in the auditory–oral system. Another difference deals with the level of grammatical complexity. The semantic–syntactic level used in the auditory–oral system is generally less complex than that found in the visual–graphic system once one progresses beyond the early learning stages. Still another difference relates to the amount of context available. Reading and writing are more decontextualized modes of communication than listening and speaking. That is, fewer cues to decipher and impart meaning are available in reading and writing compared to listening and speaking. We cannot point or use facial expressions to communicate in reading and writing, although graphs, illustrations, and pictures are attempts to supplement written material. Additionally, speech consists of sounds that occur over time, and these are generally temporary and fleeting. Writing consists of marks in space that are relatively permanent and can be referred to repeatedly. However, it is faster to speak than to write. Another difference is the fact that most children acquire the auditory–oral system without formalized instruction, whereas carefully planned instructional processes are typically offered in schools in order to teach most children to read and write. And, while use of the auditory–oral system can develop independently of the visual–graphic system, proficiency with the visual–graphic system is exceedingly difficult to achieve without first acquiring some proficiency with the auditory–oral system. This point will be reiterated in later parts of this text.

Visual–Gestural Systems

Consistent with our earlier discussions, the visual modality combined with gestures, body postures and movements, and/or facial grimaces can be used as communication modes. Here we introduce readers to two forms of visual–gestural communication systems: manual communication and other forms of augmentative/alternative communication (AAC). Another form of a visual–gestural communication system, nonverbal communication with its nonlinguistic elements, was discussed previously, and that discussion will not be repeated here. We do include brief discussions of manual communication and other AAC systems because these are sometimes used with children who have language and/or speech disorders.

Manual Communication.   One of the more familiar visual–gestural systems is manual communication, or sign language, sometimes used by people who are deaf or severely hearing impaired. Children with other speech and/or language problems also sometimes use manual communication. There are many forms of manual communication. Some use manual signs that correspond closely to or match exactly the sequence of morphemes in English syntax. Other forms are actually languages different from English. One is American Sign Language (ASL), which, as the name implies, is a language communicated through the visual–gestural modalities used in the United States. However, other English-speaking countries, for example, England and Australia, have different signed languages, e.g., Auslan in Australia. Just as speakers of one language, such as Greek, will not understand speakers of another language, such as Cantonese Chinese, users of ASL cannot be expected to understand users of Auslan and vice versa.

Understanding that ASL is a language raises several questions about the education of children who are hearing-impaired. For example, are we, in teaching reading and writing to children who already know ASL, attempting to teach them to use a visual–graphic system of a language (English) for which they have little background? Is this a second-language visual–graphic system for them? For those children who acquire some oral communicative skills, are these oral skills based on a different language than the one they may already know (ASL)? We really do not yet know all the answers to these questions.

Augmentative/Alternative Communication (AAC).　　In addition to manual communication, a number of AAC systems rely primarily on visual–gestural modes for communication. With professionals' increased understanding of and emphasis on communication, greater acceptance and use of AAC for individuals with speech and/or language problems has occurred. Advances in technology in general have also facilitated the development of a wide variety of more sophisticated, efficient, and flexible AAC systems. Later in this text we will discuss AAC in more depth as an intervention for some children with language disorders.

Biological, Cognitive, and Social Bases of Human Communication

Communication is a complex linguistic, biological, cognitive, and social phenomenon. All of these factors are involved in language functioning, but the ways in which they interact are not fully understood. Earlier in this chapter we discussed some of the linguistic and social bases of language. Here, we introduce some of the biological and cognitive bases of language and include some additional discussion of social bases of language. Volumes have been written on each of these topics. We cannot hope to cover them in depth in one chapter. Rather, this chapter provides an overview or, for some readers, a refresher.

Biological Bases of Communication

In the previous section on communication modes, we read that hearing and speaking were identified as the primary modalities used in spoken languages. Although other modalities, such as vision and gesture, may contribute to the total communicative process, our discussion here provides an overview of the major physical bases of auditory–oral language: the ear, the speech mechanism, and the nervous system.

Hearing and Listening

Basic Anatomy and Physiology of the Ear.　　The ear is the sensory mechanism that receives sound waves and converts them into mechanical, hydraulic, and finally electrical/electrochemical energy (neural impulses). If the ear is not adequately sensitive to a variety of sound frequencies (the psychological parallel is pitch) and intensities (the psychological parallel is loudness), auditory information needed to receive and understand the spoken code of others is prevented from being converted to neural impulses and reaching the brain.

The ear consists of three main parts: the outer ear, the middle ear, and the inner ear. Together these are the peripheral hearing mechanism (Figure 1.3). In the *outer ear,* the auricle

Outer Ear   **Middle Ear**   **Inner Ear**

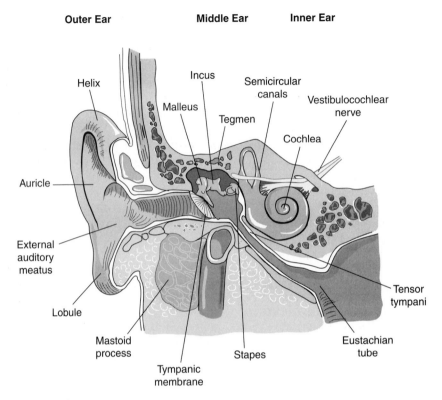

FIGURE 1.3   **The Ear**

and ear canal (external auditory meatus) collect sound waves and funnel them toward the middle ear, where the waves hit the eardrum (tympanic membrane) and make it vibrate. The movement of the eardrum, now mechanical energy, is transferred to three small bones of the *middle ear*—the malleus, incus, and stapes—which pass the movement to the inner ear. The major structure for hearing in the *inner ear* is the cochlea. The *cochlea* contains a membranous structure suspended in fluid. As the mechanical energy in the middle ear reaches the inner ear, the fluid is set in motion. Mechanical energy now becomes hydraulic energy. As the fluid moves, it impinges on a membranous structure in the cochlea that also contains fluid and the end organ of hearing, the *organ of Corti*. Rows of inner and outer cells that contain protruding hairs (*inner hair cells, outer hair cells*) extend from the organ of Corti to the membrane so that as the fluid moves it causes the membrane to move and the result is a rubbing or shearing action on these parts of the organ of Corti. This rubbing converts the hydraulic energy to neural energy, which travels to the brain via cranial nerve VIII (the vestibulocochlear, or auditory, nerve). The brain interprets the neural energy it receives.

Biological Basis for Listening to Speech.   According to Owens (2001), the middle and inner ears reach their adult size at 20 weeks gestation. The auditory nerve is developed by the 24th week of gestation. Newborn infants thus enter the world having listened to their internal environment (e.g., mother's blood flow and heart beat) and external environment (e.g., mother's speech, music, environmental noises) for some months. They enter the world with some idea of what it sounds like. Researchers have shown that infants can in fact discriminate between a variety of speech sounds and linguistic boundaries within the first few weeks and months of life (Vihman, 1996). Infants as young as 4 weeks old have also been found to attend longer to facial (lip) movements that match the vowels being heard than those that do not match the vowels being heard (Kuhl, 1990; Kuhl & Meltzoff, 1988). Apparently, infants' attending skills are intermodal in that they associate lip movements with the appropriate speech sounds. These findings support the idea that infants have a biological basis for attending to speech. How infants and toddlers actually learn to process incoming auditory stimuli, however, and understand the speech they listen to, is a more complex phenomenon.

Speech and Talking

Basic Anatomy and Physiology of the Speech Mechanism.　　The anatomical structures used to produce speech are actually parts of the respiratory and digestive systems (Figure 1.4). The exhaled air from the lungs provides the basic source of energy for speech. It is this air that is modified by the vocal folds in the larynx ("voice box") and/or the vocal tract—pharyngeal (throat), oral (mouth), and nasal (nose) cavities above the vocal folds—that results in speech. The physical production of speech requires four processes: respiration,

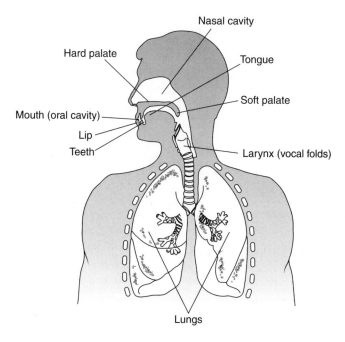

FIGURE 1.4　The Speech Mechanism

phonation, resonation, and articulation (McLaughlin, 1998). Let's now take a brief look at the main structures involved in these processes.

The *larynx,* located in the front of the neck, houses the *vocal folds.* The function of the larynx is not solely or primarily the production of sound. Rather, the larynx and vocal folds serve to stop foreign objects (such as food) from entering the airway and as such keep us alive (McLaughlin, 1998). If we want the larynx to produce voice, then respiration and phonation are needed in addition to the functioning of the larynx. *Respiration* involves the inhalation and exhalation of air from the lungs. *Phonation* involves the use of the exhaled air from the lungs in conjunction with changes in subglottic air pressure to create vibrations of the vocal folds (Boone & McFarlane, 2000).

During the production of approximately one-half of the English consonants, the vocal folds do not move to phonate, or produce voice. Hence, these sounds are termed *voiceless consonants.* The production of voiceless consonants merely requires the air from the lungs to pass unobstructed through the vocal folds into the vocal tract. If a hand is placed lightly against the front of the neck (where the larynx is located) and the consonant /s/ is produced with no accompanying vowel, no vibration is felt. However, during production of all vowels and the remaining consonants, the vocal folds vibrate to create a voiced sound. Thus, phonemes that require vocal-fold vibration are termed *voiced sounds.* Vocal-fold vibration, or phonation, can be felt when a hand is held lightly on the front of the neck as a sound such as /z/ is produced. The size of the vocal folds and the rate at which they vibrate are primary factors in determining the pitch of a person's voice. Generally, the faster something vibrates, the higher is the pitch.

After the exhaled air passes through the larynx, it travels through the vocal tract (including the pharyngeal, oral, and or nasal cavities), as shown in Figure 1.4. When the vocal folds have vibrated and therefore vibrated the air, a sound wave is produced and the vocal tract acts like a resonator, much like the main body of a cello. *Resonation* involves the modification of the sound generated at the vocal folds through changing the shape and size of the spaces in the vocal tract (McLaughlin, 1998), which emphasizes some parts of sound waves and dampens others. The outgoing air (whether or not the vocal folds are vibrating) also hits barriers in the form of the palate (the roof of the mouth), the tongue, lips, and teeth. These movable barriers are the articulators and the different positions they take give the outgoing air (vibrating or not) certain characteristics, that is, articulation.

The *impedance* (obstruction, barrier) of the air is greater for consonants than vowels. Some obstructions for consonants are complete and are then released (e.g., /p/, /t/, /k/), while other obstructions allow for an obstructed but continuous flow of air (e.g., /s/, "sh"). The type of obstruction is called the *manner of formation.* The place in the mouth where obstruction occurs for consonants (e.g., lips–teeth for /f/, or back of the tongue for /k/) is termed the *place of articulation.* The different positions of the articulators cause sound energy to be concentrated in different frequencies. For example, /s/ and /z/ have sound energy concentrated in higher frequencies, whereas /f/ and /v/ have sound energy concentrated in lower frequencies. If a consonant is voiced, such as /z/, the mouth noises created by the articulators are superimposed on the vibrations of the vocal folds. Therefore, voiced sounds have a fundamental frequency from the vocal-fold vibrations, which is comparatively low, and concentrations of sound energy in certain other higher frequencies (mouth noises) because of the obstructions of the articulators. For most English vowels and consonants, the exhaled air is directed into the oral cavity, or mouth. However, production of three

English phonemes ("m," "n," and "ng") requires that the air be directed into the nasal cavity to create a nasal resonance (*nasalization*). The effect of the air in the nasal cavity can be felt if an index finger is placed lightly along the bony side of the nose while saying a prolonged /n/. As all three nasal sounds are voiced, the nasal resonance is superimposed on vocal-fold vibration.

For vowels, all of which are voiced as we have noted, the articulators place few obstructions in the way of the exhaled air. Instead, movement of the articulators changes the internal shape of the mouth cavity in order to give each vowel its unique sound. These changes concentrate sound energy in different frequencies. For each vowel, energy concentration occurs in identifiable bands at different frequencies, including the low-frequency one associated with the vocal-fold vibrations. The frequency location of the higher frequency bands of energy gives each vowel its unique acoustic features. The bands of energy are called *formants,* which are particularly important for receiving and perceiving speech and play important roles in what children with hearing impairments might be able to detect and perceive.

Biological Basis for Speech Production.   Infants' vocal tracts become adultlike over the first three years of their life (Kent, 1999). Unlike the ear, which is born ready to listen to speech, the infant vocal tract differs from the adult and so is not in such a ready state for producing speech. Hillis and Bahr (2001) note the following differences between the newborn's vocal tract and that of the adult:

1. The oral space of the newborn is small.
2. The lower jaw of the newborn is small and somewhat retracted.
3. Sucking pads are present in infants but not in adults.
4. The tongue takes more relative space in the newborn, because of the diminished size of the lower jaw and the presence of sucking pads in the cheeks.
5. The tongue shows restrictions in movement, partially because of the restricted intraoral cavity in which it resides.
6. Newborns are obligated mouth-breathers. They do not breath through their noses.
7. The epiglottis and soft palate are in approximation in the newborn as a protective mechanism.
8. Newborns can breathe and swallow at the same time.
9. The larynx is higher in the neck of the newborn than in the older infant or adult. This eliminates the need for sophisticated laryngeal closure to protect the airway during swallowing.
10. The Eustachian tube in the infant lies in a horizontal position. It assumes a more vertical angle in the adult. (pp. 17–18)

Over the first three years of life, the vocal tract anatomy and function of a child change. For instance, tongue muscle tone increases, tongue movements become dissociated from jaw movements, lip closure improves, the larynx moves farther down the vocal tract, and more sophisticated movements (including elevation) of the larynx occur during swallowing (Hillis & Bahr, 2001). Together, these changes coincide with an improvement in the child's ability to articulate. Thus, although the speech-production mechanism is devoted primarily to breathing and swallowing, it develops into a marvelous platform for speech production.

The Controller and Interpreter: The Nervous System

Basic Anatomy and Physiology of the Nervous System.   Two major divisions of the nervous system are integrally involved in communication: the central nervous system (brain and spinal cord) and the peripheral nervous system (cranial and spinal nerves). A third division, the autonomic nervous system, regulates the presumably involuntary bodily functions, such as stomach and bowel contractions and heartbeat. Since this last system affects speech and language only indirectly, it will not be discussed here.

The Central Nervous System (CNS).   At its superior end, the spinal cord forms a structure known as the *brain stem* (Figure 1.5). The cerebrum (often referred to as the *brain*) sits on top of the brain stem and surrounds it, much as a mushroom top surrounds the upper stem of a mushroom. The wrinkled outer surface of the cerebrum is the *cortex*. The cerebellum is located below the cerebrum and behind the brain stem. Like the cerebrum, the cerebellum also has a wrinkled outer surface called a cortex. The wrinkles of both structures are the result of folds in the surfaces. Each ridge created by these folds is known as a *gyrus,* or *convolution,* and each indentation caused by the folds is called a *sulcus,* or *fissure.* These convolutions and fissures provide us with landmarks in order to describe the brain.

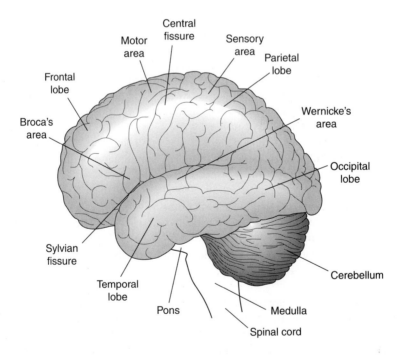

Lateral View

FIGURE 1.5   **The Brain**

Both the cerebellum and the cerebrum are divided into left and right hemispheres. Each cerebral hemisphere is further divided into four lobes. The most anterior lobe is known as the *frontal lobe.* The *parietal lobe* lies behind the frontal lobe and is separated from it by the *central fissure.* Behind the parietal lobe is the *occipital lobe.* The *temporal lobe* is on the side and separated from the frontal lobe by the *Sylvian fissure.* The area around the Sylvian fissure is known as the *perisylvian area,* which contains the *planum temporale* in the upper portion of the temporal lobe in the perisylvian area. The planum temporale is well implicated in language function.

The cells that make up the nervous system are referred to as *neurons.* Most neurons contain a nucleus (contained within a cell body), an array of dendrites extending from one side of the nucleus—which conduct impulses toward the nucleus—and an axon extending from the other side of the nucleus—which conducts impulses away from the nucleus. When a neural impulse is generated by the nucleus of a neuron, the impulse travels along the axon until it reaches another cell. The point at which one neuron meets another is referred to as a *synapse.* The neural impulse then crosses the synapse and continues its journey onto adjacent cells, via chemicals known as neurotransmitters. Curiously, the power and complexity of the human brain is not due to the sheer number of neurons, but rather to the rich array of inter-connections (particularly, dendritic connections) between neurons (McLaughlin, 1998).

As the result of studies investigating the effects of damage to parts of the brain on neurological functions and, more recently, studies using newer neuroimaging techniques, we know that certain functions in adults are generally related to different parts of the cerebral cortex. The *motor area* is located in the frontal lobe in front of the central fissure. Neural impulses are sent from the motor area to various muscles of the body, including those involved in speech production, in order to produce movement. For most adults, regardless of which hand is dominant, the left cerebral hemisphere is the primary controller of speech and language. In fact, only 40 percent of left-handers, which in turn is only 2 percent of the population, are right-hemisphere dominant for speech and language (Owens, 2001). For the majority of the population, the left frontal lobe in front of the motor area and above the Sylvian fissure is a region known as *Broca's area.* This area programs speech production. It coordinates neural signals that then travel to the motor area (also located in the frontal lobe but in front of the central fissure) and subsequently to the articulators. Congruent with the left hemisphere's dominance for speech and language, Broca's area in the left frontal lobe is typically described as more convoluted than the corresponding area in the right hemisphere. Furthermore, for adults, damage to Broca's area in the left hemisphere impairs speech production, whereas damage to the same area in the opposite hemisphere typically results in no discernible disturbance of speech production. The sensory area of the cerebrum is located in the parietal lobe just behind the central fissure. This area receives neural impulses from various parts of the body and uses this information to help control functions in those parts of the body.

Many of the functions of the temporal lobe are involved in receiving and processing auditory stimuli. For example, the auditory (vestibulocochlear) nerve, which transmits neural impulses from the ear to the brain, courses toward the temporal lobe. An area in an adult's left hemisphere especially important for the comprehension of oral language—Wernicke's area—is located partially in the temporal and partially in the parietal lobe. The left Wernicke's area is dominant for understanding spoken words. In contrast, processing of other types of sounds, including music, takes place largely in the right hemisphere. However, there is some evidence that in adults, both the right and left temporal-parietal areas are active when they listen to speech.

Although certain functions can be attributed to specific parts of the cerebral cortex, Boone (1985) reminds us that "there is far greater appreciation today of the interplay among all parts of the brain as a requisite for normal function" (p. 374). One way in which the structure of the cerebrum provides for functional interrelationships among cortical areas is via its association fibers. These fibers, located in the interior of the cerebrum, interconnect various cortical areas, including lobes and hemispheres. The largest and most important interhemisphere fiber is the *corpus callosum,* containing approximately 200 million neurons (Owens, 2001). Another particularly important association fiber connects Wernicke's area with Broca's area.

The cerebellum is the last structure of the CNS to be discussed. This structure is integrally involved in analysis and coordination of motor activity, although it does not initiate any of the activity. Its analytic and coordinating functions result in the ability to produce well-timed, smooth movements.

The Peripheral Nervous System (PNS).   The PNS is made up of 12 pairs of cranial nerves and 31 pairs of spinal nerves. The cranial nerves extend from the brain stem primarily to the neck and head areas, and the spinal nerves extend from the spinal cord to the remaining lower parts of the body. Many of the nerves contain both sensory fibers (which travel to the CNS and provide it with information) and motor fibers (which transmit commands from the CNS to various parts of the body). Cranial nerves are identified by both Roman numerals and names. Seven of these twelve pairs of cranial nerves are especially important for speech and language functions (see Table 1.6). These nerves carry the command signals originating in the CNS to the specific muscles of speech production that they innervate. Their sensory fibers then feed back to the CNS information about the performances of muscles. This allows the CNS to monitor the activities and send corrective signals if necessary. Furthermore, information about the acoustic characteristics of a speech signal, sent to the CNS via the auditory nerve, augments other sensory data about an organism's speech and language performance.

Neurological Basis for Human Communication.   Much of our discussion thus far has centered on the adult nervous system. Care must be taken when attempting to draw parallels between adult and child neurological functioning. The nervous systems of children are immature. Like the speech-production mechanism, the newborn's nervous system, particularly the CNS, has further anatomical and physiological advances to come. This can be seen by the sheer difference in weight of the human brain. At birth, the infant's brain weighs only 25 percent of the adult brain weight (McLaughlin, 1998). So what needs to develop? More neurons? No. Neuron formation is complete by birth. In fact, the human brain is thought to contain a complete set of neurons by 5 months' gestation (Kent, 1999). What does need to occur is an increase in the interconnections between the neurons. If we focus on the areas of the brain dedicated to communication development, according to Hillis and Bahr (2001), by about 3 months of age dendritic branching becomes "more advanced in the oral area of the cortical motor strip than in Broca's area and in the right hemisphere than in the left hemisphere" (p. 3). By around 2 years of age, dendritic branching is thought to become

TABLE 1.6   Seven Cranial Nerves Involved in Language and Speech

Number of the Nerve	Name	Functions
V	Trigeminal	*Sensory*—face; jaw; mouth
		Motor—jaw; soft palate
VII	Facial	*Sensory*—taste; mucous membrane of soft palate and pharynx
		Motor—face; lips
VIII	Vestibulocochlear (auditory)	*Sensory*—hearing; balance
IX	Glossopharyngeal	*Sensory*—taste; mucous membrane of pharynx, middle ear, and mouth
		Motor—pharynx
X	Vagus	*Sensory*—mucous membrane of pharynx, larynx, soft palate, tongue, and lungs
		Motor—larynx; pharynx
XI	Accessory	*Motor*—soft palate; larynx; pharynx; neck
XII	Hypoglossal	*Sensory*—tongue
		Motor—tongue

more complex in the Broca's area and throughout the rest of the left hemisphere, and by 6 years of age, dendritic branching in the Broca's area is more advanced than the oral region of the motor cortex (Hillis & Bahr, 2001). Thus, children are born with the neurological *potential* for speech and language acquisition. With exposure and experience, children's brains change and learn to understand and produce speech and language.

Having noted that certain parts of the adult brain are dedicated to linguistic functions, and that children's brains gradually develop the rich array of interconnections seen in the adult brain, children's brains differ in one particularly important aspect. Children's brains are described as having much more *plasticity* and much less cerebral *localization* and specialization than those of adults. Consequently, the effects on language seen from focal CNS damage in adults may not be seen in children. Damage limited to left hemispheric areas in children appears not to account fully for the presence of developmental language disorders, as opposed to language disorders in children who have acquired language problems as a result of childhood trauma or disease.

Thus, while we have certainly come a long way in understanding how the brain works and how infants are born with the neurological potential for learning speech and language, we still have a lot more to learn and understand. As Kent (1999) states, "neural development is far from well understood, and only fragmentary information is available on many of the structures and processes thought to be involved in speech production" (p. 46).

Cognitive Bases of Language

What Is Cognition?   Consider the newborn infant for a moment. For months he or she has been curled up in a protective and nurturing environment. The day of birth brings with it a whole new environment to get to know and understand if he or she is to survive. This task of "getting to know" is what cognition is about (Carlson, 1987). The newborn infant needs to learn how to process incoming stimuli and make sense of them. According to Piaget (1954), infants have psychological structures (schemas or schemata) that allow them to process and organize incoming stimuli. Over time, these schemas adapt or change in response to incoming stimuli. In Piaget's pursuit to understand the development of cognition he proposed a series of stages that children progress through as they learn to "get to know" the world in which they live. Specifically, Piaget proposed four stages of cognitive development: (1) the sensorimotor stage from birth to about 2 years, (2) the preoperational stage from about 2 to 7 years, (3) the concrete operations stage from about 7 to 11/12 years, and (4) the formal operations stage from about 11 years to 14/15 years. These are described in more detail in Table 1.7.

Within the first year of infancy, specifically during the sensorimotor stage of cognitive development, children develop a particularly important cognitive ability that enables them to learn more about the world in which they live—they learn to create symbolic mental representations (Bernstein & Levey, 2002). Why is this ability important? Earlier in this chapter we defined language as a code in which we make specific symbols stand for something else. Thus, it would seem that cognition and language are related. However, there is no universal agreement concerning the nature of the relationship. Does cognitive development for specific mental processes occur *before* the acquisition of language structures? Does language influence cognition? Are the developments of language and cognition separate entities that become entwined at some point? If so, when? Finally, how do language and cognition influence each other? We have no definitive answers to these questions yet, although a number of theoretical positions regarding the relationship of language and cognition have been advanced.

The Relationship between Cognition and Language

Dependency of Language on Cognition.   According to one view of the relationship between language and cognition, language use is a function of cognition and its acquisition is dependent on underlying cognitive processes. Proponents of this position strongly support the notion of cognitive precursors to language, that is, prerequisite cognitive abilities that children need to develop before learning various language skills. This viewpoint is sometimes referred to as the *strong cognition hypothesis.*

Piaget is one of the best-known advocates of this position. According to Piaget, children progress through each of the cognitive developmental stages he proposed (see Table 1.7) in order, without skipping any of them, and each stage of development is the foundation for each succeeding stage. As children progress through the stages, they acquire the necessary cognitive operations that lead to the development of successively higher levels of language. Piaget, therefore, believes that thought precedes language. Language use is a reflection of underlying cognitive skills.

A related view of language functioning as dependent on cognition is the *weak cognition hypothesis.* This position proposes that cognition accounts for many of a child's lan-

TABLE 1.7   Characteristics of Piaget's Stages of Cognitive Development

Sensorimotor (0–2 years)

Substage 1: 0–2 months
Reflexive sensorimotor behavior
Reflexive vocal/prelinguistic behavior

Substage 2: 2–4 months
Coordinated hand–mouth movements
Coordinated eye–hand and auditory orienting
   movements
Anticipatory gestures

Substage 3: 4–8 months
Begins to act otorically on objects
Searches for objects
Babbles and imitates sounds

Substage 4: 8–12 months
Begins to recognize own ability to cause objects to
   move
Early stages of walking
Searches for objects based on memory of last
   location
Uses first word

Substage 5: 12–18 months
Experimentation with objects' functions and
   properties
Imitates models' behaviors when models present
Walks
Evidence of object permanency

Substage 6: 18–24 months
Represents objects internally
Problem solving with thought
Acquires basic cause–effect relations
Uses memory for deferred imitations
Uses words when referents not present

Preoperational (2–7 years)

Preconceptual: 2–4 years
Experiences difficulty with sub- and
   supraclassifications
Uses transductive reasoning (inferences from one
   specific to another specific)
Over- and underextends word meanings

Intuitive: 4–7 years
Thought guided by perceptions
Deals with only one variable at a time
Lacks conservation and reversibility
Employs improved but still inadequate classification
   skills
Egocentric
Concreteness of thought

Concrete Operations (7–11/12 years)
Uses effective classification skills
Acquires conservation and seriation skills
Uses coordinated descriptions
Employs logical causality
Reasoning limited to concrete operations
Less egocentric

Formal Operations (11/12–14/15 years)
Uses hypothetical and prepositional reasoning
Demonstrates lack of egocentricity
Employs adequate verbal reasoning and logical
   "if . . . then" statements
Can deal with the abstract
Uses deductive and inductive thought processes

guage abilities, but not all of them. There remain some aspects of language that do not derive directly from cognition. Rice (1983) referred to this as a partial "mismatch" between language and cognition and presented, as examples of the mismatch, "language acquisition not rooted in parallel change in meanings, linguistic competence exceeding the supposed cognitive base, and language-specific difficulties with the expression of meanings" (p. 353).

Language and Cognition as Separate (but Sometimes Related) Entities.   A differing point of view concerning language and cognition is that although language and cognition are related, cognitive activity without language and language without underlying cognitive bases are both possible. For example, a composer or a sculptor at work is not necessarily directed by language processes (Langacker, 1968). Langacker suggested that if cognitive processes were not possible without language, we would never encounter situations in which we know the ideas we wish to convey but are unable to find the right words to express them. Whereas Langacker (1968) suggested that cognition without language is possible, Vygotsky (1962) proposed that language without appropriate underlying cognitive bases also occurs. He cited examples in which children correctly use conjunctions, such as *because, but,* and *if,* before they fully understand the logical relationships expressed by the terms.

Vygotsky (1962) also suggested that the developments of language and thought stem from different roots. A child progresses independently through a "preintellectual language" period and a "prelinguistic thought" phase. Although these lines of development are separate for some time, the two developmental processes do eventually merge. The child's thought then becomes verbal and language rational. According to Vygotsky (1962), once the union of language and thought has occurred, language becomes the foundation of further cognitive development:

> The speech [language] structures mastered by the child become the basic structures of his thinking. . . . The child's intellectual growth is contingent on his mastering the social means of thought, that is, language. (p. 51)

The *local homology model* offers a different point of view (Bates, Benigni, Bretherton, Camaioni, & Volterra, 1977, 1979). Some have observed that certain cognitive and linguistic skills develop at the same time, but not necessarily in a predetermined order. That is, a specific language ability sometimes emerges first, and in other instances a cognitive ability appears. This perspective suggests a correlative relationship between language and cognition for some skills at certain points in time, but the particular correlation between cognitive and language skills may not be maintained over time. Language and cognition are seen as distinct functions that both derive from a common but separate source. This model has found considerable favor with a number of professionals and researchers in the child language area.

Language Mediation of Cognition.   Although there may not be agreement on the exact nature of the early relationship between language and cognition, many suggest that, once acquired, language does mediate many of our cognitive processes. Although Piaget believed that in the earlier stages of a child's development thought precedes language use, he stressed the importance of language in the acquisition of conceptual thinking in the later stages of a child's development.

Both Vygotsky (1962) and Luria (1961) have proposed that language mediates cognitive activity. They used their concepts of *inner speech* and language as a *second signal system* to explain. Vygotsky (1962) and Luria (1961) viewed inner speech as thought processes that take place in the forms of words. Once language and thought have merged (as previously discussed), thinking occurs in terms of language or word meanings.

Vygotsky's concepts of inner speech led him to disagree with Piaget on the role of children's *egocentric* speech. Piaget described the egocentric speech of young children as speech that occurs with no intent to communicate with others, whether or not others are present, or with no attempt to consider the informational needs of others in communication. It is speech emanating from children who see themselves as the centers of the universe, without communicative concern for others. According to Piaget, egocentric speech disappears as children develop, and socialized speech—speech aimed specifically at interpersonal communication—emerges. Vygotsky, however, proposed that the egocentric speech of children is a forerunner of inner speech. He viewed the function of egocentric speech as an overt act of thought, or putting thought into expressed words. According to Vygotsky, the acts of expressing cognitive processes in words are children's ways of guiding and regulating their actions and thoughts. He suggested that as children develop, they are able to turn the overt expressions of thought inward into language, which is used for the same purposes of regulating and guiding thoughts and actions but is not heard by others, that is, inner speech. In contrast to Piaget, Vygotsky described egocentric speech as evolving into inner speech rather than disappearing and being replaced by socialized speech.

The discussion of egocentric speech functioning to regulate and guide thought and action, and then evolving into inner speech for the same guiding and regulating purposes, leads us to Luria's view of language functioning as a second signal system. As children interact with the environment and the verbalizations of adults, complex connections between perceived phenomena and words are formed (Luria & Yudovich, 1971). Initially, adult verbalizations in the presence of stimuli serve to guide children's behaviors, either to focus the children's attention on specific, essential features of stimuli or to modify and direct their actions in certain directions. That is, in the early developmental stages, the regulation (or direction) of children's cognitive activities and behaviors is externally controlled by the verbalizations of adults, which occur simultaneously with perceived phenomena. Because of the connections between these perceptions and others' verbalizations, children eventually begin to use the verbalizations internally to regulate their own behaviors. Through this process children learn to use language to direct their own thoughts and actions. Language becomes a mediator of cognition and purposeful behavior. For Luria, language is the basis of the development of higher mental processes because of the second signal function it plays in mediating experiences.

We have seen here several different views on the relationship between language and cognition, but we really do not know what the relationship is. What we generally agree on, however, is that there is a relationship and that the relationship is different at different stages of development.

Information Processing.   Information processing refers to the ways in which we deal with incoming stimuli and what we do in our heads to figure them out. There is currently considerable discussion in the literature about the role of various aspects of information processing in children's language learning and language disorders (Bishop, 1997; Gillam, Cowan, & Marler, 1998; Gillam, Hoffman, Marler, & Wynn-Dancy, 2002; Leonard, 1998; Marton & Schwartz, 2003; Montgomery, 2000, 2002a; Windsor, Milbrath, Carney, & Rakowski, 2001). A number of information processing models have been proposed, but in comparing models it is not unusual to find that they include different component processes, label the processes differently, and use different definitions for what appear to be similar processes. Furthermore, no one information processing model has been universally adopted. Ellis Weismer and Evans (2002) suggest that information processing accounts related to children's language disorders mostly fall into two broad groups—those emphasizing generalized processing and those focusing more on specific aspects of processing. Among the specific processing accounts, two aspects of processing are frequently discussed—phonological processing, which deals with the processes involved in the ability to mentally manipulate phonological aspects of language such as word rhyming or breaking words into their component phonemes (Baddeley, 1986; Just & Carpenter, 1992), and temporal auditory processing, which deals more specifically with the ability to perceive brief acoustic events that comprise speech sounds and track changes in these as they occur quickly in others' speech (Merzenich et al., 1996; Tallal, 1976). Among the generalized processing accounts, speed of processing (Miller, Kail, Leonard, & Tomblin, 2001; Montgomery & Leonard, 1998) and overall processing capacity (Ellis Weismer, Evans, & Hesketh, 1999; Montgomery, 2000) are prominent in discussions.

Processing linguistically based (verbal) information involves such functions as

- Selecting the elements of a verbal message to attend to
- Temporarily storing the representations of those elements in memory
- Keeping those representations active in our short-term memory so that they do not fade, disappear, or decay before we are finished working with them
- Organizing our cognitive functions and directing them to undertake particular tasks with the representations, that is, our analysis of the representations
- Choosing where and how to store the analyses of the representations in longer term memory for future use—or in some cases not sending the analyzed information to long-term memory store

It can also involve how and when we access the stored information at a later date, the form in which it is available to us, and the degree to which the original elements are or are not distorted as a result of all the processing. On a small scale, it is not unlike what we do when someone tells us a new telephone number and we need to walk into another part of the house to dial it. Most of us attend carefully to presentation of the number and then make a conscious (cognitive) effort to keep the number rumbling around in our heads so that we can actually "hear" the number silently in our heads as we move to the other room. We do not want any part of the auditory representation of the complete number to disappear on us. If the number is one we believe we need only once, many of us promptly let the auditory representation of the number in our heads decay after dialing it. That is, we forget the phonological representation, "phonological" because the numbers are words to us and the words are made up of phonemes. If we believe we will need the number again at a later time after we dial it, we undertake different processing strategies to move it into our long-term memory or we record it somewhere else in a different form. If we do the latter, we need to be able to find it when we need it—another memory process. If we decide to store it in our heads, we still need to be able to find and retrieve it when we need it—a different processing and memory process. Some of the associated terms encountered in information processing literature are *verbal working memory, working memory, short-term memory, auditory short-term memory, auditory processing, phonological processing, phonological memory,* and so on. Different terms are obviously associated with different accounts of information processing.

If we have inefficient or slow processing, smaller temporary storage capacities or resource limitations, poor working memories, problems dealing with fleeting auditory stimuli, or poor executive override and control of our processing, the elements we need to retain for processing incoming stimuli will decay in our heads before we have a chance to go through all the other processes we need to do with them for them to make sense, be usable, or learn from them. Something we need to keep in mind is that while we are trying to process one thing, other information is coming our way. "System overload" is possible if tasks to be processed are too hard or too fast for us and/or our systems are too fragile to deal with what might be quite easy tasks for another individual with a more robust system. These ideas find their way into concepts about children and their language impairments when we talk about trade-offs between different aspects of language performance, children's repetition of nonsense words as a way of assessing their information processing of phonological aspects of language, rehearsal strategies, central auditory processing dysfunction, and many other topics related to children's language learning or their problems with language. These are among the concepts associated with information processing ability that readers will encounter later in this text. In fact, our upcoming discussion of metacognition is not devoid of notions related to information processing.

Metacognition. Earlier in this chapter, we introduced the concept of metalinguistics. Like metalinguistics, metacognition relates to the ability to stand back from what we know and the cognitive skills that we have and consciously analyze, control, plan, and organize them. This has parallels with Vygotsky's concepts of inner speech that we encountered earlier. As adults, we can think about our thinking and can decide what learning and cognitive strategies we might want to use in specific situations. We can even monitor our performance and may decide to employ different learning or cognitive strategies. For example, if we need to memorize a list, we might choose to use any of several types of rehearsal strategies—saying the list over and over, writing the list over and over, or making up sayings (associations). If one strategy does not work, we may choose to abandon it for another or to use several strategies simultaneously. In other instances, we may ask ourselves: "What else do I know with which I can associate this new piece of information?" or "How can I organize this information so it makes sense?" These are all metacognitive activities.

In order to engage in metacognitive activities, we need to *decenter,* that is, be less egocentric, to use a Piagetian term. Like metalinguistics, true metacognition in children is a later-developing skill, with some suggesting a shift to metacognitive abilities occurring sometime in the early elementary grades. These grades tend to correspond to about the time children enter Piaget's concrete operations stage (Table 1.7). Another shift to higher-level, more refined metacognitive skills is generally seen at about grade 6, or 11 to 12 years of age, about the time children enter Piaget's formal operations stage.

Not surprisingly, metacognitive skills are important in school success. Expectations for how children are to solve problems and approach learning increase as children progress through school. By high school, students are expected to monitor and plan their own learning and to think and reason with adultlike abilities. We suspect some relationship between metacognitive and metalinguistic skills, but as with the relationship between cognition and language generally, the exact nature of the relationship is not clear. We do know, however, that many children with language disorders evidence problems with metacognitive tasks, as well as problems with metalinguistic tasks.

Social Bases of Human Communication

Even before babies are born, they are part of a social world. They spend months listening to their mother's voices and the voices of the people around her. They sense the rhythms of the mother's routine, including the quiet times and the busy times (Murray & Andrews, 2001). At birth, they seem to have an inborn tendency to seek social interaction (Solter, 2001). For instance, newborns are attracted to faces, despite never having seen one. Murray and Andrews (2001) describe the newborn's fascination with the face.

> A baby just a few minutes old, if content and alert, will gaze intently at the face of another person, watching them seriously. If the adult clearly and slowly moves her own face, for example, opening her mouth wide, or protruding her tongue, the baby will watch intently and then imitate the adult expression. It is as if the baby can already sense that she and the other person are in some way the same. (p. 21)

As we will see in this section, the social influences in children's language-learning environments play a major role in their acquisition of language and the rules that govern how the code is used in context. What follows is a short discussion on the social bases of communication. We look at infant–caregiver attachment and the nature of infant–caregiver interactions. We also look at two skills that are integral to social interaction and language learning: imitation and reinforcement.

Infant–Caregiver Attachment.   According to McLaughlin (1998), attachment is "the close, nurturing, long-term relationship that develops between the caregiver and the infant" (p. 84). During the first few months of an infant's life, he or she does not appear to mind being held by strangers or being briefly separated from caregivers. However, as infants get older they begin to show definite signs of attachment. They may cry or become distressed when separated from familiar caregivers. By the time infants learn to crawl, they may display attachment by following their parents and actively seeking to maintain contact with them (Solter, 2001). Why do infants become attached to their caregivers?

Certainly, taking care of basic needs is part of the answer, but the answer seems to be more complicated that this. According to Solter (2001), healthy infant–caregiver attachment may be the result of parents and infants sharing a unique system of communication. Caregivers become familiar with the ways their infants communicate needs and wants. The relationship is reciprocal. Infants learn that their caregivers are the ones who "understand" them and meet needs. Let's take a look at the nature of the infant–caregiver interaction and the social basis on which children learn how to communicate with other human beings.

Infant–Caregiver Interaction.   Infants and caregivers both have behaviors that are conducive to communication development. As we read earlier, infants have a preference for looking at the human face. Caregivers actually reciprocate by spending time gazing at their infant's face while producing a wide array of facial expressions that in turn sustain the infant's interest. Such early interactions provide a social foundation for speech and language development.

Infant Behaviors during Infant–Caregiver Interactions.   Certain infant behaviors appear to stimulate adults to respond in specific ways. One of the main behaviors or attributes of an infant that seems to motivate adults to attend to them and respond to their needs is their helplessness. As we have also seen, infants prefer looking at the face. This is helped by the fact that an infant's best visual acuity is around 22 cm, or the distance from the adult face to the infant being cradled in an adult's arms (Murray & Andrews, 2001). Infants also show a preference for their mother's voice. Other infant behaviors that seem to act as positive reinforcers of adults' language stimulation include eye gaze, smiling, and reciprocal touch and vocalization. As children become capable of producing some speech, they provide verbal feedback to adults in terms of what has and has not been comprehended, as well as signal understanding by increasing their attention to the adults. As Hubbell (1981) states, "In this way children regulate the input they receive and hence the language models that they learn from" (p. 276).

Caregiver Behaviors and Language during Infant–Caregiver Interactions.   Think back to the last time you interacted with an infant. How did you talk? What distance did you keep between you and the infant? What sorts of facial expressions did you use? What did you talk about? Your communication style probably (hopefully!) differed from the way you talk with your peers. Some of the behaviors you engaged in during an interaction with an infant probably included:

- Vocalizing in response to an infant's smile
- Moving in closer to an infant
- Engaging in eye gaze with an infant
- Holding and cuddling an infant in your arms
- Imitating an infant's behavior
- Waiting for an infant to respond to your behavior such as a smile or vocalization, and as such engaging the infant in turn taking
- Engaging in rituals such as "peekaboo"

Caregivers have also been shown to tune in to and respond to the different types of cries produced by their infants (hunger, pain, anger cry) (McLaughlin, 1998). The caregiver's responses may, in fact, teach infants that a cry provides attention, and therefore if they want attention, they initiate a cry.

In addition to the array of adult behaviors listed previously, the speech and language used by adults when conversing with infants and young children differs. Most investigations of adults' communication with young children have focused on mothers. Consequently, results tend to focus on discussions of *motherese,* a term used to describe the unique characteristics of maternal language patterns to children (Berko-Gleason & Weintraub, 1978). Table 1.8 summarizes a number of the characteristics of motherese.

As infants become young children and begin to use speech and language, not only do adults appear to modify their verbal input, they also appear to alter the ways they respond to children's utterances. For example, corrections of young children's inaccurate utterances

TABLE 1.8   Characteristics of *Motherese*

Short utterances

Syntactically simple but grammatically well-formed utterances

More concrete nouns and verbs and fewer modifiers in utterances

Proper nouns replacing pronouns

Length and complexity varied as a function of children's ages and language skills

Higher pitched than speech addressed to adults

Rising intonation patterns, rather than falling patterns, at the ends of the utterances

Duration of spoken words longer

Overall rate of speech slowed

Obvious pauses occur between individual utterances in mothers' speech

More than one stressed word in utterances

Stressed words typically substantive words rather than function words

Sources: Berko-Gleason & Weintraub (1978); Broen (1972); Brown (1973); Mahoney & Seely (1977); Moerk (1976); Phillips (1973); Snow (1972, 1977).

tend to be corrections of content (semantics) rather than morphosyntactic or phonological corrections. As children get older, however, mothers begin to correct these latter aspects of their children's utterances. During parent–child communicative interactions, adults have been found to respond to what the children say by using expansions and recasts of the children's utterances, with semantically contingent responses that may be paraphrases of the children's comments. Furthermore, adult responses tend to consist of frequent repetitions of messages.

Thus, it would seem that infant–caregiver interactions lay the foundation for speech and language acquisition. Infants seem to be prewired for social interaction. They also engage in certain behaviors that elicit responses from the adults around them. They become attached to caregivers who understand and respond to the ways in which they communicate. Primitive as these early communicative attempts may be, they pave the way for more complex symbolic communication. Caregivers also seem to have an ability to respond to infants that not only meets their needs, but provides them with a sociolinguistically rich environment that fosters speech and language acquisition.

Infant–Caregiver Interactions and Language Disorders: A Possible Link?   Infants' responses to adult inputs can either motivate the adults to continue their language-facilitating behaviors, discontinue them, or modify the behaviors to some that are less beneficial for language learning. It appears that children with a disability may not respond to parents' attention in ways that positively reinforce the parents to provide appropriate language stimulation.

Parents of children with language disorders have sometimes been criticized for not providing adequate and appropriate language stimulation for their children. This may not be a totally fair judgment. For the most part, parents of children with language disorders have been found to provide language stimulation similar to the stimulation that parents of younger children with normal language acquisition provide. However, in other instances, parents of children with language disorders may engage in some types of child–adult inter-actions that are less conducive to language learning. We must be careful, however, not to overgeneralize. In light of our previous discussion, it may be that the children, because of their disorders, do not provide the reinforcement for the parents to engage in appropriate language stimulation activities.

Imitation and Reinforcement.   The roles of imitation and reinforcement in language acquisition have been debated. Much of this debate has probably resulted from differing definitions of the terms. Imitation, if viewed as children's exact reproductions of adults' utterances, cannot account fully for the language-learning process. If that were the entire basis of language and speech acquisition, children would not produce novel utterances. On the other hand, if we view imitation in light of Bandura's (1971) concept of social, obser-vational learning, in which adults provide numerous models from which children abstract the key elements to form rules for behavior, then imitation that encompasses the rules, not exact duplications of the models, may well be involved in language learning.

This discussion does not imply that imitation in the form of exact duplications has no role in language learning, although its role may change as a function of age and/or language skill. Young children approaching the end of the sensorimotor stage of cognitive develop-ment have been found to produce a high percentage of imitative utterances. However, as productive language skills develop, the number of imitative responses decreases as children begin to use a higher proportion of unique, spontaneously generated utterances.

The role of reinforcement in language acquisition is also unclear. Reinforcement, as it is used in conditioning or stimulus–response theories of learning (Skinner, 1957), is not totally sufficient for language learning. Not all of children's early utterances are reinforced, and those that are may not be reinforced in a manner conducive to learning to talk. Yet chil-dren do learn to talk. Humans are social beings. If infants find that their early vocalizations, and toddlers discover that their early words, establish and maintain adults' interactions with them, then we may consider that reinforcement is operating. Furthermore, adults' expan-sions and paraphrases of children's utterances, in addition to providing language models, probably serve to reinforce verbal behavior, because they also maintain the adults' interac-tions with the children and support language production.

Summary

In this chapter we have seen that

- Communication refers to the sending and receiving of messages. It can be as simple as a sigh or as complex as a spoken word.
- Extralinguistic aspects of communication include paralinguistics, nonlinguistics, and metalinguistics.
- Language consists of a system of phonological, semantic, morphological, syntactic, and pragmatic rules that are used to put ideas and thoughts into a code in order to communicate them to others and to relate to others. Language is the code; speech is one of several sensorimotor processes that can be used to produce the code.
- Communication involves both comprehension and production, but the relationship between comprehension and production is not fully agreed on.

- Communication can be accomplished through several modes: auditory–oral (hearing and speech), visual–graphic (reading and writing), and visual–gestural modes.
- Communication has biological, social, and cognitive bases.
- Metacognition involves conscious analysis, control, planning, and organization of our thinking
- Infants have a tendency to seek social interaction, such as a preference for looking at the face, and engage in certain behaviors that make them active partners in their own language learning.
- Caregivers engage in an array of behaviors that facilitate social interaction with infants.

Communication refers to the sending and receiving of messages. For humans, language is the major vehicle for communication. Language comes about as a result of complex interactions among cognitive, physiological, psychological, and sociological factors. Numerous approaches have been taken in attempting to explain these interactions. None alone is sufficient to describe how children learn language. Language is a complicated human behavior that has yet to be explained by any single theory or approach.

2 Normal Language Development

A Review

VICKI A. REED   **ELISE BAKER**

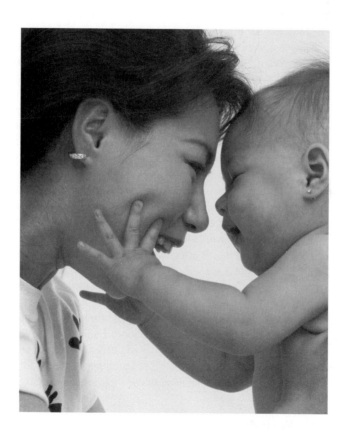

OBJECTIVES

After reading this chapter you should be able to discuss

- Prelinguistic communication development and types of vocalizations produced by infants during the prelinguistic period

- Language skills of children aged 1.0 to 2.0 years, including semantic, morphological, phonological, and pragmatics abilities
- Types of two-word utterances produced by children, as well as their pragmatic characteristics
- Many of the major features of the language development of preschool and school-aged children in terms of their phonological, semantic, morphological, syntactic, and pragmatic development
- How oral language relates to literacy and education and general expectations for children at different stages of their education

Learning to talk is a relatively orderly process, although not all children acquire all language abilities in precisely the same order and at identical speed. There is individual variation. Nevertheless, as a general pattern, newly acquired skills are used to modify and augment existing language abilities, and these new abilities are based on earlier learned skills. The process is one of refinement, expansion, and extension. Language learning is synergistic in nature. All components of language—syntax, morphology, semantics, phonology, and pragmatics—interact to evolve gradually into adultlike competence. Although there is variability in individual children's language acquisition, there is also a great deal of consistency. What may be the most amazing aspect of this process is that by about 7 to 8 years of age, most children have learned to use oral language to communicate in basically adultlike fashion. This does not mean, however, that language development stops at these ages. We need to be careful not to fall into the trap of thinking that only uninteresting and minor language development occurs beyond 8 years of age. As we shall see in Chapter 5, some important language skills are not fully acquired until the adolescent years and possibly beyond. Nevertheless, 7- and 8-year-old children typically produce a wide variety of well-formed sentences containing large numbers of different words with only rare speech-production errors. Moreover, they use these sentence types and words effectively and fluently for many different purposes.

In this chapter we will take a quick trip through some of the language achievements of younger children. The discussion is by no means complete, and much more has been written about children's language acquisition. An extensive discussion is well beyond the scope of this book. What this chapter does provide is an overview of some of the major language milestones during early childhood. Language development in adolescence will be discussed in Chapter 5, which also addresses teenagers with language disorders. In this chapter, we also take a brief look at language and emergent literacy and the educational sequence in which children need to use their language skills to achieve.

The Prelinguistic Period: The First 12 Months

From the moment of birth, newborns communicate. Sucking movements may indicate that a newborn is ready to feed, squinting may indicate a dislike for bright lights, and crying may indicate a dislike for the coldness of a delivery suite (Solter, 2001). This period during which an infant communicates, but does not use language, is known as the *prelinguistic period.* To the casual observer, the prelinguistic period may seem quite uneventful

(Hulit & Howard, 2002). To the trained observer, however, the prelinguistic period is a hive of developmental activity. An incredible amount of learning takes place prior to an infant's first birthday in order for the "first word" to be uttered. The term *infant* is used in this section, in keeping with the Latin form of the word *infans*, which means "one unable to speak" (McLaughlin, 1998).

Prelinguistic Communication Development

To appreciate the communication development of the prelinguistic infant, an understanding of the basic "pragmatic" elements of a speech act are needed. These basic elements include (1) the speaker having an intention to communicate—known as *illocution*, (2) the speaker expressing intention—known as *locution*, and (3) the listener interpreting the speaker's intended utterance—known as *perlocution* (Bates, 1976). During the first 8 months of an infant's life, the focus is on the perlocutionary element of the speech act and this is therefore known as the perloctionary period. During this period, caregivers have a vital role to play in facilitating learning, because the infant's behaviors are not intentionally communicative but need to be interpreted as communicative. Some of the infant's behaviors that caregivers interpret as communicative include:

- Different cries that reflect hunger, pain, or anger (Reich, 1986)
- Facial expressions including displeasure, fear, sorrow, anger, joy, and disgust (Owens, 2001)
- Eye-gaze patterns, including mutual gaze (prolonged eye contact), gaze coupling (infant and caregiver looking at each other, looking away, and looking back), and deictic gaze (infant looking at an object of interest) (McLaughlin, 1998)
- Moving limbs and making mouth movements such as opening the mouth, pushing the tongue forward, and smiling, when in a settled state (Murray & Andrews, 2001)

By about 3 months of age, the infant and caregiver engage in protoconversations. According to Owens (2001), these "conversations" typically consist of the caregiver initiating an interaction, followed by the infant and caregiver engaging in greeting behaviors (mutual smiles and eye gazes). Play dialogue follows the greeting. During play dialogue, the caregiver talks, then pauses to allow the infant time to vocalize during the pause. The dialogue continues until the infant or caregiver looks away. These are sometimes also referred to as reciprocal interactions between adult and child. Protoconversations are an important experience for the infant, as they teach the infant the basic ingredients of a conversation, including greeting and taking turns. By 6 months of age many infant–caregiver interactions become triadic, as they include an object or toy (Owens, 2001).

By about 8 months of age the infant begins to show signs of communicative intent, and thus enters the illocutionary period of communication development. This period typically spans 8 to 12 months of age (Hulit & Howard, 2002). Gestures such as showing objects to adults, requesting items by pointing to them, and giving objects to adults are considered to be the hallmark of the illocutionary period. During this period, infants are able to follow the eye direction of an adult to locate the object at which the adult looks when the object is present in the infant's visual field (Delgado et al., 2002). This ability to use joint attention or mutual gaze is important because it provides a basis for pairing words with objects. Another important communication milestone occurs around 8 to 9 months, specifically, the comprehension of spoken first words (Benedict, 1979).

By 12 months of age, the infant enters the final stage for the development of the speech act, known as the locutionary period. Between 12 and 18 months of age, children become gradually able to use joint attention to locate objects outside their immediate visual field (Delgado et al., 2002). Also at about the time of the infant's first birthday, he or she begins to use words to accompany or replace gestures (Owens, 2001). True language or symbolic representation thought expressed in words has begun. A major milestone in language development has been achieved. The infant is no longer "unable to speak," has typically begun to walk, and is therefore considered a toddler.

Prelinguistic Vocal Development

The sounds that infants make change in the first year of life from reflexive vocalizations to babbling to the emergence of the first word at approximately 12 months of age. This section reviews the vocal development of the infant over the first 12 months, using five stages proposed by Stark (1980) and Oller (1980) to guide discussion.

Stage 1 (Birth to 2 Months): Reflexive Vocalizations. From birth to approximately 2 months, the infant has a relatively small repertoire of reflexive vocalizations and vegetative sounds. The first reflexive vocalization is the birth cry, which is produced in response to the first breath. Subsequent cries signaling hunger, pain, and anger are considered a reaction to internal stimuli (McLaughlin, 1998). Other types of reflexive vocalizations include coughing, grunting, and burping (Bauman-Waengler, 2000). Vegetative sounds include sighs, vowel-like sounds, and grunts associated with an activity, in addition to lip and tongue clicks and other noises associated with feeding (Bauman-Waengler, 2000; McLaughlin, 1998; Paul, 2001; Proctor, 1989).

Stage 2 (2 to 4 Months): Cooing and Laughter. From 2 to 4 months, the infant's range of vocalizations changes with the appearance of cooing, sounds associated with pleasure, and laughter. *Cooing* refers to vowel-like sounds (often "oo") preceded by velar consonant-like sounds such as "g" or "k" (McLaughlin, 1998). Infants are thought to coo when they are in a comfortable state. Infants have also been observed to produce pleasure-like sounds such as "mmmm" during this stage (Paul, 2001). Laughter emerges around 16 weeks (Gesell & Thompson, 1934). Crying and primitive vegetative sounds are thought to reduce from about 12 weeks onwards (Bauman-Waengler, 2000).

Stage 3 (4 to 6 Months): Vocal Play. From 4 to 6 months, the infant's repertoire of vocalizations expands to include a greater number of vowel-like and consonant-like sounds (including front plosives and nasals), to make way for marginal babbling (Paul, 2001). According to McLaughlin (1998), marginal babbling refers to "infant sound productions with a variety of vowels and consonant-like productions that approximate syllables" (p. 434), which may contain sounds that are both representative and not representative of the infant's native language. The infant's fascination with sounds produced at the front of the mouth sees the introduction of raspberries and lip smacks. Intonation contours also emerge, along with yells, squeals, and low-pitched growls (Paul, 2001).

Stage 4 (6 Months and Older): Canonical Babbling.   From 6 months onwards, canonical babbling emerges. Canonical babbling is a collective term for the production of reduplicated and nonreduplicated (or variegated) babbling (Bauman-Waengler, 2000). Put simply, babbling refers to well-formed syllables that consist of at least one vowel-like sound and one consonant-like sound that are connected in quick transition (Oller, Levine, Cobo-Lewis, Eilers, & Pearson, 1998). Descriptions of the two types of babbling observed during this stage are found in Table 2.1.

Stage 5 (10 Months and Older): Jargon Stage.   The final stage of prelinguistic vocal development coincides with children's production of first words. According to Menn and Stoel-Gammon (2001), the jargon stage is characterized by "strings of sounds and syllables uttered with a rich variety of stress and intonation patterns" (p. 82). Other names for this type of jargon include conversational babble and modulated babble. During this stage, parents are often convinced that their infant is trying to say something. First words may in fact be produced among a string of jargon.

   The types of consonants produced in jargon include stops, nasals, and glides, and these are also typical of children's first words. Consonant types that do not appear in babbling include fricatives, affricates, and liquids. Predictably, these are not typical sounds of children's first words. These observations provide support for the continuity hypothesis, which, according to Menn and Stoel-Gammon (2001), suggests that "the phonological

TABLE 2.1   Types of Canonical Babbling Seen in Infants from about Age 6 Months and Older

Type of Babbling	Description
Reduplicated	■ Repetitive string of consonant-vowel productions ■ Consonant sound remains constant ■ May exhibit slight vowel changes ■ Example: "mamamama" ■ Tends to predominate in earlier period (i.e., from about 6 months)
Non-reduplicated or variegated	■ Repetitive string of consonant-vowel productions ■ Both consonant and vowel may change ■ Example: "mabameba" ■ Tends to emerge somewhat later than reduplicated babbling and becomes frequent about 12–13 months of age

Sources: Adapted from Bauman-Waengler (2000) and Menn & Stoel-Gammon (2001).

patterns in early meaningful speech are directly linked to the patterns that they [children] use in babbling" (p. 84).

The First-Word Period

Phonology

Children typically produce their first word around their first birthday. To be considered a true word, it needs to be used consistently in a specific context, and it needs to have a recognizable phonetic form (Owens, 2001). That is, although the word may not match the adult pronunciation, it needs to closely resemble the adult target. During the beginning stages of phonological acquisition, children show great individual variation. For example, although most children use plosive and nasal sounds, one child may favor labial sounds such as /b/ and /m/ while another child may favor alveolar sounds such as /d/ and /n/. According to Menn and Stoel-Gammon (2001), some children first learn to pronounce words as whole items, rather than treating them as being made up of individual sounds. Once children have a single-word vocabulary of about 50 words, they adopt a new, more efficient strategy of treating each word as being made up of individual sounds and as such consider the phonological rules of the language they are learning (Bauman-Waengler, 2000).

Semantics

Recall from Chapter 1 that children from birth to about 2 years of age are in Piaget's sensorimotor stage of cognitive development. One of the resulting cognitive achievements is the concept of object permanence, or object constancy, that is, that objects exist in the environment even though they may not be immediately visible. Object permanence is a basis for internal representations of the environment, mental images, or symbols of those objects and events that exist around the children. Many suggest that these internal representations are related to children's ability to use verbal symbols—words.

Lahey (1988) identifies three broad categories of the types of single words that children use to represent what they learn about the environment: *substantive, relational,* and *social.* Children use *substantive words* to name objects. Many of the words are used to refer to classes or categories of objects. As children learn about the perceptual or behavioral consistency of objects, they learn that objects with similarly identified characteristics have the same names. Many of these early words are names for objects on which children can act and produce changes, such as *cookie, ball,* and *shoe.* Children at this stage use fewer attributives, words such as color and size words, than names for objects. Other types of substantive words refer to objects that children believe exist only as one of a kind. There is only one "Mommy", one favorite blanket, and, to the child, one bottle. In a child's mind, these are unique instances of objects and do not belong to a class of objects.

The second broad category of single-word utterances identified by Lahey (1988) consists of relational words. *Relational words* describe the relationships or characteristics among objects, including movements of objects, or relationships of an object to itself, such as an object that has suddenly disappeared (McLaughlin, 1998). Some children may use more relational than substantive words (Bloom, 1973; Gopnik, 1981). The types of relational words include existence, nonexistence/disappearance, recurrence, rejection, denial, attribution, possession, action, and locative action (Lahey, 1988). Table 2.2 lists and explains the types of relational words that children use in the single-word stage. It is important to realize that the same word may actually be used to express several different relations. For example, *no* can be used to indicate rejection, denial, or nonexistence/disappearance. *No* is a very functional, versatile, and important word for children. A noun, such as *ball,* can be used to mean existence or recurrence or to label the object.

The last broad category of single-word utterances consists of *social words*, such as *hi* and *bye.* These are important words in a child's early repertoire, as they provide a foundation for establishing and maintaining human relationships according to the culture's social code. Although they are important, these words, unlike substantive and relational words, do not lead to later grammatical complexity.

During the single-word-utterance stage, there also seems to be a relationship between a child's phonological and semantic development. Children appear to learn more easily and quickly new words that begin with consonants they have used previously in other words than they do words that begin with consonants they have not yet used (Leonard, Schwartz, Morris, & Chapman, 1981; Schwartz & Leonard, 1982), and children exhibit greater

TABLE 2.2   Relations Expressed in Single-Word Utterances

Relation	Explanation
Existence	An object is present in a child's immediate environment and the child is attending to it. Examples: *this, that, there*
Nonexistence/disappearance	An object is expected to be present but is not. An action is expected to occur but does not. An object has been present but disappears. Examples: *all gone, no, bye-bye*
Recurrence	An object reappears. Another object like the one the child is attending to is placed with the first one. An event happens again. Examples: *more, another*
Rejection	The child does not want an object or an event to occur. Example: *no*
Denial	The child rejects the truthfulness of a previous utterance. Example: *no*
Attribution	The child mentions a characteristic of an object or event, usually not shape or color in this stage. Example: *big, little*
Possession	The child identifies ownership of an object. Examples: *mine, my*
Action	The child identifies or requests an action. Examples: *go, open*
Locative action	The child refers to a change in an object's location. Examples: *here, there, in, up*

Source: Adapted from Lahey (1988).

phonetic accuracy in saying object words than action words (Camarata & Schwartz, 1985). These findings support the notion of synergism among the various components of language in children's development (Reed, 1992; Storkel, 2003).

Pragmatics

Halliday (1975) described seven purposes, or functions, of communicative attempts that occur between approximately 9 to 16 or 18 months of age. Table 2.3 lists and explains these seven functions. Because these functions emerge during part of a period in which children have few, if any, words, much of the communication may be accomplished in nonverbal ways. Halliday's (1975) view of communicative functions considered the listeners' responses. On the other hand, Dore (1975), who concentrated on the period during which children are using single words (approximately 12 to 18/24 months), focused on children's intention to use these single-word utterances, with less emphasis on the listeners' reactions to the intents. Dore's (1975) intentions are also shown in Table 2.3. As Prutting (1979) explains, Dore provides a way of identifying children's reasons (intentions) for communication, while Halliday furnishes a way of describing how well the reasons worked or functioned.

During the stage from about 16 or 18 months to 24 months, children use language for different functions. According to Halliday (1974), the earlier instrumental and regulatory functions combine with part of the interactional function to form a new function—the pragmatic function. The *pragmatic function* is basically a controlling one used to satisfy desires and needs while interacting with people at the same time. Some response from the listener is expected. The newly acquired mathetic function is derived from the more basic personal and heuristic functions in combination, again, with part of the interactional function. The *mathetic function* focuses on language as a tool for learning more about the environment (e.g., asking the names of objects) and for commenting on the environment. In contrast to the pragmatic function, the mathetic function does not always require a response from the listener. Children use a third function during this period: the informative function. In employing the *informative function,* children actually convey information to the listeners. An important achievement occurs by the end of this stage: children learn that language can be multifunctional. That is, one utterance can serve more than one function at a time, a characteristic of most adult communications.

Two aspects of engaging in effective dialogues involve taking one's turn appropriately and helping to maintain the topic of conversation. It appears that children even before the age of 9 months demonstrate rudimentary turn-taking skills in the form of reciprocal interactions (Bochner, Price, & Jones, 1997). By the time children are 18 to 24 months old, they have learned to participate in dialogues and demonstrate ability in applying rules of turn taking in their dialogues (Bloom, Rocissano, & Hood, 1976; Halliday, 1975; McLaughlin, 1998).

The Period of Two-Word Utterances

Semantic–Syntactic Development

In the second year of life, children gradually expand their single-word vocabularies until they have learned to combine two words in one utterance. This first two-word utterance

TABLE 2.3   Children's Functions and Intentions of Their Early Language

Halliday's Functions (9 to 16/18 months of age)		Dore's Intentions (approximately 12 to 18/24 months)	
Function	*Description*	*Intention*	*Description*
		Labeling	To name objects; no response expected
Instrumental	To receive material needs, desired objects, or assistance from others	Answering	To respond to adult's request
Regulatory	To control the behavior of others	Requesting action	To get adult to do something
Interactional	To make interpersonal contact with others in their environment by initiating and/or sustaining contact with other people	Requesting an answer	To get adult to respond to request verbally
Personal	To demonstrate awareness of self and express one's own feelings and individuality	Calling/addressing	To address adult; to get adult's attention
Heuristic	To attempt to have environments or events in the environments explained	Greeting	To acknowledge adult's or object's presence
Imaginative	To pretend or playact	Protesting	To resist or deny adult's action
Informative	To communicate experiences or tell someone something	Repeating/imitating	To model utterance after adult's; no response expected
		Practicing (language)	To rehearse language to self; no response expected

Sources: Adapted from Dore (1975) and Halliday (1975).

usually occurs around 18 to 26 months of age. A child's expressive vocabulary at 18 months is about 50 words. Between 18 and 24 months, children experience a lexical growth spurt, and at 24 months of age they typically have a single-word lexicon of 120–300 words (Dale & Thal, 1989; Reich, 1986; Rescorla, Alley, & Christine, 2001). A vocabulary of at least fifty words is generally considered the minimum prerequisite to beginning to combine two words into one utterance, but most 2-year-old children have expressive single-word vocabularies four to six times greater than 50 words at 2 years of age. Children need a variety of words in order to allow them eventually to use two-word combinations that, in turn, evolve into sentences.

The development that occurs from the single-word to the two-word stage is not haphazard. Children demonstrate an increase in the number of verbs, a reduction in other types of relational words, and an increase in the number of object-class words used in their language as they approach the two-word stage (Bloom, 1973; Bloom & Lahey, 1978). Some have also suggested that children begin to produce chained single-word productions shortly before they use two-word combinations (Bloom & Lahey, 1978; McLaughlin, 1998), although not all agree with this suggestion (Branigan, 1979; Owens, 2001). *Chained single-word utterances* are two single words that children use in very close succession to each other but, based on stress and intonation patterns, use as individual words. These utterances appear to demonstrate children are beginning to see more than one aspect of an event. That is, the children seem to identify and talk about relations within one event, such as *ball/roll* or *cookie/gone*. These successive single-word utterances may form a base for the two-word utterances about to occur, such as *ball roll, no cookie,* and *more juice* (McLean & Snyder-McLean, 1999).

Types of Two-Word Utterances

The two-word utterances that children typically begin to use about their second birthday are often described as reflections of *semantic relations* (Bloom, 1970; Brown, 1973). These two-word productions reflect meaning based on different relationships among the words in the utterances. Children can use the utterance *baby ball* to signify possession ("baby's ball") or to signify the actor and the object of an action ("baby [rolls] ball"). An utterance can indicate two different meanings or two separate relations between the words. Table 2.4 lists a number of the more common semantic relations that Brown (1973) identified in children's two-word productions. As we can see, different semantic relations can be expressed in the same grammatical form, such as noun + noun (N + N) to signify possession, agent–object, and entity–locative. Another significant characteristic of this stage of language use is the absence of morphological endings on the words used. Children do not use the possessive word endings even though their intent is to indicate possession, nor do they use any endings on verbs. Instead, only lexical, or root, forms of words are used.

Brown (1973) has termed this semantic relations period of language development Stage I. During this period, children use about an equal number of one- and two-word utterances. If we average the number of words in many of their utterances, we obtain a mean length of about 1.5. The average lengths of young children's utterances are frequently used as measures of their language growth (Eisenberg, Fersko, & Lundgren, 2001; Miller, 1996). Although we can average the number of words that children use in their responses, such an approach does not tell us whether the children are using more complex word endings, such as plural markers. A more common method of arriving at average length is to count the number of morphemes, both free and bound, that occur in the utterances. When children are in Stage I, this averaging procedure also results in a *mean length of utterance* (MLU) of about 1.5, because children are not yet using grammatical inflections or bound morphemes. In the early periods of language learning, as MLU increases, the complexity of children's utterances generally increases. However, when children begin using more complex sentence forms, this relationship between length and linguistic maturity does not remain as closely associated as in the earlier stages of language acquisition, because there are ways other than length to increase syntactic complexity (Bernstein & Tiegerman-Farber, 1997; Eisenberg et al., 2001).

The Preschool Years and Beyond

From the two-word utterance stage at about 2 years of age, children's language development grows in leaps and bounds. The ability to produce complete and even complex sen-

TABLE 2.4   Common Semantic Relations

Relation	Example	Structure
Nomination	"That ball"	Demonstrative + N
Nonexistence	"No ball"	No (allgone) + N
Action–object	"Roll ball"	V + N
Agent–action	"Baby cry"	N + V
Recurrence	"More cookies"	More (another) + N
Action + locative	"Jump [on] chair"	V + N
	"Roll here"	V + Loc.
Entity + locative	"Ball [in] chair"	N + N
	"Mommy here"	N + Loc.
Possessor–possession	"Baby ball"	N + N
Agent–object	"Baby [roll] ball"	N + N
Entity–attributive	"Pretty ball"	Att. + N
	"Ball pretty"	N + Att.
Notice	"Hi ball"	Hi + N
Instrumental	"Cut [with] knife"	V + N
Action–indirect object	"Give [to] doggie"	V + N
Conjunction	"Coat hat"	N + N

Source: Adapted from Brown (1973).

tences is acquired, speech becomes intelligible even to unfamiliar listeners, and vocabulary size explodes. Particularly noticeable is the period leading up to 8 years of age, when the changes in language abilities become subtler—but the changes do continue.

Phonology

Children learn some sounds before others. This means that the words they say do not always match the adult pronunciation. For example, a child may say *moon* correctly at 2 years, because the word contains early-developing sounds; however, words such as spaghetti and spoon may be pronounced as "detti" and "poon," respectively.

Mastering Production of Speech Sounds.   Stoel-Gammon (1987) has reported that at approximately 2 years of age, children use a repertoire of nine to ten different consonants in the initial position of words. In the final position of words, these children use five to six different consonants. Between 24 and 39 months of age, children use an average of 2.2 consonant clusters (i.e., two or more consonants together acting liking one, such as "sky") in the initial position and 1.7 clusters in the final position of words. With advancing age, children's phonological repertoires increase, in terms of both the number of different sounds used and the word positions in which they are used. Most researchers agree that by age 7 or 8, children have fairly well mastered the English phonemes and are producing them correctly in their speech. However, some speech development may continue into fifth grade, or approximately age 10/11 (Ingram, 1989b; Sax, 1972; Stoel-Gammon & Dunn, 1985).

Numerous investigations have contributed significantly to our knowledge of when children learn to produce specific sounds (McLeod, van Doorn, & Reed, 2001a, 2001b; Poole, 1934; Smit, 1993a, 1993b; Smit, Hand, Freilinger, Bernthal, & Bird, 1990; Templin, 1957). Although differences in research designs and criterion levels prevent exact comparisons among results, several similar trends have emerged from the studies. Generally, children learn to master the production of nasal sounds, such as /m/, /n/, /ŋ/,[1] stop consonants, such as /d/, /k/, /g/, /p/, and /b/, and glides, such as /w/, between 2 and 3 years of age. These phonemes are typically considered early-developing and relatively easy sounds. In contrast, fricative sounds, such as /s/, /z/, /ʃ/, and /ʒ/, and affricates, such as /tʃ/ and /dʒ/, are mastered later, often not until age 7 or 8. As Bauman-Waengler (2000) points out, there is a great deal of variation across the studies that have examined children's mastery of speech sounds, both in terms of the methods used to collect, collate, and report the data and in the ages of mastery reported across the studies. However, despite the differences across the research, two clear points emerge. First, children demonstrate variability in the ages at which they acquire individual phonemes (McLeod et al., 2001a, 2001b); and second, there are trends in terms of when children master the production of the various manners of articulation. For the most part, stop consonants and nasals are typically learned before fricatives and affricates. Furthermore, children often continue to have difficulties with /r/ and /l/ after they begin school.

So far, we have only discussed consonant sound development. Children generally learn to produce the vowels correctly before they acquire the consonant sounds. In fact, vowel production may be mastered by the time a child is 3 years old. It is unusual to see school-aged children making more than occasional errors in their vowel productions.

Producing Words without All the Speech Sounds.   Children's simplified pronunciation of words follows patterns known as *phonological processes* (Bauman-Waengler, 2000). For example, if a child regularly substitutes consonants produced in the front of the mouth (e.g., /t/, /d/) for those that are supposed to be produced in the back of the mouth (e.g., /k/, /g/), and so says *tea* for *key,* the child might be said to be using a fronting process. Or, if a child regularly omits one or more consonants when they occur together as clusters, and so says "poon" for *spoon,* the child might be described as using a cluster reduction process.

Ingram (1989b) has listed several of these processes under the three broad classifications of syllable structure, assimilation, and substitution processes. In *syllable structure* processes, young children tend to omit consonants in the final position of words or syllables ("bi" for *bite*), delete unstressed syllables in polysyllabic words ("jama" for *pajamas*), and reduce the number of sounds produced in consonant clusters, such as /bl/ ("bu" for *blue*). *Assimilation* processes are those in which one sound in a word affects the production of

---

[1]See Table 1.1 for the International Phonetic Alphabet (IPA).

another sound so that its production is modified. Examples of assimilative processes are "gog" for *dog* or "mam" for *lamb*. When children use both a syllable duplication and an assimilative process simultaneously, an utterance such as "gaga" for *doggie* may be produced. Finally, *substitution* processes are employed when children use one group of sounds, such as stops, in place of another group, such as fricatives. It is not uncommon to hear children say "toap" for *soap*.

As children get older they discontinue using early phonological processes so that their productions of words approximate those used by adults. Because this learning process takes time, however, any one word may go through several stages in pronunciation. Consequently, just because a child is capable of saying a sound correctly in one word, this does not mean that the sound will be said correctly in all words that contain it, if different phonological processes are operating in the production of the other words.

Semantics

Table 2.5 illustrates what happens to expressive vocabulary size from the first word at about 12 months of age to first grade. In terms of receptive vocabulary, children comprehend their first words at about 8/9 months of age (Benedict, 1979); at about 13 months of age, children comprehend about 50 words (Benedict, 1979). By 6 years of age their comprehension vocabulary is between 20,000 and 24,000 words, and by 12 years of age it is 50,000 words or more (Owens, 2001). The size of a child's vocabulary depends, in part, on the experiences and words to which the child is exposed (Rescorla, Alley, & Christine, 2001), which after the early years leads to considerable variability in vocabulary composition as well as size.

Rescorla and her colleagues (2001) write that "young children are highly consistent in the words they acquire in their early lexicons" (p. 605). There seem to be patterns to what

TABLE 2.5 Expressive Vocabulary Growth from the First Year to First Grade

Approximate Age	Approximate Number of Words in Expressive Vocabulary
15 months	10
18 months	50
20 months	150
2 years	120–300
3 years	1,000
4 years	1,600
5 years	2,100–2,200
6 years	2,600–7,000

Sources: Dale, Bates, Reznick, & Morisset (1989); Owens (2001); Reich (1986); Rescorla et al. (2001); Wehrebian (1970); and Zintz (1970).

words children acquire and the sequence in which they add words to their lexicons (Pan & Berko-Gleason, 2001):

- Overextension and underextension of the meanings of words (e.g., overextension such as all four-legged animals being *dogs;* underextension such as *bottle* applying only to the baby's bottle)
- Acquiring words that occur more frequently in their environments
- A general tendency to label first objects and actions, then words that attach attributes to objects or events (*big*), and finally, words that express temporal, spatial, conditional, and causal relationships
- A shift from classifying words on the basis of perceptual or functional characteristics (concrete classifications) to classifying words according to abstract properties such as temporal–spatial features or animate–inanimate characteristics

There are several ways in which young children are believed to be so good at learning (Rice & Watkins, 1996). One way is with a process known as *fast mapping* (Crais, 1992; Dollaghan, 1985; Heibeck & Markman, 1987). Dollaghan (1987) describes fast mapping as a lexical acquisition strategy in

> . . . which a listener rapidly constructs a representation for an unfamiliar word on the basis of a single exposure to it. This initial representation might contain information on the semantic, phonological, or syntactic characteristics of the new lexical item, as well as non-linguistic information related to the situation in which it was encountered. (p. 218)

This first meaning may or may not be complete and/or accurate. It does, however, create a basis for further refinement as additional experiences with the word in context occur. Children seem to be able to fast map meaning by having only "incidental" exposures to new words. That is, new words occur in context in a child's ambient environment, and the child is able to discern what the new word means. This is referred to as *quick incidental learning* (QUIL) (Rice, 1990; Rice, Huston, Truglio, & Wright, 1990; Rice & Woodsmall, 1988). However, McGregor, Friedman, and colleagues (2002) remind us that the quick, partial learning of the meaning of new words only starts what is the longer-term, slow mapping process of vocabulary learning. Any new word and its partial meanings need to be remembered, and over time as new contexts are encountered in which a child is exposed to the word, refinements in the meaning need to be made. These authors comment that the "process can take weeks, months, or years, depending on the semantic complexity and frequency of the word to be learned" (p. 332).

In addition to fast mapping and QUIL, a number of propositions have been advanced that also help children figure out labels for and meanings of words. Some of these are the whole object-versus-object components proposition, the mutual exclusivity proposition, and the novel name–nameless category proposition. The *whole object-versus-object components* proposition (Golinkoff, Mervis, & Hirsh-Pasek, 1994) suggests that children will focus on an entire object as the most likely referent for a new word before thinking about one of the parts of the object or an attribute of the object as the possible referent. According to the *mutual exclusivity* proposition (Markman, 1989; Markman & Wachtel, 1988), a child will assume that a new word applies to an object that does not yet have a name (from the child's perspective) and will not be inclined to give an already-named object a second label, that is, one item, one name, or mutually exclusive labels. Therefore, in a context where a new word occurs and the names for all things are known except one, the new word will be assumed to apply to the unnamed item and will not be another word for one of the other items. The third, the *novel name–nameless category* proposition (Golinkoff et al., 1994; Mervis & Bertrand, 1994), is similar to the mutual exclusivity proposition but adds that children will consider other possibilities, including another name for an object whose label is already known.

The strength of these three propositions as well as others in explaining how children go about figuring out what new names go with what referents is still a matter for discussion. What is certain, however, is that the context in which children encounter words and their referents is central to their word learning. What is also necessary for full knowledge of a word and its referents is multiple exposures of the word in multiple contexts (Hoff-Ginsberg & Naigles, 1999).

Spatial and Temporal Terms. Children's comprehension of spatial (location in space) and temporal (location in time) words develops gradually from about 2 years for *in* as a preposition (Bangs, 1975) to about 11 years for terms such as *before* and *after* (Wiig & Semel, 1974), with children's understanding of selected spatial and temporal relationships developing throughout Piaget's concrete operational period (about grades 1 to 5 and approximately 7 to 11 years old). In grade 1, children's ability to interpret temporal terms has been found to be greater than their comprehension of spatial relationships (Wiig & Semel, 1974). However, in grade 2, according to Wiig and Semel's results, the children were able to understand the spatial terms better than the temporal ones. This difference in skills, in favor of spatial relationships, continued to grade 5.

Many conjunctions involve temporal concepts (e.g., "She will leave *when* it is convenient" and "We ate breakfast *before* we went to school"), as does the "wh-" question word *when.* And a number of these same terms occur as prepositions (e.g., "We ate breakfast *before* school). Children generally use these temporal terms as prepositions before using them as conjunctions. Additionally, terms expressing order of events (e.g. *before* and *after*) appear to be learned prior to terms expressing simultaneity (e.g., *while* and *at the same time*) (Feagans, 1980).

Spatial relationships are also often expressed by *prepositions. In* and *on* are among the first of these word types to be acquired. Some words that function as prepositions also occur as part of a *verb particle,* that is, a multiword construction that functions as a verb, as in "She *put up* a good argument." Like prepositions, these words as verb particles emerge early in children's language and by about 4 to 5 years of age are used with reasonable accuracy (Goodluck, 1986; Wegner & Rice, 1988). However, Wegner and Rice (1988) suggest that certain words seem to be used more as prepositions (*in, on,* and *over*) and others (*up, down,* and *off*) more as verb particles.

Other spatial prepositions (e.g., *in front of* and *next to*) are more difficult for children. The referents for these prepositions vary, depending on the children's relationships to objects and the characteristics of the objects. When an object has a front, such as a person, *in front of* relates to the object's front (Owens, 2001). For an object without a front, such as a ball, *in front of* derives its meaning from the relative positions of the speaker and the object—positions that can vary. Furthermore, *next to* can mean *beside, in back of,* or *in front of,* all of which can be very confusing for a child. As might be expected, these types of spatial prepositions develop later.

Deictic Words.   Deictic words are terms that have changing referents, depending on who in a communicative dyad is speaking, on the respective locations of objects and people, and on the temporal relationships relative to the speaker and listener (Pan & Berko-Gleason, 2001). The spatial prepositions discussed in the preceding section are deictic in nature. As another example, the referents for *I* and *you* shift as the speaker–listener relationship changes. The terms *here* and *there,* and *this* and *that,* vary depending on the location of the speaker, listener, and/or objects. Among the deictic verbs are *come, go, bring,* and *take.* Such words must be confusing for young children, although the literature suggests that children demonstrate some use of deictic shifts for first- and second-person pronouns (*I, you, me*) sometime between approximately 1 and 2 years of age (Bloom et al., 1976; Morehead & Ingram, 1973). Third-person pronouns appear later in children's language, between approximately 2 and 3 years of age, and their development may even continue to 5 years of age and possibly beyond. Bloom and her colleagues (1976) indicate that, when children's MLUs approach 4.0, they evidence deictic shifts for the terms *here, there, this,* and *that.* Other deictic words, such as *come, go, bring,* and *take,* tend to be learned later (Pan & Berko-Gleason, 2001), and complete acquisition may extend into children's school years.

Morphology

One way in which young children increase their utterance length is to begin to use grammatical morphemes in their utterances. Recall that in the early two-word combination stage (Brown's Stage I), a child's MLU is 1.5 but no grammatical morphemes are attached to words. Children begin to use grammatical morphemes when their MLUs reach about 2.0. At this point children progress into Brown's Stage II, acquiring the present progressive *-ing* ending for verbs ("ball rolling") and the prepositions *in* and *on* ("kitty in chair" and "cup on table"). It is important to note, however, that acquisition of a grammatical morpheme, as used in relation to Brown's stages, means that a child uses it correctly in at least 90 percent of the situations in which it is required by adult standards, that is, in 90 percent of the obligatory contexts. Children may use morphemes such as *in* and *on* before this stage, but not at the criterion level set by Brown. Table 2.6 summarizes Brown's (1973) findings about the sequence in which children acquire fourteen selected grammatical morphemes and indicates the corresponding stages determined by MLU at which the morphemes are acquired. The process of learning these morphemes occurs over several years, and children are developing other language skills during that time. For example, by the time children are 3 years old, they typically demonstrate the use of negative and interrogative sentences, as well as basic declarative sentences.

Of the other verb forms Brown (1973) investigated, irregular past-tense words such as *ran* and *saw* appear in children's language before regular past-tense verb markers. In learning morphological rules, children typically acquire a more general rule first and then they gradually modify and refine the rule to account for the more specific applications and exceptions, so this initially appears a bit strange. It may be that children simply acquire these irregular verb forms as vocabulary words instead of word-form variations derived from lexical verbs. Support for such an interpretation comes from the observation that after

TABLE 2.6   Sequence of Acquisition for Fourteen Grammatical Morphemes

Morpheme	MLU	Maximum Length in Morphemes	Stage
1. Present progressive ending (-*ing*)			
2. 3. *In* and *on*	2.25	7	II
4. Noun plurals			
5. Past-tense irregular verbs			
6. Possessive nouns	2.75	9	III
7. Uncontractible copula ("Here I <u>am</u>")			
8. Articles			
9. Past-tense regular verbs	3.50	11	IV
10. Regular third-person singular present-tense verbs			
11. Irregular third-person singular present-tense verbs			
12. Uncontractible auxiliary ("He <u>was</u> running")	4.00	13	V
13. Contractible copula ("She<u>'s</u> big")			
14. Contractible auxiliary ("The boy<u>'s</u> eating")			

Source: Adapted from Brown (1973).

children begin to use regular past-tense verb forms correctly, they often incorrectly apply the rules to irregular verbs previously used accurately—so that utterances such as "He runned" and "I seed a dog" are not uncommon (Tager-Flusberg, 2001). This is not inconsistent with research that suggests even some regular past-tense verb endings are first used with specific verb words, that is, as vocabulary items (Pine, 1999).

When regular past-tense forms ("She jumped") appear, not all variations of regular past-tense verbs are acquired at the same time. Learning to use the variety of verb forms that occur in English is especially problematic for many children with language disorders. For this reason we will take a somewhat closer look at normal verb morphological acquisition. Verbs to which the past-tense allomorph /d/ is added (*played*) appear to develop slightly before those to which the allomorph /t/ is attached (*jumped*) (Berko, 1958; Moran, 1975; Newfield & Schlanger, 1968; Wiig, Semel, & Crouse, 1973). Acquisition of the /əd/ allomorph (*painted*) occurs somewhat later. There are also different ways in which irregular past-tense verbs are formed. Some use an internal vowel change (*swim* → *swam*), whereas others use both a vowel and final consonant change (*catch* → *caught*). The former types seem to emerge somewhat earlier for children. In one study, 7- and 8-year-old children gave fewer than 75 percent correct responses for irregular verbs with internal vowel changes, and only about 40 percent gave correct responses for irregular verbs formed by changing both a vowel and a final consonant (Moran, 1975). Such data indicate that children are continuing to refine some of their morphology in the early school years.

According to Brown (1973), the regular forms of third-person singular present-tense verbs ("She jumps" and "He swims") emerge after past-tense regular forms (see Table 2.6). Shortly thereafter, children begin to use irregular forms of third-person singular present-tense verbs (*do* to *does* and *have* to *has*). Of the fourteen grammatical morphemes in Brown's investigation, the verb forms involving the contractible copula and auxiliary ("We're big" and "She's running") and the uncontractible auxiliary ("He was running") were the last ones the children acquired.

Table 2.6 indicates that children begin to use regular noun plurals after present progressive verb endings and before irregular past-tense forms (Brown, 1973). Again, there are various forms of regular noun plurals, and there appears to be a developmental sequence for acquisition of these variations. Children's utterances with the plural allomorph /z/ (*pigs*) tend to be more accurate before their utterances containing plural nouns with the /s/ allomorph (*boats*) (Berko, 1958; Solomon, 1972; Wiig et al., 1973), whereas accurate use of the /əz/ plural allomorph (*houses*) is achieved after the /s/ and /z/ plural forms. Although children begin to use some noun plurals early in their language-learning process, the complete acquisition of plural forms takes several years. In fact, 6- and 7-year-old children may still demonstrate problems with plural nouns that require use of the /əz/ ending (Berko, 1958; Solomon, 1972). The learning of irregular noun plurals (*child* to *children*) seems to lag considerably behind the acquisition of regular forms.

Brown (1973) indicates that children begin to use possessive forms of nouns shortly after the appearances of noun plurals and irregular past-tense verbs (see Table 2.6). Possessive forms of nouns are derived in basically the same ways as noun plurals, and their sequence of acquisition appears to be essentially similar. Correct use of the /z/ allomorph (*bug's*) tends to be achieved somewhat before that of the /s/ allomorph (*duck's*) which, in turn, tends to be acquired before the /əz/ ending (*horse's*). We notice that regular forms of noun plurals, possessives, and third-person singular present-tense verbs all use the same word endings, /z/, /s/, /əz/. Therefore, it is not surprising that Brown (1973) found that once the children in his study correctly added the endings to form any one of the three word types (plurals, possessives, or third-person verbs), they used the other two types within 1 year.

Other morphological forms include comparatives (*bigger*) and superlatives (*biggest*), noun and adverb derivations (*painter, fireman, violinist, gently, quickly*), and prefixes (*preheat, undone, miscue*). The results of Berko's (1958) classic study indicated that, even by age 7, children had not yet fully acquired the rules for forming comparative and superlative adjectives and for deriving nouns and adverbs. Prefixing also is a difficult skill to acquire because it requires knowledge of the meanings for both the prefix form and the root word. As we can see, refinement of several morphological rules continues well into the school years.

Syntax

Syntactic complexity increases both in terms of length and the types of syntactic structures children learn. Consequently, children extend their previous two-word utterances into multiword utterances and begin to use different sentence forms.

Expanding Two-Word Utterances. Children learn to expand their utterances by combining previously separate semantic relations, such as "baby ball" (possessive) and "ball roll" (agent–action) to form "baby ball roll "(Brown, 1973; Lahey, 1988). Children do not, however, use any new relations in forming these longer utterances. Only previously expressed two-word semantic relations are combined and expanded. The production of the first true sentences is also derived from this combining process. Agent–action ("baby roll") and action–object ("roll ball") combine to form agent–action–object ("baby roll ball"), the subject + verb + object basic English syntactic rule discussed in Chapter 1. With gradually increasing skill in producing the basic sentence form, the child is acquiring the foundation abilities to begin to manipulate that syntactic form to make other types of sentences. As McLean and Snyder-McLean (1999) summarize:

> Between 3 and 4 years of age, typically developing children are able to produce well formed, declarative sentences with generally appropriate grammar. . . . They can ask simple questions using *wh-* words. . . . Future learning will allow children to alter . . . declarative structures to produce interrogative forms. . . . (pp. 170–171)

Acquisition of Negatives. In our discussion of the types of single words that children use, we saw that negative words occur very early in the developmental process. When children begin to combine words, negative utterances are produced by placing the negative marker *no* in front of an element that occurs in the predicate of a sentence, such as a verb or direct object. Utterances like "no milk" and "no go" are typical. Even though children at this stage may produce affirmative sentences with a subject and predicate ("boy roll ball"), the subject is deleted when a negative marker is added. It appears that the use of negation increases the length and complexity of an utterance, which, as a result, can exceed children's linguistic capacities. Perhaps to accommodate these limited capacities, the overall length and complexity of an utterance are reduced to a manageable unit by omitting the subject when a negative is added ("no roll ball"). Furthermore, the subject of a sentence is usually the information shared most between speaker and listener, so its omission tends not to affect communication. Meaning can still be conveyed despite the omission.

Children gradually learn to re-add the subjects to produce negative sentences such as "boy no roll ball." However, before children's negative sentences can evolve into more complex forms, the children need to learn that *no* is the negative word used with nouns and *not* is the negative for verbs. The occurrence of later negative sentences also depends on the use of a copula or auxiliary verb ("The ball is not big" and "The boy is not running"). For sentences in which an auxiliary verb does not occur ("The boy eats"), an auxiliary in the form of *do* must be added ("The boy does not eat" or "The boy doesn't eat"). Although the use of *do* plus a negative is generally considered to be a reasonably complex language skill, the negative words *don't* and *can't* do appear in children's early language productions. These early occurrences of *can't* and *don't,* however, are typically viewed as vocabulary words indicating negation rather than as evidence that children have acquired the operation of adding *do* when an auxiliary is absent. The negatives *won't* and *isn't* also occur in children's early productions, although less frequently than *don't* and *can't.*

Negatives can be used to express a number of different concepts (Tager-Flusberg, 2001). For example, with negative utterances, we can reject ("I don't want any"), deny ("That's not a red car"), or signify nonexistence ("It's not here"). Table 2.7 presents six

TABLE 2.7   **Suggested Developmental Sequence for Negative Functions**

Negative Function	Example and Explanation
Nonexistence/disappearance	"No ball" (The ball is not in the toy box where it belongs.) "No milk" (The milk is all gone.)
Nonoccurrence	"No pull" (The toy is stuck and cannot be pulled.)
Cessation	"No turn" (The top has stopped spinning and has fallen over.)
Rejection	"No juice" (I do not want any more juice.)
Prohibition	"No go" (The child is telling Mommy not to leave.)
Denial	"No doggie" (Having been told the Great Dane is a dog, the child does not believe it belongs to the same class as the toy poodle at home.)

Source: Adapted from Bloom and Lahey (1978).

functions of negatives in a suggested developmental sequence and provides examples of each (Bloom & Lahey, 1978). The syntactic representation of these negative functions appears to follow this same sequence. That is, children at a specific developmental level will express nonexistence in a fairly complex way ("It isn't here") while at the same time signifying denial in a less sophisticated manner ("That not a ball").

Acquisition of Questions.   Preschoolers' acquisition of interrogative, or question, forms tends to lag somewhat behind their negative utterances. However, before discussing the development of questions, we need to review two types of question forms that can occur in English:

1. Yes/no interrogatives, which
   - Are labeled as such because the answer to such a query is *yes* or *no*
   - Involve moving, or transposing, a copula or auxiliary verb to the beginning of the sentence, as in changing the basic sentence "The boy is running" to "Is the boy running?"
   - If there is no auxiliary or copula verb in the basic sentence to transpose, as in the sentence "The girl rides the bike," one must be added in the form of *do;* then transpose to form the question, "Does the girl ride the bike"?
   - Transposing reverses the usual sequence of subject and verb; the term *interrogative reversal* is also used to refer to this process

2. "Wh-" questions, which
   - Request information; require a "wh-" word, such as *what* or *who,* be added to the beginning of an utterance
   - With a "wh-" word, is a process called *preposing*
   - Usually involve both a transposing operation and a preposing process ("The boy is riding" → "What is the boy riding?")

- Need to use "wh-" words that reflect the correct meanings of the utterances
  What is the boy riding?
  Where is the boy riding?
  When is the boy riding?
  How is the boy riding?

In the early stages of learning to ask questions, children mark their yes/no queries only by using rising inflections, such as "mommy go↗." These children may also use a limited set of "wh-" questions, although the utterances are not yet in adult form ("What that?" and "Where Mommy going?"). Children learn to prepose with "wh-" words before they learn to transpose verbs. This is a particularly logical pattern, because children are not yet using copula and auxiliary verbs in these early stages; therefore, they have nothing in their utterances to transpose.

Although children learn to add copula and auxiliary verbs to their basic sentences, their yes/no questions may continue to be marked by rising intonations ("Mommy is gone↗"), although some children may begin with correct transposing. The children do prepose for their "wh-" questions, but they still do not transpose, so their queries sound something like "What Daddy is doing?" or "Where Mommy is going?" If we examine these forms, we see that the children are using a basic sentence that includes the auxiliary *is* and are simply adding the preposed "wh-" word to the beginning. Gradually, the children begin to transpose for their yes/no questions ("Is the girl eating?"). At this stage, however, they may still fail to transpose copula or auxiliary verbs in their "wh-" questions ("What the girl is eating?"). Children's attempts at negative questions demonstrate the same patterns. Transposing occurs in yes/no questions ("Can't we go?") but not in "wh-" questions ("Why Daddy can't go?"). Finally, children learn to transpose in their "wh-" questions ("What is the girl eating?" and "Why can't Daddy go?").

The choice of which "wh-" word to use in "wh-" question forms requires children to apply semantic concepts (Tager-Flusberg, 2001). *What* and *who* reflect concepts that differentiate between people and things; *where* involves the concept of location. These semantic concepts develop fairly early in children and, not surprisingly, the "wh-" words reflecting them are among the first to be used in "wh-" questions. Children use *when* and *how* in their questions somewhat later, since time and manner concepts are acquired after the three early developing concepts. Causal relations develop even later. As a result, "wh-" questions with *why* are among the last to be used meaningfully. The word "meaningfully" is used here because children may ask "Why?" as an attention-getting device before they truly understand the concept of causality and use it accurately in "wh-" questions.

Acquisition of Compound and Complex Sentences. The use of a *compound sentence* (a sentence containing more than one independent clause) or a *complex sentence* (a sentence that contains at least one independent clause and at least one dependent or subordinate clause) involves the expression of two or more ideas or propositions in the one sentence. (A clause, in contrast to a phrase, contains a subject and verb.) These more advanced sentence forms are created by joining two or more clauses together, often with a linguistic form such as a conjunction or a relative pronoun. This clausal joining process usually begins sometime between 2 and 3 years of age, when a child's MLU reaches about 3.0 morphemes. This approximates Brown's Stage IV (Brown, 1973). The first conjunction that children learn to use is *and*. Bloom, Lahey, Hood, Lifter, and Fiess (1980) indicated that the first appropriate use of *and* appears when a child is about 25 to 27 months old, but it may initially be used for serial naming ("baby and kitty"). For clausal joining, some data suggest that this conjunction is initially employed to conjoin two independent clauses in utterances such as "You do this and I do that" and "The boy runs and the boy jumps" (Tager-Flusberg, 2001). These types of sentences simply require the children to add on to existing utterances in their language. This addition operation is among the earlier transformations that children acquire. However, because a number of coordinated sentences with *and* contain redundant information, as in "The boy runs and the boy jumps," the redundant elements can be deleted to form sentences like "The boy runs and jumps."

Utterances that contain object complements appear to be the first types of complex sentences that children use (Limber, 1973). In sentences with object complements, a second basic sentence or clause is used as the object of the verb in the first sentence or clause. For example, in the sentence "I think I have it," the clause "I have it" operates as the object of the verb *think* in the clause "I think." Often included in discussions of object complements are sentences that contain certain types of infinitives. (An *infinitive* is a form of a verb that typically appears with *to*, e.g., "to run," "to go.") In these sentences an infinitive and its associated words are used as an object of a verb, as in "I want to run fast." Both object complement forms—those with a second basic sentence and those with an infinitive—appear in children's utterances at about the same time. Complex sentences in which a second clause is introduced with a "wh-" adverbial word are acquired shortly after object complement sentences (Limber, 1973). Examples of these sentence types are "I remember where Mommy is" and "Daddy knows when Mommy comes home." Children tend to use clauses conveying time and location before other "wh-" clauses.

Relative clauses, which are clauses serving as modifiers for nouns (and are therefore a type of adjectival clause), develop somewhat later (Bloom et al., 1980; Limber, 1973; Tager-Flusberg, 2001). A relative clause is often introduced by a relative pronoun, such as *what, who, which, whose,* or *that* ("I see the boys who are running" or "The dog that has the bone is growling"). However, in some instances the relative pronoun may be omitted ("That's the bed [that] we sleep in"). Children initially use relative clauses to modify predicate nouns ("That is the balloon that I like") and objects ("I see the boy who wears glasses"). They later begin to modify subjects with relative clauses ("The girl who wears glasses sees better"). We see a pattern in which children add to the ends of their sentences before rearranging or adding elements within the sentences (Tager-Flusberg, 2001). The latter process, termed *embedding,* is one of the later-developing transformational operations. Other terms that are used in the literature to refer to the locations of clauses are *left branching* (toward the end of a main or independent clause) and *right branching* (toward the beginning of a main clause or embedded near the beginning).

Although Limber (1973) indicates that 3-year-old children demonstrate the use of clauses with object complements, "wh-" adverbials, and object relatives, Paul (1981) suggests that the use of all of these clause types may not be demonstrated until children are closer to 4 years of age. Embedded relative clauses (subject relatives), having already been identified as later-developing, are not used by children at these ages. In one study (Hass & Wepman, 1974), the embedding operation was shown to be a continuing developmental process in children 5 to 13 years old. Embedding appears to emerge somewhat later than other types of clausal operations, and it continues to develop into adolescence. Furthermore, the use of various types of dependent clauses, as found in complex sentences, continues to increase through twelfth grade (Loban, 1976), with a major shift to the use of clausal constructions occurring at 10 years of age.

The construction of many compound and complex sentences requires the use of connective devices such as conjunctions. The accurate use of these sentences involves both the syntactic operations to combine clauses and the selection of appropriate conjunctions to express the correct meanings. In some instances, the semantic task may be more difficult than the syntactic task. We indicated earlier that the conjunction *and* is the first to be acquired by children. Beyond *and,* the exact sequence in which children learn other conjunctions and the ages at which they acquire them are difficult to report. Authors have investigated the use of different conjunctions by children at varying ages and have reported their data in different ways. However, we do know that the frequency with which children use different conjunctions may be related to their knowledge of and facility with the different conjunctions. Thus, the frequency with which conjunctions occur in children's language may provide a clue to their developmental sequence.

In addition to the studies focusing on preschoolers' acquisition of conjunctions, the use of conjunctions by first graders has been examined (Menyuk, 1969). As might be expected, 95 percent of these children produced well-formed sentences with the conjunction *and.* In contrast, 35 percent of them used adequate sentences with *because.* The conjunctions *if* and *so* were more difficult. Only 20 percent and 19 percent of the first graders produced well-formed sentences with *if* and *so,* respectively. These results certainly suggest that children continue their acquisition of conjunctions past the first grade and into middle and late childhood.

Pragmatics

There are many factors involved in how people use language and what influences their communicative choices in various speaking situations. In this section, we look at children's developing skills in several of these areas—their changing abilities in the functions for which they use language and what they intend to accomplish by its use, their competencies in maintaining a topic and taking turns during a conversation, their uses of presuppositions, their fluency in delivering their messages, and their evolving narrative skills.

Functions of Language. By age 3, children's utterances consistently contain more than one function. This is the third, adultlike stage, and the functions that Halliday (1975) has identified in children's communications in this period are the *interpersonal purpose* (used to relate to other people), the *textual purpose* (used to relate to preceding and following utterances in a dialogue), and the *ideational-experiential purpose* (used to express ideas or events to others).

As we know, the true intentions and functions of some speech acts do not always match the forms of the utterances or their propositional content. As noted in Chapter 1, these are the indirect functions and intentions of speech, and common uses of these indirectives hide the true purposes of utterances in syntactic forms created for the sake of politeness (the interrogative, "Can you open the door?," instead of the imperative, "Open the door") or hint at a purpose by employing content different from the true intent (a child's utterance to a babysitter, "My mommy always lets me stay up late on Fridays," or an adult's remarks, on wishing to have a window closed, "My, it's chilly in here," with no direct reference to the window) (McLaughlin, 1998). In some ways, children's ability to understand and use these indirect speech acts depends partly on their skills in making presuppositions about communicative situations, a topic we discuss in the next section. However, intentions and functions of speech acts are certainly involved.

After about age 3½, children employ these polite devices and hints in their utterances, and they steadily improve with age in their ability to regard requests that contain *please* as more polite than those without it. However, their skill at judging interrogative forms as polite (e.g., "Could I have some candy?") develop later than their skill with *please.* When the children are asked to determine whether a request in the form of an interrogative with *please* ("Could you give me a nut, please?") is more polite than a request in the form of an imperative with *please* ("Give me a nut, please."), even 7-year-olds can have difficulty, although their performance is better than that of 3- and 5-year-olds (Nippold, Leonard, & Anastopoulos, 1982). Use of the polite form—interrogative with *please*—increases steadily between 3 and 7 years, the age at which the children's use of this form approximates that of the adults (Nippold et al., 1982). These findings suggest that although children may begin to use indirectives and polite forms sometime after age 3, it takes at least 4 years more for their use to have many adultlike elements (Bryant, 2001).

Presuppositions.   Speakers make presuppositions about what knowledge is shared between speakers and listeners and about what information listeners need to understand messages, and effective speakers modify the form and content of their utterances based on their presuppositions (McLaughlin, 1998). From this perspective, the use of indirectives, hints, and polite forms can be viewed as part of the presupposition aspect of language use.

It was previously believed that children's egocentricity would prevent them from taking a listener's needs into account as they formulated their messages. Surprisingly, however, there is some evidence that, even at the single-word stage, children adapt what limited language they have for their listeners (Greenfield & Smith, 1976). Normal-hearing 2-year-old children of deaf parents have been found to alter the amount of their oral language, the length of their utterances, and the degree to which they use manual communication depending on whether they are talking with a normal-hearing adult or one of their hearing-impaired parents (Schiff, 1979). Furthermore, children between ages 3 and 4 change the amount of information they give to listeners relative to their listeners' prior knowledge of communicative topics and ability to share in immediate communicative contexts. The ages of children's communicative partners also influence how 4-year-old children encode their messages. Children at this age use shorter and less complex sentences when talking to younger children than when speaking to their peers or adults (Shatz & Gelman, 1973).

How children differentially encode new and old information in their utterances is another aspect of presupposition. When this occurs through the use of pronouns, it is referred to as *anaphoric reference* (McLaughlin, 1998; Tager-Flusberg, 2001). The following example of sequential utterances illustrates what happens as new and old information occur in the content of a message:

I got new shoes. They're brown and white. But Billy doesn't like them. He liked the black ones.

New information is linguistically emphasized (i.e., named, as in *shoes*), while old information is linguistically deemphasized (i.e., pronominalized). Children in the single-word to approximately the three- or four-word-utterance stages of language learning omit old information in their speech and verbalize information that is new or changing about a situational context (Greenfield & Zukow, 1978; Weisenberger, 1976). As children increase the length of their utterances to approach five words or morphemes, they begin to use pronouns in referring to old information and to name specifically new information (Skarakis & Greenfield, 1982).

Use of the definite (*the*) and indefinite (*a* and *an*) articles is also related to the ways in which new and old information is encoded. Although we see children using articles when their MLUs are about 3.5 and they are approximately 2½ to 3 years old (Brown, 1973), accurate use of articles varies, depending on the contexts in which they occur, the amount of shared information between listener and speaker, and whether or not the information is new or old. In a sequence of utterances, the indefinite article is used to introduce a new referent and the definite article is employed to encode a previously introduced referent. The following example illustrates this variation:

I bought a new dress. The dress is red with ruffles.

Because of the shifting use required for articles, we might anticipate that complete acquisition evolves over a number of years. Warden (1976) investigated the developmental changes that occur in the use of articles in children 3, 5, 7, and 9 years old and compared their performances to those of adults. All of the children and the adults showed a consistent preference for using the definite article to refer to previously introduced referents. However, the 3-year-old children randomly used either the definite or indefinite article for introducing initial referents. From 3 years on, there was an increase in appropriate use of the indefinite article for initial referents, but it was not until 9 years of age that the children demonstrated a true preference for using the indefinite article for initial referents. In contrast, adults consistently introduced initial referents with the indefinite article.

Turn Taking, Topic Maintenance, and Revisions. Two aspects of engaging in effective dialogues involve taking one's turn appropriately and helping to maintain the topic of conversation. It appears that children even before the age of 9 months demonstrate rudimentary turn-taking skills in the form of reciprocal interactions. By the time children are 18 to 24 months old, they have learned to participate in dialogues and demonstrate ability in applying rules of turn taking in their dialogues. However, a number of years are necessary to refine these skills. In contrast to children younger than 4½ years who have a fair amount of overlap in their conversations with others, 6- to 8-year olds have learned to time their turns so that they occur at appropriate places in dialogues so there are few overlaps (Leonard, 1984).

Beyond turn taking, a person's response must relate in some way to a speaker's previous utterance if a topic of conversation is to be maintained. Sometime before age 2, approximately 40 percent of children's responses to adults' utterances were found to maintain a topic of conversation (Bloom et al., 1976). This proportion increased steadily during approximately the next 12 months, and at about 3 years, approximately 50 percent of children's responses in a conversational dyad continued the topic. However, children at these ages tend not to maintain topics with a series of several successive related utterances, and it is not until approximately age 3½ to 4 that children demonstrate skills in maintaining topics through a number of adjacent comments in a dialogue (Bloom et al., 1976). Brinton and Fujiki (1984) reported that the average number of utterances even 5-year-old children produced on a single topic during a conversational interchange was five. Additionally, these children covered, on the average, fifty topics in fifteen minutes of conversation. The type of activity/context may, however, influence children's ability to maintain topics. Schober-Peterson and Johnson (1989) found that 4-year-old children were able to maintain one topic over as many as 13 to 91 utterances during activities that involved enacting, describing, and problem-solving conversations. Although these children demonstrated considerable topic maintenance skill during activities that promoted these forms of text, 75 percent of their topic maintenance utterances were still relatively short.

Not only do children show developmental patterns in their turn-taking skill and topic-maintenance ability, they also demonstrate changes with age in the devices they use to maintain topics (McLaughlin, 1998). As children grow older, they increasingly add new information to a topic to maintain it. Before age 3, children tend to use *focus/imitation* topic maintenance devices (Bloom et al., 1976; Keenan, 1975). That is, they attend to one or more of the words in a previous utterance and repeat or imitate those portions in their succeeding responses. As children approach age 3, their use of focus/imitation devices decreases while their use of substitution/expansion operations increases (Bloom et al., 1976; Keenan, 1975). In *substitution/expansion,* children add information to the topic of a previous utterance or modify the previous utterance in some way.

Unfortunately, not all utterances in a conversation are understood by listeners. When this occurs, effective speakers revise their messages. Children between the ages of 21 and 29 months have been found consistently to modify their original utterances when their listeners misunderstand (Gallagher, 1977). Initially, children use phonetic modifications (changing word pronunciations) in attempts to clarify their messages. As children mature, they change their revision strategies and use more word substitutions to modify their communicative attempts. However, at 4½ years of age, children tend to increase the length of subsequent utterances when they know their listeners have not received the messages adequately (Iwan & Siegel, 1982). Conversely, they also decrease the length of utterances when they are aware that their message has been understood. The intent of children's messages when there has been a communication failure may affect how successfully the children resolve the communication breakdown. For example, children between the ages of 3½ and 5½ years of age may be more successful at resolving their communication failure when the intent of their message was a request than when it was an assertion (Shatz & O'Reilly, 1990).

Fluency.   All speakers revise phrases, repeat words, hesitate, use fillers such as "uh," and make false starts in the delivery of messages. These disruptors are often referred to as *mazes.* In fact, preschool children typically go through a period of normal disfluency. However, most children outgrow this period of normal disfluency, and once they enter school, the degree to which messages are delivered with a smooth, easily flowing series of words often becomes one of the factors people use, consciously or unconsciously, to evaluate the language proficiency of children (Loban, 1976).

Contrary to what we might expect to see, the overall occurrence of mazes in children's spoken language seems not to decrease with age (Loban, 1976). In fact, as length and complexity of utterances increase with age, so does the number of maze behaviors, although there may be erratic increases and decreases in the number of maze behaviors at different times and during different tasks.

Narratives.   Narratives are a common part of language use and are not limited to relating information about movies or storybooks. We use narratives when we describe to officials what happened in an automobile accident or when we recount events that occurred during our summer vacation. Narratives are monologues that place heavy demands on logical structure, temporal and causal sequencing, cohesion, and presuppositional abilities. As such, successful narrative ability is a later-developing language skill in children. Children generally are not successful at producing full narratives until the early school years. However, preschoolers pass through several stages in developing the ability to produce true narratives.

Applebee (1978) proposed six levels of narratives; from least to most complex, these are heaps, sequences, primitive temporal narratives, unfocused temporal chains, focused temporal or causal chains, and proper narratives. Although children between the ages of 2 and 3 years begin to tell fictional narratives and briefly describe what has happened to them (Hughes, McGillivray, & Schmidek, 1997; Sutton-Smith, 1986), these narratives are considered to be protonarratives and are characterized by what Applebee (1978) refers to as *heaps.* These are series of unrelated, unsequential statements. Little, if any, concern for the listener's informational need is present, and beginnings and endings are not obvious. These heaps gradually evolve to sequences (Applebee, 1978). The information in *sequences* is presented in an additive but not temporal fashion.

From about 3 to 5 years of age, children begin to relate narratives that show some concern for temporal sequencing of events (McLaughlin, 1998). Initially, children's narratives represent what Applebee (1978) terms *primitive temporal narratives.* Although these narratives still do not contain plots or evidence causality, they do present information in a rudimentary temporal sequence and are focused around a central event. These primitive temporal narratives are gradually replaced with narratives characterized by *unfocused temporal chains.* Narratives of this type contain concrete relationships chained in temporal order. Applebee (1978) suggests that the next narrative level is that of *focused temporal or causal chains.* Narratives of this type typically have a main character and events are presented in a chained manner around the character. Initially, events are chained in a temporal order (Lahey, 1988). Causal chaining generally does not emerge until the early school years, or about 5 to 7 years of age. Focused causal chain narratives are the forerunners of true narratives, which appear at about 7 to 8 years of age (Lahey, 1988).

True narratives not only have central themes and/or characters but generally include multiple causal chains, as well as temporal organization (Lahey, 1988). When children achieve the true narrative level, the narratives have defined episode structure(s) made up of the multiple focused causal and temporal chains referred to above (Stein & Glenn, 1979). Typically, by about 9 years of age, children produce narratives that conform to story grammar structure (Stein & Glenn, 1979). This means that their stories include:

- Setting statements
- Initiating event(s)
- Internal responses of characters
- Internal plan(s) to resolve the dilemma(s) in the story

- Attempts at resolution
- Direct consequences
- Reactions

However, children continue to develop in their ability to include more multiply embedded episode structures. We see, then, that children's narratives evolve from those presented at about 2 years of age, which are characterized by heaps of unrelated statements, to those produced in the first 2 or 3 years of school, characterized by several embedded episodes containing causal and temporal patterns (Hughes et al., 1997).

Metalinguistics.   Young children who are initially learning language do not understand that what they are saying can be something separate from what they are doing. They do not know that they can talk about language, analyze it, see it as an entity separate from its content, and judge it. They are simply learning language to communicate. When they begin to ask what an object's name is, comment that they have forgotten the word for something, repair their utterances spontaneously, practice words or sounds, rhyme words spontaneously, or say that somebody did not say something correctly, they are showing the early glimmers of metalinguistic awareness.

True metalinguistic skills do not, however, appear until the early school years, or about 7 to 8 years of age (McLaughlin, 1998; Owens, 2001; Saywitz & Cherry-Wilkinson, 1982). Metalinguistic skills develop well into, if not throughout, high school and possibly even into adulthood. Two aspects of oral language that are related to the development of metalinguistic skills are the ability to detect ambiguities in utterances and the intentional use of figurative language and jokes. Because these are relatively late-developing skills, they are discussed in Chapter 5.

Language, Literacy, and Education

Language and language-related skills comprise the majority of the curricula in the early grades, which emphasize learning to read and write and, later, improving reading and writing skills. In the upper grades, the language and language-related skills acquired earlier become the modes through which the content areas are learned. Students are asked to do independent reading in content areas and to write about what they have learned. Language is, therefore, a fundamental aspect of literacy and the educational process.

As we have seen, when children enter school, often at the kindergarten level, they typically bring with them a solid base in the auditory–oral language system. This is not to say that their oral language system is wholly developed by age 5, but children beginning kindergarten have usually had 5 years of listening experiences and 4 years of talking experiences. We know that they use fairly well-formed, complex sentences to express their ideas and needs and to ask questions, have a large expressive vocabulary, and understand between 20,000 and 24,000 words. This competence in the auditory–oral language system is a significant factor in learning to read and write. In Loban's (1976) longitudinal investigation of language skills of school children, children whose listening and speaking skills were well developed had better reading and writing skills than those whose auditory–oral language systems were less advanced. Conversely, elementary school children described as "low-achieving" (but not receiving special education services or diagnosed as language-disordered) have been found to have poorer language skills than their academically achieving peers (Hill & Haynes, 1992). Oral language development in the preschool years prepares the child for formalized education, and it is integrally related to literacy. According to Scarborough (1998), children's ability to decode printed words at the end of second grade was predicted by the sizes of the children's receptive and expressive vocabularies when they were 3½ years old.

Emergent Literacy and Preliteracy

Achieving literacy in Western societies is no longer seen as just acquiring the abilities to read and write, that is, having literacy skills. Rather, literacy is viewed as engaging in literate behaviors. These include reading spontaneously for pleasure and learning, writing to convey analyzed and synthesized thoughts and ideas, listening and speaking to argue, discuss, and plan, and even using computers to communicate and acquire information. Recent views of literacy have also discarded the notion that literacy begins when children go to school and learn to read and write (Justice & Ezell, 2002). The acquisition of literacy is now seen to begin basically at birth, and toddlers and preschool children are considered to be in the process of becoming literate. *Emergent literacy* and *preliteracy* are terms that have been applied to the development occurring during the preschool years in the child's early environments that leads to literacy. These are prereading and prewriting behaviors and skills that develop into conventional reading and writing abilities.

Several factors have been associated with emerging literacy skills in children. One of these is what goes on in preschoolers' homes and their family environment (Justice & Ezell, 2000; Justice, Weber, Ezell, & Bakeman, 2002; Lonigan et al., 1999; Snow, Burns, & Griffin, 1998; van Kleeck, 1998; van Kleeck, Gillam, Hamilton, & McGrath, 1997; Whitehurst & Lonigan, 1998). Characteristics of home and family environments that promote literacy include:

- A variety of print materials in the environment
- Writing instruments (crayons, pencils) and paper easily available
- Adults who are responsive to the child's attempts to read and write
- Reading and writing as integrated and embedded activities in daily family routine as regular activities of living
- Adult–child storybook reading that
  - Is a social, interactive event
  - Contains routinized dialogue cycles
  - Varies differentially to allow children to take more responsibility for the reading as their language skills grow

Factors such as these are seen as helping to prepare young children for the more formal learning activities they will experience during their elementary and secondary school years. These young children begin school knowing that print represents oral language and, therefore, that it is meaningful and serves a variety of functions. They may even know something about the visual–graphic symbols associated with printed material. Combined with metalinguistic skills, these developmental factors play important roles in children's learning the literacy skills (reading, writing, spelling) that allow them to engage in literate behaviors, that is, to become literate individuals.

School

The educational system is divided into the elementary and secondary school grades. The primary emphasis of the elementary grades is acquisition of basic learning skills (reading, writing, spelling, arithmetic abilities), although as children progress into the upper elementary grades somewhat more importance is placed on using basic skills for content learning. In secondary school, emphasis shifts dramatically to acquiring content-area information, with gradually increasing expectations for independent learning. At this level, basic skills are assumed to have been acquired.

The Elementary Grades

Kindergarten.   Kindergarten is often considered as a "readiness" grade, to prepare children for the learning experiences to come in first grade. Because of the influence that listening and speaking skills have on reading and writing abilities, kindergarten learning activities frequently focus on further developing the children's oral language skills. Although kindergarten may emphasize the listening and speaking skills, most children are also introduced formally to reading and writing skills. Kindergartners may learn to recognize the printed words for the days of the week, their classmates' printed names, or the names of printed letters. Learning activities may involve having the children formulate their thoughts and dictate them to the teacher, who writes them on the board. Such an activity emphasizes the relationship between the spoken and printed word and is an initial stage in the development of written composition skills. The children's early experiences with the sensorimotor processes of the visual–graphic language system typically include learning to write the letters of the alphabet and their names and matching sounds to graphemes. The children may also be shown how to improve their drawings of circles and lines, the elements of writing. An important feature of kindergarten is acculturating children to the scripts and routines of formal group instruction, that is, learning to listen in groups, knowing when to talk and when to be quiet, knowing how to ask and answer questions, and learning how to work quietly alone and to cooperate in groups. In some schools, limited formal instruction in reading and writing may be introduced in kindergarten. In other schools, formal instruction in reading and writing is not introduced until first grade.

First Grade.   Formal reading and writing instruction most typically begins in first grade. Children learn to use word-recognition skills, acquire information from printed words, distinguish among beginning sounds of spoken words, and read for meaning. In writing, children learn to form both lower and uppercase letters and to print short words. Skill levels in writing, however, usually lag behind reading. Although the primary emphasis on language skills in first grade may shift from the auditory–oral system to the visual–graphic system, learning activities continue to involve listening and speaking skills. The children are encouraged to dictate letters and stories; because their writing skills are still limited, the teacher acts as a scribe. Such experiences further demonstrate to children the relationship between the spoken and written word and encourage them to learn to write the words they say.

Second Grade.　　Second-grade curricula emphasize increased skill in listening, speaking, reading, and writing. Children may be asked to rhyme words, follow sequences of orally presented directions, write short stories, increase their spelling vocabularies, and improve printed forms. In reading, the emphasis turns to independence. Students are expected to develop independent word-recognition and reading-comprehension skills; typically, the curriculum also encourages the children to spend time in independent reading. Learning activities move from concrete, hands-on experiences to abstract, language-related experiences.

Third Grade.　　Third grade is a transition grade. Increased attention is given to independent reading, with emphasis on reading more complex, longer stories. Instruction in cursive writing typically begins, although printed forms may continue to be used in situations where speed is expected. If we look at the demands of cursive writing, we see that we are asking children to recode previously learned printed symbols, which were themselves coded symbols for the auditory code. Children are asked to answer questions by writing sentences and to write increasingly complex paragraphs. Continued emphasis is placed on increasing spelling vocabularies. Children in third grade are also typically expected to proofread and correct their written work. Oral activities include participating effectively in group discussions and making presentations.

Fourth, Fifth, and Sixth Grades.　　The curricular emphases in these grades continually shift from learning activities directed to building skills in the auditory–oral and visual–graphic language systems to using these language skills for acquiring content-area information. Students gain information through class discussions and short teacher lectures and demonstrations. Students may even be given independent reading assignments and be asked to write short reports about what they have read. They are expected to use their language skills to seek out information from resources. Without the necessary underlying basic skills in both the auditory–oral and visual–graphic systems, we can see how children may be at risk for failure.

The Secondary Grades.　　The shift from elementary to secondary education generally occurs somewhere around sixth or seventh grade. Lectures as the means of instruction become more common, and students are increasingly expected to be able to take written notes on the lecture content. Additionally, students may have different teachers for different subjects. This means that students need to adjust to varying lecture delivery. Independence in all forms of learning is stressed, and teachers expect students to be able to seek out and organize information for themselves. The emphasis is on learning content and on demonstrating what information has been acquired. There is a significant increase in the use of the written mode for demonstrating knowledge, and performance on written tests of content knowledge takes on greater importance.

　　Children's language skills evolve dramatically from kindergarten on. Although the development is a complex process, with listening, speaking, reading, and writing skills closely related to and interacting with one another, a large part of the early educational achievement in reading and writing depends heavily on the children's abilities with the auditory–oral language system. Later educational achievements depend on both the auditory–oral and visual–graphic language systems.

Summary

In this chapter we have seen that

- Babies are born communicating, and before infants use their first words, they engage in many behaviors (e.g., smiling, laughing, gazing) that convey communication intent and exhibit a range of prelinguistic vocalizations.
- In the one- and two-word stages, children learn the names for objects and relations in their environment; vocabulary growth begins slowly, spurting ahead between 18 and 24 months of age.
- Children's early utterances systematically develop into basic kernel, negative, and question sentences, and later into compound and complex sentences.
- Semantic as well as syntactic factors are involved in sentence development.
- Several patterns influence word learning, and there seem to be several principles that apply to children's word learning.
- Children acquire specific grammatical morphemes in a developmental sequence related to increasing mean length of utterance (MLU).
- The functions and intentions of language use change as children get older; utterances change from those containing one function to those containing more than one function.
- Young children adapt the form of their language for their listeners; this ability to adapt grows more refined as children become better able to make accurate presuppositions about their listeners; turn-taking, topic-maintenance, and revision skills improve gradually throughout the preschool years and into the school years.
- Children's narratives develop from those produced at about 2 years of age, characterized by heaps of unrelated statements, to those produced in the first 2 or 3 years of school, characterized by multiply embedded episodes with causal and temporal patterns.

As this review of normal language development illustrates, there are a great many skills that children must acquire in the process of learning to talk. We have seen, however, that the process follows developmental patterns. Often these developmental patterns become a basis for planning intervention programs for children who have impaired language skills. These same developmental sequences also provide one way of identifying children who are not progressing appropriately in acquiring their language.

CHAPTER

3

Toddlers and Preschoolers with Specific Language Impairment

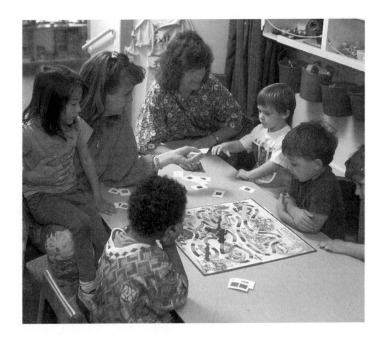

OBJECTIVES

After reading this chapter, you should be able to discuss

- Issues related to characterization of specific language impairment in children
- Whether subgroups of children with specific language impairment exist given the heterogeneity of the language characteristics of the children
- Various labels that have been used to describe this population of children, identify the issues related to causation, and discuss the relationship between these issues and the various labels
- Possible causal factors and potential clinical markers of specific language impairment
- Prevalence figures that have been presented for youngsters with specific language impairment and the implications of the figures

- Factors that may allow us to know which youngsters might outgrow early language problems and which might not
- The relationship between language problems in the preschool years and later academic difficulties
- Various language and related characteristics of toddlers and preschoolers with specific language impairment
- Assessment and intervention considerations for toddlers and preschoolers with specific language impairment

This chapter is about toddlers and preschool children who evidence language problems in the apparent absence of other clearly identifiable problems, such as those indicated in the titles of many of the chapters that will follow in this text. These include intellectual disability, autism, hearing impairment, or acquired language impairment. The children we will discuss in this chapter appear on the surface to be essentially normal, except for their language acquisition, which does not match that of their peers. Because we cannot attribute their language-learning problems to an identifiable condition we, and others, have chosen to use the term *specific language impairment* (SLI) to refer to these children, hence the chapter title. Leonard (1998) describes these children as those

> . . . who show a significant limitation in language ability, yet the factors usually accompanying language learning problems—such as hearing impairment, low nonverbal intelligence test scores, and neurological damage—are not evident. This is a real curiosity, especially in light of the many language acquisition papers that begin with a statement to the effect that "all normal children" learn language rapidly and effortlessly. The only thing clearly abnormal about these children is that they don't learn language rapidly and effortlessly. (p. 3)

Part of the decision to use the term specific language impairment in the chapter title was guided by a desire to distinguish as much as possible the topic of this chapter from other chapters in this text. Using the phrase was not, however, a completely easy choice, because of several unresolved issues about these children. Among these are whether the children's language problems are, in fact, specific only to language and whether the language problems of these children reflect language delay or disorder. Another is the possibility that there may be subgroups of these children. How we approach these issues affects what we label the problem. Here is the dilemma about the chapter title. Other issues concern the prevalence data for preschool children with language impairments without obvious concomitant problems, how we identify children who have these language-learning problems, our abilities to predict who will outgrow early language problems, and the intervention implications of these issues. These are topics we address in this chapter. We also discuss language characteristics seen in some of these young children and introduce assessment and intervention considerations. There is no longer any question that language problems of children in their preschool years signal the real likelihood of later academic, vocational, and social failures, topics taken up further in the two subsequent chapters.

However, before moving too far into discussion of toddlers and preschoolers with specific language impairment, some consideration of the issue of identifying children with language impairment more generally is appropriate. This topic is relevant for many of the children with language disorders whom we will discuss in this text, as well as the children with specific language impairment who are the focus of this chapter.

Identification of Children with Language Impairment

It may seem strange to think of identifying children with language problems as a major issue. One might think that identifying these children would be straightforward. Certainly, a child whose language performance does not correspond to that of children the same age might be considered to have language problems. However, several questions arise. We know that children who are acquiring language normally can show marked variability in language development. If a child's performance does not correspond to that of other children of the same age, does the difference reflect normal variation or a problem? How do we determine if the difference is normal variation or problematic? If the difference is considered not to be a reflection of normal variability, how much of a difference from expectations constitutes a real problem versus a slowed pattern within normal limits? If a child demonstrates above-average development in areas other than language, such as cognition/intelligence or motor skills, but only average development in language, should we consider the child to have a language impairment? A related issue is how do we think about infants who are preverbal, so that oral language performance cannot be observed, or about children who at a particular point in time seem to demonstrate adequate language skills but who have intrinsic factors that may place them at risk for later language problems? Should these children be considered to have language impairments? These are only a few of the questions. The answers to these questions influence which children, as Lahey (1990) writes, "shall be called language disordered" (p. 619), who may and may not, therefore, receive intervention, and what the forms of intervention might be.

Given normal variability in children's language development and in their language performances from one communicative context to another, the standard to which we compare an individual child's performance and the conditions under which we observe that performance are important factors in identification. This latter factor requires that a child's language performance be observed in a variety of contexts, a topic that will be discussed later in this book. Although language developmental milestones provide relevant information about whether a child's performance is similar to or different from these milestones, they provide very little information about the significance of any variations that might be observed. It is the significance attached to the variations that leads to identification of a child as having a language problem. However, deciding on the significance of the variations depends, in part, on the standard to which we compare the performance.

Mental Age, Chronological Age, and Language Age

The two standards of comparison that have commonly been used are mental age (MA) and chronological age (CA). MA refers to the age level at which a child is functioning on cognitive/intellectual tasks. In using MA as the standard, children's language performances are compared to those of children with similar MAs. The assumption is that normal children's language performance does not generally differ markedly from their nonverbal cognitive abilities. When language performance is lower than MA, a language impairment is presumed to be present. That is, there is a gap between MA and language age (LA). There are, however, several problems with this approach (Bishop, 1997; Cole, Mills, & Kelley, 1994; Cole, Schwartz, Notari, Dale, & Mills, 1995; Fey, 1986; Johnston, 1994; Lahey, 1990; Leonard, 1983, 1998; Plante, 1998):

1. The exact relationship between cognition and language has not been established (see Chapter 1). Therefore, it cannot be assumed that cognitive abilities will necessarily set the limits for or determine language performance.
2. Some, but not many, children may have language skills higher than their cognitive skills.
3. There may be different types of intelligence, and a theoretical relationship between these and language has not been demonstrated.
4. It is possible that many children with intellectual disabilities would not be identified as having a language disorder because there may be no gap between their MA and LA. As a result, these children may not receive language intervention services even though they might benefit from intervention.

One advantage of this approach is that children who have above-average cognitive skills but language skills below their cognitive levels could be identified as language impaired.

The second approach uses CA as the standard to which language performance is compared. Fey (1986) writes that "with CA referencing, language impairment is defined as a clinically significant departure from what is expected for children of the child's own CA" (p. 36). That is, there is a gap between CA and LA. Although this approach resolves the concern about the still unestablished relationship between cognition/MA and language performance, it has certain problems:

1. Children whose cognitive levels exceed their CA but whose language performances correspond to their CA may not be identified as having language problems.
2. These might be very bright or gifted children whose language abilities may prevent achievement at the level that might be expected from their cognitive level.
3. The number of children identified as having language problems may be so large that it strains the professional resources available to serve them. This approach implies, as Fey (1986) explains, that the ultimate goal of intervention for any child identified as language disordered "would be to bring the child's communicative abilities to an age-equivalent level. . . . Unfortunately, this is frequently an unrealistic expectation for many of the children" (p. 36).

Despite the problems associated with the CA–LA gap approach to identifying the children, these may be less serious than those related to the MA–LA comparison. Of these two, CA is generally the preferred standard for comparison.

We now return to the issue of what constitutes an important variation from the standard we use. Even in light of our previous discussion, there is justified concern about using age-equivalency measures, such as LA referred to in the preceding discussion (Bishop,

1997; Lahey, 1990; McCauley & Swisher, 1984; McCauley & Demetras, 1990; Paul, 2001; Rice, 2000). One reason for this concern is that the same delay in terms of age-equivalent performance may not have the same importance for children of different ages. For example, a 1-year delay in language performance for a 10-year-old child may not likely carry the same significance as a 1-year delay for a 3-year-old child. Lahey (1990) argues that a more appropriate approach describes a child's "relative standing with peers" (p. 615), so that normal variability from an average is considered.

Normal Variation, Normal Distribution, and a Statistical Approach

The approach of using normal variability to decide which children's language performances are sufficiently different from their peers' to constitute an impairment is based on concepts surrounding the normal distribution of performance in samples of children of the same age with particular demographic characteristics. It is rooted in statistical approaches to distribution, so that the metrics of mean and standard deviations (SD) are considered. We know, for example, that if we measured the receptive vocabulary size of lots of 3-year-old children, about 64 percent of them would have scores falling between –1 standard deviation (SD) below the mean score and +1 SD above, with approximately half on either side of the mean. This –1 to +1 SD range is generally considered to be the "normal" range of performance, and a score below the –1 SD point is often the point at which some unease about a child's performance might occur. Approximately another 13.5 percent of the children would have scores between –1 SD and –2 SD, leaving about another 3 percent of the children having scores below –2 SD. Concern about a child's performance generally escalates the greater the child's score is below the –1 SD point.

The question is, which cutoff tells us that a child's receptive vocabulary (or any other aspect of language we measure in this way) is sufficiently poor to indicate language impairment? What cutoff tells us when the child's performance will cause academic and social difficulties for the child? In essence, the cutoffs that are frequently used are relatively arbitrary because, as Rice (2000) explains, "there is no intrinsic criterion for where to draw the line between 'normal' and 'affected'" (p. 20). Recall also that if we make the cutoff –2 SD below the mean, there will only be 3 percent of children who will be considered to have impaired language. Bishop (1997) reminds us of the "inherent circularity of statistical definitions" because "if you define a language impairment as a score in the lowest 3%, then 3% of the children will be language-impaired" (p. 23). Besides standard deviations, other descriptions of language performance based on normal variation, normal distribution, and related statistics include standard scores, percentile ranks, and stanine scores.

To provide some point of reference as to how these metrics correspond to each other, a –1 SD deviation cutoff is commonly about equal to a standard score of 85, a 17 to 18th percentile rank, and a stanine of 3. With regard to identifying children with SLI, a standard of comparison or cutoff at the 10th percentile has been considered as a plausible cutoff for identifying a child's language to be sufficiently problematic to be language impaired (Fey, 1986; Lee, 1974; Paul, 2001). A 10th-percentile rank equates to about –1.25 SD and a standard score of 80. This standard of comparison has been shown to have good agreement with speech–language pathologists' judgments of children's language abilities as being impaired or normal (Tomblin, Records, & Zhang, 1996).

Social Standard

Scores such as percentile ranks and standard scores still do not tell us how much a child's language abilities might interfere with academic and/or social achievements. Using the above cutoff of the 10th percentile rank, a child whose language performance is at the 10th percentile would be considered language disordered, whereas one whose performance is at the 15th percentile rank might not. However, it could be that the child at the 15th percentile rank will experience just as many or more difficulties because of language problems as the one at the 10th percentile. An approach that focuses on variance scores also has the danger of leading professionals to depend too heavily on norm-referenced, standardized tests of language for identifying language-disordered children, a topic discussed in Chapter 13.

There may be a third standard of comparison to consider, that is, a social standard. In using this standard, societal values placed on the degree of language facility and on the degree of success for life functions that are dependent on language facility (e.g., educational success, social success) become important in identifying children (Bishop, 1997; Brinton, Fujiki, & McKee, 1998; DeKroon, Kyte, & Johnson, 2002; Gertner, Rice, & Hadley, 1994; Goodyer, 2000; Johnson et al., 1999; Leonard, 1998; Redmond & Rice, 1998; Stothard, Snowling, Bishop, Chipchase, & Kaplan, 1998). Children whose language performances are evaluated as being sufficiently poor to cause potential problems in succeeding within the conditions of societal values could then be seen to have language impairments. Although this standard is harder to measure in numerical terms, it may overcome some of the difficulties inherent in the other standards for identification discussed so far. This may be particularly true if a social standard is used in combination with one of these more traditional standards. It also has the potential to provide a framework for approaching language and language impairments in linguistically-culturally diverse children.

Challenging and Changing the Child's Language Performance

None of the preceding discussion addresses the identification of children who appear to be able to communicate adequately but who have less obvious language problems that potentially interfere with academic performance or social interactions. These children may attain scores on standardized language tests that place them within normal limits (although the scores may be at the lower end of the normal limits and their scores may be significantly lower than those of their normally achieving peers) (Girolametto, Wiigs, Smyth, Weitzman, & Pearce, 2001; Paul, 1996; Stothard et al., 1998). They may also be able to engage in casual, relaxed conversational interchanges (Lahey, 1990; Owen & Leonard, 2002), but they may experience difficulties with academic skills closely related to oral language abilities, such as reading, spelling, and writing, and with high-level, demanding discourse language skills such as narratives (Beitchman, Wilson, Brownlie, Walters, & Lancee, 1996; Girolametto et al., 2001; Johnson et al., 1999; Paul, 1996; Stothard et al., 1998). These factors have implications for the procedures we use in identifying the children. For this reason, Lahey (1990) suggests that identification should be made under conditions that include stressing or challenging the child's language performance, "so that difficulties with performance would most likely be evident" (p. 618).

Children with language disorders should also have more difficulty acquiring particular language skills under conditions of instruction than their peers without language problems. Degree of difficulty in learning language targets can be measured in terms of the speed with which new language skills are learned, the amount of teaching effort that is needed, or the accuracy of performance, that is, the quantity of learning. Children with language disorders should therefore require more tries to learn a language target, and/or need more and varied stimuli to learn the targets, and/or use the targets correctly less often than their typically developing counterparts. These suppositions suggest that another way in which children with language disorders can be identified is by determining how well or poorly they respond to "trial language instruction," or, to be consistent with the terminology currently used in the literature, how well they respond to dynamic assessment.

Risk Factors for Language Problems

Identification also involves predicting which children will ultimately experience problems related to language. There are very young, and therefore primarily nonverbal, children (e.g., below 1 or 1½ years of age) who may be at risk for language development problems, and there are preschool and school-age children who may not have observable language problems at a specific time but who have a history or other problems that place them at risk for the emergence of later language difficulties. Tomblin and his colleagues (1991) suggest that it might be possible to assign neonates to an "at risk for language problems" category based on criteria related to prenatal and perinatal events. The children's development could then be monitored and intervention begun as soon as any problems with language emerged. It might also be possible to institute "preventive intervention" for these children, even before actual language problems are identified, through parent/caregiver training programs. For older children who have histories or other problems that place them at risk for the emergence of language difficulties, preventive intervention through parental and/or teacher training programs might also be effective.

These approaches depend, of course, on determining what factors place children at risk for language disorders. Some birth factors (e.g., anoxia, hyperbilirubinemia, kernicterus), chromosomal syndromes (e.g., Down syndrome), and known neurological or physical conditions (e.g., cerebral palsy, hearing loss, cleft palate) have been linked to potential language problems. Additionally, risk for language problems has been associated with socioeconomic factors and environmental deprivation, although these are not always independent of other factors, such as familial or genetic factors. Although some have suggested that prematurity may place an infant at risk for later language problems, this has not been fully substantiated in the research (Aram, Hack, Hawkins, Weissman, & Borawski-Clark, 1991; Menyuk, Liebergott, Schultz, Chesnick, & Ferrier, 1991).

When these more obvious factors are absent, there may be other factors that can place children at risk for later language problems. Among those suggested in the literature are (1) a family history of communication problems and/or literacy problems, particularly among members of the immediate family; (2) birth order, with later birth indicating a greater risk; (3) parents' levels of education, particularly mother's level of education; and (4) gender of the child, with males appearing to be more at risk than females (Bishop, North, & Donlon, 1995; Choudhury & Benasich, 2003; Dollaghan et al., 1999; Entwisle & Astone, 1994; Felsenfeld & Plomin, 1997; Hart & Risley, 1995; Paul, 1991; Plomin, DeFries, McClearn, & McGuffin, 2001; Plomin, Fulker, Corley, & DeFries, 1997; Rice, 1996; Tallal, Ross, & Curtiss, 1989;

Tomblin & Buckwalter, 1998; Tomblin et al., 1991). Caution is important in interpreting these possible risk factors. It is likely that not all factors have been fully determined, that the factors just listed are not invariably associated with later language difficulties, and that their interrelationships with other factors have yet to be explained. Language learning and language performance are complex human behaviors influenced by multiple factors, so the factors that place children at risk for language impairment are more than likely going to reflect complex interactions. However, in their study of a variety of prenatal and perinatal risk factors (e.g., parental education, family history of language and/or learning problems, tobacco smoking) for SLI, Tomblin and his colleagues (Tomblin, Smith, & Zhang, 1997) found that, in contrast to risk factors considered to occur during the perinatal period of the children or during their fetal development, SLI in children was more likely to be associated with factors related to their parents that were present before the children were conceived.

Despite the limits on the current information, Tomblin and colleagues (1991) suggest that using an at-risk procedure that places children in a developmental monitoring program in combination with a language screening procedure may aid the identification process. However, if we apply Lahey's (1990) idea, the screening procedure should include tasks that stress the child's language performance. The notion of using high-risk factors with monitoring combined with screening programs is consistent with her suggestion that perhaps two identification categories should be devised. One would be for those children who show problems with language, and the other for children at risk for language problems. Using the findings from Tomblin and colleagues (Tomblin, Smith, & Zhang, 1997) above, it might be possible to begin considering weighting the degree of risk associated with various risk factors.

Table 3.1 summarizes some of the issues we have raised with regard to identifying children with language problems. Although the issues remain, Fey (1986) has offered a practical definition of "who shall be called language disordered" (Lahey, 1990) that is based on one presented in 1983 by Tomblin:

> A child may be viewed as language impaired when the pattern of communicative performance exhibited enables a clinician to predict continued deficits in language development *and* in the social, cognitive, educational or emotional developments which rely heavily on language skills. Furthermore, infants who have biological or behavioral conditions that are commonly associated with future impairments in communicative functioning (e.g., Down's syndrome, profound hearing impairment, autistic symptoms) may be viewed as language impaired even before the age at which language forms typically begin to appear. The degree of confidence that a clinician can place in this prediction will determine the severity rating for the child's impairment. (p. 42)

We would add that children with other factors that may place them at risk for language impairment would be identified as, as Lahey (1990) writes, "at-risk for language-related problems" (p. 618) and placed in language developmental monitoring programs.

An Overview of Specific Language Impairment

Delay versus Disorder

To say that a child demonstrates a *language delay* implies that language skills are slow to emerge or develop but that the order in which the child acquires the skills corresponds to the

TABLE 3.1   Issues in Identification of Children with Language Problems

Issues	Explanations	Problems
Standards of comparison	Mental age (MA): language performance compared to expectations for child's mental (cognitive) age	Children with language performance higher than MA
		Relationship between cognition and language not fully established
		Different forms of intelligence and relationship with language not established
		Mentally retarded children excluded from being considered language impaired
	Chronological age (CA): language performance compared to expectations for child's chronological age	Excludes children with above-normal cognitive abilities but average or below-average language performance
		Too many children identified as having language problems for resources available
		Implication that goal of intervention is always to achieve age-equivalent language performance
	Social standard: degree of social value attached to verbal ability and aspects of performance linked to verbal ability (e.g., academic achievement, social relationships) and degree to which language problems therefore negatively affect achievement	Hard to measure numerically
		Not a 1:1 relationship between variance score (e.g., standard score) of language performance and degree of impact on child's current and future life
		Involves prediction with regard to future problems child might have
Measures of performance	Age equivalency (language age, LA)	Same amount of delay in terms of age equivalence not equally important at different CAs
		Normal variation in language performance not considered
	Variance measures (e.g., standard scores, percentile ranks, standard deviations, stanines)	Cutoff point not descriptive of actual problems in real-life language functioning
		Danger of excessive dependence on norm-referenced, standardized language tests
Identifying subtle language problems	Stress/challenge language performance	Casual language performance and/or standardized language performance may appear normal unless performance stressed to reveal subtle problems
		Subtle problems can affect language-related academic skills (e.g., reading, spelling)
Predicting future language problems	Identifying children at risk for language difficulties; supplement with screening programs	At risk factors not completely identified
		Relationships between factors not understood

sequence seen in normal children. It also usually implies that the degree of delay is basi-cally the same for all features or aspects of language, so that a child's profile in the differ-ent areas of language is relatively flat. There is sometimes the implication that a child with a language delay might overcome the delay and catch up. In contrast, the term *language dis-order* denotes a deviation in the usual rate and/or sequence with which specific language skills emerge. This deviation can include differences in the rate of acquisition for skills within one aspect of language (e.g., semantics or syntax), inordinate difficulties with cer-tain features within one aspect of language (e.g., grammatical morphology), differences in the rate of acquisition among various aspects of language (e.g., pragmatic development related to syntactic development), and/or age-appropriate skills in one or more aspects with lags in acquisition of one or more other aspects of language. Because of asynchrony in rate of acquisition within and across various language parameters, normal developmental sequence is disrupted. With the term *language disorder* there may be less of an inference that children might just catch up with their language.

Despite the differences in these definitions, some have referred to these children with language-learning problems as having a *language delay,* while others have used the term *language disorder* to refer to children with similar language characteristics*,* frequently without justifying why one phrase has been used over the other. And the research involving various aspects of language (pragmatics, semantics, syntax, and morphology) has often yielded conflicting interpretations and certainly has not clarified the issue for us (Bishop, 1997). Consistent with Paul's (2001) explanation, we have tended to use *impairment* and *disorder* interchangeably, but have been more careful to use *delay* to mean a lag in devel-opment without necessarily implying a disorder.

One reason for these conflicting interpretations of whether language-impaired chil-dren show us delay or disorder in their language behaviors is that a problem with any one aspect or component of language will negatively affect other aspects so that the entire lan-guage performance appears disturbed. Although we may talk about the components of lan-guage separately, in actuality all components interact at one time, with one component affecting others (Ellis Weismer & Evans, 2002; Gershkoff-Stowe & Smith, 1997; Lahey & Bloom, 1994; Leonard et al., 1981; Masterson, 1997; Reed, 1992; Storkel, 2003). A num-ber of years ago, Carrow-Woolfolk and Lynch (1982) reminded us that "a simplification of the language code is the expected result of a problem in any specific language area" (p. 297). What we typically see, however, in children's language is their total performance, and trying to factor out the many aspects of language that can be interacting at any one time is exceedingly challenging.

In light of issues surrounding delay versus disorder, the usefulness of specific lan-guage impairment as a construct has been called into question. In promoting debate about SLI as a diagnostic entity, Leonard (1987, 1991) posited that the language abilities seen in children with SLI might simply represent abilities that are at the lower end of a continuum of normal variation. Rather than having a language disorder, the children simply are not as good at learning and using language as other children, in the same way that other children might not be as good at learning and using musical skills, for example. Children on the low end of language-skill performance would not be seen to have a disorder, but rather to reflect the con-cept of normal variation within and across individuals. Some children are just better at some things than other things, and different children are different in what they are good or weak at learning and doing. From this perspective, it is only because language abilities are so highly regarded in Western societies and because language abilities are so intimately tied to the Western process of formal education and academic success, which are also highly regarded in Western societies, that weaker skills in language could be seen to represent a disorder.

Most researchers and practitioners who work with toddlers and preschoolers who have inordinate language-learning problems in the absence of explicable conditions for language problems reject this position. Lahey (1988) writes that

> . . . some children who fit this syndrome [specific language impairment] have such severe difficulties with language learning that if this same degree of difficulty were apparent in motor impairment, for example, they might well be classified as having a disorder or disability. (p. 54)

Since Lahey's comment, both the 1993 *International Classification of Diseases* (ICD-10) (World Health Organization, 1993) and the 1994 *Diagnostic and Statistical Manual of Mental Disorders,* 4th Edition (DSM-IV) (American Psychiatric Association, 1994) include conditions (e.g, [Specific] Developmental Language Disorder) that could be considered descriptive of and similar to SLI. The position that SLI is a condition differentiated from other conditions that include disruptions of language performance suggests that the exceptional problems that some children have in learning and generalizing certain language skills and the continuing difficulties with language that they demonstrate simply cannot be viewed as anything but a disability. However, one of the problems that confounds the discussion of delay versus disorder is the variety of language problems these children can display, that is, their heterogeneity.

Subgroups of Young Children with Specific Language Impairments

Children with SLI are generally described as a heterogeneous group because of the variation in language performance seen from child to child. It may be that, to understand young children with specific language impairment more fully, we need to consider the possibility that subgroups of these children exist. If this is the case, we need to ask what the relevant subgroups might be.

Some children described as specifically language impaired have difficulties with both language comprehension and expression (Tombin, Zhang, Buckwalter, & O'Brien, 2003). Other children have problems with language expression but relatively unimpaired comprehension, although the areas of expressive language that pose the more serious difficulties (e.g., lexical retrieval, syntax, and morphology) might vary from child to child. Still others may have comprehension problems in the absence of language expression difficulties. . Three likely subgroups are therefore implicated:

1. Both comprehension and expression difficulties
2. Expression difficulties only
3. Comprehension difficulties only

This model for subgroups may, however, be too simplistic (Bishop, 1997; Evans, Viele, & Kass, 1997). Phonological problems have been found to co-occur frequently with syntax problems. Additionally, gestures representing symbolic play or for communicative purposes have been associated with early language difficulties (Thal & Tobias, 1992, 1994; Thal, Tobias, & Morrison, 1991; Thal, Oroz, Evans, Katich, & Leasure, 1995). Paul, Looney, and Dahm (1991) also found a relationship between early language deficits and socialization characteristics. On the basis of their findings, Paul and colleagues (1991) proposed four subgroups:

1. Deficits in expression only
2. Deficits in expression and socialization, with normal comprehension
3. Deficits in expression, comprehension, and socialization
4. Deficits in expression and comprehension, with normal socialization

Of the subjects in this study, one-third fell into the first category (expressive deficits only) and about 38 percent fell into the second (deficits in both expression and socialization, with normal comprehension). Together, these two categories accounted for approximately 70 percent of the children in their study. There are also other ways to classify children into subgroups, such as the six groupings proposed by Rapin and Allen (Rapin, 1996; Rapin & Allen, 1987).

If we consider only the five potential deficit areas mentioned thus far (comprehension, expression, phonology, socialization, symbolic play gestures), we can see in Table 3.2 some, but not all, of the combinations that might lead to possible subgroups of children. If we break down expression into the possible specific aspects of language (e.g., semantics, pragmatics, syntax, morphology) that might be problematic, we see even greater complexity in the combinations that could be possible. However, it might not be valid to separate some of these factors because of the overlaps, interrelationships, and associations that are known to operate across linguistic components and among and across other behaviors (e.g., relationships

TABLE 3.2   **Examples of Areas of Deficit Leading to Some Possible Subgroups of Children with Specific Language Impairments**

Subgroups	Expression	Comprehension	Phonology	Socialization	Gesture
1	X	X	X	X	X
2	X	X		X	X
3	X	X	X		X
4	X		X	X	
5	X		X		
6	X	X			X
7	X			X	
8	X				
9		X			X
10		X	X	X	X
11		X		X	X

between measures of socialization and use of communicative intentions/functions). Our factors or areas of deficit might not be correct and/or discrete. Other factors and associations have also been implicated with specific language disorders (e.g., behavioral difficulties). Additionally, we would likely need to take account of the relative degree of skill (or deficit) in each of the possible areas. It is possible that the combinations could change in an individual child as chronological age changes (Conti-Ramsden & Botting, 1999b). The syndrome we refer to as specific language impairment may be too large and nondiscrete to account for the heterogeneity seen in the children. As Aram (1991) writes, it may be that "children with specific language impairment do not represent a single clinical entity, but rather are a cluster of subgroups whose overlapping and defining feature is that of a language impairment" (p. 84). In clearly summarizing the current state of knowledge, Leonard (1998) explains that "the task of identifying distinct and reliable subgroups has proven to be a formidable one. And we still don't have it right" (p. 23). Our present knowledge has not yet allowed us to overcome the complexity of the task of identifying valid subgroups, although as Leonard (1998) also reminds us, there are some themes that keep popping up with regard to possible subgroups: a group of children with similar degrees of depressed comprehension and production abilities, a group with a considerable gap between production and comprehension with production being the lower area of ability, and a group with particular difficulty with aspects of language form (syntax, morphology, phonology). We are still searching for what the subgroups, if they exist, might be.

A Label for It and Reasons for It

In the introduction to this chapter, the dilemma regarding how to title the chapter was raised. Many terms have been used in the literature to label the condition in which language difficulties appear to be the sole problem of these children. Among these terms are specific language impairment (SLI), specific language disability, specific language disorder, developmental aphasia, developmental dysphasia, congenital aphasia, language delay, developmental language disorder, expressive and/or receptive language delay, clinical language disorder, language disorder, and slow expressive language development (SELD), although this last term tends to be used with toddlers more frequently than with older preschool children. When these children go to school and their language problems begin to cause academic difficulties, a situation that is more likely to occur than not, the children may be referred to as learning disabled or language-learning disabled.

Without obvious hearing, intellectual, emotional, neurological, or notable environmental deficits, the question of why these children have such a hard time acquiring language is an important one. The search for explanations has sometimes turned to other, less explicit reasons for the existence of the language difficulties.

Neurological Bases. Some authors and researchers have proposed that, in the absence of gross neurological problems, the children's language difficulties must stem from mild central nervous system dysfunction, and the terms *minimal brain dysfunction* and *minimal brain injury* have been suggested, terms that we will see in the next chapter have also been associated with learning disabilities. There has in the past, however, been no conclusive link between abnormal findings of brain function measurements and the language problems exhibited by children. The general superiority of the left cerebral hemisphere over the right in adults' language functioning has been well established, but we know that early damage to the left hemisphere in children has not been shown to account for the severity or persistence of their language impairments (Aram & Eisele, 1994). However, there are many ways in which brain structure and function can vary to disrupt language acquisition, and approaches that look at focal damage to particular areas may not be fruitful.

Most scholars working in the area of SLI agree that there must be neurological correlates and/or substrates for these children's difficulties in language learning and performance (Leonard, 1998). Advances in technology leading to continuing improvements in neuroimaging (e.g., *f* MRI) and event-related electrophysiological procedures have resulted in some of these techniques beginning to be used with children with language impairments (Lincoln, Courchesne, Harms, & Allen, 1995; Plante, 1996b; Plante, Swisher, Vance, & Rapcsak, 1991; Tomblin, Abbas, Records, & Brenneman, 1995), and these approaches seem to hold some promise in unraveling the puzzle. Using these technologies, some differences with regard to event-related potentials between normally developing children and children with SLI during auditory processing tasks have been identified (Lincoln et al., 1995; Neville, Coffey, Holcomb, & Tallal, 1993), and some differences in brain morphology of the left and right perisylvian areas and/or planum temporale (see Chapter 1) have also been implicated in children's specific language impairment (Jackson & Plante, 1996, 1997; Plante, 1996b; Plante et al., 1991). It is also possible that higher than expected levels of the hormone testosterone might be associated with left–right perisylvian asymmetries in brain morphology (Plante, 1996b; Plante, Boliek, Binkiewicz, & Erly, 1996).

In thinking about these possibilities, it is important to realize that such conditions can be related to other findings about possible causes and associations presented in the literature. For example, testosterone is a male-associated hormone, a point that leads us to wonder about the many findings suggesting a greater prevalence of SLI among boys than girls. A particular disorder, congenital adrenal hyperplasia, is a genetic, and therefore heritable, disorder characterized by elevated testosterone levels. Recent research suggests that there is increased prevalence of language problems in children with this condition, as well as the presence of the atypical left–right perisylvian asymmetry. We have already seen that a family history of language impairment is a factor that puts a child at risk for a language impairment. We will take up the point about genetic transmission of SLI later in this chapter, but certainly the implication of a genetic disease involving elevated testosterone levels possibly affecting prenatal brain morphological development (Plante, 1996b; Plante, Boliek et al., 1996) would not be inconsistent with findings that SLI tends to run in families. The state of the science is such that we have not unraveled the relationships among prenatal neurological development, genetics, postnatal brain morphological development, and endocrinology, so our discussion about the links is speculative, but these are several of the speculations that are guiding some of the current research.

Language Knowledge and Access to Language Knowledge.   Another proposition as to why these children have language problems is that the children have difficulties abstracting from their language-learning environment the requisite implicit language rules, demonstrate incomplete learning of rules, and/or have problems accessing language information that they already know (Clahsen, 1989; Connell & Stone, 1992; German, 1982; Gopnik, 1990; Leonard et al., 1983; Rice & Wexler, 1996). That is, the children can take in, process, and acquire at least part of the requisite language information, but they have trouble getting to it and bringing it forward to use it consistently, or they acquire incomplete knowledge of the language rules. The observations that children with SLI are often inconsistent in what they can do with their language lend support to this proposition. For example, children can use appropriate tense-marking morphemes sometimes but not always, or they may sometimes have difficulty retrieving a word to use but at other times are able to use the same word quickly and easily, with no latency. Again we see a difficulty, which involves the question about what causes the possible problems with their language knowledge in the first place.

Cognitive Deficits.   Cognitive abilities of children with SLI have also been the subject of investigation as to the reason for the children's language problems. As we have seen previously, a criterion of SLI is the absence of intellectual disability as the reason for children's language problems. A common way in which the intellectual level of these children is established is via tests of nonverbal intelligence, referred to as nonverbal IQ (NVIQ), or tests of performance IQ. These types of tests are used so as not to contaminate IQ measurement with measurement of language ability. Because the classification of SLI excludes children with intellectual disabilities, children with SLI generally demonstrate normal nonverbal intelligence skills.

Nevertheless, deficits in particular aspects of cognitive functioning, such as symbolic play, hypothesis formation and testing, and representational thought have been associated with SLI in children (Ellis Weismer, 1991; Johnston, 1994; Leonard, 1998; Rescorla & Goossens, 1992). If the language impairment of these children is, in fact, linked to deficits in their cognitive functioning, the terms *specific* language impairment, *specific* language disability, and *specific* language disorder may be inappropriate (Leonard, 1982). However, deficit cognitive functioning has also not always been substantiated in language-impaired children (Casby, 1997). The question also arises as to how testing of cognitive ability, particularly NVIQ, can be completely devoid of the influences of language ability (Johnston, 1994). While it might be possible to separate some intelligence measures from language ability in young children (Leonard, 1998), it appears, in fact, that as children with SLI mature, effects of their language problems on their measured NVIQ do emerge. The measured NVIQ of older children, adolescents, and even adults with SLI has been shown to decline from the previous levels seen in their younger years (Johnson et al., 1999; Stothard et al., 1998; Tallal, Townsend, Curtiss, & Wulfeck, 1991; Tomblin, Freese, & Records, 1992). Of course, if there are cognitive deficits associated with SLI in children, there is the recurring question about the underlying reasons for the deficits.

Information-Processing Deficits.   Although somewhat related to the notion of cognitive deficits presented above, another direction that the explanation for a causal factor has taken has involved how children process information, that is, an information-processing account of SLI (Ellis Weismer & Evans, 2002; Evans et al., 1997). The basic premise of this explanation suggests that SLI in children stems from problems in how well the children can deal with (process) incoming stimuli and/or use the stimuli in order to acquire information. There are generally two themes within the information-processing account. One focuses on more generalized information processing limitations, such as reductions in the speed with which information can be processed and constraints on what the children can hold in their working or short-term memories in order to process and make sense of it (Ellis Weismer et al., 1999; Miller et al., 2001; Montgomery, 2000; Montgomery & Leonard, 1998). A second theme proposes that the children's information-processing problems are more specific to particular processes, such as the temporal processing of rapidly changing auditory stimuli or phonological processing (Gathercole & Baddeley, 1990; Gathercole, Hitch, Service, & Martin, 1997; Gillam, Hoffman, Marler, & Wynn-Dancy, 2002; Merzenich et al., 1996; Tallal, 1976; Tallal et al., 1996). Although evidence seems to be mounting that implicates information-processing issues in SLI, the ways in which information-processing might affect language learning are not fully understood. Additionally, the question of the underlying reasons for information-processing problems, if they exist, suggests the possibility of neurological dysfunction, and the reasons for neurological dysfunction, if it exists, are also unanswered, as we have just discussed.

Language-Learning Environment.   Children's exposure to language in their environment, or rather the lack or type of exposure, has been suggested as a reason for the language problems of children with SLI. However, we need to be explicit about what we mean about the language-learning environment, because we can think of the environment for learning language in terms of quantity or quality of exposure. With regard to quantity of input, Bishop (1997) and Harris (1992) both point out that children can acquire language without a lot of language stimulation. The point is made fairly clearly with hearing children of deaf parents; most such children seem not to have difficulties acquiring spoken language if there is a relatively small amount of regular exposure to it. On the other hand, we noted previously that maternal education is sometimes considered a possible risk factor for language disorder. This is presumably because of the reportedly greater amount of language stimulation that mothers with more education provide to their children (Hart & Risley, 1995). However, if there are impacts with regard to quantity of maternal input to children's language development, these appear to affect semantic (vocabulary) development rather than other aspects of language ability that are particularly problematic for children with SLI, such as grammatical morphology (Dollaghan et al., 1999; Entwisle & Astone, 1994; Harris, 1992; Huttenlocher, Haight, Bryk, Seltzer, & Lyons, 1991; Rice, Wexler, & Hershberger, 1998; Rice, Spitz, & O'Brien, 1999). Quantity of language exposure in the environment seems insufficient by itself to account for SLI in children (Bishop, 1997), although it might affect children's performances, both those with and without SLI, on common measures of language, such as those involving lexical density (size of vocabulary) and length of utterances (Dollaghan et al., 1999). And, we need to keep in mind that one of the several criteria that are used to exclude children from being identified as having SLI is severe environmental deprivation such that the deprivation can account for the disruption in language development. Children with SLI generally do not live in environments where insufficient amounts of stimulation for learning language alone can be deemed to cause the children's problems. And many of the studies on preschoolers with SLI have been conducted on children with middle and upper-middle socioeconomic status.

In contrast, results of studies looking at the quality of language interactions between mothers and children with SLI give a somewhat mixed picture as a potential reason for the children's problems, at least at first glance (Leonard, 1998). There have been suggestions that mothers of SLI children do not engage in as many of the language interactions with their children that are known to facilitate children's language learning—that is, many of the characteristics of "motherese" and other behaviors such as responses to questions, imitations, or self-repetitions. However, mothers of children with SLI have been found to talk in the same manner to their younger children whose language is developing normally (Conti-Ramsden & Dykins, 1991), so attributing the cause of children's language learning problems to mothers' interaction styles seems not to stand up consistently to empirical scrutiny. It appears that where differences have been identified, these may be because mothers have adjusted their language levels to those of the children. That is, because the language of children with SLI seems more like that of younger, normally developing children, mothers seem to modify their language and interactions to accommodate their less language-able children. In this way, characteristics of the children are probably affecting the language input they receive.

There has been, however, one finding that might point to children with SLI having different language-learning interactions with their mothers than other children. This deals with mothers' use of recasts. *Recasts,* as we will see elsewhere in this book, are responses to a child's utterance that are semantically contingent and include language elements the child used but add or modify the child's utterance in some way that makes it more complex or complete, as in:

CHILD: Go now?

MOTHER: Yes, we'll go now.

Mothers have been found to use recasts with children with SLI differently, including using them less frequently (Conti-Ramsden, 1990; Conti-Ramsden, Hutcheson, & Grove, 1995; Nelson, Welsh, Camarata, Butkovsky, & Camarata, 1995). However, even here it is not clear that the direction of influence is from mother to child as opposed to from child to mother. Mothers of normally developing children reduce their use of recasts as children get older. It could be that, for use of recasts specifically, mothers are responding to the greater ages of their children with SLI or their nonverbal cognitive levels rather than the children's lower language levels (Nelson et al., 1995). Again, there is the possibility that characteristics of the children affect their language-learning environment as much as, if not more than, their language-learning environment leading to their language problems. However, this does not rule out a reciprocal interaction in which some of the modifications that mothers make to their children's impaired language inadvertently become less facilitating for the children's language development.

Genetic/Familial Bases.   Previously we noted that a family history of language, communication, and/or literacy problems is a risk factor for a child having a language impairment. Recall also the findings from the study by Tomblin and his colleagues (Tomblin, Smith, & Zhang, 1997) that suggested SLI in children was more often associated with risk factors related to their parents' status before the children were even conceived than with various fetal or perinatal risk factors. Among the parental factors were levels of education and family histories of language and/or learning problems, two factors that are not independent of each other.

There is now no question that language impairment has a tendency to run in families and that language-learning environmental influences alone are insufficient to explain the children's language-learning problems (Bishop et al., 1995; Bishop, Price, Dale, & Plomin, 2003; Choudhury & Benasich, 2003; Crago & Gopnik, 1994; Felsenfeld & Plomin, 1997; Flax et al., 2003; Lahey & Edwards, 1995; Lewis & Thompson, 1992; Plante, Shenkman, &

Clark, 1996; Rice, 1996; Tallal et al., 1989, 1991; Tomblin & Buckwalter, 1998; Viding et al., 2003). That is, in many cases there is a heritable, genetic basis for the impairment. However, it is implausible that we are looking at a single gene effect and more likely that multiple genes are involved (Plomin & Dale, 2000). Twin and adoption studies, along with advances in multivariate genetic analysis, behavioral genetics, and molecular genetics, are moving our knowledge ahead rapidly in this area, and we anticipate that the work in the next several years will add considerably to our understanding.

It is important, however, that we be careful to note that not all children with SLI have positive family histories. Rice (2000), in referring to her study with co-workers (Rice et al., 1999) in which they followed the language development of children who, when born, were placed in neonatal intensive care units, writes that there is emerging "explicit evidence of the very reasonable assumption that biological risk and inherited risk can lead to similar symptoms from diverse etiologies" (p. 28). Nevertheless, positive family histories of language and/or literacy problems do increase the odds of the children having language problems. On the other hand, not all children in families with a history of language problems will themselves have problems. These situations have several possible causes, which can be consistent with genetic principles but also implicate other variables. As Bishop (1997) points out, "genes do not act in isolation to cause behaviour" (p. 49), and notions of genetic determinism are, according to Plomin and Dale (2000), "based on misconceptions about genetic research, and on a lack of appreciation of the way complex traits and common disorders are influenced by multiple genes as well as multiple environmental factors" (p. 49).

There are several ways to conceive of environmental factors in combination with genetic transmission of SLI. On one hand, a child with inherited SLI might grow up in a family in which one or both parents also has a language impairment, associated literacy problems, difficulties with psychosocial aspects of behavior (which we will see later are often a part of language impairment), and resulting lower socioeconomic (SES) conditions. For this child, the environment may exacerbate the inherited trait, or at least, not serve to counter it. Goodyer (2000), in discussing "psychosocial disadvantages" (p. 232) related to the family environment of children with SLI and "environmental adversities" (p. 232) that can therefore impact on the children, writes that:

> It may be that there are common genetic components that will be expressed as a familial effect. Also, language and cognitive deficits in a parent may limit the direct help they can give their children. (p. 232)

Figure 3.1 illustrates how these factors might come together to affect a child's language abilities and even continue to have effects in subsequent generations. Plomin and Dale (2000) remind us of the concepts of assortative mating and additive genetic variance. They explain that:

> Assortative mating, the tendency for like to mate with like, is much greater for cognitive abilities, especially verbal abilities, than for any other physical or behavioral traits. . . . Assortative mating increases genetic variance cumulatively generation after generation. If one parent is high in ability, the other parent is also likely to be high in ability, which means that the offspring are likely to be higher in ability than if they just had one parent high in ability. . . . Second, assortative mating increases a particular type of genetic variance called

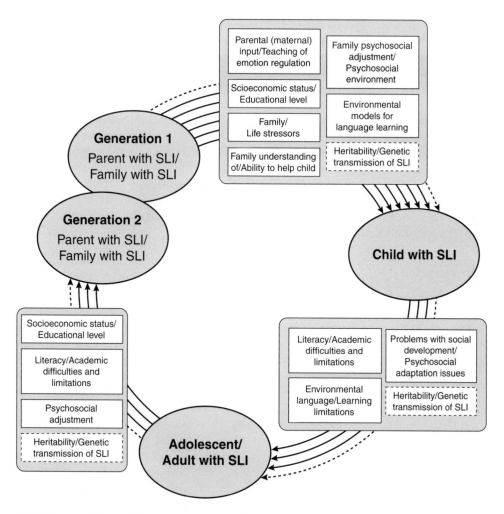

FIGURE 3.1   Schematic Representations of Some of the Interactions and Effects of Genetic/Familial and Environmental Factors in SLI

additive genetic variance, which is caused by the independent effects of alleles[1] that "add up" to affect the trait. (pp. 47–48)

On the other hand, for another child with inherited SLI, the environment might differ, perhaps by introducing into the environment the feature of intervention that could serve to counter the inherited trait and lessen its influence (Bishop, 1997). Where SLI is concerned, it is probably a mistake to think of the effects of nature (genetics) and nurture (environment) separately and more accurate to consider them as interacting.

[1]Any of alternative forms of a gene, e.g., either the wrinkled-pea gene or the smooth-pea gene, that can occur at a given locus.

This brings us to the question of whether any of the preceding discussion about the various possible causes should be disregarded. The answer is no. Even if SLI has a genetic basis, we do not yet know what in the human system and at what stage in human development the effects occur that are manifested as the language-acquisition problems we see in children with SLI. For example, perhaps the genetic effects lead to changes in fetal brain development that we might see later as differences in brain morphology of the left and right perisylvian areas and/or planum temporale (Jackson & Plante, 1996, 1997; Plante, 1996b; Plante et al., 1991), or maybe the genetic influences lead to production of high levels of testosterone, which might be associated with left–right perisylvian asymmetries in brain morphology (Plante, 1996b; Plante, Boliek, et al., 1996). Any or all of these could be manifested as inefficient or impaired processing of information, either more generally or more specifically for particular areas of functioning that are especially important for language learning (Ellis Weismer & Evans, 2002). The next several years in research should be very interesting indeed as we begin to sort out some of this with more advanced techniques and technology.

Prevalence

Some young children start off slowly in their language development and then appear to catch up. Other children start off slowly and continue to lag behind and to have problems. Still other children start off slowly, seem to catch up for a while and then either fall behind again or show problems in different areas related to language. Therefore, we may see different prevalence figures at different ages, and these may also be affected by what we are measuring.

Vocabulary development is one of the first obvious indices of language growth in very young children. One of the earliest signs that a child may have problems with language is that the first word is used late or that not very many additional words are acquired after the first word. Between 18 and 24 months of age, signs that a child may have language problems include absence of a vocabulary growth spurt, failing to combine words into two-word utterances, and generally talking very little. About 10 to 15 percent of 2-year-old children fit this latter picture (Klee et al., 1998; Rescorla, 1989; Rescorla, Hadicke-Wiley, & Escarce, 1993), and for children at 24 months of age concern generally focuses on an expressive single-word vocabulary of less than fifty words and no two-word combinations. Yet some of these toddlers do catch up later. The children who catch up are often referred to as *late bloomers.* However, some of the toddlers who demonstrate *slow expressive language development* (SELD)[2] in their first 2 years continue to lag behind in their language development as they grow older. How many of these children continue to lag behind in their language throughout the preschool years and into the school years is a matter of considerable debate.

At 3 Years of Age.   In reviewing her work and that of others, Paul (1991, 1996) suggests that between about 20 and 75 percent of children who were slow in language development at 2 years of age moved into the normal range on measures of expressive language at 3 years of age (Paul, 1991, 1993; Rescorla, 1993; Whitehurst & Fischel, 1994), the age at which language skill begins to be measured as much by syntactic and morphological abilities as

---

[2]The current literature on toddlers has so far refrained from using the term specific language impairment to refer to these young children. Rather, slow expressive language development (SELD) has been the preferred descriptor. In keeping with this trend, SELD will be used in this section of the chapter.

by vocabulary. From the opposite perspective, Dale and his colleagues (2003) report that about 45 percent of 2-year-old twins with language delays showed persisting language difficulties at 3 years of age. Together, these results mean that 25 to 80 percent of these 2-year-olds continued to show expressive language delays at 3 years of age.

The difference between 25 percent and 80 percent is very large. One of the reasons for the big range is the wide variance in what is "normal" in very young children. For example, one parent report measure of young children's expressive language at 2 years of age has a mean of 300 words but a standard deviation of 175 (Fenson, Dale, Reznick, Hartung, & Burgess, 1990), more than half the mean. Consequently, any vocabulary size above 125 would certainly be considered normal or above, and a vocabulary size of zero or more would place a child at or above the –2 SD deviation point. Other reasons for the big range are the different tools that have been used to assess the children's language, the aspects of language measured, the degree to which language performance has or has not been challenged in the children, and the varying degrees of specificity and sensitivity of the tools in identifying language delay. Other reasons are the heterogeneity of the groups studied and the children initially being identified at 2 years of age on the basis of their expressive vocabulary size, with some but not all of them having normal comprehension abilities (Ellis Weismer, Murray-Branch, & Miller, 1994; Girolametto et al., 2001; Kelly, 1998a; Olswang, Rodriguez, & Timler, 1998; Paul, 1997b; van Kleeck, Gillam, & Davis, 1997). As we saw previously, children with expressive language problems without language comprehension problems may represent a different group from children with both expressive and receptive language problems.

Of particular note is that vocabulary size of some 2-year-olds with SELD who continue to have language problems may have moved into the normal range by 3 years of age (Paul, 1993; Rescorla, 1993; Whitehurst, Fischel, Arnold, & Lonigan, 1992), even though this was the primary criterion used to identify the children as having delayed language at age 2. What this also means is that at 3 years of age expressive language skills other than vocabulary are being considered to be below normal expectations. These are often aspects of language related to form, that is, syntax, morphology, and/or phonology.

Others have provided different estimates of continuing language delay in 3-year-olds. Klee and colleagues (1998) suggest that one-fifth (20 percent) to one-third (33 percent) of 2-year-old children who could be considered as having SELD at 2 years of age continue to be clinically concerning at age 3 years. Paul (1991) reports that 40 to 50 percent of 2-year-olds may continue to have expressive language delays at age 3 years. If we calculate 40 to 50 percent of the 10 to 15 percent figure given for the proportion of 2-year-olds with SELD, we arrive at a 4 to 7.5 percent prevalence figure for expressive language problems in the 3-year-old group. If we use Klee and colleagues' (1998) 20 to 33 percent figure to calculate the proportion of the 10 to 15 percent of 2-year-olds with SELD who have problems at 3 years of age, we arrive at a 2 to 5 percent prevalence figure, and if we use the 25 to 80 percent figure, we arrive at a 2.5 to 12 percent prevalence figure for language delay at 3 years of age.

At 4 Years of Age.   What is the language of 2-year-old children with SELD like when they are age 4? In compiling the results from her study (Paul, 1991, 1993) and others (Rescorla, 1993; Whitehurst & Fischel, 1994), Paul (1996) has reported that about 45 to 85 percent of 2-year-olds with SELD received scores within normal limits on measures of expressive language at 4 years of age. In another study, at 4 years of age 71 percent of children who had been late talkers had MLUs above the 10th percentile rank (Rescorla, Dahlsgaard, &

Roberts, 2000). Reversing the figures from both of these reports, this means that 15 to 55 percent of the 2-year-olds did not move into the normal range at 4 years of age. We need to keep remembering that these figures are proportions of a proportion of the population of 2-year-olds, that is, the 10 to 15 percent of 2-year-olds who have SELD. Therefore, to estimate general prevalence of language impairment at age 4, we need to look at 15 to 55 percent of 10 to 15 percent, or 1.5 to 8.5 percent, which we see is still a considerable range. From a slightly different perspective, in tracking 28 toddlers who had previously been slow to develop their expressive language, Paul and Smith (1993) found that 57 percent of these children had persisting expressive language deficits related to narrative skills at 4 years of age. As Paul (1991) points out, this "finding is particularly significant because narrative skills in preschoolers have been shown to be one of the best predictors of school success" (p. 8). Extrapolated to the general 10 to 15 percent of 2-year-olds with SELD, this estimates that 6 to 9 percent of 4-year-old children might have problems with their narrative skills, a possible portent of coming academic difficulties for these children. Readers might want to keep this 6 to 9 percent estimated prevalence figure in mind.

The language status of preschoolers at 4 years of age, and even more so between 4 and 5 years of age, likely foreshadows their later language and literacy outcomes. Several authors have noted that children whose language abilities are behind those of their peers at 4 years of age may be in for long-term problems. By "long-term," we mean problems that extend into the elementary and secondary school years and even into adulthood (Rescorla & Lee, 2001; Stothard et al., 1998). It is possible, but not confirmed, that these children will have demonstrated language comprehension problems in addition to their expressive language weaknesses when they were 4. Expressive syntax and morphological abilities are two areas that frequently show particular weaknesses if language problems persist in children to the age of 4, often more so than a vocabulary deficit, which was used to first identify the children as SELD.

At 5 Years of Age.   How many of these SELD children will continue to show language problems at 5 years of age? From the results of one study, 5-year-olds who had been slow in their early expressive, but not receptive, language development evidenced expressive vocabulary performances and general verbal fluency skills that were not obviously different from normally developing 5-year-olds (Whitehurst, Fischel, et al., 1991). Given that syntax and morphology are particular problems for most children with SLI and, as we will see later, that many of these children also have problems in interpersonal interactions and psychosocial difficulties, it is unfortunate that this study did not include measures of syntactic or pragmatic abilities. However, the authors reported that, if any problems in the areas of syntax at 5 years of age did exist, they were "subtle and not apparent" (p. 67). These findings could suggest that the children had caught up to their normally developing peers. However, while Bishop and Edmundson (1987) found that many preschool children with language deficits (without nonverbal intelligence deficits) appeared to catch up by 5½ years of age, Conti-Ramsden and her co-workers (1997) pointed out that about an equal proportion (40 percent) did not. Paul (1996) reported that, in kindergarten, 75 percent of her 2-year-old toddlers with SELD had moved into the normal range on most measures of language, including achieving syntax scores on samples of their spontaneous language (i.e., their Developmental Sentence Score [DSS]) that placed them above the 10th percentile rank. However, 25 percent still exhibited delays in their syntax, as well as with other aspects of language. In Rescorla's (1993) study of toddlers with SELD, whom she followed for several years, 15 percent of the children performed poorly on a test of expressive grammatical ability at 5 years of age and were therefore considered to show impaired language, compared to the 85 percent who demonstrated more age-appropriate language performance (Rescorla, 2002). Girolametto and his colleagues (2001) reported that when their 21 children who had expressive vocabulary delays at 2 years of age reached 5 years of age, three of the children (14 percent) scored below the normal range on standardized measures of language. We need to remember that these studies differed on the proportions of the children in the groups who had receptive language problems in combination with their expressive language impairments.

It could seem that most children who have early histories of language delay seem to catch up by the time they are 5 years of age. There may, however, be some real dangers in accepting these findings without more information. Although most of the SELD children in Paul's (Paul, 1991, 1996; Paul, Murray, Clancy, & Andrews, 1997) research scored within normal limits on standardized tests of language at 5 years of age, most of their scores were in the lower range of normal and were significantly lower than their peers who did not have a history of slow language development. Their narrative performance both in kindergarten and grade 1 continued to be notably poorer than that of the children without histories of language problems (Paul, 2000; Paul & Smith, 1993; Paul, Hernandez, Taylor, & Johnson, 1996). Recall from our previous discussion that Lahey (1990) has suggested that our identification procedures need to examine children's language abilities under conditions that stress the language system. Narrative tasks do just that. The 5-year-old children in the study of Girolametto and colleagues (2001), most of whom scored within normal limits on standardized measures of language, also performed significantly poorer on these tasks than their peers and had particular problems on higher-level language tasks such as narratives and perspective-taking language tasks. The SELD children in Rescorla's (2002) research, too, generally performed within normal limits on most language measures at age 5, but their performance was significantly poorer than their peers and they continued to show poorer performance through to 9 years of age. There was also evidence of emerging reading problems at ages 8 and 9. The children in the Bishop and Edmondson study (1987) who had appeared to "resolve" their early language problems by 5½ years of age had measurable and noticeable academic and language at 15 years of age, and their skills with the higher level language skills of narratives at age 5½ seemed particularly important in terms of what their outcomes were. All may not be rosy for these SELD children as they mature, even though some of the their test scores place them in the normal, albeit often lower normal, range.

These outcomes seem to reinforce the concerns expressed by some that early expressive language delay portends the likelihood of future language- and language-learning-related problems and warrants early intervention (Girolametto, Pearce, & Weitzman, 1996; Nippold & Schwarz, 1996; van Kleeck et al., 1997). Those who adopt this position stress the importance of early intervention that tries to take advantage of the neurological plasticity of brains of children younger than 5 years. Rice (2000), in summarizing the work of Dale and his colleagues (1998) on genetic contributions to slow vocabulary development in 2-year-old children and speculating on its implications for later language development, writes that

> the children whose early vocabularies are small, compared to other children, in effect have a
> qualitatively different status than the children with more robust vocabularies; they are not

just at the low end of the normal distribution. In other words, the emergence of first vocabulary items may function much like a clinical marker in affected [i.e., having language impairment] children, although whether or not vocabulary status retains this marker function for older children remains to be seen. It may be that first vocabulary acquisition serves as a valuable indicator of the fact that affected children's language emerges late relative to unaffected children. (p. 28)

Others have suggested that such children should be monitored closely and intervention provided if the children do not appear to be catching up well and early (Paul, 1996, 2000), that is, a "watch and see" policy (Paul, 1996, p. 15). From this perspective, SELD should be viewed as a risk factor for SLI but not a disorder (Paul, 1996, 1997b; Whitehurst & Fischel, 1994).

Some of the findings about 5-year-olds who as toddlers and preschoolers had slow language development could be interpreted as suggesting a relatively low prevalence rate for children of kindergarten age. However, the experience of professionals who have worked with young children tells us that this may not be true (Johnson et al., 1999). In a large-scale and well-controlled study of kindergarteners, Tomblin and his research team (Tomblin, Records, et al., 1997) reported that the prevalence of SLI among children in their first year of school, between about 5 and 6 years of age, was 7.4 percent. (This is why readers were earlier asked to keep the estimated prevalence figure derived for 4-year-olds in mind.) As Leonard (1998) comments, "there is no reason to believe that the prevalence of 7.4 percent is artificially high" (p. 20). In fact, Johnson and her colleagues (1999) arrived at an estimate of 6.7 percent. Because children's language abilities at 4 and 5 years of age are quite predictive of what their language will be like as they mature (Catts, Fey, Tomblin, & Zhang, 2002; Rescorla & Lee, 2001; Stothard et al., 1998; Tomblin, et al., 2003), we might be able to believe that about 6.5 to 7.5 percent of students during their school years, including high school, will have SLI.

Considerations and Implications.   One consideration about trying to determine prevalence is that language deficits may become more selective or narrow as children get older (Scarborough & Dobrich, 1990; Whitehurst, Fischel, et al., 1991), thereby affecting language performance less globally and instead more specifically for certain aspects of language behavior. As we indicated previously, syntax and morphology may be problematic, as might higher-level language skills such as narrative, even when delays in early vocabulary size might seem to have resolved. These factors suggest that tasks, such as complex sentence usage and narrative skill in situations that challenge children's language performance, need to be utilized with older preschool children to tap their levels of language competency (Lahey, 1990; Paul, 1991).

Another concern relates to a pattern of normal language development in which 5-year-old children seem to plateau in their language but show a growth spurt again between ages 6 and 7 (Scarborough & Dobrich, 1990). These authors propose that, because normally developing peers may plateau at about 5 years of age, 5-year-old children with histories of SELD may appear to catch up, at least on the surface, in language use in unchallenging situations. However, when their peers' language skills move ahead again a year or two later, the children with SELD histories may be left behind at a time when acquisition of literacy skills, which are heavily dependent on oral language abilities, becomes critically important in school for future academic success. Certain aspects of language behavior may also plateau at different ages (Scarborough & Dobrich, 1990), thereby creating the illusion of recovery for different language skills at different times, that is, "illusory recovery." This would create the impression of differing profiles of language adequacy in different children at different ages.

An additional concern relates to what other skills children with SELD may not be learning while they are catching up that their normal language-learning peers have the opportunities to learn because their learning resources are not having to be directed to learning more basic language skills. A "Matthew" effect might operate (Stanovich, 1986), in which case those children who are better at language are able to take advantage of language-learning opportunities to learn more language, but those who are not good, fall further and further behind, and the gap between the language able and language impaired widens with time. It is possible that (1) children with histories of SELD give the illusion of recovery and then relapse; (2) if subgroups of young children with language difficulties exist, children in different subgroups will evidence different patterns of language growth, recovery, and relapse; (3) some language skills may "catch up" but others do not, and findings may depend on which skills have been measured; and (4) SELD children expend learning resources and learning time on catching up, and therefore they "miss out" on other learning—learning that may eventually affect their school performances. Paul (1991) writes that the interpretation of findings suggesting these children "catch up" by 5 years of age needs to consider

- Whether the full range of language skills that are important at this age—and not detectable in measures of expressive vocabulary size, general verbal fluency, or unstructured conversation (such as complex sentence use and narrative skill)—is evaluated
- Whether any recovery that does appear to be completed by age 5 is stable or will again be outpaced by development in normal children over the course of the next year or two, when their rate of language growth accelerates, in conjunction with the acquisition of literacy skills
- Even if oral language skills do appear to remain eventually within the normal range by the end of the preschool period, whether the underlying processes that slowed them down at first continue to operate, now influencing primarily the learning of reading, writing, and spelling, as seems to be the case for so many youngsters with a history of language delay (pp. 9–10)

Preschoolers with continuing language problems in the apparent absence of other problems run the risk of encountering academic difficulties when they enter school (Aram, Ekelman, & Nation, 1984; Catts et al., 2002; Johnson et al., 1999; Stothard et al., 1998; Tomblin et al., 1992). In fact, in Chapter 5 we shall see that the difficulties created by language problems first evident in the preschool years can continue into and through adolescence and even into adulthood. Prevalence data on the occurrence of language problems in school-aged children are, however, conflicting, with some suggesting a fairly dramatic decrease in the prevalence of language impairments in school-aged children (U.S. Department of Education, 2001b). Academic difficulties stemming from language deficits frequently lead to school-aged children being referred to as "language-learning disabled" or "learning disabled," a topic taken up in more detail in the next two chapters. As well as an apparent false recovery period for oral language skills in the early school years, this relabeling may account for what Snyder (Snyder, 1984) has termed the "great disappearing act" (p. 129). That is, once in school, children with SLI may no longer be seen as language impaired in "head counts" of children having disabilities. Rather, they are counted in a different category. To support her position, Snyder notes that the prevalence figures for learning disabilities are higher in states where language problems and learning disabilities are combined into one label that is used in lieu of the label *learning disability,* and lower in states where the term *learning disability* is used separately from *language disorder.*

The implications of these prevalence figures raise several questions about intervention for school-aged children with SLI that will arise in the next two chapters. Two of these are worth noting here. One is the legalities and ethics of providing appropriate intervention for these children. If a child demonstrates language deficits with resulting academic difficulties, intervention for both problematic areas will likely be more effective than intervention for either problem alone. Unfortunately, funding issues and definitional criteria for categorizing children with disabilities that some educational systems use mean that such a combined approach is not always the case for these children. A second question concerns professional territorialism. Instead of the question about which professional group should serve these children, we take the position that when the children receive intervention for both their learning problems and underlying language deficits, professional territorialism becomes a nonissue. There is really an issue only when intervention for one of their problem areas is provided. This may, however, be as much of an ethical and legal issue as a territorial one. Children for whom language problems underlie learning problems need to have their language impairments accurately identified and deserve intervention for both their language deficits and resulting academic difficulties.

Predicting Spontaneous Recovery from Early Language Delay

Which of the children we have been discussing in the previous section are the ones who seem to "outgrow" their early language delays, that is, spontaneously recover from their early delay without intervention, and which do not? This is an important question because, given the insidious and potentially long-lasting effects of language impairment, we want to provide early intervention to those children who need it but do not want to waste professional resources providing intervention to those children who will "outgrow" their delays and with no residual negative effects. Intervention with toddlers and preschoolers has positive effects on their language and accelerates their language growth (Fey, Cleave, & Long, 1997; Fey, Cleave, Long, & Hughes, 1993; Girolametto et al., 1996; Jacoby, Levin, Lee, Creaghead, & Kummer, 2002; Lee, Koenigsknecht, & Mulhern, 1975; McLean & Cripe, 1997; Rice & Hadley, 1995; Rice & Wilcox, 1995), although we do not yet know if intervention can result in children with SLI closing the gap between their language performance and that of their peers. The situation may be much like many medical conditions or other disabilities; they do not go away even with the best of practice and intervention, but the effects of the conditions can be moderated with intervention so as to lessen negative impact.

Professionals who work with children with SLI become concerned about advice to parents of 2-year-olds who are not talking very much not to worry about it because the child will outgrow it. From the previous discussion we know that such advice might have about a 50/50 chance (splitting the difference on the range of estimates) of being right. For the children for whom the advice was wrong, valuable intervention time has been lost. For 3-year-old children whose language does not match that of their peers, we become even more concerned about such advice, and by 4 years of age, the odds of spontaneous recovery are against the child. However, predicting which children will eventually outgrow their early language delay is not an exact science because we do not yet have all the factors that affect spontaneous recovery pinpointed (Kelly, 1998b; Olswang et al., 1998; Paul, 2000), although as Olswang and her colleagues write, "we know a lot" (p. 23) that can be used to help us make educated predictions so that we lower the odds of being wrong. Table 3.3 lists several of the factors that might provide predictive information about toddlers and preschoolers at risk for continuing language problems.

Comprehension skills are conspicuously absent from the Table 3.3. One might think that youngsters who have both expressive and receptive deficits would be more likely to have continuing language problems as they mature than those with only expressive deficits, and that the greater the gap between expressive and receptive language abilities, the greater the likelihood of continuing language problems. The reason comprehension skills are missing from the table is that the research findings for young children are conflicting (Bishop & Edmundson, 1987; Bishop, 1997; Ellis Weismer et al., 1994; Paul, 2000; Paul et al., 1991; Scarborough & Dobrich, 1990; Thal et al., 1991). However, when the abilities of adolescents who had language problems identified in their early years have been examined, those adolescents who had language comprehension problems in addition to expressive language problems have been reported to generally fare more poorly (Beitchman, Wilson, Brownlie, Walters, & Lancee, 1996; Beitchman, Wilson, Brownlie, Walters, Inglis, et al., 1996). Even with preschoolers, receptive language deficits may have more impact on peer interactions or parents' reports of their young children's conversational skills than expressive language problems (Gertner et al., 1994; Girolametto, 1997). In summarizing the literature, Olswang and her coauthors (1998) comment that:

> The consensus suggests that toddlers with significant expressive and receptive language delays of 6 months or more are more at risk for continued language delay. Further, for those children delayed in both comprehension and production, the larger the comprehension–production gap, the poorer the prognosis. (p. 25)

It is also probably worth a bit more discussion of the early vocabulary of toddlers with early language delay. Although the criterion of using fewer than fifty single words at 24 months of age has been a major guideline for identifying toddlers with SELD, the work of Dale and his colleagues on the heritability of early vocabulary development suggests that we might need to be more specific about vocabulary size. In this discussion we need to keep our perspective with regard to the single-word vocabulary size of 2-year-olds, which is somewhere around 130 to 300 (Fenson et al., 1990; Rescorla et al., 2001). When the vocabulary size of at least one of 2-year-old twin pairs was in the lowest 5 percent of the distribution on a parent report measure, the MacArthur Communicative Development Inventory (MCDI) (Fenson et al., 1994), there was a substantial genetic contribution to the vocabulary size, but the influence of shared environment was found to contribute very little to the vocabulary size (Dale et al., 1998). A vocabulary size of 0 to 8 words placed the 2-year-old children in the lowest 5 percent. What this suggests is that very low vocabulary size at 2 years

TABLE 3.3   Some Factors Potentially Predicting Continuing Language Problems

Factors	Explanation
Extrinsic	
Family History (Bishop et al., 1995; Dale et al., 1998; Felsenfeld & Plomin, 1997; Plomin & Dale, 2000; Rice, 1996; Tomblin & Buckwalter, 1998)	Greater risk for children with family member with a history of language, speech, or literacy/learning problems
Mother's Education/Family Socio-economic Status (SES) (Dollaghan et al., 1999; Rice et al., 1998)	Lower SES, but large proportion of SES reflected in mother's education
	Lower educational level of mother implicated in slower vocabulary development but maybe not syntactic complexity and grammatical morphology
Intrinsic	
Communicative Intentions, Symbolic Gestures, and Play (Olswang, Johnson, & Crooke, 1992; Paul, 1991; Rescorla & Goossens, 1992; Thal & Tobias, 1992; Thal et al., 1991)	Production of symbolic gestures in familiar script routines (e.g., bathing a teddy bear) reduced
	Ability to produce symbolic gestures positively related to comprehension vocabulary level
	Less frequent use of gesture generally (may be related to reduction in frequency of communicative intentions produced gesturally)
	Range of communicative intentions used appropriate, but frequency with which they are used is reduced
	Reduction in frequency with which comment/joint attention communicative intentions used
	Less use of representational, communicative gesture
	Greater use of complementary gesture (same meaning as word) and less use of supplementary gesture (add meaning)
	Grouping and manipulation of play objects but less thematic/combinatorial play
Babbling and Phonology (McCarthren, Warren, & Yoder, 1996; Oller et al., 1999; Paul, 1991; Paul & Jennings, 1992; Rescorla & Ratner, 1996; Stoel-Gammon, 1991; Whitehurst, Smith, Fischel, Arnold, & Lonigan, 1991; Whitehurst, Fischel, et al., 1991)	Less language growth for children with higher occurrences of vowel babble and greater language growth for children with consonantal babble
	Greater language growth related to greater babble complexity
	Less complex syllable structure (e.g., CV versus CVC versus C_1VC_2V)
	Fewer consonants in phonetic repertoire, with less than 4–5 at 24 months and limited vowel repertoire
	Phonological patterns at 36 months that include vowel errors, glottal stops or /h/ substitutions for consonants, a lot of initial consonant and final consonant deletion, back-consonant substitutions for front consonants
Socialization and Behavior (Fischel, Whitehurst, Caulfield, & DeBaryshe, 1989; Hadley & Rice, 1991; Paul, 1991; Paul et al., 1991; Rice et al., 1991)	Possible deficits in social skills (e.g., smiling appropriately, playing social games)
	More passive communicators who initiate communication and nonverbal interactions less
	Possibly overactive and difficult to manage
	Less language growth in children with behavior problems

of age may have genetic contributions operating that then decrease the probability of spontaneous recovery of the early delay. Professionals might be wise to treat a 2-year-old with very low vocabulary development differently from one with a vocabulary size closer to the fifty word criterion.

Another aspect of early vocabulary that might inform about probability of spontaneous recovery is the composition of the vocabulary, particularly verbs. In summarizing the work of several researchers (Loeb, Pye, Redmond, & Richardson, 1996; Olswang, Long, & Fletcher, 1997; Rice & Bode, 1993; Watkins, Rice, & Moltz, 1993), Olswang and her colleagues (1998) identified several "red flags" (p. 25): (1) a relatively small verb vocabulary compared to other types of words, particularly nouns; (2) reliance on GAP (general all-purpose) verbs, such as *look* or *want,* rather than more specific verbs, such as *walk* or *clap;* and (3) fewer intransitive (not requiring a direct object) and ditransitive (able to either have or not have a direct object) verbs than transitive verbs.

Research attempting to identify clinical markers of SLI in young children may help us in knowing which children have SLI and which have an early language delay that they will outgrow without residual effects. A *clinical marker,* or *phenotype,* is a characteristic or feature of children with SLI that is independent of the normal distribution of language skills and correctly identifies those children with SLI (affected children) and does not incorrectly identify other children as affected. An analogy might be that people with a particular medical condition have a unique combination of hormones in their bodies (that is, the hormone combination is the clinical marker or phenotype) that people without the condition do not have. Having or not having the hormone combination is not dependent on a normal distribution in the population.

Grammatical morphology and nonword repetition are two of the directions that the search for an SLI clinical marker has taken. English-speaking children with SLI are renowned for their persisting difficulties with grammatical forms, and in particular those related to marking verb forms (Leonard, Eyer, Bedore, & Grela, 1997; Leonard et al., 2002, 2003; Redmond, 2003; Redmond & Rice, 2001; Rice & Wexler, 1996; Rice et al., 1998). Rice and her colleagues (Rice, 2000; Rice & Wexler, 1996; Rice et al., 1998) have reported that tasks examining 5-year-olds' verb form marking abilities correctly identify 97 percent of children with SLI and 98 percent of children without, and that the longitudinal course of development of verb tense marking for SLI children is protracted and does not reach adult-like levels of accuracy, unlike normally developing children, who make almost no errors by 8 years of age. Verb morphology may emerge as a clinical marker.

The second of the directions that the search for a clinical marker of SLI has taken, nonword repetition, focuses on aspects of children's information processing and requires children to repeat nonsense words of varying length and phonological complexity (Campbell, Dollaghan, Needleman, & Janosky, 1997; Conti-Ramsden, 2003; Dollaghan & Campbell, 1998; Edwards & Lahey, 1998; Ellis Weismer et al., 2000; Gathercole, 1995; Gathercole, Willis, Baddeley, & Emslie, 1994; Gray 2003a). Children with SLI generally perform much worse than normally achieving children of the same age and younger children with similar levels of language, with children's performances on the tasks generally separating them with good accuracy into groups with known language impairments and those without. It is possible that nonword repetition will also emerge as a clinical marker of SLI. As promising as nonword repetition might be for identifying SLI in children, tasks designed to assess this ability in children have mostly been restricted to children 5 years of age and older because of the complexity of the tasks involved, although some attempts have been made to use nonword repetition tasks with preschoolers (Gray, 2003a). This situation contrasts with the various tools (spontaneous language sample, standardized tests, and contrived probes) that are available to test preschoolers' grammatical morpheme abilities. To really be helpful in knowing which young children have language that is only slow to emerge but is not impaired and which have slow developing language because of SLI and, therefore, to be helpful in predicting the children who will spontaneously recover from their early language delays and those who will not, the tasks tapping children's nonword repetition abilities will need to be "toddler and preschooler friendly."

Two other factors may assist us with the task of determining which children will spontaneously recover from early language delay. Previously in this chapter we noted that children with language impairments would be predicted to be relatively slower to respond to trial language instruction than children without language impairment but with delayed language development. We have also mentioned stressing a child's language ability via narrative production tasks. Narrative skills of children with language impairments have regularly surfaced as one of the areas of considerable and persisting difficulty. Tracking children's developing abilities in narrative production may also help in predicting spontaneous recovery. Chapter 13 includes several narrative tasks that could be useful.

A few caveats are in order. Although a considerable body of literature is available to support the factors discussed here as having predictive value for spontaneous recovery, Paul (2000) has reported that only three of the many variables she examined in her 2-year-olds with SELD predicted their syntactic level at or above the 10th percentile rank in grade 2. These were SES, expressive communication score on a parent report measure, and gross motor score on the same parent report measure. Again, it is important to keep in mind methodological differences across studies with different findings. Additionally, Paul (2000) reports significantly lower performances of the grade 2 children with histories of SELD than of normally developing peers on a number of language and language-related measures. We continue to amass information about toddlers and preschoolers with SELD (or SLI) that will help us refine our predictions. In the meantime, we think the way Olswang and her colleagues (1998) summarized the current level of knowledge and the implications gets it about right for now:

> Research has revealed robust trends about language learning in toddlers who are typical and atypical in their language development. These trends have brought to light characteristics that allow us to decide whether we should be seriously concerned about a toddler's actual and potential language growth. The argument being made from this literature is that the magnitude of our concern should directly translate to our recommendations. To our way of thinking, and the thinking of others (Thal & Katich, 1996; Whitehurst & Fischel, 1994), this is not only a reasonable position, but also an ethical and intellectually defensible one. (p. 29)

Borrowing the medical profession's risk-factor model is suggested as a way to judge the "magnitude of our concern" (Thal & Katich, 1996; Whitehurst & Fischel, 1994). This is an additive approach in which the degree of risk for the occurrence of a condition increases with an increase in the number of different known risk factors that are present. The more factors present in or associated with a young child that point to the possibility of future language problems for the child, the greater the magnitude of concern and, therefore, the more likely that intervention is an appropriate recommendation for the child.

Language Characteristics of Children with Specific Language Impairment

In this section, we review a number of the language characteristics observed in toddlers and preschool children with specific language impairments. We need to be aware that not all children will necessarily demonstrate all of these problems and that a problem with one aspect of language can result in problems with other aspects. These potentially diverse patterns reemphasize the fact that specifically language-impaired children are heterogeneous. Additionally, we need to be aware that some of the same types of problems can be observed in school-aged children and adolescents with language disorders, albeit at different levels.

Some Language Precursors

Recognition of and attention to environmental change are important to language acquisition, because without these a child will not develop the underlying concepts of language. Furthermore, children need to learn that they can be the agents of change. Unless children realize that what they do results in modifications of objects or people's behaviors, they will be unlikely to learn that language is one of the most effective ways of producing change.

Several of the factors listed in Table 3.3 referred to or involved concerns about behaviors and abilities that can be considered precursors to language development, for example, use of symbolic gesture and communicative intentions. As well as participating in reciprocal interactions, establishing joint reference with an adult appears to be important for language acquisition (Delgado et al., 2002). Early child–adult behaviors of give-and-take play routines and repetitive games such as patty-cake may be prerequisites of conversational turn-taking skills. Some preschoolers with SLI seem to have difficulty participating in these reciprocal routines. These children may also not engage frequently in joint attention or learn to utilize cues provided by joint reference with an adult. With regard to communicative intents, some have suggested that communicative intents, in general, may be encoded by specifically language-impaired children more via gestures and vocalizations than by verbal means (Caulfield, 1989; Coggins, 1991; Wetherby et al., 1989), and in particular, as we see from Table 3.3, reduced ability to produce *symbolic* gestures reflecting script routines may predict longer-term language problems.

The relationship between babbling and the production of first words is not fully understood, although the phonetic content of babbled vocalizations likely affects children's early lexicons and may even be a distinguishing feature of some children with language problems. In order to produce a variety of single words, one might anticipate that children would need to have several different consonants in their repertoires and use these consonants in different distributions and in combinations with different vowels. In this way, the syllable structure of babble might be a precursor to use of first words. When we review Table 3.3, we see that reduced occurrences of certain types of babbling and particular patterns of early phonology might be early indications of language impairment. The impact of limited forms of babbling on language ability beyond 12 months of age was described in a large-scale study of Oller and colleagues (1999). In their study of 3,400 infants at 10 months of age, the "infants with delayed canonical babbling had smaller production vocabularies at 18, 24 and 36 months than did infants in the control group" (p. 223).

Phonology

Given the preceding discussion, it is probably not surprising that toddlers and preschoolers with SLI frequently have concomitant phonological problems. The reverse is also true. For example, Shriberg and Kwiatkowski (1994) have reported that about 80 percent of children identified as having phonological problems also have language impairments. Normally developing children are moderately intelligible by about 2 years of age. In contrast, it is not unusual to find 3- and 4-year-old children with SLI who are difficult to understand. However, phonological problems are more likely than language problems to resolve as children mature, and children with speech-sound difficulties have been reported as having better long-term academic, social, and vocational outcomes than those with language impairments (Beitchman et al., 2001; Hall & Tomblin, 1978; Johnson et al., 1999; Shriberg, Gruber, & Kwiatkowski, 1994; Whitehurst, Fischel, et al., 1991).

Some have proposed that problems with phonological acquisition are simply reflections of more general language-learning problems. Others suggest that phonological problems may be characteristics of subgroup membership within the larger, heterogeneous group of specifically language-impaired children. Whatever the relationship between SLI and phonological problems, we know that young children with SLI acquire more quickly single words that begin with consonants they use correctly in other words than words that begin with consonants not yet produced correctly (Leonard, Schwartz, et al., 1982). This relationship between phonology and lexical acquisition is consistent with a developmental pattern seen in normally developing toddlers (Schwartz & Leonard, 1982). We also know from one study that about 20 to 30 percent of the preschool children who experienced phonological difficulties apparently not related to concomitant problems in other areas received special education services when they entered school, even though many of the children no longer showed obvious evidence of phonological difficulties at the time of entering school (Shriberg & Kwiatkowski, 1988). This may reflect what we know about phonological problems in the preschool years affecting children's abilities to achieve academically in areas related to linguistic skills, possibly because of phonological processing difficulties.

Semantics

We have indicated that a delay in using the first word (usually emerging at about 12 months of age) and being slow to add lots of words to their vocabularies are frequently the first signs of possible language problems. We have also indicated that vocabulary may be one of the areas in which children who are slow to talk seem to catch up first. However, we must be clear that this does not mean that children with SLI do not have semantic difficulties, because many, if not most, have some degree of problems with words and their meanings, although sometimes these are seen most clearly with words and expressions with abstract, nonliteral meanings and those related to the more literate aspects of semantics. Several areas of semantic acquisition that characterize some of the problems young children with SLI exhibit have been identified in the literature and are presented in Table 3.4.

TABLE 3.4   Several Areas of Semantic Difficulties Experienced by Children with SLI

Areas of Semantic Difficulty	Problems
Size of the lexicon	Smaller vocabularies
Rate of growth of the lexicon	Slower vocabulary acquisition
	Less lexical diversity
Robustness of word meaning	Less depth of knowledge about word meanings
	Less known about the meaning of individual words
	Only partial meanings of a word known
Speed of new word learning	Difficulties learning new lexical items quickly
	More exposures to a new word in context needed to abstract the meaning of the word
Word finding	Difficulties retrieving words from the cognitive store to use them in quick flow of connected speech
	The word on the "tip of the tongue"

With regard to vocabulary size, we have seen that a delay in using the first word (usually at about 12 months of age) and failing to show a spurt in single-word lexical acquisition after emergence of the first word are possible early signs of SLI. Other early delays in semantic development have also been described. Examples of some of the delays that have been reported for young late talkers and children with SLI are

- On average, using their first word at about 23 months of age (Trauner, Wulfeck, Tallal, & Hesselink, 1995), almost a year late in this report compared to normally developing children
- At 24 months of age, an expressive vocabulary size of about 17 words compared to 128 to 193 for normally developing children, and at 36 months, a vocabulary size of 197 words, similar to that of normally developing children at 24 months (Rescorla et al., 2001)

Rescorla and her colleagues (2001) also reported on the composition of the vocabulary of 3-year-olds who were late talkers and whose expressive vocabulary size was approximating that of normally developing 2-year-olds. These authors comment that although the children seem to acquire many of the same words as normally developing children, they also learn some different words that seem to reflect that they are older and, therefore, are experiencing different events in their environments, for example, words associated with toilet training. Children with SLI also seem to have more difficulty acquiring a wide variety of verb words than noun words (Conti-Ramsden & Jones, 1997; Kelly & Rice, 1994; Rice & Bode, 1993; Rice, Oetting, Marquis, Bode, & Pae, 1994; Watkins et al., 1993; Windfuhr, Faragher, & Conti-Ramsden, 2002). These findings raise a point that we need to keep in mind. Early delays in vocabulary acquisition may well result in children with SLI having qualitatively different, as well as quantitatively different, vocabularies. This possibility has important implications for what we might be able to assume about their continuity of language development compared to that of children without language problems, about what concepts and world knowledge these young children are building up along their developmental way, and about what the cumulative effects of what might be somewhat unusual concepts and knowledge might have on later academic and language learning.

As we saw early in this text, when words and their meanings join with other words and their meanings in multiword utterances, composite meanings evolve. Similar to their delay in early vocabulary, young children with SLI are typically slower to begin to use two-word semantic relations (Brown, 1973). Trauner and colleagues (1995) reported that their children with SLI did not begin to use two-word combinations until about 3 years of age, which compares to normally developing children beginning to use these combinations sometime between 18 and 24 months. Although children with SLI may be slower to acquire the range of semantic relations expressed in two-word combinations than normal language-learning children, they seem generally to acquire the same range expressed by their language-normal peers (Freedman & Carpenter, 1976; Leonard, Bolders, & Miller, 1976).

In the previous chapter, we discussed normal children's abilities to learn a lot about a word's meaning from very few and fleeting exposures to the word in context. We referred to this ability as "fast mapping" or "quick incidental learning." Young children with SLI have been found to demonstrate some abilities to fast map the meanings of words, particularly in structured learning situations, but they have been found to comprehend meanings of fewer new words when the learning task involved challenging tasks of discerning the meanings embedded in ongoing narratives (Dollaghan, 1987; Rice, Buhr, & Nemeth, 1990; Rice, Buhr, & Oetting, 1992; Rice et al., 1994). Overall, preschool children with SLI seem to learn new words more slowly than their normal-language peers and "may need to hear a new word twice as many times as a child with [normal language] before comprehending it" (Gray, 2003b, p. 56) and may need twice as many chances to use it before the word becomes a permanent part of their vocabulary (Gray 2003b).

Even if children with SLI are successful in gleaning meanings of words, this does not necessarily result in them using the words. One suggestion for this limitation is that the children have difficulties accessing or retrieving the words for production rather than a failure in storing the words in memory (Dollaghan, 1987). Another reason proposes that difficulties using words that seem to be known in the lexicon are a result of knowing only incomplete or partial meanings of the words. McGregor and her colleagues (McGregor, Friedman, Reilly, & Newman, 2002) suggest that the children may have a mental representation of a word, but it may not be a fully developed representation and may therefore be fragile. The fragileness of the meaning makes the word more susceptible to "retrieval failure" (p. 332).

The observation that many children with language problems have difficulties in retrieving known words (word-finding problems) is not new (German, 1979; German & Simon, 1991; Kail, Hale, Leonard, & Nippold, 1984; Leonard et al., 1983; MacLachlan & Chapman, 1988). In fact, many specifically language-impaired children are described as having word-finding problems. These difficulties can show up when children are asked to name pictures, particularly in timed naming tasks, and in their connected speech (German, 1991, 2000; McGregor, 1997). The connected speech of children with language problems is often characterized by hesitations, dysfluencies, reformulations, word substitutions, and fillers, features that are often interpreted as being related to word-retrieval difficulties. Additionally, the children may use a substantially higher number of words without clear referents, such as *thing, this, that, here,* and *there.* Consistent with the discussion above about incomplete, fragile representations of word meanings, some have proposed that these difficulties in accessing known words may be related to a less elaborate and extensive knowledge of the word meaning (Kail et al., 1984; McGregor, Newman, Reilly, & Capone, 2002) rather than, as McGregor and Leonard (1989) write, the use of "less efficient algorithms for retrieving word names" (p. 141).

It does not appear that children with SLI have semantic difficulties in the absence of problems with other aspects of language, although some children may have greater semantic weaknesses than others. In describing the children they had followed from 2½ to 5 years of age, Scarborough and Dobrich (1990) have written that when the children reached age 5, "no child ever showed a purely lexical deficit. Instead, residual phonological and syntactic problems, in combination and in isolation, were seen in most cases" (p. 80). To the extent that these findings are correct, we suspect that most, if not all, children with SLI with semantic difficulties will also have deficits with syntax and morphology.

Syntax and Morphology

Children with SLI are known to have inordinate difficulty with the morphosyntactic aspect of language, and it is doubtful that any child with SLI escapes at least some problems in this area. Deficit syntactic and morphologic skills are almost "classic" characteristics of preschoolers with language impairments. Lahey (1988) has written that "By far the most outstanding characteristic of this group of children and one that they all share, is late and slow development of form with better development of content and use interactions. . . ." (pp. 59–60).

It is at about 3 years of age that evidence of syntactic and/or morphological problems can usually be first identified, as children's MLUs, sentence complexity, and use of morphological markers are expected to increase. As examples of the difficulties that are observed in these children in the preschool years, we tend to see (1) shorter length of utterances (MLU) than same-age peers; (2) syntactically simpler sentences, including limitations in the types of transformations used and limited use of subordination; (3) omissions and/or confusions of grammatically obligatory elements, such as articles and noun plural morphemes; (4) subject case marking problems, as in *him* for *he* and *her* for *she* when the pronouns are to serve as subjects of sentences; and (5) failure to consistently mark verbs for tense and number, with particular difficulties with both regular and irregular past-tense marking (Leonard et al., 1997; Rice et al., 1998; Rice, Wexler, Marquis, & Hershberger, 2000). Table 3.5 provides a list of some of the common problematic morphemes for children with SLI (Leonard, McGregor, & Allen, 1992).

Because verb morphology is particularly vexing for children with SLI, their abilities in this area have been the subject of considerable study. One consistent but frustrating observation about the morphosyntactic performances of these children is the inconsistency in their use of morphological markers, especially with regard to their use of verb morphology (Leonard et al., 2003; Miller & Leonard, 1998; Rice, Wexler, & Cleave, 1995). Their inconsistency means that sometimes they treat a finite verb (one that needs to carry tense and number, such as "The girl run<u>s</u>" or "The boy jump<u>ed</u>") as a nonfinite verb (an infinitive form or bare stem form, such as "The girl run" or "The boy jump"). Other patterns with regard to

TABLE 3.5   Some Troublesome Grammatical Morphemes for Children with SLI

Morpheme	Examples
Plural -s	boys; coats
Possessive 's	baby's; cat's
Regular past -ed	played; liked
Third person singular -s	plays; likes
Articles a and the	a boy; the cat
Copula	The baby is big
On	on the floor; put on the coat
Auxiliary be	The baby is crying; The girls are playing
Irregular past tense	ate; went; drank
Complementizer to	I'm going to (go); gonna (go)

Source: Adapted from Leonard, McGregor, et al. (1992).

their use of grammatical markers for verbs have also been observed. These, along with the pattern of inconsistent use, are shown in Table 3.6.

Two alternative explanations for why these children demonstrate inordinate difficulties with verb morphology have featured prominently in the literature. One is referred to as the *surface account* (Leonard, McGregor, & Allen, 1992; Leonard et al., 1997) because it focuses on the phonetic features, that is, the morphophonological characteristics, of the problematic grammatical morphemes. Leonard and his fellow researchers (Leonard, McGregor, & Allen, 1992) point out that these morphemes have "low phonetic substance" (p. 1077). The morphemes have shorter durations in connected speech than adjacent morphemes. They are also unstressed, nonsyllabic segments. Some of them also have lower fundamental frequencies and amplitude, which means they may seem to be lower pitched and less loud. These features mean that they may be auditorily less salient than surrounding morphemes. This account suggested by Leonard and colleagues (1997) "assumes a general processing capacity limitation in children with SLI but assumes also that, in the case of English, this will have an especially profound impact on the joint operations of perceiving grammatical morphemes and hypothesizing their grammatical function" (p. 743). That is, the children with SLI have inefficient processing mechanisms that interfere with their abilities to take in these particularly brief, often faint elements of the language and analyze them fast enough during the ongoing flow of language and environmental activity in order to figure out what they mean and what the patterns and rules are in order to use them.

The second, the *extended optional infinitive account* (EOI) (Rice & Wexler, 1996; Rice et al., 1995, 1998, 2000), is a knowledge-based account. According to this account, children with SLI, like normal children, do not know that marking verb tense and number is obligatory and treat it as a rule of language that is optional to use. Where children with SLI differ from their normal counterparts is that they continue to treat verb marking as optional for an extended period of time, whereas normal children by about the age of 5 years figure

TABLE 3.6 Patterns of Verb Morphological Problems of Children with SLI

Patterns	Descriptions and Examples
Inconsistent errors	Bare stem verbs ("The girl run") used frequently but not always
	Sometimes verb marked correctly ("The girl run<u>s</u>")
Errors of omission common	Likely to omit grammatical markers ("Baby sleep<u>s</u>" or "Baby sleeping")
	Likely to omit auxiliaries, which mark the number and tense ("Baby sleeping")
Errors of commission infrequent	When verbs marked for tense and number, they tend to be marked correctly ("Baby is sleeping" not "Baby are sleeping")
Regular past-tense verbs problematic	Inconsistent use of finite or infinitive (bare stem) verb when finite form required ("[yesterday] Boys jump" instead of "Boys jumped")
	Perform at level worse than younger normal children matched for overall language level
Irregular past-tense verbs problematic	Frequently overgeneralized ("Kitty runned" instead of "Kitty ran")
	Bare stem used ("Kitty run" instead of "Kitty ran")
	Perform at levels similar to younger normal children matched for overall language level when percent correct versus percent incorrect metric used ("Kitty run" correct vs. "Kitty runned" incorrect)
	Perform at levels similar to those for regular past tense (i.e., worse than younger, language-matched children) when percent correct marking for knowledge of past tense used as the metric (percent correct for finiteness) ("Kitty runned" credited as correct for knowledge of need to mark tense)
	More likely than CA-matched peers to judge bare stem forms as correct ("[yesterday] Birdie fly off" deemed okay)
	More likely than CA-matched peers to judge overgeneralized forms as correct ("[yesterday] Birdie flied off")
Case marking on pronouns related to verb marking	*An early suggestion:*
	■ A potential developmental link between verb form acquisition and pronoun case development
	More recent suggestions:
	■ Incorrect use of objective case pronouns (*him, her, them*) as subjects (*he, she, they*) related to occurrence of verb tense marking
	■ Greater likelihood of objective case when verb unmarked for tense/number ("Her jump" more likely than "Her jumps") or auxiliary omitted ("Her jumping" more likely than "Her is jumping")
Inclusion of auxiliary verbs potentially susceptible to structural priming effects	■ Likely to include rather than omit auxiliary if child used an auxiliary in immediately preceding utterance ("Mommy is sleeping" instead of "Mommy sleeping" if previous sentence included auxiliary, e.g., "Babies are crying")

Sources: Bishop (1994); Connell (1986); Leonard, Bortolini, Caselli, McGregor, & Sabbadini (1992); Leonard et al. (1997, 2002); Loeb & Leonard (1991); Marchman et al. (1999); Montgomery & Leonard (1998); Oetting & Horohov (1997); Rice & Wexler (1996); Rice et al. (1995, 1998); Wexler, Schütze, & Rice (1998).

out that they need always to mark tense and number on finite verbs (main verbs in clauses) rather than treat them as infinitives (bare stem verbs). While children with SLI know about finiteness of verbs, and they know about the concepts of present and past tense, they do not know they are obligated to mark tense on verbs in main clauses. It is unknown if children with SLI finally ever learn and consistently apply verb marking, but we know that by 8 years of age, while the frequency of failure to do so has declined considerably, they still are inconsistent— some suggesting about 10 to 15 percent of the time (Rice et al., 1998)—whereas normal children achieve this level of consistency at 5 years of age and by age 8 almost always use appropriate verb marking. We also know that older children with language impairments also continue to have more difficulty with verb morphology than their peers (Marchman, Wulfeck, & Ellis Weismer, 1999; Reed & Evernden, 2001). This account of the verb morphological difficulties of children with SLI is silent about the reasons the children do not learn the obligatory aspect of verb marking as soon as or as well as normal children.

There are several other accounts of the reasons children with SLI have such inordinate difficulties with grammatical morphology and verb morphology in particular. One of these accounts is based on limited linguistic knowledge. This account proposes that children have difficulty abstracting the implicit rules that govern grammatical morphology (Gopnik, 1990; Ullman & Gopnik, 1994), hence the term *implicit rule deficit account* (Leonard et al., 1997). A variation on this account suggests that children with SLI learn the rules about verb marking but have difficulties accessing them (Connell & Stone, 1992). While this account has less empirical support than the surface or extended optional infinitive accounts as far as verb morphology is concerned (Leonard et al., 1997), it is still considered among the various possible reasons children with SLI have language-learning difficulties more generally. Two other accounts, the *dual mechanism account* (Oetting & Horohov, 1997) and the *connectionist account* (Marchman et al., 1999), have more recently been proposed, but these have been subjected to comparatively less empirical study in trying to explain the grammatical morpheme problems, and in particular the verb morphological difficulties, of children with SLI.

One question that has been raised is that if children with SLI have weaknesses in their verb vocabularies, as indicated previously in this chapter, then it might be possible that their difficulties with verb morphology might relate to their vocabulary problems rather than reflect primarily morphosyntactic problems. The work of Watkins and Rice (1991), in part, explored one aspect of a possible relationship between vocabulary and verb morphology in their study of verb particles and prepositions. Certain prepositions (e.g., *in, up*) also occur as part of a verb (e.g., a multiword construction that functions as a verb, such as *climb up*), that is, a verb particle. These authors proposed that since the same word (the preposition) in these two different grammatical functions has the same meaning and carries similar levels of auditory salience (phonetic substance), any differences in children's acquisition should be primarily grammatically or morphosyntactically based. In their study, children with SLI did, in fact, have more difficulty with verb particles than prepositions, leading these authors (Watkins & Rice, 1991) to suggest that "multiple sources of vulnerability for mastery of grammatical form classes" (p. 1139) may be involved. Leonard and his colleagues (1999) took a different approach to the question of the relationship between verb vocabulary and verb morphology and looked at the what children with SLI did with verb marking as a function of their lexical diversity. The findings suggested that even with greater verb vocabularies, the children's ability to deal with the grammatical marking of verbs did not keep pace, in contrast to the pattern seen for normally developing children. The findings led these authors (Leonard et al., 1999) to comment that "the lag in finite-verb morphology use in children with SLI may become more striking as vocabulary expands" (p. 687). The findings also indicated that the problems the children had with their verb morphology was "not a matter of having an inadequate number of lexical items . . . but they were simply not making use of the associated grammatical morphology" (p. 687). It appears, therefore, that children's verb morphological problems cannot be attributed wholly to vocabulary deficits. Findings such as these increase the potential of grammatical morphology and in particular verb morphology as a clinical marker, or phenotype, of SLI, as raised earlier in this chapter.

Pragmatics and Discourse

Many children with SLI have difficulties with pragmatic aspects of language. It is not clear whether these are the result of the children's problems with morphosyntax and possibly semantics or whether these difficulties are problems in their own right and simply represent another area of deficit for some of these children (Leonard, 1998; Rowan, Leonard, Chapman, & Weiss, 1983). Study of the pragmatic abilities of young children with language impairments has slowed in recent years with the surge in interest in their morphosyntactic problems, but the 1980s, prompted by some work in the mid- and late 1970s, was a particularly fruitful decade for learning about the various aspects of these children's pragmatic characteristics. This is particularly true for explorations into the functions and intentions used by these children. Somewhat later, attention turned to looking at the conversational and discourse patterns of children with SLI. A number of these findings are summarized in Table 3.7

When we look at the pattern reflected in the intentions and functions section of Table 3.7, it seems that youngsters with SLI not only demonstrate differences in their use of functions when compared to normal language-learning children, but their differences suggest a passivity in their interactions. Paul (1991) has commented that the toddlers with language problems that she examined simply appeared to be "less interested in interacting with others, even nonverbally" (p. 6). The information in Table 3.7 also suggests that children with SLI may not respond as readily as normally developing children to the initiation attempts of others. Hadley and Rice (1991) found that in the peer interactions of the preschool children in their study, the children with SLI were less likely to respond to their normal language-learning peers' initiations.

Fey's (1986) interactionist approach might be a useful way to think about what we see as pragmatic patterns for these children. Fey (1986) has proposed two continua related to conversational variables. One continuum deals with children's degrees of *assertiveness* in conversation, that is, the degree to which they initiate conversational acts or turns. The second refers to the degree of children's *responsiveness* to their conversational partners' needs. For both of these continua, children can be high (+) or low (–) on the variable, depending on the pattern they display in their interactions with others. Four patterns arise:

1. + assertiveness and + responsiveness, or children who are active conversationalists
2. + assertiveness and – responsiveness, or children who are verbal noncommunicators
3. – assertiveness and + responsiveness, or children who are passive conversationalists
4. – assertiveness and – responsiveness, or children who are inactive communicators

TABLE 3.7   A Summary of Pragmatic Difficulties of Children with SLI Compared to Normally Developing Children

Areas of Pragmatics	Sources
Functions and Intentions Fewer occurrences of communicative initiations, including gestural and vocalized initiations Fewer occurrences of functions that initiate (child-initiated) than those that involve responding Greater uses of the answering function Fewer uses of: ■ Declarative and imperative functions ■ Statement functions involving naming ■ Descriptive functions ■ Acknowledging functions ■ Joint attention or comment	Leonard, Camarata, Rowan, & Chapman, 1982; Paul, 1991; Rom & Bliss, 1981; Snyder, 1975, 1978; Wilcox, 1984
Conversation and Discourse *Initiating Verbal Interactions* Initiate conversations ■ With inappropriate/ineffective methods to gain listener's attention ■ At the wrong times Difficulty gaining access to existing conversations *Responding to Others' Verbal Interactions* Less responsive to peers' attempts to initiate conversations *Sustaining Verbal Interactions* Difficulties sustaining topics over several conversational turns, in part due to ■ Problems timing turns and interrupting ■ Inserting noncontingent, irrelevant comments ■ Switching topics abruptly *Clarifying and Repairing* Frequent breakdowns in conversational interactions, in part due to above conversational behaviors In seeking clarifications: ■ Tend not to indicate lack of comprehension overtly and/or with verbal/vocal signals ■ Eye-contact behavior may signal degree of comprehension; may look at interactant's face rather than other stimuli when a message is not understood ■ Tend not to ask for clarification even though may recognize lack of comprehension In making repairs: ■ Tend to revise previous utterances when not understood ■ Use more limited repertoire of revision strategies ■ Rarely use revisions involving substitutions of one syntactic or semantic element for an equivalent. *Adapting Messages/Code Switching* Problems seen in ■ Not verbally encoding the most informative elements of messages ■ Conveying both uninformative and informative elements of messages equally ■ Interpreting and using polite devices (indirect requests with and without *please*) Evidence of some ability to adapt by attempts to ■ Modify messages on basis of interactant's age ■ Revise messages to better suit interactant's language ability	Brinton & Fujiki, 1982; Craig, 1993; Craig & Evans, 1989; Craig & Gallagher, 1986; Craig & Washington, 1993; Donahue, Pearl, & Bryan, 1980; Dukes, 1981; Fey, Leonard, & Wilcox, 1981; Gallagher & Darnton, 1978; Hadley & Rice, 1991; Lucas, 1980; Prinz & Ferrier, 1983; Shatz, Bernstein, & Shulman, 1980; Skarakis & Greenfield, 1982; Skarakis-Doyle, MacLellan, & Mullin, 1990

The characteristics in Table 3.7 suggest that youngsters with SLI are more like the group described in #3 or #4, that is, passive conversationalists who are nonassertive in initiating but may respond if others do the initiating or inactive communicators who neither initiate readily nor respond easily.

Breakdowns in the conversational interactions of children with SLI are, unfortunately, common. Rice, Sell, and Hadley (1991) found that preschoolers with SLI tended to address their communicative attempts to adults more than to their peers in a preschool classroom, possibly because of their histories of unsuccessful communicative interactions with their peers and/or because of their histories of having had their communicative initiations ignored by their peers. Another finding of the Hadley and Rice study (1991) was that normally developing preschoolers were less likely to respond to the attempts at initiation of their classmates with SLI, a finding similar to that of Craig and Gallagher (1986). These preschoolers with SLI tended also not to be nominated by their normal-language counterparts as favored playmates and not to have, among their classmates, a friend without language difficulties (Gertner et al., 1994). Of particular note in this study was that the children with receptive language involvement in addition to their expressive language problems fared worse in their peer relationships compared to the children with only expressive language problems. Rice and her colleagues (1991) suggest that "children are sensitive to their relative communicative competence, or incompetence, at an early age" and that "as young as 3 years of age, children adjust their social interactions to take into account their communication abilities relative to those of others" (p. 1304). According to Rice and her co-workers, the early breakdowns in communicative interactions may be the beginning "of a negative interactive spiral generated by a child's history of communicative failure wherein a child becomes less likely to respond as he or she experiences failure in peer interactions and peers become less likely to attend to the child's initiations" (Hadley & Rice, 1991, p. 1315). The longstanding failures in and problems with peer interactions that have been well documented for language-impaired children and adolescents (Asher & Gazelle, 1999; Beitchman, Wilson, Brownlie, Walters, Inglis, et al., 1996; Brinton et al., 1998; Fujiki, Brinton, & Todd, 1996; Fujiki, Brinton, Robinson, & Watson, 1997; Fujiki, Brinton, Hart, & Fitzgerald, 1999; Jerome, Fujiki, Brinton, & James, 2002; Nippold, 1993) seem to have their roots in early childhood.

Findings about the friendships of preschoolers who have *not* been identified as language impaired provide some support for this proposition. Communicative characteristics of preschoolers less well liked and/or rejected by their young peers include (Black & Hazen, 1990; Black & Logan, 1995; Hazen & Black, 1989)

- Making more irrelevant comments
- Making fewer contingent responses
- Being less responsive to peers
- Taking longer turns in conversations
- Interrupting more
- Engaging in more talking over or talking simultaneously

These characteristics sound remarkably similar to the problematic pragmatic characteristics of children with SLI listed in Table 3.7, and the discussion provides a good transition to the next topic.

Socialization and Psychosocial Factors

Recall that at the beginning of the previous section on pragmatic characteristics, we noted that we could not be certain whether pragmatic problems are the result of children's linguistically based deficits or whether they are separate components. Similarly, it is difficult to separate pragmatic difficulties from socialization and psychosocial factors that are associated with SLI and to know "what's what" when we look at how youngsters with SLI behave. Although SLI has been described as occurring in the absence of *severe* emotional disturbances, there is clear recognition of a relationship between some degree of psychosocial involvement and language impairment (Baltaxe & Simmons, 1988; Beitchman et al., 2001; Beitchman, Brownlie, et al., 1996; Mack & Warr-Leeper, 1992; Prizant et al., 1990; Wilson, Brownlie, Waters, Inglis, et al., 1996). Examples of findings from some of the older well-known research studies illustrate this point:

- Of forty consecutive admissions to a child psychiatric unit, 50 percent of the children had language problems (Gualtieri, Koriath, Van Bourgondien, & Saleeby, 1983).
- Of approximately 300 successive intakes of children to a community-based speech and language clinic, 95 percent of the children with expressive language problems had some form of psychosocial difficulties according to 1980 criteria used by the American Psychiatric Association (Baker & Cantwell, 1982).
- Sixty-seven percent of the children consecutively admitted because of behavioral/emotional problems to an inpatient facility failed a speech and language screening (Prizant et al., 1990).

In some respects we may have a "chicken-and-egg" dilemma. Communicative failures may result in psychosocial difficulties, psychosocial difficulties may be a part of the syndrome of specific language impairment, or early psychosocial difficulties may manifest themselves in terms of language problems. We would, at least, suspect a reciprocal, if not a cyclical, relationship. As Rice and her colleagues (1991) write:

> To the extent that experiencing success in social interactions is central to a child's sense of self-esteem and social role, children with communication limitations are at risk for the development of social competencies. Limited social interactions would in turn limit their opportunities to learn communication skills from their peers, especially in the development of discourse skills. (p. 1305)

Findings from four studies may shed some light on the issue. In the research of Rescorla and Achenbach (2002), no significant association was found between toddlers about 2 years old who were evincing slow expressive language learning (i.e., fewer than 50 single words or no two-word combinations) and scores in the problematic range on a parent-rating protocol of their child's behavior, the Child Behavior Checklist for Ages 2–3 (Achenbach, 1992), thereby suggesting "no link between expressive language delays and behavioral/emotional problem" (p. 742). These authors suggest that "significant behavioral/emotional problems may be more likely when children have been delayed in language for many months (i.e., after 36 months)" (p. 742). Redmond and Rice (1998) might agree with the view that any behavioral/emotional problems of children with SLI are likely the result of their language problems, that is, a social adaptation explanation of psychosocial difficulties exhibited by these children. The children in this study were rated as being within the normal range on the Child Behavior Checklist (Achenbach, 1991a) by their parents and on the Teacher Report Form (Achenbach, 1991b) by their teachers, but their ratings were significantly poorer than those of their age-matched peers without language impairment. Recall that this is a pattern we saw earlier in this chapter for some other outcomes for children identified with SELD as toddlers. Teachers tended to identify more behavioral/emotional problems in the children than parents did, which the authors attributed to the situations in which the children were observed. According to the researchers (Redmond & Rice, 1998), a social adaptation model would expect "differences between teacher and parent ratings of sociobehaviors when children with SLI go to kindergarten and are experiencing the extensive social adjustments that appear at the time" (p. 696). The social and emotional behaviors reflect an overlay associated with their struggles with their language skills. Paul (2000), in reporting on the outcomes of the 2-year-olds with SELD when they were in second grade, noted that the children with histories of early language delay were significantly more shy than their normal counterparts, a finding basically consistent with that of Fujiki and fellow researchers (Fujiki, Brinton, Morgan, & Hart, 1999) in their investigation of withdrawn and sociable behaviors of children with SLI. Although not part of any of these studies, one wonders, assuming that a social adaptation model is accurate, if preschool experiences for these children in which they need to interact regularly with their peers might accelerate an onset of an overlay of psychosocial issues, a thought not wholly disassociated from a position raised in a somewhat different way by Paul (Paul, 2000; Paul et al., 1996).

Together, these studies hint at one possible scenario, one in which children with SELD or SLI begin life with their socioemotional systems basically intact, but their difficult and/or negative experiences trying to interact with their environments and others in their environment lead them to adopt less than positive social behaviors and acquire negative emotional responses. The relationship between socioemotional development and language impairment is complex, and this is, admittedly, a simplistic scenario. It fails to consider the many other important factors that affect development, such as children's basic temperaments, heterogeneity across children, or levels of language comprehension. For example, the children in the Rescorla and Achenbach (2002) study only had documented expressive language problems, whereas the children in the Redmond and Rice (1998) study had both receptive and expressive language deficits. Keep in mind that children with receptive language impairments seem not to fare as well as those with only expressive language deficits (Beitchman, Wilson, Brownlie, Walters, & Lancee, 1996; Beitchman, Wilson, Brownlie, Walters, Inglis et al., 1996; Gertner et al., 1994). It also does not consider research on how children's emotional reactions to situations might be able to be mediated through teaching and modeling.

Studies of self-esteem and emotion regulation in school-age children with SLI (Fujiki, Brinton, & Clarke, 2002; Jerome et al., 2002) shed some light on what children with SLI face as they mature. In a preliminary study, teachers' ratings of elementary school children with SLI indicated that these children demonstrated behaviors consistent with less sophisticated management of their emotions than their typically developing counterparts (Fujiki et al., 2002). Results of another study suggested that the self-esteem of children with SLI declines with age. Younger children (6 to 9 years) with and without SLI were found not to differ in how they perceived themselves with regard to social acceptance, behavioral conduct, and academic ability. In contrast, older children (10 to 13 years) with SLI perceived themselves more negatively than their peers in each of these areas. Although the subjects in these studies were school-aged children, the findings can help us understand what might be longer-term psychosocial issues for preschool children with SLI, as well the possibility that psychosocial problems likely escalate for these children as they mature. In the next chapter, on language and children with learning disabilities, we will see more about psychosocial issues, and in Chapter 5 we will see considerable discussion of psychosocial problems of adolescents with language impairments. Baker and Cantwell (1983) summarize the discussion well for us:

> since language is a uniquely human quality, it is therefore not unexpected that a disorder in language development might have far reaching consequences for other areas of early childhood development. (p. 51)

Narratives

Skill in relating understandable, complete narratives is an important factor in school achievement, and school-aged children with language problems frequently have difficulty in telling good narratives. Despite the fact that narratives are typically thought of as later-developing language skills, preschoolers do engage in early forms of narration. They relate rudimentary accounts about things that have happened to them, and they retell favorite stories from children's books that they have been read.

There is evidence that preschoolers with SLI demonstrate difficulties with narrative skills. We have previously indicated that the quality of language-impaired preschoolers' narrative skills is a strong predicting factor for their later school success (Bishop & Edmundson, 1987; Stothard et al., 1998). The narratives of children with SLI tend to contain less information than those of preschoolers with normal language skills and, according to Applebee's narrative stages (1978), are less mature (Paul, 1996; Paul & Smith, 1993). One explanation for youngsters' limitations on the information they encode may relate to the linguistic features the children are able to bring to the task. An efficient method to encode more than one proposition per utterance is complex sentence usage. Children whose language is limited to simple sentences or even to compound sentences are not efficient in their expression of multiple pieces of information. Contrast "When he hit the water, he started to sink so he closed his mouth" with "He hit the water. He started to go down in the water. He closed his mouth." Good, tightly composed narratives also depend on the use of high-content words with appropriate semantic choices to signal old and new information. Children with difficulties with certain abstract words, such as temporal words and deictic words, or children who have difficulties retrieving words quickly and who instead use low-content words (e.g., *thing*) will also encounter problems in producing narratives.

Production of narratives generally challenges most aspects of a language-impaired child's language system so that difficulties with one aspect of language may overload the child in such a way that other aspects of language break down or the whole system breaks down. For this reason, preschoolers who to the "naked ear" may appear to have adequate conversational language skills or who score within normal limits on standardized language tests may evidence even quite severe language problems when they are asked to relate narratives.

Implications for Intervention

Assessment

SLI in toddlers and preschoolers appears to be manifested in different ways at different times. It follows, therefore, that assessment considerations may need to differ at different times.

Toddlers

Predictive Factors in Assessment. Previously in this chapter, we reviewed several of the factors that can place infants and toddlers at risk for language impairment and those that can place a toddler with slow expressive language development at risk for continuing language problems (Table 3.3). The presence of any of these needs to be considered as part of an assessment process (Kelly, 1998a; Olswang et al., 1998). These predictive factors suggest aspects of toddlers' performances that professionals need to assess in addition to the children's language: (1) socialization; (2) phonological composition of vocalizations and babbling, as well as verbalizations; (3) use of gestures, particularly symbolic play gestures expressing script routines and those associated with joint attention; and (4) behavior. Assessment of toddlers needs to be multifaceted.

Language comprehension skills were not included in Table 3.3. However, the increasing evidence makes us suspicious that comprehension skills need to be included as an important part of an assessment process. There is also evidence that a substantial number of toddlers with expressive language problems have comprehension problems even though on superficial observation they may appear to understand quite well (Miller & Paul, 1995; Paul et al., 1991; Thal et al., 1991). Information about a toddler's comprehension skills not only helps inform about possible long-term language and learning outcomes, it is important in planning intervention as well as providing additional assessment documentation of language problems.

Young children's uses of communicative intentions produced through gestures and vocalizations can be assessed even before they use their first words. Coggins (1991) provides ideas about how to manipulate the assessment environment to identify children's uses of linguistic and nonlinguistic communicative intentions. He suggests that the children's performance should be assessed under conditions of both minimal and maximal support for producing intentions:

1. *Cuing (linguistic):* Manipulate for minimal support using indirect model; manipulate for maximal support using elicited imitation
2. *Activities (nonlinguistic):* Manipulate for minimal support using novel activities; manipulate for maximal support using known event routines and scripts
3. *Interactor (nonlinguistic):* Manipulate for minimal support using clinician; manipulate for maximal support using mother/caregiver
4. *Materials (nonlinguistic):* Manipulate for minimal support using no toys or props; manipulate for maximal support using familiar objects/toys and those with thematic base (e.g., doll, bottle, diaper)
5. *Interaction (nonlinguistic):* Manipulate for minimal support using naturalistic child–adult interactions; manipulate for maximal support using contrived tasks (e.g. desired food item in transparent, tightly sealed container)

Differences in the children's performances under these conditions can be identified, with differences possibly indicating the children's potential for change (Coggins, 1991; Platt & Coggins, 1990). A toddler's ability to modify behavior quickly under various conditions of support often has prognostic value, as we know from dynamic assessment practices, discussed more fully in Chapter 13, and can provide valuable insights about strategies that might be included in intervention plans.

Early Language Milestones.   Early language developmental milestones provide additional guidelines for assessment. Many of these were highlighted in the previous chapter and even in earlier parts of this chapter. Of particular import for assessing toddlers are milestones related to prelinguistic developmental behaviors, early expressive vocabulary development, early and later multiword utterances, and early sentences.

Tracking toddlers' progress from single-word to multiword utterances requires assessment measures that are sensitive in picking up what are important developmental patterns. Of particular importance is knowing that toddlers are moving toward productive, rule-based combinations so that these become generative in order that novel utterances using the rules can be produced as context and meaning warrant. A normally developing toddler takes about 4 to 5 months to move from the emergence of the first two-word combination to the use of many new and unique word combinations (Ingram, 1989a). Ingram's (1989a) work indicates that during these months, when the toddler manages to have produced about a hundred novel two-word utterances, the child is likely to demonstrate a "syntactic spurt," suggesting that the child has learned about grammatical productivity, that is, the generative basis of syntax. This typically happens at about 2 years of age. At this point the toddler is, in essence, "off and running" with regard to syntax and grammar. Two assessment procedures can be particularly helpful in tracking toddlers' progress toward their use of productive two-word utterances. Long and his colleagues (1997) developed a procedure to observe and analyze the generative productivity of the types of two-word utterances showing up in young children's language as they move from using single-word utterances to word combinations, that is, MLUs slightly over 1.00.[3] Their procedure looked at "utterance level productivity (ULP), which reflects general positional rules for word combinations; and grammatic level productivity (GLP), which reflects specific rules based on semantic consistency" (p. 36). These authors (Long et al., 1997) reported that the children with SELD in their study who achieved grammatic-level productivity as a result of intervention were the ones who showed greater progress. Hadley's (1999) approach was to analyze the spontaneous language of children with MLUs between 1.00 and 2.00 (Brown's Stage I) over time for changes in the number of *unique syntactic types* (UST) the children use. A UST is "a combination of two or more words with syntactic status that could fit into the phrase structure of a more grammatically complete adult utterance" (p. 263). Hadley (1999) found that her procedure was highly correlated with children's performances on the Index of Productive Syntax (Scarborough, 1990) and their MLUs. As Hadley (1999) states, the procedure was designed for "tracking the progress of children in this early stage of grammatical development" (p. 269). Both of these procedures appear to help professionals

---

[3]Recall that an MLU of 1.00 means only single words without any grammatical morphemes attached, whereas an MLU of 1.50 suggests single words with grammatical morphemes and/or equal numbers of single-word utterances with no grammatical morphemes and two-word combinations with no grammatical morphemes.

more precisely distinguish between toddlers who are displaying progress toward using generative, productive multiword combinations and those whose word combinations seem stalled and/or nonproductive for expansion.

Assessment Instruments and Parental Report.   A number of developmental instruments have been available for several years to assess infants and toddlers. Among these are the Bayley Scales of Infant Development—Revised (Bayley, 1993), the Denver Developmental Screening Test—II (Frankenburg et al., 1990), and the Vineland Adaptive Behavior Scales (Sparrow, Balla, & Ciccetti, 1984). This list is by no means complete, and new instruments are regularly developed and existing ones updated. These instruments examine a range of developmental areas (e.g., gross motor, fine motor, personal-social), including items that address communication skills. In addition to these more general assessment tools, several tools that focus specifically on the assessment of early communication skills have been published. Among these are the Early Language Milestone Scale (2nd ed.) (Coplan, 1993) and the Clinical Linguistic and Auditory Milestone Scale (Capute et al., 1986). These instruments are screening tools that have been used most often for identifying severe developmental delays in children (Rescorla, 1991).

The use of parental reports of young children's communicative behaviors has recently increased in popularity as a means of assessing toddlers' language abilities. Although there were initial concerns about validity and reliability when instruments based on parental reports were first developed, findings from subsequent research have largely, although not completely, allayed many of the concerns. Parental report has several inherent features that make it an attractive method of assessment. These include: (1) the parents have had more opportunities to observe their children's language, so they typically know more about what the children do with their communication than a professional can learn in an assessment session; (2) parental report can be obtained prior to professionals seeing the children and can, therefore, help professionals plan assessment sessions; and (3) it is cost-effective.

Parental report procedures can be systematized, standardized, and structured, which reduces some of the problem about accuracy of the procedure. A common approach, therefore, is a recognition format that presents parents with communicative behaviors and asks them to identify those that apply to their children. Two such parental report instruments using this technique that are designed specifically to tap toddlers' communication skills are the Language Development Survey (LDS) (Rescorla, 1989) and the MacArthur Communicative Development Inventories[4] (CDI) (Fenson et al., 1993). The CDI has two versions, one for earlier-developing language and focusing primarily on gestures and single-word vocabulary and a second that focuses more on word combinations in addition to vocabulary. Of the two instruments, the CDI is the more extensive, taking parents about 30 minutes to complete. In contrast, the LDS, according to its author (Rescorla, 1991), was designed "as a quick and efficient . . . screening tool for the identification of language delay in 2-year-old children" (p. 17). The LDS takes about 10 minutes for parents to complete. Both instruments provide parents with a list of vocabulary items (or phrases) and ask them to indicate which of the words their children use. Both have been used in the early identification of toddlers with language delays.

---

[4]Earlier versions were known as the Early Language Inventory.

A slightly different approach to parent report was taken by Girolametto (1997) in his development of a parent report measure to profile the conversational skills of children between the ages of 1 and 3 years of age. This protocol is based on Fey's (1986) assertiveness–responsiveness continua used to describe children's conversational interactive style, discussed previously in this chapter. It asks parents to rate the degree to which each of twenty-five statements, reflecting various responsive or assertive conversational behaviors, describes their child. Advantages of the tool are its ease of administration and speed of completion and its ecological and social validity. According to Girolametto (1997), "The rating scale profiles the strengths and weaknesses of individual children and provides unique information that is unavailable from other assessment sources" (p. 32).

Several instruments that focus on communication skills are available for professionals to use during assessment sessions with toddlers. Space precludes providing a comprehensive list of these. Additionally, any such list would be outdated as soon as it was compiled. However, some of the more commonly used instruments over the years are: Communication and Symbolic Behavior Scales (CSBS) (Wetherby & Prizant, 1993), Sequenced Inventory of Communication Development (SICD) (Hedrick, Prather, & Tobin, 1975), Preschool Language Scale-4 (PLS-4) (Zimmerman, Steiner, & Pond, 2002), Receptive-Expressive Emergent Language Test-Second Edition (REEL-2) (Bzoch & League, 1991), Reynell Developmental Language Scales-III (Edwards et al., 1999), and Rossetti Infant and Toddler Language Scale (Rossetti, 1995). The procedures for a number of these instruments include some degree of parental report, as well as direct professional–child interaction. General aspects of assessing children's language and factors involved in selecting and using standardized instruments are discussed in Chapter 13.

Parent/Caregiver–Child Interactions.   An important part of assessment involves the interactions between primary caregivers and their children. As we know, parents'/caregivers' interactions with their language-impaired children are, for the most part, not terribly different from the interactions of other parents/caregivers with younger normal language-learning children. That is, the parents/caregivers seem to respond more to the child's language level than the child's chronological age. The few problematic areas that have sometimes been noted generally relate to (1) the degree of directiveness in the parents'/caregivers' interactions, with parents/caregivers of language-impaired children tending to use more directive language to their children, such as commands, rather than responses to their children's initiations; and (2) the frequency with which parents/caregivers provide semantically contingent responses (recasts) to their children's utterances. Somewhat related to this latter factor is the quickness with which parents/caregivers respond. Roth (1987) has suggested that a 1-second interval between a child's production and the parent's/caregiver's response is the time frame in which a 1-year-old child can pick up on the contingency of the parent's/caregiver's response.

There need to be caveats on interpreting these findings. Recall we have indicated that a child's language behavior itself may modify an adult's mode of communicative interaction, so that interactions may be less appropriate and stimulating. The communicative interactions likely have reciprocal effects. However, some of these adult behaviors, once established possibly because of previous adult–child interactions, may maintain slowed language development in a child. The purpose of assessing parent/caregiver–child interactions is not to judge the adult. Rather, it is to identify possible factors in the interactions that can be modified or included in interactive routines to enhance and facilitate a child's language learning.

Preschoolers

General Guidelines. For preschoolers, many more standardized language instruments are available. It is also easier to obtain reliable assessment results from preschoolers than from toddlers. However, professionals still need to be alert to the fact that considerable variability can occur in preschoolers' communicative performance. As with toddlers, it is also important with preschoolers to assess caregiver–child interactions and a variety of behaviors. Language developmental milestones continue to be important guidelines, although as preschoolers mature much beyond 3 years of age, MLU may no longer be a consistently reliable indicator of language growth (Klee, 1985; Klee & Fitzgerald, 1985; Scarborough, Wyckoff, & Davidson, 1986; Wells, 1985). Additionally, gross measures of expressive vocabulary size may also be less reliable indicators of language skill with preschoolers than with toddlers. Recall we previously suggested that delays in expressive vocabulary acquisition may appear to resolve during the later preschool years. This is not to say expressive vocabulary should not constitute part of the assessment process. Rather, care should be taken to ensure that procedures include assessing a child's use of words with more abstract meanings. Comprehension vocabulary would also constitute part of the assessment process. Again, however, abstract vocabulary words need to be included in the assessment.

Because syntax and morphology are especially troublesome areas for preschoolers with SLI, children's performances in these areas should be thoroughly assessed. Of particular importance are children's uses of complex sentences and the emergence of grammatical morphemes, especially their use of verb-tense grammatical marking. Children's developing skills with both micro and macro aspects of narrative production are also major parts of assessment. These areas for assessment are consistent with our previous discussions in this chapter, so none of this should be surprising. However, all measures need to be fine-grained rather than global and general (Paul, 1991). Chapter 13 has information that applies to the assessment of preschool children.

An area of assessment of preschool children that is increasingly more common is their ability in areas associated with literacy development, given the greater understanding of the relationship between children's early language levels and their learning to read (Boudreau & Hedberg, 1999; Justice & Ezell, 2002; Justice et al., 2002). Catts (1997) suggests that many of the problems associated with reading disabilities can be observed in children before they begin formal reading instruction. This means that, in addition to preschoolers' language and their abilities with narratives and phonological processing, as discussed below, their knowledge about letter names, print concepts, literacy terms, and rhyme can be assessed. Results can assist in identifying those children at risk for reading difficulties so that early intervention aimed at reducing reading failure can be provided (Catts, 1997; Fey, Catts, & Larrivee, 1995).

Illusory Recovery. If preschoolers can appear to recover from deficits in certain aspects of language behavior at different times, this has implications for assessment. Language performance needs to be assessed in such a way that overcomes the possibility of obtaining *false negative* results—that is, results indicating no problem exists when, in fact, it does.

One way to address the problem of illusory recovery is to ensure that assessment is comprehensive, that is, that many aspects of communication are assessed, as well as behavioral aspects known to be associated with SLI, such as those listed in Table 3.3. It may be appropriate to assess over several sessions and in a variety of settings, including in a child's home and in situations where the child interacts with other children (Hadley & Schuele, 1998).

Another way to address the problem is to stress or challenge the child's language performance (Lahey, 1990). It is not enough to know what a child *does* with language. We need to know what a child *can do* with language. Earlier we indicated that narrative production particularly challenges a child's language performance. Asking a child to relate a narrative should probably be a standard part of a preschooler's language assessment, not only to stress the system but for its predictive value as well. However, professionals should avoid basing any decisions about a child's language abilities only on production of stereotyped narratives such as fairy tales. These may be "rehearsed" narratives for a child because they have occurred frequently in the child's environment. Rather, novel narratives should be elicited using one or more of the several ways described in Chapter 13 and considering the various advantages and disadvantages of the various methods.

Previously in this chapter we discussed the work that has been emerging with regard to grammatical morphemes and nonword repetition as possible clinical markers of SLI. This work points to other important areas for assessment. These are two areas, therefore, that are essential to include in assessment and that can help to overcome some of the issues related to illusory recovery. The various formal and informal methods available to assess children's abilities in these areas are presented in Chapter 13.

Social Communicative Interaction.   Part of assessing language performance involves assessing children's communication in social, interactive situations. For preschoolers, this goes beyond assessment only with the primary caregiver. Ideally, children should be assessed as they interact in a group with other children, some of whom are normal language-learning children (Hadley & Schuele, 1998). As Rice and her colleagues (Rice, Sell, & Hadley, 1990) point out, however, most systems designed to measure children's social communicative interactions are sufficiently complex and cumbersome to render them impractical for routine assessment.

To provide "a quick way of obtaining clinically relevant information about the use of language in natural settings along the social dimension" (p. 7), Rice and colleagues (Rice, Sell et al., 1990) developed the Social Interactive Coding System (SICS). This instrument focuses on Fey's (1986) assertiveness/passiveness conversational dimension and examines a child's interactions with peers during a variety of activities that typically occur in preschools, such as art, dramatic/symbolic play, and free play with toys. Each turn a child takes in an interaction, the nature of each turn (e.g., initiation, response—verbal, response—nonverbal, ignore), and the number of turns in the interaction are recorded on a standardized protocol, which also allows for the addressee of the child's interactions to be recorded. The tool incorporates an on-line observational technique in which the professional records all of the child's interactions in a 5-minute period and then takes a 5-minute break to update notations on the protocol. The "5 minutes on/5 minutes off" procedure is repeated three times, for a total of four observational segments. The advantages of the Social Interactive Coding System include: (1) it can be completed in the classroom, (2) it is easy to learn,

(3) minimal equipment is necessary, and (4) results are immediately available for interpretation. The authors caution, however, that the SICS should not be used as a sole assessment procedure, but rather as a supplement to other forms of assessment.

Chapter 13 provides additional information about assessment of children's language in general. The information in that chapter is relevant to language assessment of toddlers and preschoolers and should be used in conjunction with the information presented here.

Intervention

Decisions about Intervention.   The issue of predicting which toddlers and preschoolers will outgrow their early delays in acquiring language without assistance and which will not leads to a main consideration for intervention. That is, under what conditions is intervention recommended, when is intervention recommended, and what is the nature of the intervention—monitoring, indirect intervention, or direct intervention carried out by a professional? There are no hard-and-fast answers to these questions (Olswang & Bain, 1991b; Olswang et al., 1998; Paul, 1996, 2000). The philosophical and theoretical positions of the professional, the philosophical and procedural positions of the organization in which the professional works, and the attitudes and wishes of the caregivers affect the decision. Professionals' decisions are influenced by information about identification of language impairment and standards to which a child's language performance is being compared, predictive and risk factors relevant to a specific child, and the long-term implications of unresolved language impairments. To this, information about a child's potential for language change and the factors important in facilitating the change are added.

A word of caution is warranted. The quality of input into decision making about recommending or not recommending intervention, whether it is the professionals' or parents' input, is only as good as the information and understanding that these individuals have about associations among language, literacy, and socialization. The results of one study (Zhang & Tomblin, 2000) are both informative and disturbing. These researchers explored which of three categories of communication problems (speech-sound production problems, expressive language problems, or receptive language problems) were associated with 5-year-old children receiving intervention, as well as which of these categories of communication problems had a greater effect on the children's academic and social functions. Speech-sound production problems were more closely associated with children having received intervention services than language problems. According to these researchers (Zhang & Tomblin, 2000), of the children with language problems, "intervention receipt was more closely related to expressive language than to receptive language" (p. 352). In contrast, language problems had the greater negative effect on academic and social variables compared to speech-sound production problems. These findings suggest that the aspect of communication (speech-sound production) less likely to affect the important areas of academic and social success is the aspect more likely to lead to children receiving intervention. Conversely, the aspects of communication most closely associated with personal and school success (language) are less likely to be related to children's receipt of intervention. Speech-sound production problems are more obvious to listeners—whether the listeners are professionals in speech and language, professionals in other areas of education or health, or lay individuals such as parents—than expressive language problems, and expressive language problems are more obvious than receptive language problems. Zhang and Tomblin (2000) write that the "aspect that is most available to the listener has the greatest effect on the child's receipt of clinical services" (p. 354). This is despite the fact that the most available aspect is the one least likely to affect a child's academic and social achievement. These results indicate that professionals need to be alert to what factors of children's communication abilities they are judging with regard to intervention recommendations. The results also indicate that professionals need to provide individuals who have had fewer opportunities to know about the potential impact of language ability on other areas of children's development and achievement with the information they need to participate in deciding what to recommend about intervention.

An important principle is that, whatever initial decision is made, it is reassessed regularly as a child's behavior does or does not change (Bain & Dollaghan, 1991; Olswang & Bain, 1991a, 1991b). If direct intervention administered by a professional is not recommended initially, it is possible to implement indirect methods, such as parent training and/or preschool enrollment, and monitor the child's progress. If the anticipated progress is not seen in a specified period of time, a decision to intervene directly can be made. If direct intervention is the initial decision, the child's progress is also monitored regularly. If progress is rapid, the professional and parents may decide to discontinue direct intervention, implement indirect intervention programs to maintain the level of progress, and monitor the child's behaviors at regular intervals. If progress is not continued, direct intervention can be reinstated. Ongoing monitoring, regular measurements of a child's language performance across many parameters, consistent follow-up, and flexibility in moving from one form of intervention to another are critical in providing effective intervention.

Indirect Intervention.   As indicated above, one aspect of intervention is deciding on the way in which services for a specific toddler or preschooler are delivered, that is, direct intervention provided by a professional interacting with the child or indirect intervention provided through consultation and collaboration with others. Both methods may also be employed either simultaneously or consecutively. The decision will differ for each child. No one service delivery model is suitable for all youngsters with SLI or SELD. However, parents/caregivers play a large role in the early language learning of toddlers and preschoolers, and their participation in intervention is essential. Furthermore, a common recommendation for youngsters with SLI is placement in a preschool program.

Parents/Caregivers.   Toddlers and preschoolers spend most of their time interacting with parents/caregivers. Therefore, these adults are potentially powerful sources of change in children's communicative behavior. Involving parents/caregivers in intervention is not only mandated by federal education laws but generally makes good sense as well. As Olswang and Bain (1991a) point out, the "question is not should the parent be involved in the intervention process, but how" (p. 77). The "how" usually takes one of two approaches. The parents/caregivers can augment, expand, and supplement the intervention provided directly by a professional, who is the primary agent of change, or they can serve as the primary agents of change, with the professional serving to develop the initial directions and methods for change and to monitor both the process and the progress (Cleave & Fey, 1997; Fey et al., 1993, 1997; Girolametto et al., 1996; Girolametto, Weitzman, Wiigs, & Pearce, 1999; Robertson & Ellis Weismer, 1999). Whichever strategy is chosen for an individual child, the parents/caregivers need education and training. This generally focuses on two objectives: (1) creating or enhancing the child's environment to facilitate change in the child's language and (2) responding within that environment in a manner that most optimally facilitates language change.

At least two primary aspects are involved with regard to changing or enhancing the child's language-learning environment. One aspect focuses on helping the parents/ caregivers recognize and take advantage of language-learning opportunities that occur in a child's daily activities. This approach stresses seizing opportunities and capitalizing on language-teaching moments. These moments can occur during dressing, interactive play, meal or snack time, story time, or any other time during a day when the child's attention is focused on a specific action, object, or event. The parents/caregivers are shown how to identify these moments and how to structure their language and gestural input accordingly. The second aspect involves creating opportunities for language learning. The parents/caregivers are shown how to set up moments in the environment to facilitate a child's use of specific language behaviors and how to encourage the child to use these behaviors during those periods. These moments may or may not be specified, allocated periods. In some instances, the parents/caregivers may be able to observe a situation and know that if they make an immediate and sometimes small change, they will be able to facilitate a desired language behavior. In other instances, short periods may actually be set aside for creating the opportunities to facilitate certain communicative behaviors in the child. As with the "opportunistic" approach, the parents/caregivers are shown how to structure their communicative behavior so as to enhance the child's learning.

In helping parents/caregivers respond to the children in ways that best promote language learning, it is important to remember that the aim is likely to help them do more of some things they already do and perhaps less of others (Conti-Ramsden, 1990; Conti-Ramsden & Dykins, 1991; Fey et al., 1997; Fey, Krulik, Loeb, & Proctor-Williams, 1999; Girolametto et al., 1996, 1999; Proctor-Williams, Fey, & Loeb, 2001). In most instances, it may simply be a matter of changing the frequency of certain behaviors, such as increasing how often they use expansions and recasts of the children's utterances and encourage imitation. These are language-facilitating techniques described in Chapter 14, where more specific information about intervention is presented.

Earlier we indicated that most parents/caregivers of specifically language-impaired children provide language interactions that are similar to those of parents of normally developing children, but there may be two, or perhaps three, adult behaviors that are worthy of particular attention. One may involve helping the parents/caregivers reduce the frequency with which they use directive speech acts, including commands and demands for responses from the children, and increase their use of (1) responsive speech acts, (2) information-seeking questions for which the information presumably is not known to the adult, (3) confirmation requests that are used to affirm that the adult understood the child correctly, and (4) simple recasts and expansions of the child's utterances that serve to maintain the content of the child's utterances but do so in a form that modifies slightly that used by the child. Both Fey and his colleagues (Cleave & Fey, 1997; Fey et al., 1993, 1997, 1999) and Girolametto and his co-workers (Girolametto et al., 1996, 1999) describe parent-training programs that teach parents how to engage in these behaviors with their children. Both groups of researchers have reported positive effects of their programs in helping to advance the language of toddlers and preschoolers with SELD and/or SLI.

Another area in which parents/caregivers may be able to facilitate children's language learning is to increase the frequency with which they respond to what the child says and to do so with semantically contingent statements (Girolametto et al., 1996). These responses again maintain the content of the child's utterances and serve as comments about the content of the child's utterance. For example, to the child's utterance "big doggie" the adult might say "Yes, it is a big doggie." A third possibility for enhancing further a child's language learning may focus on helping parents/caregivers provide quicker responses to the children's utterances, that is, reduce latencies in parents'/caregivers' responses.

There is not a large body of research to help us know if parent-implemented intervention or clinician-implemented intervention or a combination of both is the most effective for accelerating children's language growth both in the short- and long-term. One study, however, found that, while parent-implemented intervention following parent training was effective, preschool children with SLI made greater and more consistent gains in clinician-implemented intervention (Fey et al., 1997). The clinician-administered intervention was, of course, more costly than the parent-implemented program (Cleave & Fey, 1997; Fey et al., 1997). It is not known what differences, if any, there may be in long-term outcomes for the children in terms of different intervention programs. That is, we do not know the cost–benefit ratios associated with clinician-implemented and parent-implemented intervention.

Preschools.   Preschool experiences are often recommended for youngsters with SLI in order to provide a stimulating language-learning environment and opportunities for social communicative interactions for the children. Peers have been shown to be able to facilitate the language development and social interaction skills of children with SLI or SELD (DeKroon et al., 2002; Robertson & Ellis Weismer, 1997). However, the simple presence of normal language-learning children in a preschool does not guarantee that these children will be effective facilitators for children with SLI. Special attention may have to be given to how the aims of such an approach can be achieved (DeKroon et al., 2002; Hadley & Schuele, 1998; Robertson & Ellis Weismer, 1997).

One problem that has been observed is that normal and language-impaired youngsters together in preschools do not particularly spend very much of their time in communicative interactions with each other (Hadley & Rice, 1991; Hadley & Schuele, 1998; Rice et al., 1991; Weiss & Nakamura, 1992). As Hadley and Rice (1991) point out in their study on the conversational interactions of normal and language-impaired preschoolers,

> The implications for intervention are somewhat sobering. It seems that placement of these children [with SLI] in an integrated setting, even one in which adults are highly responsive to and encourage the children's initiation attempts, does not necessarily ensure peer interactions. . . . Preschoolers behave as if they know who talks well and who doesn't, and they prefer to interact with those who do. Therefore, placement of communicatively impaired children in an integrated setting, with normal-language peers and facilitative adults, will not in and of itself establish successful peer interactions in spontaneous interactions. (p. 1315)

It seems, therefore, that the facilitative adults in these settings need to develop strategies that specifically target encouraging successful peer interactions. It cannot be assumed that these will occur without professionals' direct attention and planning.

These adults, too, might benefit from assistance in how to make their interactions more facilitating for children's language learning. Girolametto's research team (Girolametto & Weitzman, 2002; Girolametto, Weitzman, van Lieshout, & Duff, 2000) examined the degree of responsiveness and directiveness in the language of day-care teachers with training in early childhood education. To track, categorize, and analyze teachers' interactions, the researchers used the Teacher Interaction and Language Rating Scale (Girolametto, Weitzman, & Greenberg, 2000). Results indicated that although many of the teachers' interactions with the children were characterized by language-facilitating behaviors and demonstrated some sensitivity to children's different language levels, there were aspects of their verbal interactions that the researchers identified as directive and less language facilitating. Different instructional contexts (e.g., book reading, play dough activity) resulted in different levels of directiveness. The researchers suggested that training to help teachers reduce some types of directiveness where it is not necessary for direct instruction might enhance children's language learning (Girolametto, Weitzman, van Lieshout, 2000).

A final note relates to the involvement of parents/caregivers as part of children's preschool experiences. Marvin and Privratsky (1999) found that, when preschool children left school at the end of a day with "remnants from recent school events, toys, or child-produced art products" (p. 231), the children's talk with their parents in the car on the way home or when they arrived home contained more references to events that had transpired at preschool than when no materials were sent home with the children. These authors suggest that sending child-centered materials home with children at the end of a preschool day may help facilitate their ability with what is a more difficult discourse situation, that is, to talk about events in the past in situations where there is no shared knowledge between narrator (the child) and listener (the parent). In developing preschool plans, part of the routine might be regular child-centered "take-home" materials that parents realize are important to talk about with their children. Another part of involving parents in their children's preschool or day-care experience considers the advantages of including parent training in conjunction with their children's attendance at preschool. For example, in one study (Roberts et al., 1989), children who attended a preschool that included regular parent/caregiver education achieved better conversational skills by 5 years of age than either children who did not attend preschool but whose parents/caregivers did receive education or children who neither attended preschool nor whose parents/caregivers received education. This finding suggests that the combination of parent/caregiver education and preschool programs provides more powerful opportunities for enhancing children's language performances than parent/caregiver education alone.

Direct Intervention. Direct intervention for youngsters with SLI can be conducted individually with a child, via group sessions, or a combination of both. However, much of what is discussed in the literature describes group intervention, with or without adjunct individual sessions. Consistent with our discussion, groups have a greater potential to facilitate children's peer interactions, assist them to use language appropriately in social interaction, provide opportunities for generalization of language skills, tend to have more naturalistic environments for language use, and are likely to include more events and experiences to talk about and more people to talk with (Bunce, 1995; Hadley & Schuele, 1998; Rice & Wilcox, 1995; Robertson & Ellis Weismer, 1997). When it comes to characterizing group intervention for toddlers and preschoolers, there are many variations on the theme. Some of these are:

- Some programs have smaller numbers of children in them (e.g., four) (Robertson & Ellis Weismer, 1999); others are larger, with as many as 18 to 20 (Bunce, 1995; Rice & Wilcox, 1995).

- Some consist only of children with language delays or impairment (Cleave & Fey, 1997; Robertson & Ellis Weismer, 1999); others have a mix of children with and without language problems (Bunce, 1995; Rice & Wilcox, 1995).
- Some place greater emphasis on acquisition of grammatical forms (Cleave & Fey, 1997), others on vocabulary and early word combinations (Robertson & Ellis Weismer, 1999), and others on a wide variety of aspects of language based on individual children's needs (Bunce, 1995; Rice & Wilcox, 1995).
- As indicated above, some include individual intervention sessions with children as part of the total intervention program (Cleave & Fey, 1997); others use group sessions exclusively (Robertson & Ellis Weismer, 1999).

Despite these variations, there seem to be some commonalities. One is that most of the programs recognized the importance of peer interaction and socialization for the children and and addressed these in varying degrees in the intervention programs. Another was the inclusion of routine events and scripts to help children scaffold their language and reduce processing demands for them.

One point that came through from the results of Long and his colleagues' (1997) study and Hadley's (1999) work was the need to be alert to what particular types of word combinations toddlers are and are not acquiring. Recall that a positive indication is acquisition of word combinations that reflect generative, rule-based, grammatical principles. When facilitating the acquisition of word combinations is a goal of intervention for children, Long and his co-workers (1997) recommend that specific grammatical rules that carry "syntactic status" and can "fit into the phrase structure of a more grammatically complete adult utterance" (Hadley, 1999, p. 269) be targeted directly. These can be equally targeted in group or individual intervention sessions.

Summary

In this chapter we have seen that

- Characterization and understanding of SLI as a condition is far from complete.
- Some suggest that youngsters with SLI represent a large, generic grouping of children and that there are subgroups of children with SLI. If there are subgroups, these have not yet been satisfactorily identified.
- A number of different labels to describe these children have been used; SLI has gained some acceptance, but is not universally agreed on.
- Causal factors remain elusive, but information processing, neurological factors, and genetics are receiving considerable attention.
- Some children outgrow early delays in acquiring language; others do not. Predicting who will and who will not catch up is currently an important area of research. Issues related to possible "illusory recovery" need to be addressed. Issues of illusory recovery and prediction impact on assessment strategies and intervention decisions.
- Two aspects of performance, grammatical morpheme use and nonword repetition, are being looked at as potential clinical markers of SLI.

- Children with SLI can exhibit different combinations of communication problems that can involve some or all parameters of language. One common feature is difficulty with syntax and morphology and, in particular, verb morphology.
- Parental/caregiver involvement is important in obtaining assessment information, and parental/caregiver education is an important aspect of intervention.
- Placement of children in preschools will not necessarily ensure successful social communicative interactions unless these are specifically addressed within the preschool situation.
- A number of different intervention models are available, and which model is used should depend on the needs of individual children and their parents.
- Intervention is a process of ongoing monitoring, regular measurements of the children's language performances, consistent follow up, and flexibility in moving from direct to indirect intervention modes and vice versa.

Toddlers and preschoolers with SLI are at risk for academic failure when they begin school. They are also at risk for early social failure. Proper and early identification and intervention are critical if a potential cycle of social and academic failure is to be prevented.

4

Language and Children with Learning Disabilities

STEVEN H. LONG

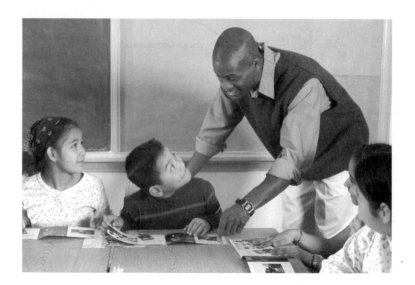

OBJECTIVES

After reading this chapter, you should be able to discuss

- Definitions of learning disabilities and other etiological categories with which learning disabilities overlap

- Relationships between language disorders and learning disabilities

- Differences between oral and written language and how these can contribute to learning disabilities

- General characteristics of the language of children with learning disabilities

- Principles of language intervention for children with learning disabilities

Although it now sounds familiar, the phrase "children with learning disabilities" is of fairly recent origin. The first use of the term by professionals in education was in 1962. It did not appear in federal legislative documents until 1968 (Hammill, 1990). This does not mean, of course, that children with learning problems did not exist until the 1960s. Rather, it reveals a change that has occurred since then in how we think about and label the problems. It also reflects the influence of the federal government. To a large extent, research on and educational practice with learning disabilities have been guided by actions taken in Washington, D.C. The single most important action was passage of the Education for All Handicapped Children Act (Public Law 94-142) in 1975, which provided an official definition of children with learning disabilities. Another important federal action, beginning in the 1980s, was the Regular Education Initiative (REI), which led the movement in favor of mainstreaming children with learning disabilities, that is, placing them in regular education classrooms for much of their schooling. These directions have since been continued and extended in federal legislation known as IDEA (Individuals with Disabilities Education Act).

Unfortunately, legislation alone cannot solve educational problems. The relationship of learning disabilities to other types of behavioral and learning problems is still unclear. Research has not yet determined what is the best model for representing the relationship among various types of language, speech, reading, writing, and learning impairments. Are they the same problem or different problems? If they are different, where is the line drawn between one type of disorder and the next? Because we do not fully understand the nature of the disabilities, it is not surprising that we lack a universally accepted plan of how these children should be assisted. Currently, it is a responsibility shared by a number of professionals.

An Overview of Children with Learning Disabilities

Professionals have struggled for years to develop a definition of learning disabilities that would be satisfactory to everyone. They have not succeeded, though some believe that a consensus view, if not a unanimous one, has evolved. Which definitions we use are important, inasmuch as they

- Determine how children are placed in our educational systems and the professionals who work them
- Influence government decisions about funding
- Influence funding decisions by local school districts
- Guide professional preparation programs and curriculum design
- Assist or hinder discussions among parents, physicians, psychologists, teachers, and other professionals

If, for example, a specialist attends an educational planning meeting, it must be clear what qualifies a student to receive special assistance for children with learning disabilities. It must also be clear what is meant by terms such as attention deficit hyperactivity disorder, specific language impairment, or central auditory processing disorder, all of which are used by certain professionals to describe some children who have learning disabilities.

Labels and Terminology

Various diagnostic labels have been used to refer to children who have trouble learning. Like clothing fashions, labels tend to have a period of general popularity, after which they retain this popularity only with certain professional groups or in certain regions. Some labels are intended to be purely descriptive, whereas others refer to what is presumed to be a cause of a child's learning problems. Following is a list of several terms that are commonly applied by educators and other professionals. We will briefly discuss the meaning of each of these labels.

> ### Descriptive
> Learning disabilities
> Dyslexia
> Slow learner
> Attention deficit hyperactivity disorder
> Phonological processing disorder
>
> ### Etiological
> Central auditory processing disorder
> Minimal brain dysfunction
> Developmental apraxia of speech

Learning Disabilities.   Over the years, different definitions of learning disabilities have enjoyed some degree of support by professionals. The two most influential definitions, however, have been those put forward by the National Joint Committee on Learning Disabilities (NJCLD) and the U.S. Office of Education (USOE). These are cited in Table 4.1.

How do the two definitions differ? A careful reading of the two finds that the NJCLD definition is different on three points:

1. It shifts away from the position that underlying perceptual-motor difficulties ("basic psychological processes") are at the root of all learning disabilities. This change more accurately reflects research findings.
2. It emphasizes the heterogeneous nature of learning disabilities and the fact that they are not limited to children.
3. It revises the interpretation of concomitant conditions. The USOE definition is often referred to as exclusionary in that it stipulates conditions that cannot coexist with learning disabilities, such as intellectual disabilities or economic disadvantage. Under a strict interpretation, this means that children from backgrounds of poverty cannot be diagnosed as having learning disabilities. The wording of the NJCLD definition makes such a diagnosis possible.

Both the NJCLD and USOE definitions make it plain that children with learning disabilities may show problems across a range of skills. What the definitions do not state, but is of intense interest to researchers and practitioners alike, is whether all children with learning disabilities have a single underlying problem or whether they should be regarded as falling into subgroups. A number of researchers have attempted to classify learning dis-

TABLE 4.1   Two Major Definitions of Learning Disabilities

National Joint Committee on Learning Disabilities (1991a)	U.S. Office of Education, as contained in the Individuals with Disabilities Education Act (IDEA) (P.L. 101–476) [34 CFR 300.7(c)(10]
Learning disabilities is a general term that refers to a heterogeneous group of disorders manifested by significant difficulties in the acquisition and use of listening, speaking, reading, writing, reasoning, or mathematical abilities. These disorders are intrinsic to the individual, presumed to be due to central nervous system dysfunction, and may occur across the life span. Problems in self-regulatory behaviors, social perception, and social interaction may exist with learning disabilities but do not by themselves constitute a learning disability. Although learning disabilities may occur concomitantly with other handicapping conditions (for example, sensory impairment, mental retardation, serious emotional disturbance) or extrinsic influences (such as cultural differences, insufficient or inappropriate instruction), they are not the direct result of those conditions of influence.	A disorder in one or more of the basic psychological processes involved in understanding or in using language, spoken or written, that may manifest itself in an imperfect ability to listen, think, speak, read, write, spell, or to do mathematical calculations, including conditions such as perceptual disabilities, brain injury, minimal brain dysfunction, dyslexia, and developmental aphasia. The term does not include learning problems that are primarily the result of visual, hearing, or motor disabilities, of mental retardation, of emotional disturbance, or of environmental, cultural, or economic disadvantage.

abilities into subtypes, using a variety of statistical and analytical methods. Generally, there have been two approaches to classification (Lyon & Risucci, 1988). In the *clinical-inferential approach,* investigators have examined batteries of test scores and identified groups of children with common profiles. Following this method, three subgroups of children with learning disabilities have been distinguished (Mattis, French, & Rapin, 1975):

1. Those with difficulty on language and language-related tasks (40 to 60 percent of the population)
2. Those with articulatory and graphomotor (handwriting/drawing coordination) deficits (10–40 percent)
3. Those with visuospatial perceptual deficits (5 to 15 percent)

The second approach, used in more recent studies, has been to identify subgroups from *statistical analyses.* For example, researchers have studied children who score poorly on achievement tests despite average or above-average intelligence (Satz & Morris, 1981). By examining the statistical interrelationships among scores from a battery of neuropsychological tests, five types of children with learning disabilities have been revealed:

1. Those with global language impairment (30 percent of the population)
2. Those with selective impairment of naming (16 percent)
3. Those with a mixed deficit of language impairment and difficulty on visual-perceptual-motor tasks (11 percent)

4. Those with impairment only on nonlanguage visual-perceptual-motor tests (26 percent)
5. Those with normal performance on all the neuropsychological tests (13 percent)

Children with learning disabilities can also be differentiated by the age at which their problems are first observed—a *historical* approach. Three patterns have been identified in these children's language-learning histories (Donahue, 1986):

1. Children diagnosed during the preschool years with obvious language learning problems or evidence of attention deficit hyperactivity disorder (ADHD) (Blackman, 2000; Connor, 2002)
2. Children who enter school with adequate interpersonal communication skills but who soon show poor performance
3. Children who initially fare well in school but eventually exhibit problems

Each of these three approaches—the clinical-inferential, the statistical, and the historical—offers insights into the factors that can distinguish one child with learning disabilities from another. None, however, represents a canonical view of the disorder that can be used to classify children, place them into different educational settings, or identify particular intervention strategies.

Dyslexia (Reading Disabilities).   Of all the basic skills affected in children with learning disabilities, reading is the most often impaired. Some 80 percent of this population shows some impairment in reading decoding or comprehension (President's Commission on Excellence in Special Education, 2002). The term *dyslexia* (or other terms, such as *reading disability* or *specific reading disorder*) is usually used to describe a specific problem of children with learning disabilities—learning to read. Thus, a child with dyslexia is presumed to be of normal intelligence and without any serious sensory or emotional disorders. One would not refer to a child with intellectual disabilities or autism as also exhibiting dyslexia.

Although problems in reading are found in the majority of children with learning disabilities, the relationship between dyslexia and other kinds of learning deficiency is not fully understood. Some scholars have argued that children with language impairment and children with reading impairment should be regarded as subgroups of children with learning disabilities. There may be extreme subgroups in both categories, that is, children with marked language impairment but relatively good reading skills, and children with reading impairment but mild language impairment (Kamhi & Catts, 1986). Longitudinal studies show individual variation. In the main, however, it appears that children who are failing to read by the end of first grade almost never catch up in elementary school (Catts, Fey, Zhang, & Tomblin, 2001).

Early research into the causes of dyslexia tended to focus on visual perceptual skills. That perspective dimmed, however, as researchers failed to find evidence of significant perceptual differences in children with dyslexia. In place of the perceptual deficit model has come what has been called the *developmental language perspective* (Kamhi & Catts, 1991), which emphasizes the connection between reading deficits and problems in other language skill areas: speech production, grammatical morphology, vocabulary learning, spelling, composition, and so on.

However, while the majority of recent academic research into dyslexia has concentrated on issues of language competence, some public and media attention has focused on reports about a supposedly simple but effective optical remedy for the problem. Beginning in 1983, psychologist Helen Irlen began to treat adults and children with dyslexia by providing them with colored lenses and spectacles (Irlen, 2002). These lenses, it was claimed, served to stabilize the visual images on a page, making the perceptual component of reading less taxing. For some individuals, the lenses appeared to have a markedly beneficial effect. Research suggests that "scotopic sensitivity" runs in families and that these individuals may have cellular deficits in the portion of the brain that is responsible for low-contrast vision (Livingstone, Rosen, Drislane, & Galaburda, 1991; Robinson, Foreman, & Dear, 1996). The use of colored lenses may compensate for this inherent defect and permit the visual system of the impaired reader to function in a more normal manner. Further work is needed to confirm the reported findings, to explore the generality of this visual deficit (do all children with dyslexia have it?), and to study its relationship to other kinds of language impairment that children with dyslexia are known to have.

Slow Learner. It is obvious to any observer that children with learning disabilities do not acquire certain skills easily. However, this cannot be taken to mean that difficulty in learning always signals a learning disability. Learning disability should not be confused with either low achievement or underachievement (National Joint Committee on Learning Disabilities, 1989). *Low achievement,* the simple failure to learn, may be due to other causes, such as intellectual disability, sensory impairment, or adverse emotional, social, and environmental conditions. *Underachievement,* the failure of a child to learn up to the level suggested by cognitive ability (IQ testing) is a necessary but not sufficient criterion for the diagnosis of learning disabilities. It, too, can result from conditions in a child's environment that reduce the opportunity or motivation to learn.

Behind these definitional distinctions lies a major issue of diagnosis that can determine which children receive services. In the majority of states today (see the section on "Prevalence"), children are identified as learning disabled by means of an ability–achievement discrepancy method. We encountered this in a slightly different form in the previous chapter in the discussion of the mental age–language age (MA–LA) gap. For example, in some states a child's achievement test scores must be two or more standard deviations (2 SD) below the child's IQ score. It has been asserted that the use of a discrepancy definition penalizes children who score poorly on IQ tests because of their cultural background and are also reading disabled and/or language impaired. Because these children will not show a large discrepancy, they will likely be labeled as slow learners rather than learning disabled. Despite its widespread use the discrepancy method of distinguishing between children who are low achieving and learning disabled has, therefore, been severely criticized. It may not be the most accurate way of differentiating between the two types of problems. For this reason, it is not always applied evenly in states where it is the official criterion for classifying a child as learning disabled.

Attention Deficit Hyperactivity Disorder (ADHD). Children who are hyperactive have difficulty in directing and sustaining attention and are therefore often impaired in their ability to learn, especially from formal instruction. They are also likely to interfere with the activities of those around them. For this reason, the American Psychiatric Association considers attention deficit hyperactivity disorder to be one class of disruptive behavior disorder. The official definition of ADHD is given in Table 4.2.

TABLE 4.2   Definition of ADHD

Symptoms of ADHD are divided into two categories:

Inattention
Often fails to give close attention to details or makes careless mistakes in schoolwork, work, or other activities

Often has difficulty sustaining attention in tasks or play activities

Often does not seem to listen when spoken to directly

Often does not follow through on instructions and fails to finish schoolwork, chores, or duties in the workplace (not due to oppositional behavior or failure to understand instructions)

Often has difficulty organizing tasks and activities

Often avoids, dislikes, or is reluctant to engage in tasks that require sustained mental effort (such as schoolwork or homework)

Often loses things necessary for tasks or activities (e.g., toys, school assignments, pencils, books, or tools)

Is often easily distracted by extraneous stimuli

Is often forgetful in daily activities

Hyperactivity-Impulsivity
Often fidgets with hands or feet or squirms in seat

Often leaves seat in classroom or in other situations in which remaining seated is expected

Often runs about or climbs excessively in situations in which it is inappropriate (in adolescents or adults, may be limited to subjective feelings of restlessness)

Often has difficulty playing or engaging in leisure activities quietly

Is often "on the go" or often acts as if "driven by a motor"

Often talks excessively

Often blurts out answers before questions have been completed

Often has difficulty awaiting turn

Often interrupts or intrudes on others (e.g., butts into conversations or games)

Based on the presence or absence of these symptoms over the previous 6 months or longer, a child is classified in one of three types of ADHD:
- Combined type (ADHD,C), which requires children to display at least six of nine Inattention and six of nine Hyperactivity-Impulsivity symptoms
- Predominantly inattentive type (ADHD,IA), which requires at least six of nine Inattention symptoms and fewer than six Hyperactivity-Impulsivity symptoms
- Hyperactive-impulsive type (ADHD,HI), which requires the presence of six of nine Hyperactivity-Impulsivity symptoms and fewer than six Inattention symptoms.

Note: In the past, other terminology has been used to describe children with ADHD. The condition was first described as *brain damage;* the next term in common use was *minimal brain dysfunction* (MBD); following this, the label *hyperactivity* was applied. In 1980, the American Psychiatric Association adopted the term *attention deficit disorder (ADD)* and described it in two forms: *attention deficit disorder with hyperactivity* (ADDH) and *attention deficit disorder without hyperactivity* (ADD without H). In 1987 the distinction between these two forms was dropped. In 1994 the three types of ADHD described above were adopted for use by the American Psychiatric Association.

Source: Adapted from American Psychiatric Association (2000).

Professionals who work with children for learning disabilities should be well acquainted with ADHD, although prevalence figures range widely. A general estimate is that 3 to 7 percent of U.S. children suffer from ADHD (American Psychiatric Association, 2000). The estimate for children of school age is comparable (Stanford & Hynd, 1994). Differentiating ADHD from specific language impairment or learning deficits may be difficult. Professionals must observe children at some length to determine whether they are easily distracted in all settings or only in those with verbal stimuli (Prizant et al., 1990). Moreover, the categories of learning disability and ADHD are heterogeneous and can co-occur in the same child (Murphy & Hicks-Stewart, 1991; Shaywitz, Fletcher, & Shaywitz, 1995). In addition to inattentiveness, impulsivity, and hyperactivity, characteristics manifested in children diagnosed as ADHD include "learning disorder" and "academic underachiever" (Marshall & Hynd, 1997; Stanford & Hynd, 1994). ADHD and learning disability are estimated to co-occur in 20 to 50 percent of cases, depending on how the conditions are defined or assessed (Javorsky, 1996; Riccio & Jemison, 1998).

Phonological Processing Disorder/Developmental Apraxia of Speech. The term *phonological processing disorder* has two senses. In some language-impaired children it is used as a variant of phonological disorder or phonological disability to describe a condition in which a child's speech is systematically simplified and, therefore, is less intelligible to listeners. In other language-learning-impaired children the term refers to an individual whose ability to process (e.g., encode and decode) phonological information is impaired, leading to problems in reading, spelling, word retrieval, and other language skills. Although older children with phonological processing disturbances may, in fact, have difficulty saying words and phrases that are phonologically complex (Catts, 1986, 1989), their speech is nearly always intelligible. The problems they exhibit at a phonological level are primarily metalinguistic and are seen most clearly on experimental tasks such as phoneme and syllable segmentation ("How many sounds are in the word *block*?" "How many syllables are in the word *caterpillar*?").

Among children with speech that is difficult to understand, some investigators have identified a subgroup of individuals who present with *developmental apraxia of speech* (DAS). There is no consensus regarding the nature or prevalence of this condition, and there is evidence that it is falsely diagnosed in the majority of cases (Davis, Jakielski, & Marquardt, 1998; Shriberg & McSweeny, 2002). However, among those children who do evidence the condition, the following symptoms are common:

- Presence of other types of apraxia, such as oral apraxia (affecting nonspeech oral movements) or limb apraxia (affecting the hands)
- Inconsistent sound substitutions that are often distant from the target, for example, /m/ for /s/
- Exceptional difficulty in producing multisyllabic words
- Unusual patterns of stress and intonation that often persist even after speech becomes intelligible
- Poor response to conventional articulation therapy methods

There appears to be some overlap between the groups of children identified with learning disabilities and with DAS. It has even been claimed that the children with DAS are identical with those identified in clinical-inferential studies as exhibiting articulatory and graphomotor coordination deficits (Wiig, 1986).

Central Auditory Processing Disorder.   The relationship between language learning and hearing cannot always be expressed in terms that are satisfyingly simple, as we will see in Chapter 8. The rather controversial set of relationships that have been identified by some professionals as constituting a *central auditory processing disorder* (CAPD) is one of these. The condition of CAPD is not well bounded clinically, and this is one of the reasons it is disputed (Keith, 1999), as discussed in Chapter 8. Nevertheless, for children identified with CAPD, their case histories often reveal that they have also been identified as learning disabled or that they display a pattern of school performance very similar to that of children with learning disabilities. As an example, a study of 64 children, 7 to 11 years of age, who were referred for CAPD, evaluation showed that 55 percent of them were receiving special services in school (Smoski, Brunt, & Tannahill, 1992). Only half of the children were reading at grade level, but the percentage of those working at grade level in science, spelling, language arts, and math was 69 percent or higher. Over 92 percent of the children were rated by their teachers as at least average in general disposition, response to discipline, enjoyment of school, and peer interaction. The only marked behavioral difference was concentration: 56 percent of the children were rated as below average.

Minimal Brain Dysfunction.   In the history of the field of learning disabilities, the term *minimal brain dysfunction* (MBD) has an important place (Kavale & Forness, 1985). The term *brain-injured* was first used by Strauss and Lehtinen (1947) to describe a child who showed "disturbances in perception, thinking, and emotional behavior" (p. 4). Later it was asserted that brain injury could be diagnosed from behavioral evidence such as perceptual and conceptual difficulties and hyperactivity (Strauss & Kephart, 1955). The notion of "soft signs" as an indication of subtle neurological dysfunction grew out of this contention. Nevertheless, some objected to the use of *brain-injured* to describe a child who had no history of injury and showed no "hard" or "frank" signs of neurological damage. Thus, the term slowly changed, first by the addition of the modifier *minimal* and then by the substitution of *dysfunction* for *injury* or *damage.* The resulting label, *minimal brain dysfunction,* was popularized within the medical community in the 1960s. Clements (1966), a physician, wrote an influential report for the U.S. Department of Health, Education and Welfare in which he described children with MBD as "of near average, average, or above average general intelligence with certain learning or behavioral disabilities ranging from mild to severe, which are associated with deviations of functions of the central nervous system" (p. 9). However, passage of PL 94–142 in the 1970s had the effect of shifting some of the responsibility for disabled children away from medicine and toward education. It did not take long, therefore, before MBD was criticized within the educational community precisely because it reflected a medical-etiological model rather than an educational model focusing on assessment and remediation. Most children who display behaviors characteristic of MBD will today be described using other diagnostic labels.

Prevalence

Federal and State Guidelines.   Federal education guidelines do not state what requirements must be met in order for a child to receive special education. Thus, it has been left to the states to set eligibility criteria and establish procedures for diagnosing learning disabilities. According to Mercer, Jordan, Allsopp, and Mercer (1996), as of 1996, almost half of the states did not include a "neurological" component in their definitions, 29 percent of the states had specified an IQ cutoff that differentiated children with intellectual disabilities and learning disabilities, and 76 percent had established specific methods for determining a discrepancy between ability and achievement. In determining the presence of a discrepancy, the most common method described was standard score comparison (e.g., a child's achievement scores must be 2 SD or more below the IQ score). Statistical analysis has indicated that the effect of these changes in definition by the various states has been to *reduce* the number of students identified as learning disabled.

General Estimates.   From 1977 to 2001, the number of children with learning disabilities receiving special education increased from 782,095 to 2,871,966, a 267 percent increase over that period. Within this range of years, the annual rate of increase from 1977 to 1983 averaged 14 percent. Since 1990, the rate has slowed to 3.4 percent per year, indicating that many states have changed their eligibility criteria, thereby stemming the flow of children qualifying for service (U.S. Department of Education, 2001b).

Male:Female Ratios.   It has long been reported that far more boys than girls are diagnosed with learning disabilities. In 1995, only 2.1 percent of girls in grades 1 through 12 were identified as having a learning disability, compared to 4.5 percent of boys (Bae, Choy, Geddes, Sable, & Snyder, 2000). It may be that boys are identified more often because they tend to exhibit more overt signs of the disorder, such as hyperactivity and behavioral disruption in school (Arnold, 1996; Gaub & Carlson, 1997). On the other hand, conditions associated with learning disabilities show certain gender differences. Reading disorders are significantly associated with hyperactivity in boys but not in girls (Willcutt & Pennington, 2000). Girls with ADHD tend to have greater intellectual impairments, lower levels of hyperactivity, lower rates of conduct disorder, and higher rates of mood and anxiety disorders (Gaub & Carlson, 1997)

Risk Factors

In the previous chapter, we referred to risk factors for specific language impairment (SLI). The term *risk factor* refers to a condition that increases the likelihood of a particular disease or injury. It is helpful to be aware of the factors that have been shown to be related to a risk of learning disabilities.

Attention Deficit Hyperactivity Disorder.   We noted earlier that a high percentage of school-aged children with speech and language disorders and/or learning disabilities also present with ADHD. It is tempting to infer a causal relationship from this finding, but it is not clear which condition is the cause and which is the effect, if either is. More to the point, ADHD is not found in all children with learning disabilities or vice versa. Even when ADHD is present in a child with learning disabilities, it does not necessarily complicate the problem. Hyperactive and nonhyperactive children with learning disabilities show few differences on tests that measure cognitive maturity and style (Copeland & Weissbrod, 1983). Children with ADHD alone perform comparably to non-ADHD children on standardized language tests (Oram, Fine, Okamoto, & Tannock, 1999).

Hearing Loss.   Hearing loss can be regarded as a risk factor for learning disabilities in two ways. First, there appears to be a subpopulation of deaf students (approximately 6 to 7 percent) who also have a concomitant learning disability (Bunch & Melnyk, 1989). These students obviously have special needs that extend well beyond those of hearing students with learning disabilities. The second and more commonly identified risk factor is conductive hearing loss. In surveys of children with learning disabilities, estimates of middle-ear pathology range from a low of 15.7 percent to a high of 49 percent (Bennett, Ruuska, & Sherman, 1980; Freeman & Parkins, 1979; Gibbs & Cooper, 1989; Masters & March, 1978). Taken as a whole, it is reasonable to expect that one in four elementary school children identified by schools as learning disabled will have experienced recurrent episodes of otitis media (ear infections). Estimates of the number of children with learning disabilities and measurable conductive hearing loss range from 7.4 percent to 38 percent. The discrepancy in findings is perhaps due to differences in screening procedures.

Heredity.   There has been a long-standing suspicion among professionals that learning disabilities run in families. If we take the view that language problems are frequently closely associated with many forms of learning disabilities, the risk factors related to a family history of language problems, as discussed in the previous chapter, may lend additional support to the suspicion of a hereditary factor in learning disabilities. Research indicates that the child of a parent with reading disability is eight times more likely to have the same disability than others in the general population. However, this increased risk is not due to genetic factors alone; environmental factors within families also appear to play an important role (Lyon et al., 2001). Paralleling our discussion of the interacting roles of heredity and environmental factors in SLI, when one or more of a child's family members have learning disabilities, the family environment with regard to learning and other features will necessarily be different than that of families without the presence of learning disabilities. For the child with an inherited learning disability in such a family environment, both the child's intrinsic learning characteristics and extrinsic family environment will contribute in varying combinations to the child's learning disability and the ways in which it is manifested.

The Natural History of Learning Disabilities

Definitions of learning disabilities do not state a minimum age for applying this diagnostic label, yet it is rare to hear the term applied to preschool children. Programs for preschool children with learning disabilities vary widely across states. Some states provide no funding for preschoolers with this diagnosis, and there appears to be a good deal of confusion nationwide over appropriate terminology for describing young children with language and learning problems.

For many years it has been recognized that the problem in terminology centers on the distinction between what we call *language disorders* and *learning disabilities.* Most definitions of learning disabilities make it clear that children with learning disabilities commonly exhibit impairments of language, and a review of the previous discussion on possible subtypes of learning disabilities illustrates how frequently language problems are seen in children with learning disabilities. In cases where the child is a preschooler, the label SLI, as we know from Chapter 3, may be applied. In school, when language problems are a significant feature of a child's learning difficulties, the term *language-learning disability* might be used. Whether children are described as having learning disabilities, SLI, or language-learning disabilities often is determined by their age, as well as funding that is available for the provision of services for the children. This confusion also means that many of these children are referred to in the literature as school-age children with language impairments, and information relevant to these children commonly applies to children referred to in the literature as learning disabled.

Most professionals now emphasize that language disorders and learning disabilities must be understood in terms of their *natural history* (Bashir, 1989; Bashir & Scavuzzo, 1992). That is, a language disorder is a lasting problem that manifests itself in different ways as a child grows older. The differences in symptoms and levels of severity are the result of changes in communicative contexts and the learning tasks that a child faces. As these children grow older, the language impairment shows up in different ways. As we saw in Chapter 3, language impairment among preschool children is typically identified when they have difficulty with the basic communicative functions of talking and understanding speech. Once the children begin school and receive literacy instruction, we begin to identify problems in other aspects of learning that have a language component. These include metalinguistic abilities, narrative and classroom discourse, and figurative language, as well as written language skills.

Although the majority position at this time appears to be that language disorders and learning disabilities represent different points on a developmental continuum, several cautions are warranted. First, the position should not be misinterpreted to mean that all children with learning disabilities are also language impaired. Research on subtypes of learning disabilities, reviewed earlier, suggests that most but not all children with learning disabilities are deficient in some language skill or skills. Second, children with learning disabilities who have no history of spoken language impairment are not immune to language-learning deficits. Thus, children might be able to perform adequately during the preschool years when only oral language is required, but find themselves overmatched once they are asked to read and write. Third, it is possible that there are subgroups among children with language-learning disabilities. The suggestion has also been made that the labels *language disorder* and *learning disability* are applied differentially by professionals, even though they have no formal guidelines for doing so.

As part of their understanding of the natural history of language disorders and learning disabilities, professionals must inevitably address the issue of recovery. Crystal (1984) has framed the question this way:

> Do you believe that, if you had all the time in the world, and all the resources that you needed, the child would be normal one day? (p. 149)

We have already noted that many preschoolers diagnosed with language impairment continue to show that impairment—in different forms—as they grow older, while others seem not to continue to show obvious signs of language impairment. However, the issue of *illusory recovery* (Scarborough & Dobrich, 1990), discussed in Chapter 3, may be relevant for these children. Recall that it has been suggested that some preschoolers appear to recover because of the stair-step nature of language development. Typically developing children, it is asserted, show spurts of growth separated by extended plateaus (Scarborough & Dobrich, 1990). Children with language impairment are able to catch up during the normal children's plateau phase, only to fall behind when the normal children spurt again in the early school years.

Another perspective on recovery from language impairment and learning disabilities can be taken at the end of a child's education. To what extent do children—now young adults—show persisting social, educational, and vocational problems as a result of their deficits? In Chapter 5 we will see evidence that language impairment and associated learning problems are persistent. At the university level, learning disability was the fastest-growing category of reported disability among students between 1988 and 2000. By 2000, 40 percent of freshmen with disabilities cited a learning disability, compared with only 16 percent in 1988 (Henderson, 2001). An extensive follow-up study was reported on students with learning disabilities who had attended vocational-technical programs (Shapiro & Lentz, 1991). The general findings of this survey were that these students

- Often did not have plans for the future when they graduated
- Received most of their help after graduation from friends, family members, and co-workers
- Often (50 to 60 percent) worked in areas unrelated to their vocational training
- Remained at low income levels

These results do little to dispel the notion that learning disabilities, often with concomitant language problems, are likely to remain life-long disabilities.

Linguistic Issues Relevant to Learning Disability

As children grow older and advance in school, they are regularly expected to expand and reorganize their language systems. They must come to understand and treat language as a set of tools, as something that can be reflected upon and consciously altered to suit particular educational or social purposes. Children must also deal with a new layer of arbitrary symbolism: the printed word. Not only must they learn to recognize units of written language and their relationship to speech, they must also appreciate the sometimes subtle differences between the written and spoken word and be able to shift smoothly from one language system to another. Upon entering school, children encounter a new world, where the rules for communication are designed to promote good conduct and enhance the learning process. And, of course, older children are expected to know more and act more responsibly. Expectations for both the form and content of language continue to rise, and learning must become an activity that is both self-initiated and self-corrected.

Metalinguistic Skills

The ability to think about and eventually talk about language is the most significant linguistic achievement of the school-aged child. Metalinguistic skill, as it is called, cuts across both spoken and written language and facilitates the child's acquisition of independent problem-solving abilities (van Kleeck, 1994a).

In school, children's metalinguistic knowledge expands at all levels of language. Once children are able to read proficiently, their exposure to sophisticated aspects of language increases dramatically (Nippold, 2002). As learners of semantics, they must be able to discover and explain word definitions, deal comfortably with components of lexical organization (e.g., oppositions and similarities), and distinguish between literal and nonliteral meanings and among various types of nonliteral meaning (e.g., word play, irony, humor, metaphor). As learners of grammar, children must be able to identify and manipulate constituent structures to clarify the meaning of what they read ("What does 'come what may' mean?"), to improve their writing ("Where should this paragraph go?"), or to learn foreign languages ("What's the imperfect form of *poder?*"). To participate fully in social situations, children must also develop *metapragmatic skills,* that is, be able to communicate about situational differences in language use in order to function adequately in peer groups ("Don't talk that way in mixed company"), in school ("That kind of language belongs on the playground, not in here"), and at work ("Don't say that to the boss"). The social penalties for using inappropriate language in any of these settings can be severe.

Differences between Spoken and Written Language

In Chapter 1, some of the similarities and differences between listening and speaking and reading and writing were introduced. When we review these and other similarities and differences between these two language forms, it may be easier to understand why some children with learning disabilities find the demands of the two forms unequal.

Children learning to read and write face much stiffer demands for lexical understanding and use. When they speak, children can take advantage of physical context and listener knowledge to patch up deficiencies in vocabulary. Deictic words such as *these* and *here* work wonderfully in speech when they are accompanied by an appropriate gesture. In writing, however, they must function *anaphorically,* that is, the items or place to which they refer must have been explicitly mentioned earlier in the text. Thus, deictic words cannot be used to overcome a lack of vocabulary. In speech, some allowance is made for the use of vague words. We all say *thing, stuff, guy,* and *sort of* and allow others to do the same. In writing, however, more precise communication is expected. Words must be carefully evaluated for subtle differences in meaning, using tools such as a dictionary or thesaurus if necessary. And since this is the expectation for writing, it follows that children will confront more sophisticated vocabulary when they read. Indeed, many words will be found only in the context of reading. To be successful readers, therefore, children must develop extensive recognition vocabularies that, for the most part, are triggered only by the visual stimulus of the word.

It is easy to observe that people do not write and talk in the same way. Beyond the differences in vocabulary, however, it is not always simple to identify the formal differences between the two. First, we must ignore those instances of writing masquerading as speech, such as dramatic conversations (in plays, soap operas) or television news, when the reporter reads from the teleprompter while looking into the camera. *Real* speech is characterized by relatively high rates of formulation breakdown—repetition, pauses, filled pauses, revision—while published writing is free of these disturbances. More important, though, are the differences in the *lexical density* and *redundancy* of written and spoken language (Miller & Weinert, 1998; Perera, 1984). Following is an example of the same information presented in spoken and written forms:

Spoken Language

The man came into the store and came up to the counter. He asked me for some change and I told him that we didn't make change you know because people are always asking us for change but I told him that the laundromat next door had a change machine so he could get some there.

Written Language

When the man came into the store he approached the counter and requested some change. Because of all the requests we receive for change I referred him to the change machine in the laundromat next door.

Whereas speech has a high frequency of repetition, rephrasing, and clausal coordination, the preference in writing is for conciseness characterized by single statements employing clausal embedding. These constructions, while elegant, cannot be comprehended as easily, especially by children with language impairment.

Differences between Home and School Language

A child who is new to school soon discovers that life in a classroom is different from life at home. Most people would say that the child must learn to follow a new set of *routines*. Scholars have refined this concept and relabeled it as an event script. A *script* is a generalized representation of the varied experiences that occur within an event (Creaghead, 1990, 1992). For example, as adults we have internalized a range of experiences about conducting transactions in banks. Consequently, we know what to expect when we enter an unfamiliar bank: there will be forms to fill out, a line to stand in, and tellers to serve us. We "know the routine," but we know it in a sufficiently general way that it can be adapted to any bank, not just the one we usually use.

To act appropriately in the classroom, normally achieving children must learn a number of scripts, which can be summarized as follows (Creaghead, 1990):

Arriving	Taking tests
Coming to class	Making things
Snack time	Recess
Following verbal directions	Going home
Cleaning up	Getting objects, information, help from the teacher
Completing workbook pages	Answering teacher's questions during lessons
Story time	Reading aloud
Getting homework	Following oral directions
"Show and tell"	Getting information, help from peers
Changing classes	Getting information, help from peers
Group time	Chatting with peers
Reading group	Negotiating rules for games, play
Free play	Planning, negotiating group projects
Reading for information	Explaining, defending behavior
Field trips	Relaying messages

Group lessons   Giving reports
Going outside   Pretending, role playing
Lunch   Giving directions
Going to the bathroom

Students with learning disabilities also must know the scripts, because most of them are taught in regular education classrooms for some part of their school day. Scripts serve to govern behavior in various classroom situations, but they also set the ground rules for communication. Children must know when they can speak freely and when they must request permission. They must know that the question, "Can you tell us about . . . ?" is really a request for an elaborated reply and should not be answered with a simple *yes* or *no*. They must know when it is appropriate to seek help from friends and when it is not.

Many of the language differences in school pertain to pragmatics; children learn to vary their use of language in different interpersonal and instructional contexts. We should not overlook, though, the changes in semantic and grammatical complexity that also accompany the school experience. Children are introduced to a host of new words in the classroom. Some of these words describe objects, people, and activities of the school itself (*assembly, roll call, principal, report card, grade*). Others are words that are crucial to instruction (*turn the page, skip, alike, identical, opposite*). There is also less fine tuning in the commands given in the classroom. Teachers typically must address an entire group of students and therefore cannot tailor instructions ("Pick up the scissors— the ones right next to you—on the table"), as might a parent speaking to an individual child.

Differences in Developmental Expectations for Language Knowledge and Use

Another way of viewing the changes that can affect children's school performance is simply to reflect on what we expect them to know at different ages. Both the content and method of school instruction change from grade to grade, as we saw in Chapter 2. In some cases, these changes can serve to trigger learning problems where none had existed previously. For example, children who struggle in learning to read might be diagnosed with dyslexia in grades 1 and 2. They might continue to learn normally in other academic areas because the method of instruction is the lecture and visual demonstration. Beginning in grade 3, however, these children would be asked to do more of their learning through reading and, consequently, they might begin to lag behind in several subjects.

Communication Problems in Children with Learning Disabilities

Characterizations of children with learning disabilities are based on research in which they have served as subjects. All conclusions from research should be regarded as tentative and subject to revision by future studies that replicate, refute, or reinterpret the earlier findings.

Readers should be aware that at least three general criticisms have been made of research on children with learning disabilities:

1. Most studies have selected subjects who display a significant discrepancy between achievement and intelligence test scores, the standard required by most state laws. Such criteria do not exclude children whose learning problems are due to poor motivation, poor instruction, or inadequate opportunities for learning. Thus, many investigations may have been conducted with children who are not truly learning disabled, as it is properly defined.

2. Some studies have been conducted with students attending private schools, which may not have explicit criteria for identifying children with learning disabilities. Although results from these studies may not be representative of the population of *system-identified* children with learning disabilities, quantitative comparison of these studies with ones that employed standard subject selection criteria showed no significant difference in outcome (Lapadat, 1991).

3. Studies that use samples of system-identified children with learning disabilities may produce different findings than studies in which children are identified by means of research criteria. In particular, comparison of the two types of investigations suggests that system-identified samples tend to underestimate the abilities of females with learning disabilities (Vogel, 1990).

With these reservations in mind, we can examine some of the major findings about the language skills of children with learning disabilities.

Semantics

Research on problems at the level of semantics falls into two broad categories: difficulty in organizing word meanings and difficulty in retrieving lexical items either during naming tasks or spontaneous speech. Many professionals consider word meaning and word retrieval as separate clinical problems, but, as we saw in the previous chapter and will reiterate here, at least one interpretation of the research views them as different manifestations of an underlying semantic deficit.

Word Meanings. Both clinical observation and controlled experiments indicate that children with learning disabilities have underdeveloped lexical systems. This is reflected by their impoverished vocabularies and poor metalinguistic knowledge. Clinical reports on children with learning disabilities frequently cite their difficulty with more advanced assessments of literal word meaning. For example, they are commonly found to misunderstand words with multiple meanings, such as *toast, rear,* or *catch.* They are also much less proficient at recognizing and using words that are structurally related, such as antonyms, synonyms, superordinates, and subordinates. Poor lexical knowledge is also evidenced in their inability to provide definitions of abstract nouns (e.g., *burden, gratitude, friendship*) that are precise and reflect their essential meaning (Nippold, 1999).

An even more problematic lexical task for children with learning disabilities is the comprehension and use of nonliteral meanings. Even though these students often perform comparably to other students on standardized tests of literal comprehension, they are poorer at explaining sentences consisting of metaphors or idioms, involving atypical or nonliteral description or comparison (e.g., "Spring is a lady in a new coat," "Pull up your socks") than their nondisabled peers (Abrahamsen & Sprouse, 1995; Nippold, 1991; Nippold & Taylor, 2002; Secord & Wiig, 1993). They tend to err by giving literal responses. Children with learning disabilities apparently are better at understanding similes (e.g., "David was like a thirsty puppy finding water") than metaphors (e.g., "David was a thirsty puppy finding water"), though they improve on both kinds of comprehension tasks as they get older (Seidenberg & Bernstein, 1986). This difference in comprehension has been interpreted as due to metacognitive factors—that is, a simile indicates explicitly, with the word *like,* that a comparison is being made. Children with learning disabilities apparently need this verbal cue in order to recognize that a nonliteral meaning is being expressed. Cues provided by story context or pictures have not been found to be effective in shifting these children from literal to nonliteral interpretations (Lee & Kamhi, 1990).

Word Retrieval.   There is both agreement and dispute over the so-called word retrieval skills of children with learning disabilities. Clinicians and researchers are in accord that these children show differences in verbal behavior. In both confrontation naming and spontaneous speech, children with learning disabilities produce a range of behaviors that are either different from those of normally achieving children or occur with higher frequency (Katz, 1996; Meyer, Wood, Hart, & Felton, 1998; Swan & Goswami, 1997; Wiig, Zureich, & Chan, 2000):

1. Items are described without being named directly (circumlocutions).
2. Another word is substituted for the target.
3. A previous response is repeated (perseveration).
4. Low-information words such as pronouns and indefinite adverbs (e.g., *somewhere, sometime*) are used excessively.
5. There is greater delay in producing the target word.
6. Extra verbalizations are produced (e.g., "oh, it's uh . . .").
7. Target words are preceded by initial-sound repetitions (e.g., "f, f, thumb").
8. There are greater difficulties in naming to description ("What do you call the end of your shirt sleeve?").

Different interpretations have been offered on the nature of the impairment that produces these behaviors. By analogy with the deficits seen in adults with brain injuries, some have described the impairment as one of word retrieval (German, 1982; Wiig & Semel, 1984). In this view the children are presumed to have adequately *learned* certain vocabulary but to have trouble retrieving and using that vocabulary productively. In contrast to this account is a series of experiments in which children with word-retrieval difficulty have been given various kinds of helpful cues (Kail & Leonard, 1986b; McGregor & Windsor, 1996). Based on their findings, the researchers suggest that these children do not show a specific retrieval deficit. Instead, it is argued, they are slower and less efficient at word-retrieval tasks because of their less elaborated word knowledge, which renders them less effective at using common retrieval strategies based on semantic and phonological linkages. That is, children with language impairment retrieve words in the same way as nonimpaired children, but they are less successful because the words have been learned less completely. This explanation collapses the clinical categories of word meaning and word retrieval into one problem area, which might be termed a *generalized semantic deficit.*

Grammar

For many years the general impression has been that children with learning disabilities perform at lower levels on most measures of language form. For example, between the ages of 7;8 and 12;5 years, students with learning disabilities show a very gradual linear increase in utterance length (Andolina, 1980). Over the same period, normally achieving children are consistently higher in average utterance length. Even more interesting, the normal children exhibit periods of rapid growth, whereas the children with learning disabilities maintain a constant slow rate of growth.

There is other evidence of grammatical impairment from studies employing structured communication tasks. For example, in tasks such as describing unfamiliar objects and summarizing fictional and nonfictional videos, children with learning disabilities in grades 2, 4, 6, and 8 produced fewer words per T-unit (one main clause with all the subordinate clauses attached to it) and per main clause than normally achieving students at the same grade levels (Donahue, Pearl, & Bryan, 1982; Scott & Windsor, 2000). At the level of morphology, many patterns described for preschoolers with SLI in the previous chapter continue to be seen such that school-age children with learning disabilities have been found, for example, to show poorer command of past-tense inflections than a normal language control group (Marchman, Wulfeck, & Ellis Weismer, 1999). In this study, most errors occurred with irregular forms. Elementary-school-age children with ADHD, both with and without an accompanying language impairment, exhibited particular difficulty on a sentence-formulation task (Oram et al., 1999). These kinds of findings have led many professionals to characterize children with learning disabilities as slow learners of grammatical form.

Recent research, however, indicates that among students with learning disabilities 8 to 13 years of age there is a subgroup who do not display grammatical disability, as judged by the type and accuracy of structures produced in spontaneous story telling (Roth & Spekman, 1989; Scott & Windsor, 2000). The participants in one study attended a private school for students with learning disabilities and had IQ scores that were approximately 15 to 20 points higher than those typically found in research samples of children with learning disabilities. Judging from this study, we should be careful not to assume that a child with learning disabilities will have impairments of language form, especially if the IQ is higher than the mean score of 100.

Narratives

An important area of assessment in children of school age is the comprehension and production of language units larger than the sentence. *Discourse analysis* is relevant to both spoken and written language. The analysis of spoken discourse is often conducted by asking children to produce or listen to and answer questions about narratives (stories). A body of research using these techniques has now developed, and it paints a fairly clear picture of the problems exhibited by children with learning disabilities:

- Their spontaneous narratives are shorter and contain fewer complete episodes (Garnett, 1986; Roth & Spekman, 1986).
- Their character descriptions are shallow, with few references to internal states such as fear, anger, revenge, surprise (Gillam & Carlile, 1997; Montague, Maddux, & Dereshiwsky, 1990; Ripich & Griffith, 1988; Roth & Spekman, 1986).

- They are less successful in judging the comparative importance of information in a story (Garnett, 1986).
- They give the impression of being egocentric narrators who do not consider the needs of the audience. This may be due to inadequate mastery of discourse skills such as anaphoric reference, topic maintenance, and event sequencing (Garnett, 1986; Miranda, McCabe, & Bliss, 1998).
- They may have less knowledge of the world to help them interpret events and motivations in stories (Garnett, 1986).
- In retelling stories, they reduce the amount of information contained in the original narrative (Montague et al., 1990; Ripich & Griffith, 1988).
- They show a greater rate of communication breakdowns (stalls, repairs, and abandoned utterances) in narration than in conversation, which is not true of nondisabled children (MacLachlan & Chapman, 1988; Thordardottir & Ellis Weismer, 2002).
- They are immature in their ability to answer inferential questions about stories read to them. These questions require them to reason with the facts presented in the narrative rather than simply recall the verbatim content of the story. They are more successful at making inferences about narratives they hear than narratives they read (Wright & Newhoff, 2001). Problems with inferential reasoning are especially acute for children with lower receptive vocabularies (Crais & Chapman, 1987).

Pragmatics

There is consensus that differences exist in the pragmatic language behaviors of children with and without learning disabilities. Lapadat (1991) used a meta-analytic statistical procedure[1] to compare the results of thirty-three studies in six pragmatic categories: vocabulary selection and use, topic management, use of different speech acts, paralinguistic and nonverbal behaviors, conversational turntaking, and stylistic variation. She found that there were differences in all six categories between children with language disorders or learning disabilities and typically developing children. The differences were significantly greater in the categories of lexical selection and use and speech acts than in turn taking and stylistic variation. This result suggests that so-called pragmatic deficiencies are more likely to be due to linguistic than to social deficits.

Topic Management.   Children with learning disabilities are likely to behave differently in verbal interactions with their peers and, as a consequence, often find less social acceptance (Vaughn, Elbaum, & Boardman, 2001). For example, when asked to work with a group in making a choice, children with learning disabilities are less likely to take the lead, keep the group on task, and persuade their peers to agree with their opinions (Bryan, Donahue, & Pearl, 1981). They are similarly passive in situations where they are asked to act as an interviewer of a peer (Bryan, Donahue, Pearl, & Sturm, 1981). In conversation they may seek information less often, causing them to be viewed as boring or disinterested (Mathinos,

---

[1]*Meta-analysis* is a statistical procedure that allows researchers to compare the results from multiple studies and reach conclusions about common findings. Comparison is made between *treatment effects,* a measure of the difference between the subject groups in each study.

1991). When called on to correct their peers, they may show less tact in their word selection (Pearl, Donahue, & Bryan, 1985).

Conversational Repair.   Because all conversations break down sometimes, the ability to detect and repair these disruptions is an important language competency, especially when the function of the conversation is to inform. Children with learning disabilities appear to be less effective, both as speakers and listeners, in effecting conversational repairs. As speakers, they may offer explanations that are confusing and, to compound the problem, they may have difficulty in reformulating their messages when asked to do so (Knight-Arest, 1984). When roles are reversed, they are less likely to request clarification of information that is unclear. Naturally, this can affect their performance in formal assessments (Shields, Green, Cooper, & Ditton, 1995).

Reading

To read and understand a page of text requires a number of psycholinguistic processes to operate:

- The letters on the page must be decoded to form an accurate phonological image of each word.
- The meanings of the individual words must be retrieved from memory.
- The syntactic structure represented by the words must be parsed to derive the meaning of the entire sentence.
- The meaning of consecutive sentences must be merged to create an understanding of the entire passage.
- If an individual is reading aloud, then speech production skills must also be brought to bear.

A disruption of any stage of the process will ultimately produce an impairment in reading.

Phonological awareness is the ability to think about and manipulate the sound structure of language. Together with knowledge of letter–sound correspondences, phonological awareness is a strong predictor of children's acquisition of decoding skills in reading (Adams, 1990; Treiman, Tincoff, Rodriguez, Mouzaki, & Francis, 1998). Phonological awareness begins with awareness of rhymes, alliteration, and sound play. Eventually, children learn to segment words into individual phonemes, and it is this skill that leads most directly to the onset of reading (Muter, 1998; Nation & Hulme, 1997). Children with reading disabilities show a lack of phonological awareness compared to good readers and are therefore likely to struggle at the stage of phonological decoding. They perform inferiorly on segmentation tasks that require them, for example, to divide words into syllables or syllables into phonemes (Catts & Kamhi, 1999). They also appeared to lag developmentally in the detection of prosodic cues such as pitch, stress, and pause, which signal the boundaries of sentences (Mann, Cowin, & Schoenheimer, 1989).

Semantic representations also may be difficult for children with reading disabilities to generate. Along with other types of children with learning disabilities, poor readers exhibit word-finding deficits (Blachman, 1984; Lerner, 2000; Wolf, 2000). They also have trouble identifying sentences that are grammatically ill-formed, which suggests that syntactic cues to meaning are probably not well represented (Kamhi & Koenig, 1985). On the other hand, a comparison of good readers and poor readers in the fourth grade found that although the poor readers had lower scores on a test of syntactic comprehension, there was no significant correlation between syntactic comprehension and reading comprehension when vocabulary was controlled (Glass & Perna, 1986). Thus, it is not clear whether breakdowns in forming semantic representations during reading should be attributed primarily to lexical or syntactic factors, or to other influences such as discourse referencing. A study of tenth- and eleventh-grade students with and without learning disabilities showed that the impaired students had significantly more difficulty in comprehending the referent of anaphoric pronouns that appeared in reading passages (Fayne, 1981).

Oral reading can be impaired by breakdowns at any of the previous stages and can also be affected by subtle speech production problems that may appear infrequently in conversation. Adolescents with reading disorders have been found to make significantly more errors in naming and repeating multisyllabic words and repeating phonologically complex phrases. Their performance on these speech-production tasks correlates significantly with their measured reading ability (Catts, 1986). Furthermore, when asked to speak as rapidly as possible, college students with dyslexia repeated complex phrases more slowly and had a higher rate of "slips of the tongue," that is, substitutions of sounds for phonetically similar segments that occur in similar syllable positions (e.g., "she shells" for "seashells") (Catts, 1989). This finding suggests that students with dyslexia are deficient in their ability to plan phonetic sequences and may explain many of the disruptions commonly seen in their oral reading.

What reason can be offered for the apparent speech impairments of children who are poor readers? In a study aimed at this question, Kamhi, Catts, and Mauer (1990) asked second- and third-grade children with reading disorders and their nondisabled peers to produce four multisyllabic nonsense words, a task similar to those used in nonword repetition tasks referred to in the previous chapter. The children with reading disorders needed significantly more trials to master the task. They were also significantly poorer in recognizing the correct response when they produced an error. This suggests that their problems are the result of phonological encoding deficits and not speech-production difficulties.

Writing

Without adequate skills in spoken language and reading, a student is destined to struggle with writing as well. The foundation abilities in writing—knowledge of vocabulary, syntax, and discourse structure—are derived from these same abilities in speech. Hence, certain writing problems are predictable from and will be consistent with these same problems in spoken language production.

There is also a very close and important relationship between reading and writing. Perera (1984) notes three aspects to this relationship:

1. Reading teaches the characteristic structures of written language.
2. Children must be able to read their own writing in order to evaluate and edit it to suit its intended audience.
3. Children must be able to proofread their own writing to correct superficial errors of spelling, grammatical form, and others.

The problems students meet in learning to write are varied, as would be expected for a complex activity that depends on many subskills. Studies of children and adults who are low-achieving students or who have been diagnosed with learning or reading disabilities show a range of problems in their writing, and especially in their expository writing (Espin, Scierka, Skare, & Halverson, 1999; Parker, Tindal, & Hasbrouck, 1991; Scott, 1991; Scott & Windsor, 2000; Treiman, 1997; Watkinson & Lee, 1992):

1. *Productivity:* In controlled writing tasks, such as creating a story to match a picture, poor writers produce fewer words and sentences.
2. *Text structure:* There is an overall lack of coherence and text organization. Topics are not well introduced, and conclusions are not logical. Errors occur in the use of cohesion devices such as pronouns and temporal adverbs.
3. *Sentence structure:* Sentences are grammatically less complex and contain errors of omission, substitution, and form agreement. The connective *and* is overused, and subordinating conjunctions (*if, because, since*) are often used incorrectly.
4. *Spelling:* Poor writers have a higher frequency of spelling errors and tend to produce more *nonphonetic* errors, that is, errors that are inconsistent with the pronunciation of the target word (e.g., *skool/school* is phonetic, *sookl/school* is nonphonetic).
5. *Lexicon:* The type:token ratio obtained from samples of poor writing is lower, indicating that words tend to be used repetitively.
6. *Handwriting:* Letters are poorly formed, unevenly spaced, and may contain a mix of lower- and uppercase, printing and cursive writing.

Although poor handwriting and spelling can be components of a child's writing difficulties, the source of the problem is clearly linguistic and is therefore not easily dispelled by the use of computers. Studies comparing compositions produced by word processing and by hand have shown no differences in mechanics, grammar, vocabulary, or reading (MacArthur & Graham, 1987; Nichols, 1996). Although the frequency and timing of text revisions is different when word processing is used, the overall quality of the writing remains unaffected (Grejda & Hannafin, 1992; MacArthur & Graham, 1987). Word-processed texts are not consistently longer or shorter than handwritten ones (MacArthur & Graham, 1987; Nichols, 1996; Outhred, 1989; Peterson, 1993).

Implications for Intervention

The problems experienced by children with learning disabilities are diverse and therefore require the expertise of a number of professionals (Table 4.3). Most children with learning disabilities remain in their regular, mainstream classrooms for a large portion of their instruction and services and, in many cases, the various educators and specialists collaborate in delivering services to the children in their classroom. Having a number of workers involved in the development and implementation of a child's program can lead to confusion caused by poor understanding and communication of one another's roles. There may even be situations in which professional jealousies develop over the issue of job responsibilities. The boundary lines separating psychology from speech–language pathology from special education are not clearly drawn. Moreover, they are subject to change as ideas evolve

TABLE 4.3 Professionals Involved in the Assessment and Treatment of Children with Learning Disabilities

Job Title	Job Description
Regular-education (classroom) teacher	Organizes and oversees the curriculum in the regular-education classroom.
Diagnostic-prescriptive teacher	Following a referral from the classroom teacher, observes and tests students with perceived academic or behavioral problems. Develops recommendations for individual teaching techniques and materials and then reviews and demonstrates these for the classroom teacher. Carries out periodic follow-up and evaluation.
School psychologist	Conducts psychoeducational evaluations of a child's intelligence, academic achievement, and social interactions and relationships. Consults with parents, classroom teachers, and other personnel regarding issues of cognitive style, cognitive maturity, and group and individual conduct.
Reading specialist	Evaluates problems of reading. Consults with regular-education teacher regarding students with relatively mild reading impairments who will benefit from corrective reading instruction delivered in the classroom. Provides intensive remedial instruction to students with more severe reading difficulties.
Resource teacher	Organizes and oversees instruction in a resource room, a common alternative to placement in self-contained special education classrooms. Usually instructs students with mild to moderate educational handicaps for up to half of their school day, with students spending the other portion of the time in a regular classroom. Some resource teachers are itinerant and provide services in the regular classroom.
Teacher aide	Prepares instructional materials, helps students with classroom work, and supervises students when they are outside the classroom.
Speech–language pathologist	Evaluates problems of speech and language. Consults with the classroom teacher about ways of coping with, compensating for, and overcoming a child's communication difficulties. Provides direct service to children with communication impairments.
School social worker	Provides a bridge of communication between the home and the school. Interviews parents and compiles a psychosocial history. May be responsible for handling problems of truancy. Frequently serves as case manager for the special education committee.
School physician	Evaluates a child's sight, hearing, physical development, medical needs, and physical factors that affect school progress.

within a discipline. For example, speech–language pathologists may now be more likely to work with children who are dyslexic, as a result of a conceptual shift that views reading impairment as a component of a larger language disorder (Catts & Kamhi, 1999).

Because we know that learning disabilities, typically with concomitant language problems, persist throughout the school years, many children with learning disabilities, although they do improve, can emerge from school with poorer preparation for work and, as a result, tend to have lower-paying jobs than their non-learning-disabled peers (Shapiro & Lentz, 1991). There is evidence to suggest, then, that these children may not able to compete with their normally achieving peers when their secondary education is complete. One factor that may influence the outcomes of children with learning disabilities might be the amount of language intervention that children receive. Children with language impairments identified before school age may receive intervention before they enter school, and intervention may continue during the school years. In contrast, children identified as learning disabled may not have been identified until the school years, when intervention may first begin. In these cases, it is possible that a large focus of intervention for these children will be on the academic manifestations of their learning disabilities rather than on their language difficulties. We can do nothing to change the complexity of language and the fact that demands for increased complexity increase with age. We can, however, begin to work as early as possible with language-impaired children and perhaps forestall or lessen certain types of learning disabilities. We can also improve our methods of intervention with school-age children by ensuring continuity and integration of services and investigating instructional, motivational, professional, and other variables that affect the success of our efforts.

Issues in Regular Education

Professionals need to be sensitive to the fact that learning disabilities interact with both developmental changes in children and shifts in the organization of the classroom. Language-learning problems may be manifested at different grade levels as new competencies are required. For example, word-finding difficulties may first be discovered as children attempt to join in class discussions or produce extended oral narratives. These children may be treated for the problem and develop greater oral language competence. Later in school, however, they will be required to produce written texts that demand even greater precision of expression. Word-finding difficulties are then likely to reappear. As children move from grade to grade, the structure of their formal education changes: the amount of play time decreases, and the number of different subjects and teachers increases. Children with learning disabilities will require special attention as they make major grade transitions, such as between kindergarten and first grade, between third and fourth grade, and between elementary and junior high school. These are times when professionals should be especially alert to referrals from classroom teachers, and they may want to assist in observing and identifying children who reveal new learning problems.

The move toward mainstreaming of students with disabilities was based on the perception that regular classrooms would provide better educational and social models. This practice, though generally well reviewed, has produced certain problems to which professionals need to be alert. The National Joint Committee on Learning Disabilities (1991b) has identified a number of these related to the education of students with learning disabilities in regular-education classrooms. These are listed in Table 4.4, along with the committee's proposed recommendations for solutions.

Psychosocial Problems and Reactions

An important piece of the puzzle presented by children with learning disabilities may be their psychosocial adjustment. We saw in the previous chapter, dealing with preschoolers with SLI, concerns about psychosocial issues, and we will see these raised again in the next chapter, as well as here. We expect most of these children to show some adaptation and response

TABLE 4.4   Problems and Recommended Solutions for the Education of Students with Learning Disabilities in Regular-Education Classrooms

Problem	Recommended Solution
Teachers often are required to adhere rigidly to a pre-scribed curriculum and materials, and therefore may not have the flexibility to address the unique needs of students with learning disabilities.	Establish instructional conditions and environments that allow teachers to capitalize on the strengths and remediate or compensate for the weaknesses of students with learning disabilities. These should include: ■ Appropriate materials and technology ■ Flexibility in determining the array of skills necessary for attainment of overall curricular objectives
Adequate support services, materials, and technology often are not available for either the teacher or the student with learning disabilities.	Ensure the availability of services needed to support the education of students with learning disabilities in the regular education classroom, including: ■ Appropriate related services for students ■ Consultation services for teachers ■ Direct services for students from teachers certified in the area of learning disabilities and other qualified professionals such as school psychologists, counselors, speech–language pathologists, reading teachers, audiologists, and social workers ■ Teaching assistants or aides trained to work with students who have learning disabilities
Time and support for the ongoing planning and assessment that are needed to make adjustments in students' programs and services often are inadequate.	Provide sufficient time for collaborative planning among and between professionals and parents.
Communication concerning students with learning disabilities among administrators, teachers, specialists, parents, and students is often insufficient for the development and implementation of effective programs.	

as they work to overcome or work around their disabilities. A greater percentage of children with learning disabilities tend to avoid social interaction in school (Pearl et al., 1998). Compared to their peers, they are more likely to feel rejected, neglected, and lonely in their school experiences (Margalit & Levin-Alyagon, 1994; Wiener, Harris, & Shirer, 1990). There is evidence that boys with learning disabilities react with more frustration and antisocial behavior than girls with similar impairments (Arnold, 1996; Gaub & Carlson, 1997).

One of the touted benefits of mainstreaming is that it will improve the self-image of children with disabilities by not isolating them from their nondisabled peers. However, as they go forward in school, the self-esteem of children with learning disabilities appears to worsen. In the earlier school years they may still be able to view themselves as competent and socially acceptable despite their academic struggles. By adolescence, however, and perhaps even in the later elementary school years, there is clear evidence that these children rate themselves lower on measures of scholastic competence, behavioral conduct, and global self-worth (Bear & Proctor, 1991; Harter, Whitesell, & Junkin, 1998; Jerome et al., 2002; McNulty, 2003). Findings from Redmond and Rice's (1998) study suggest that kindergarten and first-grade teachers tended to rate children with language disorders in their classrooms as having more social and behavioral problems than normally developing peers, even though the scores the children with language problems obtained on standardized sociobehavioral measurement instruments were within normal limits. Consistent with the speculation that we introduced in Chapter 3, the experiences and interactions of children with language-learning disabilities that they encounter in school may contribute to declining self-images of the children.

As we saw in Chapter 3, one view is that social skills deficits among children with learning disabilities are associated with high rates of undetected psychiatric diagnoses such as ADHD or depression (Cantwell & Baker, 1991; San Miguel, Forness, & Kavale, 1996; Treuting & Hinshaw, 2001). Another view is that these may reflect children's negative adaptations to their problems, consistent with a social adaptation model (Redmond & Rice, 1998). Though these relationships are now better understood and publicly discussed, not all teachers and other professionals may be aware of them, and some may need to be informed regarding the interactions of learning disabilities, language impairment, psychosocial development, and behavioral and emotional factors.

The Collaborative Service Delivery Model

Federal education legislation requires an Individualized Education Program (IEP) for each student and an interdisciplinary approach. Because an IEP has to be approved by all the educators working with a particular child—for example, the classroom teacher, school psychologist, speech–language pathologist, and reading specialist—educators have begun to work as part of a collaborative team, reviewing and endorsing one another's efforts (ASHA, 1991a; DiMeo, Merritt, & Culatta, 1998). In some cases, however, they still continue to work independently of the other team members in carrying out their assessments and intervention, without the direct assistance or consultation of the rest of the team.

Even though the various professionals involved in helping children with learning disabilities now work mostly in the children's classrooms and in line with the interdisciplinary IEPs for the children, there remain difficulties in overcoming professional isolationism and achieving collaborations so that what each does fits with what the others do. Features of the collaborative service delivery model include:

- Professionals work as part of a transdisciplinary team consisting of educators, parents, specialists and special educators, and the student.
- All treatment goals, assessment methods, intervention procedures, and documentation systems are planned mutually by members of the team.
- Team members share responsibility for implementation of the educational plan.
- Special education as well as regular instruction take place within the classroom to the extent appropriate for each child.

The success of the collaborative model is being increasingly documented (Farber & Klein, 1999; Hadley, Simmerman, Long, & Luna, 2000; Smith, McCauley, & Guitar, 2000;

Swenson, 2000). For language and learning, a number of advantages accrue from this model:

- Treatment occurs within genuine communicative contexts.
- Intervention is not as limited by a service schedule but can take place throughout the school day.
- Intervention can be provided by agents other than particular specialists.
- The setting is more appropriate for the use of procedures such as modeling, role playing, and group problem solving.
- There can be joint review and modification of texts and curriculum by all members of the educational team.
- Treatment time can be shared by team members.
- Self-esteem is promoted by allowing children to demonstrate to teachers their successes as well as their failures.
- Peer tutoring can take place and the strengths of one student can be used to help the weaknesses of another.

The Traditional Service Delivery Model

In the traditional service delivery model, sometimes referred to as a "pull-out" model, children leave their regular classrooms temporarily to receive services of specialists whose rooms are elsewhere in the school. Services can be provided individually to a child, or the children can be seen in groups. Though support for the collaborative service delivery model has grown, there continue to be settings and circumstances in which traditional pull-out service is provided and is appropriate. This does not mean, however, that specialists cannot or should not seek to improve lines of communication between themselves and other educators engaged in teaching children with learning disabilities. Specialists in communication should be active in suggesting ways to promote more effective language learning in the classroom. Following is a list of general recommendations.

1. Create a physical setting that promotes talk by providing workstations for collaborative learning and maintaining a set of regularly changing classroom displays to serve as a focus of conversation.

2. Promote verbal interaction in the process of learning by leading group discussions, asking children to verbalize as they problem-solve, and using cross-age and cross-ability groupings so that children explain concepts and processes to audiences other than their teachers.

3. Provide opportunities to use language for a variety of purposes other than the traditional ones of conveying information or checking on procedures. For example, children might be encouraged to persuade the teacher or their classmates to make a particular decision, to tell jokes, to discuss feelings, or to explain something they know to an unfamiliar listener. Guests invited to the classroom can serve an important role as confederates.

4. Encourage children to talk by avoiding evaluative responses ("Don't say bestest") or overly directive comments ("Now tell us how you felt when that happened") and by giving children ample time to respond to questions and prompts.

A common problem of the traditional service delivery model is that skills learned outside the classroom do not always generalize back to that setting. Hence, professionals must plan in advance to promote generalization of learning. Among the recommended strategies are the following (Calhoon & Fuchs, 2003; Hemmeter, 2000; Hughes, 1989; Kohler & Strain, 1999).

1. Select targets that meet specific classroom needs or that draw on classroom information as material for teaching specific language behaviors. For example, select vocabulary that has already been presented as part of a child's science or history lessons, or work on inferential comprehension using materials from social studies. This strategy requires professionals to be familiar with the curricular content of their students.

2. Watch in the classroom for evidence of generalization. Observations can be done by assistants, but professionals retain responsibility to ensure that the observers are given clear "recognition rules" and a simple means for recording data

3. Reduce the differences between the therapeutic and classroom environments. For the most part, this means simulating the classroom situation. By role-playing the interactions and linguistic demands that occur in the classroom, children are better prepared to use their newly learned behaviors when they leave the therapy setting.

4. Program the classroom environment to provide children with challenges, prompts, and rewards that will facilitate generalization. Teachers, assistants, and peers can be recruited to assist in different ways. Peers can help manage inappropriate social behaviors, teach skills that they have already mastered, model selected behaviors, and provide group-oriented recognition of a child's successes.

5. Teach children to monitor their own language behavior in the classroom. Helpful techniques for this purpose include physical reminders, specific homework assignments, and record keeping.

Intervention Strategies

Regardless of the service model they use, professionals teaching and intervening with children with learning disabilities must possess a repertoire of instructional methods. Students with learning disabilities are identified by their failure to achieve academically when provided with conventional instruction. Therefore, the focus of most work with these children is to find alternative ways for them to learn. Sometimes this means getting them to *do* something that normally achieving children do not need to do in order to learn. Sometimes it means getting them to *stop* doing something that is impeding them from learning.

Information Processing and Strategies for Cognitive Training.   Comparison of children with learning disabilities to normally achieving children shows that the former exhibit a less effective and sophisticated cognitive style and are inefficient at processing and organizing information. This has been described in several studies in which different kinds of learning tasks were presented. The profile of children with learning disabilities that emerges generally includes the following characteristics.

- Children with learning disabilities respond with more impulsivity and use less mature strategies in problem-solving tasks. They have more difficulty in shifting from one intellectual task to another (Douglas, 1988; Schachar, Tannock, & Logan, 1993).
- They tend to mislabel items during naming tasks. This is due to poor semantic organization but has also been interpreted as the result of hyperexcitability, an impairment in the ability to inhibit the selection of inappropriate, or irrelevant labels from the memory store (Kail & Leonard, 1986a).
- Children with learning disabilities show less mature strategies for organizing and rehearsing words for recall unless the words are presented to them in preorganized sets. They may also rehearse isolated or fragmented bits of information, such as single words, in contrast to their normal peers, who, as they grow older, begin to rehearse units of information, such as several words at a time.
- Older children with learning disabilities may not detect logical inconsistencies in stories they read unless they are cued to look for them.
- Students with learning disabilities may learn less successfully in newer curriculum frameworks that emphasize data collection, problem solving, and reporting, rather than simple mastery of facts (Carlisle & Chang, 1996).

This profile suggests that a simple approach to improving learning and language performance is to identify instances of impulsive responding. A child may then be prompted ("Take your time") and reinforced for acting reflectively, a point we will take up again in the next chapter. A more in-depth analysis is needed to uncover immature rehearsal or problem-solving strategies. Once a learning task that is difficult for a child has been identified, the cognitive and linguistic requirements of that task must be analyzed, usually through introspection. Professionals might ask themselves, "How do I perform this task? What steps do I follow?" Then the same information can be obtained from the child, either by observing while the task is performed or by asking direct questions. (Children may or may not be able to describe what they do.) If a child's strategies are different from those of the professional, then intervention may focus on introducing the new strategies through prompts and cues, which are then gradually removed to promote spontaneous use. If the child's strategies are the same as the clinician's, then alternative methods of rehearsal (e.g., visualization) or problem solving (e.g., verbalization of each step) need to be explored.

When the language behaviors giving trouble are more complex, they require more intricate methods of instruction. Use of *graphic organizers* might help (Ellis, 1994; Griffin & Tulbert, 1995; Howard, 1994; Pehrsson & Denner, 1988, 1989). As shown in Figure 4.1, students are taught to identify and use either cluster patterns, which show superordinate–subordinate relationships, or episodic patterns, which show a change or sequence of events. The clusters are drawn with circles and connecting lines, either while reading or as a preliminary organization before writing. The professional models both the thought process and the mechanical process of constructing the clusters, and then gradually turns over the responsibility for doing them to the student.

Lexical Semantics.   Not surprisingly, recommendations for the treatment of word-retrieval difficulties vary according to the manner in which the problem is analyzed. Based on their finding that word-retrieval problems are the result of less elaborated lexical storage,

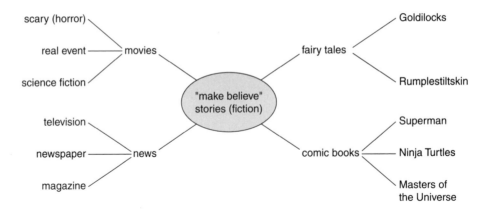

Cluster organizer for writing about "make believe" stories

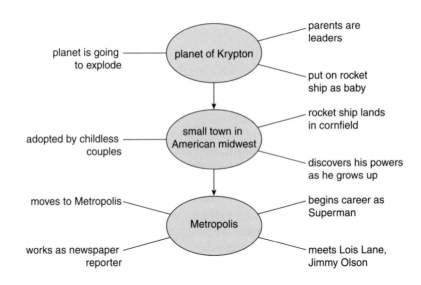

Episodic organizer for retelling the story of Superman

FIGURE 4.1 Examples of Semantic Organizers

Source: Based on Pehrsson & Denner, 1988.

Kail and Leonard (1986b) recommend the following activities to strengthen a word's paradigmatic and syntagmatic associations.

Paradigmatic

1. Teach diverse functions of a word's referent, for example, *ball* (object in a game, shape formed with modeling clay).
2. Illustrate the referent of a word with nonidentical exemplars, for example, *capsule* (a form of medicine, a conveyance for space travel, an infant car seat).

3. Compare and contrast referents from similar categories, for example, clothing (shirt, blouse, blazer, jacket).
4. Teach superordinate categories (reptiles, senses, forms of government).

Syntagmatic

1. Illustrate attribute, agent, and locative terms commonly used with the word, for example, *handcuffs* (pair of, police, wrist).
2. Illustrate the word's syntactic privileges of occurrence, for example, *desperate* precedes a noun or follows a copular verb.
3. Explain the phonetic and morphological characteristics of the word; for example, *prejudice* has three syllables, begins with a consonant cluster, and contains a prefix.

While not ignoring the issue of semantic storage, German (1982, 1992, 2001) also recommends that treatment procedures be based on an analysis of substitution types. Children who produce visually similar substitutions might be asked to concentrate on visualizing the target word. Conversely, they might be given a cue that complements the visual information that seemingly is already available to them, for example, an auditory cue such as the initial sound of the word.

Fawcett and Nicolson (1991) reported on the results of a vocabulary training program administered by parents to teenage children with dyslexia. They found that both traditional and enriched methods of instruction produced short-term improvements in both word knowledge and lexical access speed. Traditional methods consisted of worksheets, crosswords, word bingo, and missing-letter exercises, all of which aimed to help students link words with their definitions. The enriched training led to slightly better long-term effects. This program included vocabulary problems that students needed to solve, such as asking the children to decide among three choices what a *sleuth* might do (e.g., live in a cave, steal apples, climb rocks) or complete sentences with a new word such as *berate,* as in "Kathy is often berated for . . ." (p. 381). The authors recommend that for children with age-appropriate receptive vocabulary, either training approach can be used to improve lexical access speed. For children with poor receptive vocabulary, enriched training should be used, with target words matched to the child's current vocabulary level.

A specific approach to word-retrieval improvement that has been comparatively well studied is the *keyword mnemonic strategy* (Fulk, 1994; Uberti, Scruggs, & Mastropieri, 2003). Target words are recoded as other keywords that are familiar and picturable. The target and keyword are then related by means of a visual image. For example, to learn the word *celibate,* it might be related to the word *cell.* The visual image could then be a priest (who is celibate) sitting in a small room with bars on the windows (cell).

The techniques reviewed above are mostly suited for the teaching of literal word meanings. In order to understand metaphors, children must possess a set of skills:

- They must be able to remember the stimulus, for example, upon hearing of a legal verdict, a speaker might say, "That's a hard pill to swallow."
- They must have knowledge of the features being compared, that is, they must understand how legal decisions are rendered and enforced, and they must understand that pills come in varying shapes and sizes.

- They must be able to pick out the shared features of the elements being compared, that is, both the legal decision and the pill must be somehow taken in and accepted.
- They must consider the topic of conversation and extralinguistic context, that is, the conversation has up to this point *not* been concerned with drugs or vitamins, and there is no literal interpretation of the speaker's utterance that is relevant to the topic of jurisprudence.

Therefore, a teaching program for metaphors must evaluate and be able to remediate deficits in any or all of these areas.

Narratives.   Several suggestions can be made to students to improve their narrative skills. As they listen to or produce narratives, they should be asked to pay particular attention to the goals, motives, thoughts, and feelings of the characters. These children should be engaged frequently in reading or listening to and discussing stories. They can be supported in their narratives by helping them to identify explicitly the topic of their story as well as the specific structural components. Following are some questions that can be asked in preparation for producing a narrative (Garnett, 1986).

Setting	Who? Where? When?
Event	What happened to the main characters?
Goal	What are the main characters trying to do?
Attempts	What happens when they try to do it?
Reactions	What are the feelings? What are the plans?
End	How does it turn out?

Intuitively, one might think that visual aids would assist children in maintaining the sequence and organization of a narrative, but the evidence on this point is mixed. A study of children with learning disabilities found that using line drawings actually resulted in less informative narratives, perhaps because it reduced the demand on the children to supply that information orally (Ripich & Griffith, 1988). On the other hand, a simple system of "stickwriting" has been shown to improve narrative organization and detail with children at different achievement levels (McFadden, 1998). Thus, clinicians may need to experiment with a combination of visual aids and auditory cues to facilitate oral narrative production.

Reading and Writing.   Historically, the treatment of reading disabilities in children has been the responsibility of learning disabilities specialists. The approach favored by most of these specialists has been one of teaching component reading skills: word attack, word recognition, oral reading, sentence comprehension, and others (Cirrin, 1991). This contrasts with the developmental language perspective that has been taken by many speech–language pathologists who work with reading-impaired children (Kamhi & Catts, 1991). Therefore, the expertise of the two professionals may be complementary, and either or both may be asked to provide intervention to a particular child.

Earlier in this text and in this chapter, it was noted that spoken language, reading, and writing exist in a relationship that is both sequential and reciprocal. Basic language skills are learned in spoken form, and these allow reading skills to take root. Reading skills, in turn, are crucial for the development of writing. As children grow older, the interactive influence of all three skills becomes greater and greater.

Professionals must ensure that children with learning disabilities possess adequate basic language skills to support their first efforts at learning to read. Most important, children must have attained adequate levels of phonological awareness to enable them to decode letter–sound relationships (Catts, 1991). Those children who have not developed such awareness can be helped through activities that emphasize word rhyming, phoneme segmentation (such as sound blending), and sound–letter relationships (such as categorizing words by letter and then noting common sounds).

Reading skills must be supported by a variety of linguistic and metalinguistic abilities. Awareness and recognition of grammatical function words may be a critical element of some children's reading failure (Blank, 1990). In that case, metalinguistic instruction about the purpose of function words and drill to promote visual recognition of them may facilitate the child's reading efforts. Semantic skills, both literal and nonliteral, can also be key to children's ability to predict and decipher words and phrases they encounter on the page. Finally, children's familiarity with common schemas, as well as their understanding of narrative structure, can help them to unravel more complex texts (Westby, 1991). *Self-summarization* training (students asking themselves, "Who or what is the paragraph about?" and "What is happening to them?") has been shown to lead to significant improvement in reading comprehension by students with learning disabilities (Malone & Mastropieri, 1992; Reid, 1996). The addition of self-monitoring—using a card to prompt the self-summarization strategy—resulted in better transfer of improvement.

Intervention for writing problems should be contingent on students having attained sufficient spoken language and reading skills to support their efforts at writing. Once that is assured, a hierarchy of instruction, such as that proposed by Dagenais & Beadle (1984), might be used:

1. Improve students' motivation and attitudes toward writing.
2. Improve content skills.
3. Improve linguistic craftsmanship, including spelling.

Curricula developed for normally achieving students can be used in modified form with children who are learning disabled. Extra time must be provided, and directions must be translated to each student's level of comprehension. Self-monitoring strategies are effective at increasing the on-task behaviors of inattentive students (Lloyd, Hallahan, Kauffman, & Keller, 1998). As students learn to monitor their own on-task behavior, they become more aware of what triggers their off-task behavior, and they can use this information to improve work habits (Shapiro, DuPaul, & Bradley-Klug, 1998). Dictation of text can be used to develop content skills while reducing the demands for linguistic craftsmanship. Correction should focus only on the target behavior and should ignore all other errors. When spelling is targeted, intervention should be organized to address assessed deficiencies in the areas of phonological awareness, visual storage, and orthographic knowledge (Masterson & Crede, 1999).

As noted earlier in this chapter, computer use may not always have a general effect on the quality of students' writing. However, in those cases where its use is warranted for writing instruction, there may be more benefit if a student with learning disabilities is not struggling at the keyboard. Students with typing experience make more changes in word-processed compositions than students without such experience (Peterson, 1993). Another important point to be aware of is that when using a computer to write, the length, quality, and structure of students' compositions corresponds to the speed with which they type and compose (MacArthur & Graham, 1987).

Summary

In this chapter we have seen that

- Learning disabilities emerged as a diagnostic category in the 1960s and has since been redefined several times.
- There have been attempts to divide children with learning disabilities into subtypes, but there is no agreed-on scheme for diagnostic classification.
- The category *learning disabilities* includes and overlaps with several other diagnostic categories: dyslexia, underachievement, attention deficit hyperactivity disorder (ADHD), phonological processing disorder, developmental apraxia of speech, central auditory processing disorder (CAPD), SLI, and minimal brain dysfunction (MBD). Professionals should be aware of the relationships among these terms.
- Diagnostic criteria for learning disabilities are set by each state. These can differ, but a very common criterion is that a child must exhibit a discrepancy between intelligence and achievement scores.
- Nearly 3 million U.S. children are diagnosed with learning disabilities. More boys than girls are identified. There is evidence to suggest a hereditary factor.
- Most children with learning disabilities have language impairments. Language disorders and learning disabilities may be different manifestations of a single impairment, and different terms have been used to refer to these children, e.g., learning disabled, language-learning disabled, language disordered. The learning and language problems of the children tend to persist throughout the school years and beyond.
- Many learning disabilities can be understood as resulting from the demands of formal education. Children must become more sophisticated in their metalinguistic knowledge. They must learn a new set of rules and requirements for written language, which differ in many ways from those for spoken language. They must understand the scripts for language use at school.
- Lexical difficulties are common in children with learning disabilities. These children appear to be generally deficient in their lexical knowledge and organization, which leads to problems in word retrieval and word usage. Nonliteral meanings, expressed in metaphors and other figurative language, are especially problematic.
- Most children with learning disabilities exhibit problems with at least some aspects of grammar.
- Both comprehension and production of narratives may be impaired.
- Pragmatically, children with learning disabilities tend to be unassertive and have limited ability to modify their language to suit different situations or to repair conversational breakdowns.
- Reading and writing are complex language behaviors requiring a number of subskills. Consequently, difficulties occur at many different levels of processing, and children with learning disabilities present a variety of impairment profiles.

- Models for treatment of learning disabilities emphasize working with students in their classrooms. Collaborative intervention and teaching is encouraged.
- Helping children with learning disabilities to counter impulsiveness and poor task analysis offers an approach to treatment of many different learning problems. More specific intervention strategies have been applied successfully to improve lexical organization and retrieval, narrative production, and reading and writing skills.

Theories of learning disabilities are still being formed and undergo frequent revision. In this situation, professionals are likely to find varying explanations of learning problems and disparate recommendations for intervention. This makes it especially important that we critically evaluate new information and, in working with individual children, remain willing to try innovative approaches when regular methods do not succeed, but at the same time commit to assessing the value of the intervention approaches we use.

CHAPTER

5 Adolescents with Language Impairment

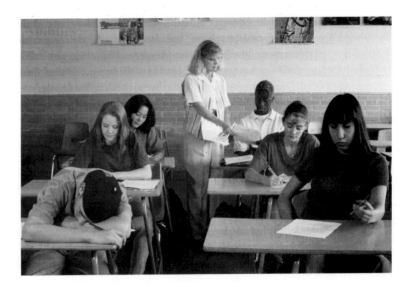

OBJECTIVES

After reading this chapter you should be able to discuss

- Academic, social, and vocational implications of unresolved language disorders in adolescence
- Reasons language-disordered adolescents remain a relatively neglected group professionally
- Aspects of language development during adolescence
- Characteristics of adolescents with language disorders
- Various strategies used to identify adolescents with possible language disorders
- Standardized and nonstandardized approaches for assessing adolescents' communicative performances
- Principles guiding the development of intervention objectives and programs for language-disordered adolescents

The developmental period known as adolescence is generally described as beginning at about 11 to 12 years of age and, in Western societies, continuing until 18 to 21 years of age, depending on which theory of adolescent development is being used. During these years, considerable cognitive, physiological, emotional, social, and educational changes occur. Language changes too, and the changes in language are affected by and affect other areas of development. When an adolescent experiences a language impairment, whether the impairment is severe, or whether it is less severe so that the adolescent's language is more likely to be shaky or, using Nelson's (1998) words, "almost but not quite" right (p. 223), the teenager is at risk for problems in all areas of development.

Much about adolescents with language disorders remains either unknown or empirically unvalidated, especially for those adolescents whose language problems exist in the absence of other conditions known to affect language, such as specific language impairment (SLI) described in Chapter 3 with regard to preschoolers. In fact, some readers may even be surprised to learn that there are adolescents with language disorders and that the extent of the problems associated with the population warrants an entire chapter devoted to this group of individuals. As we will see in this chapter, however, adolescents with language disorders do not constitute an inconsequential group, and the problems they encounter because of their language impairments are anything but inconsequential. Nevertheless, compared to the amount of work that is published regularly in speech and language journals and books about children with language disorders, much less appears in the literature about adolescents with language problems. This more limited information has some not so positive implications for those professionals trying to provide valid and accountable assessment and intervention services for these adolescents. Many adolescents with language disorders remain unidentified, unserved, underserved, and neglected (Apel, 1999a; Ehren & Lenz, 1989; Larson & McKinley, 2003). In this chapter, we discuss why this group is relatively neglected, aspects of language development during adolescence, problems related to language disorders in adolescence, and assessment and intervention factors that are particularly relevant to this group.

A Neglected Group with Significant Problems

The evidence continues to mount that problems associated with language disorders, in the absence of other conditions such as hearing loss, intellectual limitations, and physical disabilities, can persist into adolescence and even adulthood or can even emerge during adolescence (Aram et al., 1984; Beitchman, Wilson, Johnson, et al., 2001; Stothard et al., 1998; Tomblin et al., 1992). Evidence also continues to accumulate that indicates clearly adolescents' persisting language problems affect their personal relationships, academic success during junior and senior high school, choice of vocational and professional careers, and subsequent earning power (Beitchman, Wilson, Brownlie, Walters, & Lancee, 1996; Ehren & Lenz, 1989; Johnson et al., 1999; Snowling, Bishop, & Stothard, 2000; Snowling, Adams, Bishop, & Stothard, 2001; Snowling, Adams, Bowyer-Crane, & Tobin, 2000). That adolescents with language disorders typically perform poorly academically should come as no surprise because, as we have seen in the previous chapter, language ability is a well-recognized factor in students acquiring basic academic skills, skills that most obviously include learning to read and literacy (Catts & Kamhi, 1999; Westby, 1998) but that can also include mathematical abilities (Fazio, 1994, 1996). In extending the effects of language problems on learning, it should also come as no surprise that these problems affect what, if any, postsecondary education is undertaken (Hall & Tomblin, 1978), and how well an individual copes and achieves in the workplace (Johnston & Packer, 1987; Naisbitt, 1988; Rukeyser, 1988).

Socioemotional difficulties are a significant issue for adolescents with language disorders. In earlier chapters we saw how problems with social interactions and even socioemotional difficulties are associated with specific language impairment in preschool years and language-learning disabilities in the earlier school years. These problems are seen in the difficulties students have in establishing and maintaining positive interpersonal relationships (Asher & Gazelle, 1999; Fujiki et al., 1996, Fujiki et al., 2002; Fujiki, Brinton, Hart, et al., 1999; Fujiki, Brinton, Morgan, & Hart, 1999; Gallagher, 1999). There are some indications that these students have difficulties with emotion regulation, a psychosocial issue that could be expected to affect interpersonal relationships (Fujiki et al., 2002), as well as other evidence that has begun to document a decline in their self-esteem as they mature and progress in school (Jerome et al., 2002). Along with the language disorder, these can persist across childhood and into adolescence (Hyter, Rogers-Adkinson, Self, Simmons, & Jantz, 2001; Whitmire, 2000). In fact, as Wiig (1995) points out, emotional, behavioral, or mental health issues, such as "mood disorders often escalate during or immediately after puberty" (p. 17).

In one study of the relationship between socioemotional problems and language abilities in older children and adolescents, 71 percent of the students (aged 8–13 years) in a school setting who had been identified as having mild/moderate behavioral disorders had language scores between one and two standard deviations (1–2 SD) below the means for the normative sample (Camarata, Hughes, & Ruhl, 1988). (Unfortunately, none of the students had had language evaluations prior to the data collection for that research project.) In other reports focusing on students with problem behaviors, Kaufman (2001) has suggested that these pupils demonstrate difficulties in relating to peers and in making and keeping friends, and Marcon (1998) found that for a group of high school graduates, their kindergarten language abilities differentiated those who had been identified on leaving high school as demonstrating significant maladaptive behaviors from those showing no significant maladaptive behaviors. As expected, those adolescents with the lower early language skills fell mostly into the maladaptive group. A 50–70 percent co-occurrence rate of emotional or behavioral difficulties in school-age children and speech and language problems has been suggested in some of the literature (Hummel & Prizant, 1993; Prizant et al., 1990), and in one study the proportion of children who had received treatment for behavioral or emotional problems who also had language disorders ranged from 60 to 95 percent (Cohen, Davine, Horodezky, Lipsett, & Isaacson, 1993).

Not surprisingly, the problems adolescents have in establishing and maintaining positive interpersonal relationships frequently affect their relationships with their peers, teachers, and even with their parents and siblings. Difficulties with peer relationships are particularly concerning for adolescents, for whom having conversations with friends provides important sources of support and influences identity and group affiliation (Denton & Zarbatany, 1996; Hartas & Donahue, 1997). There is also evidence that, although the amount of time older children and adolescents spend talking with friends increases into the teenage years, this increase seems not to replace the amount of time they spend talking with family members (Raffaelli & Duckett, 1989). These results suggest that, overall, teenagers spend more time in discourse with others, meaning that conversational abilities take on greater importance as children mature into adolescents and can have increasing implications for the quality of interpersonal relationships.

Teenagers with language impairments often demonstrate disruptive and negative forms of behavior, both in school and in their pursuits outside school. In most cases, however, an adolescent's language impairment will have first been recognized in the early school years or even in the preschool years, when the opportunity existed to identify early signs of concomitant socioemotional issues and foresee possible future problems. The fact that the language disorders of many adolescents would have first been identified before these individuals began school led Aram and colleagues (1984) to conclude that "language disorders recognized in the preschool years are only the beginning of long-standing language, academic, and often behavioral problems" (p. 240). Some of the academic, language, and social, emotional, and behavioral outcomes for adolescents with unresolved language disorders that showed up in follow-up studies of children who were identified as language impaired either in the preschool years or the early school years are summarized in Table 5.1.

Personal and Societal Costs of Adolescent Language Disorders

While a language disorder in adolescence potentially limits opportunities for an individual's personal, vocational, and economic self-realization, the problem is not just the individual's. It is also society's problem. Undereducation and underemployment are common outcomes of a language disorder. As a result, potentially valuable human resources and contributions are wasted. In some instances, rather than contributing to society as a self-sufficient adult when the underlying potential to do so may have existed, an individual with residual language problems takes from society.

Adolescents with language disorders are at risk for leaving school before earning their high school diploma, that is, dropping out. Table 5.2 shows data from the U.S. Department of Education (2001b) indicating the percentage of adolescents with speech or language impairments in the 1997–1998 and 1998–1999 school years who left high school with a diploma, a certificate, or either dropped out or otherwise left without receiving a formal credential. Because we know that a large number of adolescents labeled as having a specific learning disability have language impairments, data for this group of adolescents with a disability are also presented. As is evident, about 80 percent of the adolescents with speech or language impairments and about 62 percent of those with specific learning disabilities either dropped out or otherwise left high school without receiving a formal credential. (It is interesting to note that a higher percentage of students with speech and language impairments left school without a formal credential than students with learning disabilities.) In Western societies, these individuals are likely to have difficulty finding gainful employment, if any employment at all. Students who are at risk for dropping out or who have dropped out are more likely to be the individuals associated with juvenile delinquency, drug and alcohol abuse, and even youth suicide.

In adolescence, juvenile delinquency, youth suicide, and drug and alcohol abuse have been linked to deficits in basic skills, including speaking and listening abilities. A relationship

TABLE 5.1 Characteristics of Adolescents at Follow-Up Who Had Language Impairments Identified in Their Preschool or Early School Years

Researchers	Age(s) of First Identification of Language Impairment	Age(s) at Follow-Up Assessment	*Language Ability*
Aram, Ekelman, & Nation (1984) [Aram et al., 1984]	3;5–6;11	13;3–16;10	90% of subjects had language scores in moderately to profoundly delayed range
Hall & Tomblin (1978)	Mean ages: 6;1 language-impaired (LI) group 6;4 articulation-impaired (AI) group	Mean ages: 22;3 LI 23;0 AI	50% of LI continued to have language problems as adults; 5.5% of AI continued to have articulation problems
Weiner (1974) (case study)	4 years old	16 years old	—Continuing semantic delay —Continuing morphological and syntax problems
Beitchman, Brownlie, Inglis, Wild, Ferguson, Schachter, Lancee, Wilson, & Mathews (1996) [Beitchman, Brownlie, et al., 1996] Beitchman, Wilson, Brownlie, Walters, Inglis, & Lancee (1996) [Beitchman, Wilson, et al., 1996] Beitchman, Wilson, Brownlie, Walters, & Lancee (1996) [Beitchman, Wilson, et al., 1996a]	5 years old	12;6 years old	Continued significant delays in receptive and expressive language performance
Tomblin, Freese, & Records (1992) [Tomblin et al., 1992]	Mean age: 8;6	Mean age: 21;6	Language-impaired (LI) young adults significantly poorer than the young adults without early LI for —Receptive single-word vocabulary —Use of well-formed sentences —Confrontation naming speed —Sentence imitation; speaking rate —Interpreting agent-action questions for semantic acceptability —Token test performance —Word fluency

Characteristics at Follow-Up

Reading and Academic Ability	Social/Emotional/Behavioral Characteristics	Other
—More than 50% of subjects below 25th percentile rank on reading and spelling measures —75% received special academic assistance*	Greater prevalence of behavior problems than peers	
From grades 3 through 12, LI scored significantly lower on composite scores of academic achievement tests than AI at each grade level except grade 3		Less postsecondary education pursued/achieved by LIs than AIs
—Second-grade reading level —Placed in work-study special education program in spite of normal nonverbal IQ	Ignored/teased by teenage peers	
—Significantly lower educational achievement test scores than subjects without language impairment —About 50% had received special academic assistance	—Increased risk/presence of psychiatric disorder in adolescence —Less participation in extracurricular non-sports activities and organizations —Behavior difficulties more apparent in school environment than at home —Rated as less socially competent —Links to externalizing and internalizing behavior problems	
LIs significantly poorer than the young adults without early LI for —Oral and written spelling —Reading comprehension	Socioeconomic status of LI subjects' families based on their fathers' occupations lower than that of young adults without early LI	LIs significantly poorer than adults without early LI for —Auditory perception of rapid temporal information —Performance IQ

(continued)

173

TABLE 5.1   Continued

Researchers	Age(s) of First Identification of Language Impairment	Age(s) at Follow-Up Assessment	*Language Ability*
Conti-Ramsden, Botting, Simkin, & Knox (2001) [Conti-Ramsden et al., 2001]	7 years old	11 years old	—Receptive and/or expressive vocabulary and/or morphology/syntax below 16th percentile rank —88.5% still had low language scores (below 16th percentile rank)
Johnson, Beitchman, Young, Escobar, Atkinson, Wilson, Brownlie, Douglas, Taback, Lam, & Wang (1999) [Johnson et al., 1999] Beitchman, Wilson, Johnson, Atkinson, Young, Adlaf, Escobar, & Douglas (2001) [Beitchman, Wilson, Johnson, et al., 2001]	5 years old	19 years old	—Continued significant delays in receptive and expressive language performance (means below –1 SD) —Only 50% had received speech/language intervention, even in early school years
Stothard, Snowling, Bishop, Chipchase, & Kaplan (1998) [Stothard et al., 1998]	3;9–4;2 Retested at 5;6 years & groups formed, among them: —"Resolved" language delay at 5;6 years —"Persistent" language impairment at 5;6 years	15–16 year olds	—Persistent language-impaired group: all measures below –1 SD and several approaching –2-SD level —Significant decrease in vocabulary between 8 and 15 years of age —"Resolved" language delay group: most measures at lower end of normal range; significantly lower than control group (normal language) on 4/8 measures

between juvenile delinquency and adolescent language disorders is only beginning to be documented in the literature, even though there has been some degree of awareness of a link between communication disorders and adult prison populations for several years (ASHA, 1973; Bountress & Richards, 1979; Castrogiovanni, 2002; Crowe, Byrne, & Henry, 1999; U.S. Department of Education, 1999). A comparison of the oft-cited characteristics of adolescents at risk for juvenile delinquency or those already in detention and the characteristics

Characteristics at Follow-Up

Reading and Academic Ability	Social/Emotional/Behavioral Characteristics	Other
—Two-thirds below the normal range on single-word reading —80% below normal on reading comprehension		~ 25% showed declines in nonverbal IQ to levels below normal
Significantly poorer reading, spelling, and maths test scores than subjects with no language impairment at 5 years of age	—Elevated rates of anxiety disorder (social phobia the most common anxiety disorder) —Likelihood of antisocial personality disorder	—For language-impaired subjects, a decline in performance IQ with advancing age into early adulthood
—Persistent language-impaired group: 95% scored below 12-year level for reading and spelling; performances at –2 SD level; 50% received no special academic assistance, 30% tutoring, and 20% placed in special classes/schools —"Resolved" language-delay group: 52% scored below 12-year level for reading and spelling; performances mostly at lower end of normal range		—For persistent language-impaired group, a decline in nonverbal IQ between "normal" nonverbal IQ in preschool years to ~50% with scores below –1 standard deviation

*"Special academic assistance" consisted of special education services, tutoring, remedial instruction, and/or special classroom/special school placement.

commonly associated with adolescents with language disorders shows considerable overlap and correspondence. For example, some of the characteristics that have been attributed to juvenile offenders, or those at risk for juvenile delinquency, include difficulties with interpersonal and social relationships, problems with emotional control, poor academic achievement including reading and writing difficulties, presence of learning disabilities, specific phonological deficits, and discrepancies between verbal IQ and nonverbal IQ scores, with

TABLE 5.2   Different Types of Credentials Adolescents with Speech–Language Impairments and Specific Learning Disabilities Left High School with in the 1997–1998 and 1998–1999 School Years

Type of Credential on Leaving High School	Types of Disability	
	Speech–Language Impairments	Specific Learning Disabilities
Left with a diploma		
1997–1998	17.5%	33.1%
1998–1999	19.7%	33.5%
Left with a certificate		
1997–1998	2.2%	4.5%
1998–1999	2.3%	4.6%
Left with no credential		
1997–1998	80.3%	62.4%
1998–1999	78%	61.9%

Source: U.S. Department of Education (2001b).

nonverbal scores better than verbal scores (Archwamety & Katsiyannis, 2000; Bigelow, 2000; Foley, 2001; Kirk & Reid, 2001; Marcus, 1996; Meltzer, Roditi, & Fenton, 1986; Schwartz-man & Ledingham, 1992; Snowling, Adams, et al., 2000; U.S. Department of Education, 1999; Williams & McGee, 1994). According to Svensson and colleagues (2001), over 50 percent of youths in juvenile detention centers have significant reading or written-language problems. Doren and colleagues (1996) examined what factors of students with disabilities predict their arrest. Their results indicated:

- Students with specific learning disabilities were almost four times more likely to be arrested than other students with disabilities.
- Students with poor social and/or personal adjustment were 2.3 times more likely to be arrested than other students with disabilities.
- Students with disabilities who left school without graduating were almost six times more likely to be arrested than other students with disabilities.

This last factor can be considered together with the information we saw in Table 5.2 about the percentages of adolescents with speech–language impairments who leave high school with no credential. The characteristics attributed to juvenile offenders are logically not independent of each other but rather interrelated, for example, poor reading and academic achievement, verbal/nonverbal IQ discrepancies, and a diagnostic tag of learning disabled. Many of these characteristics sound remarkably like attributes of children and adolescents with language disorders.

A small body of literature directly links juvenile delinquency and adolescent language disorders. A report of the U.S. Department of Education (1999) indicated that 3 percent of the young people in detention centers had speech or language impairments and another 45 percent had a specific learning disability. More specifically, Sanger and colleagues (Davis, Sanger, & Morris-Friehe, 1991; Sanger, 1999; Sanger, Hux, & Belau, 1997; Sanger, Hux, & Ritzman, 1999; Sanger, Moore-Brown, & Alt, 2000; Sanger, Moore-Brown, Magnuson, & Svoboda, 2001) have reported on various language abilities of male and female juvenile offenders. Their work has documented that the juvenile delinquent subjects in their studies

- Had poorer standardized language test results compared to nondelinquent adolescents
- Produced less complex language samples compared to nondelinquent adolescents
- Exhibited difficulties with sequencing ideas
- Showed problems with pragmatic skills that included poor topic initiation and topic maintenance, inconsistent use of politeness techniques, and variable application of rules governing conversational interactions either because there were deliberate intentions to violate the rules, or because the language resource demands required during the flow of conversations exceeded the adolescents' abilities to maintain appropriate use of rules.

Although there is evidence for an association between adolescent language impairment and juvenile delinquency, the evidence is not particularly well known, heeded, or utilized. The lack of awareness about the association of language and juvenile delinquency is demonstrated by findings, for example, that only a small proportion of incarcerated adolescents are likely to have received special education during their school years prior to their difficulties with the law, and where services were provided these tended to be for learning disabilities or behavioral disorders rather than language difficulties (Sanger, Creswell, Dworak, & Schultz, 2000; Sanger et al., 2001). None of the juvenile delinquents in these two studies had received language services prior to incarceration, even though evaluation of their language skills while in juvenile detention indicated that a considerable number of them had language impairments.

Not heeding and/or acting on evidence of the possible relationships between juvenile delinquency and language impairment can be costly. For example, Larson and McKinley (2003) reported on a 1993 speech that the then Governor of Minnesota, Arne Carlson, made in which he cited the figure of $500,000 as the cost to that state for each youth who dropped out of high school, obtained welfare for five years, then committed a major crime for which he or she was incarcerated for twenty years. He contrasted this figure with the scenario in which the same youth remained in high school and graduated, proceeded to obtain technical training, and then earned about $500,000 by working for twenty years at an annual average salary of $24,000, a level of productivity that would have contributed to the state in a variety of ways. Governor Carlson pointed out that the difference for this individual was $1,000,000, which would be the difference for each adolescent at risk for dropping out who was able to remain in school, graduate, and then work. Governor Carlson's figures were probably on the conservative side even for 1993 and would certainly be low in terms of today's dollars.

There is another potential personal and societal cost of adolescent language disorders that has also not been well documented or recognized. This is the possible relationship between language disorders in adolescence and youth suicide. Larson and McKinley (2003) reported that, of the individuals aged 10–14 years old involved with the Los Angeles Suicide

Prevention Center, about half had learning disabilities. From our understanding of language and learning disabilities, we would justifiably suspect that most of these adolescents had language impairments. Given the socioemotional problems associated with language disorders in adolescence, a possible relationship between adolescent language disorders and youth suicide should not be particularly surprising.

Although the risk factors for youth suicide are far from delineated, agreed on, and empirically validated in the literature, a number has been suggested. Among these are

- Psychosocial and socioemotional disorders, including affective disorders, and social skills problems, including low social competence disorders (Beautrais, 2000; Grosz, Zimmerman, & Asnis, 1995; King et al., 2001)
- Depression (Jones et al., 1999; O'Carroll, Crosby, Mercy, Lee, & Simon, 2001)
- Problem-solving difficulties, learning disabilities, and the correlates of learning disabilities such as impulse behaviors and, as we know, problematic social skills (Bender, Rosenkrans, & Crane, 1999; Grosz et al., 1995)
- Substance use and abuse (Beautrais, 2000; King et al., 2001)
- Unemployment issues (Gunnell et al., 1999; Lewis & Sloggett, 1998)

These factors, like the situation with juvenile delinquency, are ones frequently associated with adolescents with language disorders. There is also some evidence of a link between suicide and juvenile delinquency. In one study, 63 percent of youths who committed suicide had a record of involvement with juvenile justice (Gray et al., 2002). Social skills difficulties and peer-relationship problems that we see in adolescents with language disorders might also be implicated in the results of a study conducted by Massa and Eggert (2001), a study that was not specifically about language impairment or language ability. These investigators examined the weekly activities of adolescents at risk for suicide compared to those of non-suicide-risk peers and found that the at-risk teenagers spent more of the weekday and weekend time in solitary activities. Results such as these suggest that social isolation from peers may be a factor in youth suicide. As a possible link between teenage suicide and language problems, Asher and Gazelle (1999) suggest that youths with language impairment are at risk for experiencing loneliness as one of the "negative emotional consequences of peer relationship problems" (p. 20). Previously, we also noted emerging evidence that as school children with language impairment progress through school, their self-esteem falls. Jerome and her co-researchers (2002) found that older students with language impairment "perceived themselves more negatively in scholastic competence, social acceptance, and behavioral conduct than did children with typical language development" (p. 700). This contrasts with younger school children with and without language impairment, who did not differ in how they perceived themselves in these areas.

Figure 5.1 illustrates some of these possible links between youth suicide and adolescent language impairment. While links between adolescent language disorders and youth suicide are currently tenuous, unclear, and inexact, there seem to be sufficient cues from the literature to be suspicious that stronger links might be present but yet unexplored and unidentified. It would, however, seem worth the time and energy of professionals who work with teenagers with language disorders to be alert to signs of potential self-harm.

Links between substance (drug and alcohol) abuse and adolescent language impairment are, as with youth suicide, currently tenuous links, although there are reasons to sup-

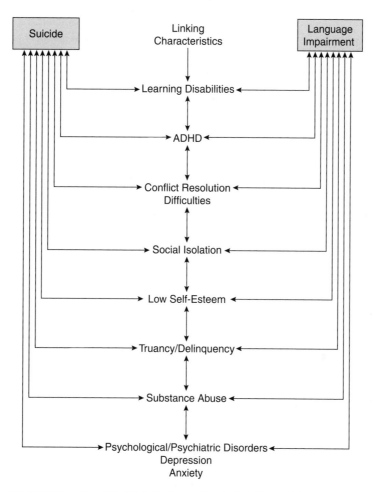

FIGURE 5.1   Possible Links between Youth Suicide and Adolescent Language Impairment

© 2002 Vicki A. Reed, Claire Ireson, and Danielle Slack

pose an association. In the study conducted by Gray and colleagues (2002), 65 percent of those youths who committed suicide had a history of substance abuse. In a follow-up study of individuals at 19 years of age who had been identified as language impaired at 5 years of age, Beitchman and his colleagues (Beitchman, Wilson, Douglas, Young, & Adlaf, 2001a) found that those with substance use disorders (SUD) compared to those without SUD were more apt to have been diagnosed with learning disabilities at 12 years of age, and this association was even stronger in cases in which the learning disability was still apparent at age 19 years. These researchers did not find a similarly strong relationship between age 5 years language impairment and age 19 years substance use problems. However, there was, not surprisingly, a strong association between children with language impairment at 5 years of age and identification of learning disabilities at age 12 and age 19 years, thus suggesting a trend but not a direct relationship. This trend prompted Beitchman and fellow researchers (Beitch-man, Adlaf, et al., 2001) to adopt a more individually focused approach using cluster analy-sis to look at the possible relationship between language impairment and substance abuse. When the co-morbidity of SUD and psychiatric disorders, such as anxiety, depression, and antisocial and personality disorders, was examined in individuals at 19 years of age, these researchers found that a statistically significant percentage of those referred to as depressed drug abusers, as well as others referred to as having antisocial behaviors, had been identified as language impaired at 5 years of age. It appears that type of psychosocial outcome, sub-stance abuse in adolescence and early adulthood, and language impairment recognized in early childhood are associated, although confirming evidence is still out (Snow, 2000).

In the past several decades there have been dramatic changes in employment profiles and the nature of work. There are now few opportunities for unskilled workers. The nature of work has increasingly required employees who can problem-solve, read well, follow instructions, integrate information, generalize knowledge to new situations, and possess good interpersonal skills in order to work effectively as members of teams (Byrne, Con-stance, & Moore, 1992; Johnston & Packer, 1987). A particularly important change has been the widespread accessibility to computers, the Internet, and e-mail. Computer-assisted teaching may help adolescents with language disorders to learn some skills, and adoles-cents with language disorders may be able to use the computer for some tasks and/or for Internet searches. However, such searching and surfing may not reflect the kinds of com-puter use that are important to employers and for personal fulfilment. Such computer use may, in fact, reflect unsystematic and inefficient strategies. Rather than decreasing demands for reading, literacy, and metacognitive skills, effective computer use and electronic com-munication modes have increased demands for reading, literacy, and problem solving. Effi-cient use of the computer and the Internet for communication and information acquisition requires skills such as increased reading speed and comprehension of printed material, meta-linguistic and semantically based organizational abilities, and critical assessment of larger amounts of information than previously experienced. Westby and Atencio (2002) write:

> In the 21st century, society has entered a new technological, information era. Where people once were valued for their ability to transform raw materials into products, now they are val-ued for the information they can possess and transmit. To be successful, individuals are expected to use technology to integrate more and more information from more and more diverse sources and communicate this information to more and more people. (p. 70)

The adolescent with a language disorder is probably at greater risk than ever before for being able to keep pace in vocational pursuits in what are increasing electronic communi-cations expectations of current work environments.

The personal and societal costs of adolescent language disorders are huge.

Reasons for Neglect

Despite the mounting evidence that language disorders do exist in adolescents and that the potential personal and societal costs associated with them are staggering, adolescents with lan-guage disorders continue to be a relatively neglected group professionally (Ehren, 2002; Lar-son & McKinley, 2003). Several reasons account for this neglect. One is the emphasis that has been placed on preschoolers and elementary school children with language disorders. Early intervention to prevent, or at least lessen, academic and personal failures is the rationale behind this emphasis on young children. It is certainly a logical and worthwhile rationale, and it can work. However, it does not always solve the problem, and ongoing support is then necessary.

An example of one way in which the emphasis on young children might be detracting attention from adolescents with language disorders can be found in the numbers of speech–language pathologists who work in secondary schools compared to those working in elementary schools and preschools. According to the American Speech-Language-Hearing Association (ASHA, 2002b), 30 percent of ASHA speech–language pathologists in 2000 worked in elementary schools and preschools, a large difference from the 2.5 percent who worked in secondary schools. Unfortunately, these data represent very little change in about a decade. In 1992, Blake (1992) reported that only 3.1 percent of these professionals worked in secondary schools. This report went on to state that the given proportion was "consistent with data from the *Thirteenth Annual Report to Congress* (U.S. Department of Education, 1991), which, according to Blake, indicate that the number of students identified as having speech–language impairments is quite high in the early elementary school years (ages 6–8) but decreases dramatically after age 9" (p. 82). Like the employment figures for speech–language pathologists, this striking decrease in the number of students with speech–language impairments being served in secondary schools continues almost a decade later and is evident in Figure 5.2. This graph shows the 1999–2000 data for percentage of these students being served in three age groups, 6 to 11 years, 12 to 17 years, and 18 to 21 years. Also shown are the data for specific learning disabilities. What is apparent is the conspicuous increase between the elementary-school-age group and the secondary-school-age group in the percentage of students with specific learning disabilities who receive special education services compared to the decrease for speech–language impairments. Given that it is unlikely that so many children with language impairments would have been "cured" prior to entering

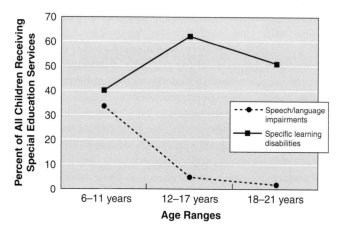

FIGURE 5.2   Students with Speech/Language Impairments and Specific Learning Disabilities as Percent of All Students Receiving Special Education Services in Public Schools in the 1999–2000 School Year

Source: U.S. Department of Education (2001b).

secondary school, and knowing what we know about the association between language impairments and learning disabilities, it is likely that many of the children with language impairments in elementary school could have been relabeled as having specific learning disabilities upon entry into secondary school.

An obvious issue with these trends for employment of speech–language pathologists and the data for numbers of adolescents being served in the secondary schools is that

■ If language disorders are not being identified in adolescents, then apparently there is no population needing the services of speech–language pathologists and, therefore, no need to employ them to serve secondary schools.

However, there is inherent circularity in this scenario:

■ If only very few speech–language pathologists are serving the secondary schools, who is available in these schools to identify adolescents with language disorders?

A related issue leading to neglect of adolescents with language disorders is that the historical lack of services at the secondary level can lead professionals serving language-disordered children who are progressing from elementary school to junior high or middle school to dismiss these children under the belief that further services may not be available (Ehren, 2002; Ehren & Lenz, 1989). Criteria for dismissal from intervention, and the tests and procedures used to determine adequacy of language functioning, may result in further neglect of language-disordered adolescents (Damico, 1988; Ehren & Lenz, 1989; Larson & McKinley, 1995). Some tests may not be sensitive to the language behaviors that can cause problems for students entering secondary schools (Nelson, 1998). The problems surrounding dismissal criteria and assessment procedures can be exacerbated by erroneous perceptions that only insignificant language development occurs beyond late childhood and that little more can be done after late childhood to help (Apel, 1999a; Ehren & Lenz, 1989; Larson & McKinley, 2003).

A failure to realize the significant, negative effects that persisting language problems have on all aspects of life is a further reason adolescents with language disorders are neglected. Another is the failure to understand that adolescents' academic, personal, or social difficulties may be related to language deficits (Comkowycz, Ehren, & Hayes, 1987; Ehren, 2002; Ehren & Lenz, 1989; Stothard et al., 1998). While some language problems of children are not resolved by adolescence, others can emerge when teenagers are confronted by the new social, vocational, and educational demands of secondary school (Ehren & Lenz, 1989; Larson & McKinley, 2003; Reed & Miles, 1989). Even academic problems not evident in the elementary grades can emerge in high school for students whose preschool language problems seemed to have resolved in the early school years (Stothard et al., 1998). These students are at risk of having their language problems neglected because of inadequate identification or misdiagnosis. If academic problems are exhibited, the student is frequently relabeled as having a learning disability, as we know, and services, if any, are provided in learning disabilities programs (Ehren, 2002; Ehren & Lenz, 1989), evidence of which we most likely saw in the data in Figure 5.2.

In light of the discussion so far, it should not be surprising to learn that we have very limited data on the prevalence of language disorders in adolescents, and this unquestionably adds to their neglect. Again, we can see how limited data can create the perception that there are no individuals with the problems. McKinley and Larson (1989) report on one of the few prevalence studies available. Results of this study, undertaken in Loveland, Colorado, indicated that 7 percent of 1,028 secondary students in a regular education program failed an adolescent language screening test. Of the students in remedial English classes for grades 9 to 12, 18 percent failed the screening test, a result that underscores the relationship between deficit oral language skills and poor academic achievement. When complete language assessments were conducted on the students who failed the screening, 35 of them were identified as language disordered and as needing intervention. This figure converts to an approximate prevalence rate of 3 percent. This study also highlighted the greater percentage of adolescents with language disorders in special services focused on reading/writing/literacy skills, that is, the remedial English classes mentioned above. Ehren and Lenz (1989), too, found high numbers in special services in their study. These authors reported that

> 73% of a high-risk population of middle school students, including students in compensatory education and special education, evidenced some degree of language disorder. This same study found a prevalence of language disorders of 80 percent for the group with learning disabilities. (p. 193)

As further documentation of prevalence, 45 percent of the students enrolled in special education programs in a junior high school in Arizona failed a screening test of language, as did 53 percent of the seventh-grade students (approximately 12–13 years of age) who had been placed in developmental reading classes because of reading problems (Despain & Simon, 1987). In this report, a disturbing finding was that only about one-half of the students in the developmental reading classes had been referred for special education services, including language intervention services. Such findings (Despain & Simon, 1987) reflect "the 'happenstance' nature of identification and composition of special education caseloads at the middle school level of education" (pp. 142–143).

At present, there is no cohesive, integrated body of knowledge regarding normal language development during adolescence. There is also (1) little knowledge about effective, efficient, and comprehensive assessment procedures for use with these teenagers; (2) a limited number of standardized assessment tools; (3) a paucity of information about what intervention strategies are most appropriate; and (4) insufficient data regarding the objectives to emphasize in intervention. In these circumstances, it may be no wonder that many professionals may feel that they are not being adequately prepared to work with language-disordered adolescents, a feeling that can lead to a reluctance to pursue assertively the implementation of services in the secondary schools (Damico, 1988). This is dangerous, because it can lead to invisibility of adolescents with language disorders and the professionals who can serve them. As Larson and McKinley (1995) point out, "Perpetuating a lack of visibility makes professionals vulnerable to being considered an expendable service" (p. 294).

Figure 5.3 summarizes various reasons language-disordered adolescents are a neglected population. These reasons are not mutually exclusive, but instead are interrelated. This has the danger of leading to circularity in thinking and circularity in the neglect of adolescents with language disorders. Ehren and Lenz (1989) have used the phrase, "self-perpetuating cycle" (p. 194) to describe the continuing problem of identifying and serving these adolescents.

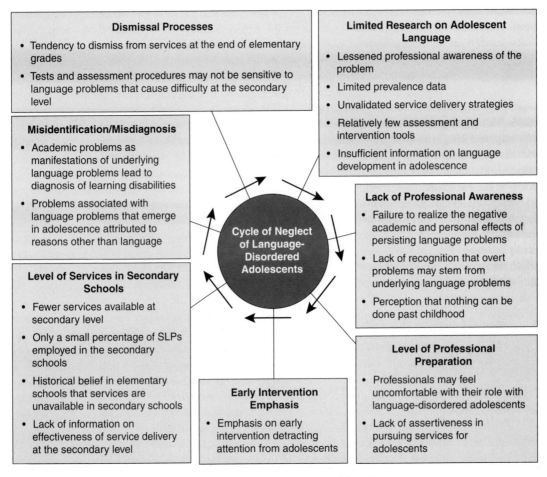

FIGURE 5.3   The Cycle of Neglect of Adolescents with Language Disorders

It is worth noting a final but disturbing thought before moving on to other topics related to adolescents and language impairment. This thought pulls together information from Figure 5.2 and Table 5.2. The data on the percentage of adolescents with language disorders who leave high school with no credential are based on the number of adolescents who are identified in the system while they are in high school. What the information in Figure 5.2 and the discussion in this section about the neglect of adolescents with language impairment tell us is that there are likely many more adolescents who have not been identified and are not included in our data, unless possibly as teenagers with specific learning disabilities, but even this is not all that encouraging. It is probable we do not have data on a considerable proportion of adolescents with language impairments. "Child Find" concepts of IDEA have yet to show up as "Adolescent Find" concepts as far as language impairment is concerned.

Language Development

In contrast to several decades ago, we now know that some very interesting aspects of spoken language continue to develop into and through the adolescent years. We also know that the changes that occur with many of these aspects of adolescent language growth may be gradual, slow, and subtle (Nippold, 2000), only become evident when "the performance of nonadjacent age groups is compared" (Reed, Griffith, & Rasmussen, 1998, p. 166), and/or show up as "spurts and regressions or fluctuations in performance" (Reed, Griffith et al., 1998, p. 176). However, as we have already indicated, compared to what is known about young children's language development, the amount of available information about language development during adolescence remains incomplete and fragmented. In the next sections, several aspects of language that show developmental growth into adolescence are highlighted. The discussion is presented using Bloom's (1988) model of language with its three components of language—form, content, and use.

Form

Length of Utterance.   Although length of utterance is one structural aspect used to estimate young children's level of language development, it has not been as widely used with older children, adolescents, or adults. An argument has been that children learn linguistic rules for embedding and deletion that can result in syntactically more complex utterances that are not necessarily longer. However, there is now considerable evidence that length of spoken utterance does continue to increase up to and during adolescence (Klecan-Aker & Hedrick, 1985; Leadholm & Miller, 1992; Reed, 1990).

Loban's (1976) longitudinal study, which remains, according to Larson and McKinley (2003), "one of the most extensive studies to date" (p. 58), examined a variety of aspects of spoken language development from first through twelfth grades (about 6–7 to 17–18 years of age), including utterance length.[1] Loban presented length data for three groups of students. One group consisted of students whom teachers identified as having advanced language skills, the second was a group whom teachers identified as having poor language skills, and the third was an artificially contrived group created by randomly selecting students from the advanced-language and poor-language groups and pooling the results of their performances. Loban suggested that this last group represented "average" or typical language users. Given what we now know about language impairment in students, knowledge that was not available during the years that Loban collected his data, it is likely that many of the students in Loban's poor-language group might today be identified as having language impairments.

With regard to utterance length, Loban's (1976) results revealed a relatively stable pattern of increasing length throughout the grades for all three groups, a pattern he discounted as resulting from simple verbosity, that is, "an increased use of language without any significant increase in meaningful communication" (p. 25). In his study, utterance length was closely associated with overall syntactic complexity. Additionally, those students whom teachers rated as having advanced language skills consistently used longer

---

[1]In Loban's study, an utterance was technically a C-unit, defined as one independent clause and all dependent/subordinate clauses attached to it, or a phrase if functioning as an elliptical response.

statements than their less language-proficient counterparts. By twelfth grade, the mean length of utterance (C-unit) for the average-language students was 11.70, compared to the higher mean length of utterance of 12.84 for the advanced-language students and the low mean length of utterance of 10.65 for the poor-language students.

Dependent/Subordinate Clauses. Complex sentences (which contain at least one dependent/subordinate clause in addition to an independent or main clause) are also of interest in adolescent language development, and growth in several aspects of complex sentence usage is particularly characteristic of older children and adolescents. Clearly distinguishing features of older students' language include

- Embedding (placing linguistic elements, such as a dependent clause, in the middle of utterances rather than at the end, as in "The man *who came to dinner* ate a lot," versus "The man ate a lot *when he came to dinner*") (Hass & Wepman, 1974)
- Using multiple embedding (having more than one dependent/subordinate clause) (Scott, 1988)
- Increasing use of left-branching clauses, such as "*When he came to dinner,* the man ate a lot" (placing dependent/subordinate clauses more toward the beginning of utterances), compared to right-branching clauses, such as "The man ate a lot *when he came to dinner*" (using these clauses toward the ends of utterances) (Scott & Stokes, 1995)

Loban's (1976) work also provides us with additional information about other aspects of dependent/subordinate clause usage that continue to develop into the adolescent years:

- More dependent/subordinate clauses per utterance with advancing age
- Increase in the percentage of words used in the dependent/subordinate clause portions of utterances from 12 to 35 percent between grades 1 and 12.

This last finding means that in grade 12 approximately one-third of the words in an adolescent's utterances are part of dependent/subordinate clauses. As Loban stated, "with increasing chronological age all subjects devote an increasing proportion of their spoken language to the dependent clause portion of their communication units" (p. 41). Findings that adolescents use more conjunctions in their utterances than younger school-age children, including conjunctions that conjoin clauses (Reed, Griffith et al., 1998), add support for Loban's findings.

The information above tells us that increasing use and length of dependent/subordinate clauses, especially those embedded in or starting utterances, are characteristics of language development during adolescence. There is, however, another aspect to complex sentence use that is a significant developmental characteristic of adolescent language. This relates to changes in the types of dependent/subordinate clauses used with advancing age. Loban (1976) found that for the "average" language users (i.e., randomly grouped students), the proportion of *noun clauses* (those functioning as nouns in utterances, as in "Ice cream is *what he wants*" or "*What he wants* is a job") increased from first to twelfth grade, while the proportion of *adverbial* clauses (those functioning as adverbs, as in "She will eat *when she comes home*") decreased and the proportion of *adjectival* clauses (which can also be termed *relative clauses*) remained the same from first to twelfth grade. These findings are shown in Table 5.3. By twelfth grade, about 50 percent of the clauses used were noun

**TABLE 5.3   Percentages of Different Clause Types Used by Advanced-,
Average-, and Poor-Language Students in First and Twelfth Grades**

Language Group	Noun Clauses		Adjectival Clauses		Adverbial Clauses	
	First-Grade Students	*Twelfth-Grade Students*	*First-Grade Students*	*Twelfth-Grade Students*	*First-Grade Students*	*Twelfth-Grade Students*
Advanced	46%	43%	23%	33%	31%	24%
Average (random)	41%	50%	26%	25%	32%	25%
Poor	34%	45%	19%	21%	47%	34%

Source: Adapted from Loban (1976).

clauses, with adjectival and adverbial clauses each accounting for about 25 percent of dependent-clause usage.

Also apparent in Table 5.3 is the different pattern of development for adjectival clauses for the group of students with advanced language skills. These students increased their use of adjectival clauses from first to twelfth grade, in contrast to noun or adverbial dependent clauses. This increase clearly separated language-proficient children and adolescents from those with average and poor language. Loban (1976) concluded that "the evidence seems clear that an exceptional speaker . . . will use a progressively greater percentage of adjectival clauses in oral language, whereas the nonproficient speaker . . . or average speaker . . . will show no such percentage increases in the use of adjectival clauses" (p. 48). He pointed out that the greatest increase in the language-proficient students' uses of adjectival clauses occurred mainly during grades 7, 8, and 9.

The relationship of adjectival clauses to adverbial clauses also seems particularly revealing about the language development of advanced- versus poor-language students. Although the proportion of adverbial clauses used by the poor-language users decreased from first to twelfth grade, as it did for the advanced-language users, across the grades the poor-language users maintained an overall greater use of adverbial clauses than the advanced-language students. For the poor-language users, their decrease in use of adverbial clauses was paralleled by an increase in the proportion of noun clauses they used. This contrasts with the increase in adjectival clause usage across the grades of the advanced-language users. By twelfth grade, approximately 33 percent of the dependent/subordinate clauses of the advanced-language users were adjectival clauses, compared to about 20 percent for the poor-language users, a considerable difference.

Adverbial Connectives.   Another characteristic of adolescent language development is the increasing use of linguistic structures that occur relatively infrequently in spoken language (Nippold, 1998; Scott & Stokes, 1995). Adverbial connectives are one category of low-frequency linguistic devices. *Adverbial conjuncts* (forms that indicate a logical relation between utterances, such as "*Nevertheless,* the burned cake was eaten") and *adverbial disjuncts* (forms that indicate an attitude or comment about the utterance, such as "There was, *of course,* some debate about the issue") are two types of these connective devices that link utterances but do so outside of the internal syntactic structure of clauses. The work of several researchers (Crystal & Davy, 1975; Nippold, Schwarz, & Undlin, 1992; Scott,

1984; Scott & Rush, 1985) has contributed to our knowledge of adolescents' uses of these advanced language forms:

- Adolescents use a greater variety of adverbial connectives, use them more frequently, and are more successful at metalinguistic tasks involving them than younger students.
- Teenagers use adverbial conjuncts more frequently than adverbial disjuncts.
- Disjuncts tend to be used by older rather than younger students.
- Adolescents' frequency of use of these forms is less than that of adults.
- Ability in dealing with adverbial conjuncts continues to improve from early adolescence to early adulthood.
- Not all adults achieve full mastery of adverbial conjuncts, especially in written language.

Content

In this section we will consider the content of language, that is, semantics, or words and meaning. We will take a look at some of the aspects of words, word meanings, and figurative language that continue to develop during the adolescent years.

One obvious measure of semantic development to think about is the number of words in an individual's vocabulary. Miller and Gildea (1987) have estimated that at the time of high school graduation, a typical adolescent will know about 80,000 words. However, vocabulary size is only part of the picture about adolescent's semantic development. Other parts of the picture involve what types of words they learn and what they do with the words and their meanings. For example, adolescents know more words with abstract meanings than younger children do (e.g., *oppression, simulate, divestiture*) and are able to use words in many more contexts (e.g., *hot* as in "hot food" and "hot topic" or *imperial* as in "imperial persona" and "imperial family"). There are several reasons for this semantic growth—educational exposure, life experiences, and cognitive shifts into formal/hypothetical thought levels. As Nippold (1998) points out, these mean that, compared to younger children, adolescents are better able to learn new words and their meanings by

- Picking up on cues that morphological markers provide (*piano, pianist*)
- Using context to decipher meanings of unfamiliar words ("The 80-year-old man enjoyed being referred to as an octogenarian")
- Taking in the direct instruction to which they are exposed in school and the vocabulary associated with it (e.g., *pyrolytic, trochaic*)

During adolescence, there is a continuing, qualitative refinement in lexical knowledge that is in addition to quantitative growth in the size of the lexicon.

Although vocabulary growth is an important aspect of later language development, there are other, equally important areas of semantic development during adolescence and even into adulthood. These include the characteristics of definitions provided for words, the ability to complete verbal analogies ("feet are to socks as hands are to _____"), and skill in detecting and deciphering statements that are ambiguous ("Pressing the suit led to unpredicted problems"). Adolescence is also a peak period for the use of figurative language, and a number of areas of figurative language feature in the language changes that occur in the teenage years. Among these are verbal humor, idioms, metaphors and similes, and proverbs. Table 5.4 provides a summary of these important areas of semantic growth in adolescence.

TABLE 5.4   **Important Areas of Semantic Growth in Adolescence**

Words and Word Meanings	Features
Defining words	Categorical definitions used with increasing frequency ("*Wombat:* an animal"); children's definitions more commonly consist of functions ("*Spoon:* something you eat with") or descriptions ("*Wombat*: A wombat is brown"; "*Wombat*: eats plants") or are idiosyncratic ("*Ball*: the thing Jimmy has")
	Gradually become more categorical with age
	("*Cat:* like a dog")
	More advanced forms likely to include a superordinate category and include one or more descriptors (i.e., Aristotelian definition) ("*Wombat:* a nocturnal marsupial")
	May include more than one feature or definition type ("*Ball*: a round, three-dimensional object often used in competitive games")
	Ability associated with adolescents' reading ability
	Ability for different word types may develop differently with different patterns (e.g., nouns vs. verbs vs. adjectives)
Verbal analogies *Wing to bird: Fin to _____*	Ability increases from childhood into adolescence but may be a skill not fully acquired until late adolescence or even adulthood
	Some fifth to eighth graders may approach verbal analogies as free association tasks
	("Wing to bird: Fin to <u>swim/water/scales/fish</u>")
	Ability associated with level of academic performance and word/vocabulary knowledge
	("Top to apical: Bottom to _____")
	Ability associated with world/cultural knowledge
	("Democrat to Republican: Labor to _____") (U.S. and Australian political parties)
	Increase in ability to deal with more complex relationships
	("Misfeasance to malfeasance: Misdemeanor to _____")
	Relationship between cognitive and semantic factors in these tasks not clear
Ambiguities *Playing cards can be expensive. The glasses were smeared.*	Statements with more than one meaning that, without context, may be interpreted inaccurately
	Four types: ■ Phonological ambiguity = homophones ("He saw three pears [pairs]") (Shultz & Pilon, 1973, p. 730) ■ Lexical ambiguity = words with multiple meanings ("She wiped her glasses") (Wiig & Semel, 1984, p. 343) ■ Syntactic or surface structure ambiguity = words in a statement can be grouped in more than one way; interpretation depends on recognition of subtle differences in stress and juncture ("He told her baby//stories"; "He told her//baby stories") (Kessel, 1970, pp. 86–87) ■ Deep structure ambiguity = more than one set of linguistic relationships are possible between words of a statement
	("The duck is ready to eat") (Shulz & Pilon, 1973, p. 728) (The duck is going to eat or the duck has been prepared and someone is about to eat it.)

(continued)

TABLE 5.4   Continued

Words and Word Meanings	Features
Ambiguities *(continued)*	("I find visiting relatives tiresome") (The act of going to visit relatives is tiresome or relatives who come to visit are tiresome.)
	Developmental sequence in ability to detect these types in the order listed above ■ Phonological ambiguities: greatest growth rate between 6 and 9 years of age; remains a superior skill compared to other types, at least through tenth grade, or about 15 years of age ■ Lexical ambiguities: detected at approximately 10 years of age, although some children in the early elementary grades may respond correctly; remains superior skill to later developing types ■ Syntactic and deep-structure ambiguities: marked development at age 12; little or no skill evidenced earlier 　■ Ability to detect syntactic ambiguity may somewhat precede ability to detect deep-structure ambiguities 　■ Estimated ages of acquisition: syntactic ambiguities at about 12 years; deep structure ambiguities at about 12–15 years 　■ Some 15-year-olds may continue to have difficulties with both types
	Often a basis of advertisements (ad for a new car travelling on a highway, "Designed to move you") (Nippold, Cuyler, & Braunbeck-Price, 1988, p. 473)
Figurative language	
Verbal humor	Often based on ambiguities
	Developmental pattern similar to that for ambiguities
Idioms *Raining cats and dogs* *Slap in the face*	Expressions that have both a figurative and literal interpretation
	Comprehension of the figurative meaning of idioms improves with age
	Gradual growth in understanding into and throughout adolescence
	In early grades children may understand literal meaning of idioms; some may also comprehend some of the figurative interpretations
	Ability associated with reading comprehension level
	Consistent ability to comprehend figurative meanings not evidenced until adolescence
	Even older adolescents may not demonstrate complete mastery of idiomatic interpretation
	Several factors influence idiom comprehension: ■ Frequency of exposure to specific idioms; familiarity; more familiar are more easily understood ■ Manner in which understanding is assessed ■ Degree of supporting contextual information 　■ More easily understood when presented in context (e.g., short stories) 　■ Harder to understand in isolation (e.g., pointing to pictures depicting the meaning) 　■ Providing explanation of idiom is also difficult ■ Transparency; the more transparent, the easier to understand ■ Culture ("Kangaroos in the top paddock," an Australian idiom meaning much the same as "Bats in the belfry") (Reed, 1991, p. 11)

TABLE 5.4 Continued

Words and Word Meanings	Features
Metaphors and similes *She is a hard person* (metaphor) *The wind was like an arrow looking for its bull's-eye* (simile)	Employing an attribute to describe an entity or to compare entities not literally or typically associated with the attribute or each other Requires acknowledgment of similarities between domains usually seen as dissimilar Common metaphors referred to as *frozen forms;* less common termed *novel forms* Similes: variations of metaphors; inclusion of *like* or the phrase *as (adjective) as;* makes comparison or association explicit Comprehension and use linked to age, cognitive growth, culture, the syntactic forms used to express the metaphor/simile, schooling, semantic growth, and exposure to the forms Similes sometimes thought to be easier than metaphors because of the explicit syntactic form similes employ; research has not fully supported this conclusion Metaphoric comprehension ■ At 7 years of age children understand some metaphors; appears intuitively based ■ As children enter the concrete operations stage, skill improves considerably ■ Continued improvement into adolescence and the formal thought stage ■ In one study (6- to 14-year-olds), only the adolescents understood the metaphors (Winner, Rosenstiel, & Gardner, 1976) ■ Novel forms more difficult than frozen forms Metaphoric use ■ Likely a U-shaped developmental pattern ■ Young children's metaphors generally conventional or frozen forms; any novel forms usually stem from inaccurate perceptions or limited cognitive and linguistic realizations ■ Use of metaphors increases up to the elementary grades ■ In elementary grades use declines; conforming to educational expectations? ■ Use increases again into adolescent years ■ Adolescence a peak in use of metaphoric productions ■ Frozen forms, not novel forms, predominant even in adolescence
Proverbs *A rolling stone gathers no moss* *Don't put all your eggs in one basket*	Most difficult form of figurative language Later developing than similes, metaphors, and idioms Rudimentary figurative comprehension possibly as young as 7 to 9 years of age if task provides supporting contexts or a receptive task used Proverb explanation a more difficult task Consistent ability in proverb comprehension develops during adolescence and into young adulthood Several factors affect ability: ■ Frequency of exposure; more familiar proverbs easier ("Clothes don't make the man" likely easier than "A peacock should look at its legs") (Nippold, 1998, p. 134) ■ Word knowledge and word definition ability ■ Culture ("The lion went to the jungle because it ate a deaf ear," a Masai proverb) (Wiig, 1989, p. 7) ■ Amount of formal education, including amount of postsecondary education ■ Degree of concreteness or abstractness of nouns in the proverbs; proverbs with concrete nouns easier ("Sleeping cats catch no mice" likely easier than "Sorrow is born of excessive joy") (Nippold, 1998, p. 135) Ability associated with level of reading ability

Sources: Achenbach (1970); Armour-Thomas & Allen (1990); Fowles & Glanz (1977); Gardner (1974); Gardner, Kircher, Winner, & Perkins (1975); Johnson & Anglin (1995); Kessel (1970); Nippold (1988, 1991, 1993, 1994b, 1995, 1998, 1999, 2000); Nippold, Allen, & Kirsch (2001); Nippold, Hegel, Sohlberg, & Schwarz (1999); Nippold, Hegel, Uhden, & Bustamante (1998); Nippold, Leonard, & Kail (1984); Nippold & Martin (1989); Nippold, Moran, & Schwarz (2001); Nippold & Rudzinski (1993); Nippold & Taylor (1995, 2002); Nippold, Taylor, & Baker (1996); Nippold, Uhden, & Schwarz (1997); Pollio & Pollio (1979); Power, Taylor, & Nippold (2001); Shulz & Horibe (1974); Shultz & Pilon (1973); Spector (1990, 1996); Wiig (1989); Wiig, Gilbert, & Christian (1978); Wiig & Semel (1984); Winner, Rosenstiel, & Gardner (1976).

It may seem strange to see so much information about the development of figurative aspects of language included in this chapter. Competence in figurative language use is generally not thought of as critical to everyday survival. It is, however, important to adolescents in their academic and social lives. School children across grade levels, including adolescents, frequently encounter figurative language in their classrooms and textbooks (Kerbel & Grunwell, 1997; Lazar, Warr-Leeper, Nicholson, & Johnson, 1989; Nippold, 1991, 1993), especially in the language arts. According to Lazar and colleagues (1989), as early as the kindergarten year, about 30 percent of teachers' utterances contained at least one occurrence of a multiple-meaning expression. Five percent of their utterances contained at least one idiom. By eighth grade, 37 percent of teachers' utterances contained at least one occurrence of a multiple-meaning expression and, of particular interest, the occurrences of utterances containing idioms increased to 20 percent. Success in school has also been found to be associated with students' levels of skill with aspects of figurative language, in particular their ability to comprehend proverbs (Nippold, Uhden, & Schwarz, 1997; Nippold, Hegel, Uhden, & Bustamante, 1998). Additionally, the use of slang and jargon, for which adolescents are renowned, is based primarily on figurative language. In fact, the ability to comprehend and use the slang and jargon of the peer group has been linked to peer acceptance and the ability to establish friendships during adolescence. In discussing later language development of children and adolescents, Nippold (1998) even suggests that "gaining competence with figurative language is an important part of becoming a culturally literate and linguistically facile person" (p. 8). It appears that an adolescent's ability to understand and use figurative expressions *should not be sold short* (to use a figurative expression) as a measure of language development.

Use

In Bloom's (1988) model, *use* refers to the pragmatic aspect of language. Several studies provide indications of developing pragmatic skills in adolescents, although we have less information regarding this area of development than for the other aspects of adolescents' language. Our discussion here focuses on five components of language use: (1) the ability to adapt and modify language, depending on the status of the conversational partner; (2) the various speech acts and functions occurring in communication; (3) ways in which topics are and are not maintained; (4) the paralinguistic features employed; and (5) the nonverbal communicative characteristics of adolescents.

An adolescent who is a competent communicator effectively adapts language to suit the situation (Norris, 1995; Reed, McLeod, & McAllister, 1999). That is, the adolescent uses code switching and different forms of communication based on the conversational partner's characteristics. Adolescents seem quite aware of the need to place greater importance on certain aspects of communication with particular communication partners than others. In the study by Reed and her colleagues (1999), when grade 10, normally achieving adolescents were asked to rank the order of importance of 14 communication skills in their own communication when they were interacting with their teachers or their peers, communication skills associated with discourse management (e.g., clarification or communication repair for unclear messages) tended to be ranked as more important for interactions with teachers, whereas communication skills associated with empathy and considered to be addressee focused tended to be ranked as more important for communication with adolescent peers. In

Larson and McKinley's (1998) longitudinal study, the language development of normally achieving male and female adolescents from grade 7 (12 to 13 years old) through grade 12 (17 to 18 years old) was tracked as they conversed in two situations, one with a same-aged peer and the other with an unfamiliar adult of opposite gender. In adolescent–adolescent conversations, the teenagers used more question types, engaged in more figurative language, introduced more new topics (i.e., evidenced more topic shifts), and used more abrupt topic shifts than in adolescent–adult conversations. These findings support Wiig's (1982a) observation that by 13 years of age, adolescents evidence the ability to change from *peer register* to *adult register* and from *formal register* to *informal register.* This adaptive communication skill is, however, apparently refined even more as adolescents grow older. By age 15, use of the more formal register seems to be extended to include less familiar peers as well as adults (Wiig, 1982a). The informal register is apparently reserved for use with the adolescents' close friends. Differences in adolescents' MLUs may also reflect use of formal or informal register. Wiig (Wiig, 1982b) reports that teenagers' MLUs tend to be shorter with peers than with adults. She suggests that one reason for this difference stems from the use of more names and titles when adolescents converse with adults. The extra words in these forms of address, therefore, increase MLU.

Besides being able to adapt their messages according to communicative situations, adolescents should have full use of all communicative functions and speech. The frequency with which adolescents employ different functions and acts appears to vary as a function of both the conversational partner's age and the age of the adolescent speakers themselves. When communicating with peers, adolescents have been described as using more functions designed to entertain and to persuade their peer to feel/believe/do something than when conversing with adults (Larson & McKinley, 1998). Although persuading their conversational partner was more evident with peers than adults, when their performance with both conversational partners was pooled, the teenagers showed a pattern of fluctuations in the frequency with which they used persuasion across the grades. Even with the ups and downs in the occurrences of persuasion, the frequency with which this communication function occurred in seventh and twelfth grades was actually quite similar. In contrast, the frequency of use of the function of describing an ongoing event increased from seventh to twelfth grade. This function is likely related to the discourse genre of narrative. Nippold (1998) has summarized aspects of narrative ability that improve during the school years and through adolescence. Among these are attempts by the older children and adolescents to include more information about the emotions and motivations of the individuals involved in their narratives and embed episodes or subplots within episodes of the narratives. Johnson (1995) cautions, however, that trying to identify norms for narrative skill is complicated by the fact that there are many different contextually related factors that affect what and how individuals produce narratives.

Other aspects of conversations have been found to change during adolescence. For example, in Larson and McKinley's longitudinal study (1998), the number of new topics that the adolescents introduced during their conversations decreased from seventh to twelfth grade, as did their use of abrupt topic shifts. The teenagers did, however, show increases in the number of interruptions during their conversations. For the most part, these findings are consistent with what Nippold (1998) has suggested the literature identifies as characteristics of increasing conversational expertise into adolescence. These include staying on a topic longer, engaging in extended dialogues with conversational partners, and shifting to new topics gracefully.

Although with advancing age adolescents may not increase the frequency with which they use the communication function of persuading the listener to feel/believe/do something (Larson & McKinley, 1998; Nippold, 1994a, 1998), reviews of the literature suggest that there may be refinements in adolescents' execution or application of persuasion. These include greater ability to generate several reasons, rationales, and arguments for a proposition, to control the interactions and discourse, and to use less immature persuasive approaches such as begging or whining. Other more advanced characteristics of persuasion that Nippold (1998) identified (i.e., anticipating counterpoints and arguments, adjusting the persuasive strategy to suit listener characteristics, proposing positive reasons or advantages) relate to the increasing ability of adolescents to adapt their communication to their partners and to see the world from the perspective of their communication partners, which is, in part, related to presupposition. Adolescents' recognition of the importance of being able to take their communication partner's perspective was identified in the Reed and colleagues (1999) study. These authors found that, although adolescents attached different degrees of importance to specific communication skills depending on who their communication partners were, the one skill that ranked as relatively important for communication with both teachers and peers was the ability to take the communication partner's perspective.

From Chapter 1 we recall that maze behavior of children—revisions, repetitions, hesitations, and false starts—does not decrease with age. Loban (1976) found that the proportion of maze behavior was the same for both twelfth and first graders. This was true for all three groups of students—the advanced-, "average," and poor-language users. Nevertheless, Loban noted erratic increases and decreases in maze behavior in the fourth through ninth grades. Larson and McKinley (1998) found similar fluctuations in seventh through twelfth grades and, like Loban, found a similar number of mazes used by the seventh-grade adolescents as by the twelfth graders. Of particular interest with regard to language impairment was that the poor-language users in Loban's (1976) study exhibited more maze behavior across all grade levels than the "average" language users, and much more maze behavior than the advanced-language users.

Findings such as these confirm that there is considerable growth in pragmatic language skills in adolescence. It is during adolescence that teenagers gain adultlike language competency to use in their interactions with others.

Characteristics of Adolescents with Language Disorders

In Chapter 4, the language characteristics of learning-disabled school-age children were discussed. Adolescents with language disorders can evidence language deficits similar to younger school-aged children with language disorders. That is, language-disordered adolescents may have difficulties with words with abstract or multiple meanings or figurative language expressions, exhibit word-finding problems, and/or use nonspecific, noncontent words, such as *thing* or *stuff,* or pronouns without clear referents. And, as we see from previous sections in this chapter as well as Chapter 4, language-disordered adolescents often experience difficulties in relationships with both their peers and adults, difficulties that have been attributed, in part, to problems in their communicative interactions. They may not adapt their communications appropriately for their listeners or they may use inappropriate strategies, such as an aggressive or abrupt tone of voice, to deliver their messages. Their nonverbal behaviors, such as standing too close, can make their listeners uncomfortable, or these nonverbal behaviors may communicate unintentionally hostile or negative messages. Problems can exist with both expression and comprehension.

Compared to the semantic and pragmatic problems demonstrated by adolescents with language impairments, morphology and syntax has tended not to receive as much attention. This may be because, by adolescence, teenagers with language problems generally talk in complete sentences that contain many correct syntactic and morphological features. However, there has been a growing awareness that some aspects of syntax and morphology may continue to be problematic for adolescents, even though errors may occur less frequently and the problems may be more subtle than in earlier years. For example, adolescents' use of syntactic structures can continue to reflect greater use of simpler, less complex forms, and the frequency with which language-disordered adolescents use the range of dependent clause types or adverbial connectives may be less than expected of teenagers. A particular characteristic of adolescents with language impairments may be a reduced frequency with which adjectival clauses are used, per Loban's (1976) findings.

The recent research findings regarding the persisting difficulties that preschool and school-aged children with language impairments have with verb morphology also prompt the question as to whether some problems with morphology, and particularly verb-form use, might continue to be evidenced by preadolescents and adolescents. Longitudinal data for children with SLI from 3 to 8 years of age (Rice, Wexler, & Hershberger, 1998) have shown that these children do not catch up with the path of increasing accuracy in marking verb tense demonstrated by their normally developing peers and do not reach at 8 years of age the almost 100 percent level of accuracy seen for their peers at 5 to 6 years of age. At 8 years of age, SLI children were still found to be achieving only about a 90 percent accuracy level. The difficulty is, however, that a 90 percent accuracy level might not be interpreted as an important reduction in the level of performance, an interpretation that could erroneously minimize the significance attached to this aspect of children's language performance. However, as Rice (2000) points out, morphological marking of tense in English is not optional, so that for children whose language is developing normally, "by a certain age, [use of correct] grammatical markers would show little variation" (p. 22). For older students, findings from one pilot study (Reed & Evernden, 2001) suggested that, compared to 12 normally achieving students aged 8 to 12 years, age-matched peers with reading difficulties co-occurring with various degrees of language difficulties had more errors in using verb forms during a narrative task, even though the frequency of errors overall was relatively small. Figure 5.4 shows the trend lines for number of verb errors made by the 12 normally achieving students and 12 students with reading/language problems. As can be seen, the trend line for the reading/language-impaired children is noticeably flatter than that for the normally achieving children. And 83 percent of the students with reading/language problems made one or more verb-form errors in their retelling of a narrative, compared to 58 percent of the normally achieving students. These two groups also appeared to differ in their patterns of marking tense. As one example, the students with reading/language problems used considerably more progressive verbs (*is running, were running*) than the normally achieving students, and the students with the reading/writing problems were about as accurate in their use of these progressive verb types as the normally achieving students. This comparable level of accuracy for both groups of students was not the case for other verb-tense forms, for which the students with reading/language problems generally were less accurate. Another

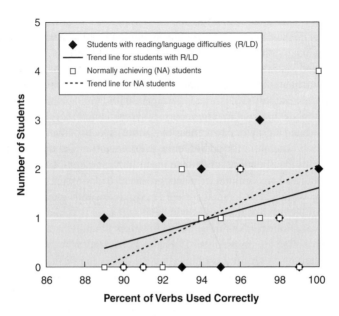

FIGURE 5.4   Percentage of Verbs Used Correctly by Students with Reading/Language Difficulties and Age-Matched Normally Achieving Students.

Source: Reed and Evernden (2001).

finding from that study suggested that the location of mazes of the students with reading/language problems included mazes on verbs, whereas none of the normally achieving students exhibited any mazes on verbs. Evidence of continuing verb errors may, along with other difficulties with syntax and/or morphology, characterize the language of some adolescents with language impairment.

We might expect, however, that some language growth as a result of intervention, maturation, or both would occur between childhood and adolescence. Therefore, the language problems of adolescents may be less obvious and more difficult to identify than those of younger children. These factors can contribute to false negatives in identification (not identifying a problem when one actually exists) or even misdiagnosis, as discussed previously.

The neglect of language-disordered adolescents means that less is generally known about their communicative characteristics than about those of younger children with language disorders. Larson and McKinley (1987) point out "that much of what is known about adolescents with communication disorders comes from related literature in learning disabilities and deaf education" (p. 8). Simon and Holway (1991) present a list of communication features that represent students' incompetent language use under the categories of form, function, and style, which these authors contrasted with a parallel list of competent communication features. For example, these authors contrasted as a competent feature, "mastery of tense reference and subject/verb agreement," with the incompetent feature, "lacks consistency in tense and number reference," "tactful deviousness used" with "tactless statements," "sustains topics of conversation" with "wanders from conversational topic," and "considers listener's infor-national needs" with "egocentric comments" (p. 152). Several authors have identified characteristics that adolescents with language problems frequently demonstrate in their classrooms (Ehren, 1994; Lenz, Bulgren, & Kissam, 1995; Schmidt, Deshler, Schumaker, & Alley, 1989). Many of these difficulties are summarized in Table 5.5. Larson and McKinley (2003) also developed a summary of problems that can characterize the communication of adolescents with language disorders. Their summary, shown in Table 5.6, contrasts expected normal skills for adolescents with problematic behaviors in seven areas: cognition, metalinguistics, comprehension and production of linguistic features, discourse, nonverbal communication, survival language, and written language. These authors (Larson & McKinley, 1987) have suggested that problematic behaviors and/or expectations, such as those listed in Tables 5.5 and 5.6, can provide starting points in determining "where a given adolescent matches or mismatches with educators', parents' or peers' expectations" (p. 15).

TABLE 5.5 Characteristics of Adolescents with Language Disorders in Classrooms

Adolescents with Language Disorders

Do not:	Recall information presented in lessons
	Participate in lessons
	Appear to listen to the teacher during lessons
	Meet minimum standards for academic work
	Define words well or use them appropriately
	Learn from other students' questions
	Get along well with peers
	Participate in group discussions
	Complete assignments on time or complete them at all
	Organize work and materials
	Prepare for class
	Work independently
	Demonstrate knowledge on tests
Do:	Need additional prompting to follow directions to complete tasks within their ability
	Demonstrate a negative attitude or approach to learning
	Ask irrelevant questions
	Violate the rules of conversational discourse (e.g., accessing conversations, taking turns, closing conversations)
	Provide irrelevant answers to questions
	Express or organize ideas illogically
	Converse in irrelevant ways with conversational partners

Sources: Adapted from Ehren (1994); Lenz, Bulgren, & Kissam (1995); & Schmidt, Deshler, Schumaker, & Alley (1989).

TABLE 5.6 Characteristic Problems of Older School-Aged Students with Language Disorders

Category	Expectations	Problems
Cognition	To be at the formal operational level	They often remain concrete operational thinkers.
	To observe, organize, and categorize data from an experience	They make chaos out of order.
	To identify problems, suggest possible causes and solutions, and predict consequences	They may not recognize the problem when it exists; if they do, they do not know how to develop alternative solutions.
	To place concepts into hierarchical order	They often cannot place concepts in a hierarchy.
	To find, select, and utilize data on a given topic	They have limited strategies for finding, selecting, and utilizing data.
Metalinguistics	To demonstrate conscious awareness of linguistic knowledge	They have difficulty bringing to awareness categories and relations in all aspects of language.
	To talk about and reflect on various linguistic forms	They do not know the labels for talking about language during formal education.
	To assess communication breakdowns and revise them	They do not have awareness of breakdowns and, if they do, they lack repair strategies.
Comprehension and production of linguistic features	To comprehend all linguistic features and structures	They misunderstand advanced syntactical forms.
	To follow oral directions of three steps or more after listening to them one time	They may not realize that they are being given directions and/or have difficulty following them.
	To use grammatically intact utterances	They often use sentences that are fragmented and that do not convey their messages.
	To have a vocabulary sufficient for expressing ideas and experiences	They have word-retrieval problems as well as a high frequency of low-information words.
	To give directions with clarity and accuracy	They often leave their listeners confused.
	To get information or assistance by asking questions and to respond appropriately to questions asked of them	They may know what questions or answers to give, but they do not know how to do so tactfully.
	To comprehend and produce the slang and jargon of the hour	They do not comprehend or produce slang/jargon, thus they are ostracized from the group to which they most desire to belong.

A determination of match and mismatch is an essential component of assessment and intervention for language-disordered adolescents (Larson & McKinley, 1995). A recurring theme throughout this book has been that individuals with language disorders do not represent a homogeneous group. Adolescents with language disorders constitute a no more homogeneous group. Each language-disordered adolescent presents a unique profile of communicative strengths and weaknesses. An objective of the assessment process is to identify each adolescent's unique profile.

TABLE 5.6 Continued

Category	Expectations	Problems
Discourse	To produce language that is organized, coherent, and intelligible to their listeners	They use many false starts and verbal mazes.
	To follow adult conversational rules for speakers (e.g., maintaining a topic, initiating a topic)	They consistently violate the rules.
	To be effective listeners during conversation without displaying incorrect listening habits	They often have poor listening skills.
	To make a report, tell or retell a story, and explain a process in detail	They often leave their listeners confused.
	To listen to lectures and to select main ideas and supporting details	They often do not grasp the essential message of a lecture.
	To analyze critically other speakers	Their judgments are arbitrary, illogical, and impulsive.
	To express their own attitudes, moods, and feelings and to disagree appropriately	They have abrasive conversational speech.
Nonverbal communication	To follow nonverbal rules for kinesics	They violate the rules and misinterpret body movements and facial expressions.
	To follow nonverbal rules for proxemics	They violate the rules for social distance.
Survival language	To comprehend and produce situational phrases and vocabulary required for survival in our society	They do not have the necessary concepts and vocabulary needed in places such as banks, grocery stores, and employment agencies.
	To comprehend and produce concepts and vocabulary required across daily living situations	They do not have the necessary concepts and vocabulary needed across daily living situations such as telling time, using money, and understanding warning signs.
Written language	To comprehend written language required in various academic, social, and vocational situations	They do not consistently and/or efficiently process information obtained through reading.
	To produce cohesive written language required in various academic, social, and vocational situations	They do not consistently and/or efficiently generate written language that conveys their messages.

Source: From *Communication Solutions for Older Students* (pp. 9–10), by V. Lord Larson & N. McKinley, 2003, Eau Claire, WI: Thinking Publications. Copyright 2003 by Thinking Publications. Reprinted by permission.

Assessment

Without a solid foundation in normal language development in adolescence, assessment is a difficult and demanding process. Summaries of problems that may characterize the communication of adolescents with language disorders such as the one compiled by Larson and McKinley (2003) (Table 5.6), can provide frameworks for assessing an adolescent's language functioning. A number of school systems have developed lists of communicative competencies for the secondary grades that can also serve as assessment guidelines.

Expectations are that adolescents can use all aspects of language to function effectively in their social, academic, and vocational contexts. These expectations imply, therefore, that in assessment, an adolescent's communicative performance in each of these contexts needs to be examined. If an adolescent is struggling in any or all of these contexts, then a language disorder should be suspected and the adolescent should be more closely assessed.

The assessment of adolescents can be divided into two parts, each serving a different function. The first part involves identifying adolescents who exhibit problematic language behaviors and who may have language impairments. The second part is a more in-depth exploration of the adolescent's language functioning to either confirm or reject the initial identification and, if the identification is confirmed, to determine the adolescent's level of functioning in a variety of areas to identify areas to be targeted in intervention and the appropriate placement for intervention, and to select the appropriate service delivery format. In the following sections, we discuss aspects of both parts of the assessment process. A few standardized tests are available to assist in the process. However, informal observation and nonstandardized assessment methods must also be employed.

Identification

Teacher referrals and language screening are two common methods of identifying language-disordered adolescents. These are not mutually exclusive methods. Both may, and probably should, be used.

Teacher Referrals.   Referrals from regular-education teachers, special educators, remedial teachers, and other specialists are effective ways of identifying adolescents with possible language problems. One critical factor in the success of this method is the degree to which these secondary school professionals understand and recognize the nature of language disorders in adolescents and know the potential sources of professional help for the adolescents. For this reason, information dissemination is important in providing services for language-disordered adolescents (Larson & McKinley, 2003).

Information dissemination includes sharing with classroom teachers and support personnel (e.g., counselors, special educators, social workers, and principals) information about the characteristics of adolescents with language disorders, the ways in which language impairments can be manifested academically and socially, and the intervention services available. Imparting this information helps to ensure that those professionals who have daily contact with adolescents or who interact with them in a variety of situations make appropriate referrals for assessment (Larson & McKinley, 1995). In-service presentations (Reed & Miles, 1989) are one way to increase school professionals' knowledge of adolescents with language disorders and the assistance that can be provided for these teenagers and to promote referrals. Another method is to contribute to school newsletters or newsletters of educators' professional groups. McKinley and Larson (1989) used this last approach to disseminate information to secondary school principals.

Asking informed educators to complete observational/behavioral ratings scales on their students is one way to obtain referrals (Wiig, 1995). Several rating scales of language and language-related skills are available for use with adolescents (Catts, 1997; Larson &

McKinley, 1987; Loban, 1976; Semel, Wiig, & Secord, 1996a). Such ratings not only aid in identifying adolescents with possible language problems, they also direct assessment to areas of communication most highly suspect in an adolescent and indicate those aspects of an adolescent's language functioning that most concern others. This latter information is particularly useful because one critical function of language is to establish and maintain positive human relations. If an adolescent's communicative behavior is interfering with human interactions, the reasons for the ineffectual or negative uses of language need to be targeted for intervention.

Screening.   Language screening tests are used to indicate in broad terms whether an individual's language skills are adequate or whether there is a discrepancy from normal expectations that is sufficient to warrant further assessment. Professionals disagree about the benefits of mass screenings of all students in secondary schools or even all students in specified grades in secondary schools, such as all seventh graders and all tenth graders. Some suggest that a more effective approach is selective screening of students who meet certain criteria, such as students in learning disabilities programs, those who received speech–language services in earlier grades, students receiving tutoring or remedial reading services, or adolescents at risk for dropping out of school.

Only a few standardized language screening tests for adolescents are commercially available. Four of these are listed in Table 5.7. Each of these is designed to be administered individually to adolescents. The tests examine a variety of aspects of communicative functioning, and the suggested estimated time to administer these ranges from about 2 to 15 minutes. Simon (1987) developed a group screening procedure, the Classroom Communication Screening Procedure for Early Adolescents (CCSPEA), to be used primarily with students in grades 5 through 9. The procedure can be administered in the students' classrooms or in other group settings and takes about 50 minutes to complete. It is a paper-and-pencil task, although the writing is limited mostly to circling answers or writing single words, so that it can be used with students who have difficulty with written language. Areas of performance examined in the screening test include content, syntax, metalinguistic comprehension, following oral and written directions, dealing with anaphoric reference, inferencing, and semantic skills involving synonyms and word definitions.

Language Assessment

Standardized Tests.   Some of the more complete language tests that are appropriate for individuals 11 years of age or older are also listed in Table 5.7. Tests that examine areas of functioning closely related to language, such as phonological processing in the Comprehensive Test of Phonological Processing (CTOPP) (Wagner, Torgesen, & Rashotte, 1999) or problem solving abilities in the Test of Problem Solving (TOPS) (Bowers, Huisingh, Barrett, Orman, & LoGiudice, 1991), are also included for reference. Most of the tests in the table are norm referenced. Some examine skills in a variety of language areas such as syntax and semantics, for example, the Oral and Written Language Scales (OWLS) (Carrow-Woolfolk, 1996) and the Test of Adolescent and Adult Language—3 (TOAL—3) (Hammill, Brown, Larsen, & Wiederholt, 1994). Others focus on one area of language such as vocabulary or pragmatics, for example, the Expressive One-Word Picture Vocabulary Test (EOWPT)—2000 Edition (Brownell, 2000a) and the Test of Pragmatic Language (TOPL) (Phelps-Terasaki & Phelps-Gunn, 1992).

TABLE 5.7 A List of Some Adolescent* Language and Language-Related Tests

Test Name	Author(s)	Year
Screening Tests		
Adolescent Language Screening Test (ALST)	Morgan & Guilford	1984
Clinical Evaluation of Language Fundamentals Screening Test—3 (CELF-3)	Semel, Wiig, & Secord	1996b
Mini-Screening Language Test for Adolescents	Prather, Brenner, & Hughes	1981
Screening Test of Adolescent Language (STAL)**	Prather, Breecher, Stafford, & Wallace	1980
Assessment Tests		
Auditory Continuous Performance Test (ACPT)	Keith	1994a
Clinical Evaluation of Language Fundamentals—4 (CELF—4)**	Semel, Wiig, & Secord	2003
Comprehensive Assessment of Spoken Language (CASL)	Carrow-Woolfolk	1998
Comprehensive Receptive and Expressive Vocabulary Test—2 (CREVT—2)	Wallace & Hammill	2002
Comprehensive Test of Phonological Processing (CTOPP)	Wagner, Torgesen, & Rashotte	1999
Detroit Tests of Learning Aptitude—Adult (DTLA-A)	Hammill & Bryant	1991
Detroit Tests of Learning Aptitude—4 (DTLA—4)**	Hammill	1998
Expressive One-Word Picture Vocabulary Test—2000 (EOWPT—2000)**	Brownell	2000
Fullerton Language Test for Adolescents—2 (FLTA—2)**	Thorum	1986
Illinois Test of Psycholinguistic Abilities—3 (ITPA—3)	Hammill, Mather, & Roberts	2001
Interpersonal Language Skills Assessment	Blagden & McConnell	1984
Language Processing Test—Revised (LPT—R)	Richard & Hanner	1995
Let's Talk Inventory for Adolescents (LTI—A)	Wiig	1982b
Lindamood Auditory Conceptualization Test—Revised (LAC—R)	Lindamood & Lindamood	1979
Oral and Written Language Scales (OWLS)	Carrow-Woolfolk	1996
Peabody Picture Vocabulary Test—III (PPVT—III)**	Dunn & Dunn	1997
Receptive One-Word Picture Vocabulary Test—2000 (ROWPVT—2000)	Brownell	2000
SCAN—A: A Test for Auditory Processing Disorders in Adolescents and Adults	Keith	1994b
Test of Adolescent and Adult Language—3 (TOAL—3)	Hammill, Brown, Larsen, & Wiederholt	1994
Test of Adolescent/Adult Word Finding (TAWF)	German	1990
Test of Auditory Reasoning and Processing Skills (TARPS)	Gardner	1993
Test of Language Competence—Expanded Edition (TLC)**	Wiig & Secord	1989
Test of Language Development (Intermediate)—3rd Edition (TOLD—I:3)	Hammill & Newcomer	1997
Test of Pragmatic Language (TOPL)	Phelps-Terasaki & Phelps-Gunn	1992
Test of Problem Solving (TOPS)**	Bowers, Huisingh, Barrett, Orman, & LoGiudice	1991
Test of Word Finding—2 (TWF-2)	German	2000
Test of Word Finding in Discourse	German	1991
Test of Word Knowledge (TOWK)**	Wiig & Secord	1992
The Expressive Language Test	Bowers, Huisingh, Orman, & LoGiudice	1998
The Listening Test (TLT)	Barrett, Huisingh, Zachman, Blagen, & Orman	1992
The Word Test-Adolescent**	Zachman, Huisingh, Barrett, Orman, & Blagden	1989
Wiig Criterion-Referenced Inventory of Language (CRIL)	Wiig	1990b
Woodcock Language Proficiency Battery—R	Woodcock	1991

* Designed for individuals 11 years of age or older.

** Listed as among the ten most frequently used tests by Oregon speech–language pathologists with individuals 13–19 years of age (Huang et al., 1997).

One exception to the normed tests is the criterion-referenced Wiig Criterion-Referenced Inventory of Language (CRIL) (Wiig, 1990b), designed to be used with individuals as old as 13 years. This instrument includes probes to assess performance in the areas of semantics, pragmatics, morphology, and syntax. Huang, Hopkins, and Nippold (1997) surveyed Oregon speech–language pathologists about the language tests they used most frequently for individuals in the age range 13 to 19 years. The ten used most often are identified in Table 5.7 by double asterisks, although in some cases the nominated tests in the Huang et al. (1997) study were earlier versions of the ones listed in the table.

Standardized tests allow those working with adolescents with suspected language problems to provide numbers that convey some notion about the presence and severity of an adolescent's language disorder (Apel, 1999b). These numbers are more often than not required by school administrators in order to qualify students for services. This is one reason that prompted Apel (1999b) to write that he is "not sure at the present time there is a way to 'beat the numbers game,'" (p. 101), even though the norms and construct validity for several of the tests have been questioned (Lieberman, Heffron, West, Hutchinson, & Swem, 1987; Stephens & Montgomery, 1985). Also, as we learned previously, Nelson (1998) has expressed concern that tests that are available are not always sufficiently sensitive to identify adolescents who struggle as a result of poor language skills. And, in comparison to the many language tests designed for use with younger children, there are many fewer for adolescents. If we proceed to eliminate any of these tests because of questionable validity and sensitivity, our choices of what to use narrow even more. These are several of the reasons that nonstandardized language assessment and informal observation are used so frequently and so effectively with adolescents. Other reasons are that many standardized tests examine only limited aspects of language behavior and usually provide for probing only small samples of any particular language skill, and these alone do not yield sufficient information about patterns of language behaviors to allow us to develop specific intervention objectives. Approximately 25 percent of the speech–language pathologists in the study by Huang and colleagues (Huang et al., 1997) expressed dissatisfaction with standardized language testing for a variety of possible reasons, including time constraints and the limited information these tests provide for intervention planning. These topics are discussed in more detail in Chapter 13. It is sufficient to say here that nonstandardized techniques are necessary when assessing the language skills of adolescents.

Nonstandardized Methods.   Damico (1993) has argued that assessment "activities used must be more *authentic,* more *functional,* and more *descriptive* than the assessment procedures previously employed with this population" (p. 29). Authentic assessment means looking at and gathering information about how an adolescent uses or cannot use his or her language in contexts that are "real" for the adolescent (e.g., in understanding what teachers say in classroom lessons, in peer interactions, in trying to apply for part-time jobs, in studying for tests, in understanding and/or explaining a movie or book). This approach to assessment, according to Paul (2001), is referred to as involving "ecological validity (goodness-of-fit with the real world)" (p. 4). A number of strategies are available to assist in undertaking more authentic assessment of adolescents. These include analyzing samples of an adolescent's language, creating contrived situations to elicit examples of specific language behaviors of interest, examining portfolios of the student's work, and assessing the educational system in which the student is expected to function.

Analysis of Spontaneous Language.   It is impractical to attempt to analyze an adolescent's entire language behavior in any one day. Therefore, one or more limited but representative samples of spontaneous language are obtained for analysis. Specific factors related to obtaining language samples are discussed in Chapter 13. There the focus is more on the younger child than on the adolescent with a suspected language disorder. However, the principles of obtaining a sample in varying communicative situations and of audio or video recording the sample apply in all instances. Here we discuss approaches that are appropriate specifically for adolescents.

A common context in which an adolescent's language is sampled is conversation. Recall that in Larson and McKinley's (1998) study of the characteristics of adolescents' conversations from grades 7 through 12, these authors obtained samples of conversations while adolescents talked with an adult and again with an adolescent's peer. To provide a guideline to analyze adolescents' conversations, Larson and McKinley (1995) have developed the Adolescent Conversational Analysis. This analysis method provides for examination of both the listener and speaker roles of an adolescent during conversational interactions. Listener abilities that are analyzed are understanding the speaker's vocabulary and syntax, following the speaker's main ideas, listening in a nonjudgmental way, and signaling lack of understanding. Speaker abilities are divided into four aspects: language features, paralanguage features, communication functions, and verbal and nonverbal communicational rules. Within each of these broad aspects, specific features of communicative functioning are noted and analyzed.

Elements of analysis for language features include the use of a variety of syntactic forms, occurrence of question forms, production of figurative language, evidence of nonspecific language, and occurrence of word-retrieval problems, mazes, and false starts. Analysis of paralanguage behavior focuses on fluency, intelligibility, and suprasegmental features such as inflection, rate, and juncture. For the broad category of communication functions, specific functions used as analysis elements are giving information; getting information; describing ongoing events; persuading; expressing beliefs, feelings, and intentions; indicating readiness for additional communication; problem solving; and entertaining. The last of the four broad aspects, verbal and nonverbal communication rules, is divided further into verbal rules for topics and turns, verbal rules for politeness, and nonverbal rules. Seven verbal rules for topics and turns are analyzed (initiating conversations, choosing topics, maintaining topics, switching topics, taking turns, repairing conversations, and interrupting). Analysis of verbal rules of politeness focuses on appropriate quantity of talk, appearance of sincerity and honesty, making relevant contributions to the topic, expression of ideas clearly, and tactfulness. Lastly, four aspects of nonverbal rules are examined—gestures, facial expressions, eye contact, and proxemics (physical distance from partner).

Each of these communicative behaviors is judged as appropriate or inappropriate each time it occurs during a language sample. The tallies or frequency counts of both appropriate and inappropriate behaviors can be transferred to a profile form that summarizes an adolescent's strengths and weaknesses. This profile can lead to the development of specific intervention objectives and can form part of the basis of a valid and defensible intervention plan. It is possible that the characteristics of adolescent conversations that Larson and McKinley (1998) identified in their study can be used to provide a framework to which the conversational characteristics of a specific adolescent in a particular grade with either an adult or peer as a conversational partner can be compared.

Larson and McKinley (1995) are not specific in identifying what "variety of syntactic forms" (p. 286) should be examined as part of their conversational analysis. However, given the information about dependent-clause development and conjunction usage in adolescence that is available (Loban, 1976; Reed, Griffith, et al., 1998), a fairly in-depth analysis of an adolescent's use of dependent/subordinate clauses is likely important. As shown in Figure 5.5, a guideline for proceeding systematically through increasingly finer-grained analyses of an adolescent's dependent/subordinate usage in a language sample can be created from Loban's (1976) findings, in combination with those of others (Hass & Wepman, 1974; Scott, 1988; Scott & Stokes, 1995). In light of Reed and Evernden's (2001) preliminary findings, another potentially important area to examine might be an adolescent's verb-form usage, including the degree to which the adolescent evidences mastery of correct verb-form use (especially past-tense verb forms), the forms by which the adolescent marks tense, and the frequency with which mazes occur on verbs compared to other aspects of morphosyntax, such as pronoun forms and nouns, or involve revisions of content.

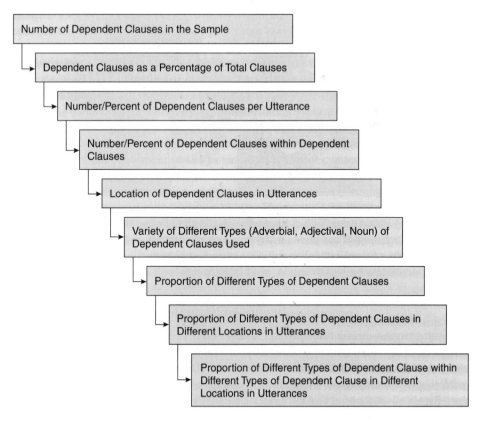

FIGURE 5.5 Increasingly Finer-Grained Analyses of Dependent/Subordinate Clause Usage in Adolescents' Language Samples

Sources: Adapted from Hass and Wepman (1974); Loban (1976); Scott (1988); and Scott and Stokes (1995).

A difficulty in using a conversational language sample with adolescents to identify language impairments and areas of language problems is that, in situations that do not require the use of particular forms, these students can avoid using aspects of language that are not well established in their repertoires or those that continue to create problems for them. A guiding principle for examining the language of an adolescent is that we need to look for what is *not* present in the adolescent's language or what the adolescent *does not do* with language as much as looking at what an adolescent does do or use. Because a conversation might not push an adolescent to use aspects of language that are difficult for the adolescent, we need to include in our assessment practices tasks that require the use of language targets of interest so that we can find out what the adolescent is capable or not capable of.

One way to do this is to take a language sample as an adolescent produces a narrative. As we saw in Chapter 3, a narrative task can often put sufficient demands on language ability to push or stress an individual's language performance. Problems with narrative production also seem to be implicated in children whose early language problems seem to persist in the adolescent years (Stothard et al., 1998). There are several types of narrative tasks, each having its advantages and disadvantages and each stressing an adolescent's language performance in different ways. In the Reed and Evernden study (2001), a story-retell task from a wordless picture book was employed to explore patterns of verb-form use. This type of narrative task reduces demands on a student's memory for a story and the influence of variables involving degrees of previous knowledge with particular stories but does not provide an auditory model of the story so that the language used is the language of the adolescent, not that recalled from an examiner's story. Retelling a story also tends to encourage the use of past-tense verbs, which means that it may trigger the appearance of verb-use patterns not evident in other types of discourse. This might explain why the students in the Reed and Evernden study (Reed & Evernden, 2001) used a greater proportion of progressive tenses (which involve a quite regular and more consistent pattern) rather than attempting to deal with the several variations of past tense (for example, regular past, irregular past involving an internal vowel change such as *swam,* irregular past involving a different word such as *did*). A further advantage of including a language sample obtained from a narrative task is that it can provide general information about an adolescent's ability to use narrative, a particularly important genre in the adolescent years. One of the more widely used computerized language sample analysis systems (Systematic Analysis of Language Transcripts—SALT) (Miller & Chapman, 2000) provides options for analyzing samples collected via conversation or through narrative. Collecting an adolescent's language sample in both contexts as opposed to just conversation or narrative is likely to provide the data needed for analyses to obtain a picture of adolescent's language abilities.

Contrived Situations.   The concepts of and push for the use of authentic forms of assessment can put professionals in a bind when assessing the language abilities of adolescents. As Nippold (1995) has indicated, "Tasks that are sensitive to later language development sometimes involve the use of language in limited or contrived contexts" (p. 320). To examine an adolescent's language performance in contrived situations seems, on the surface, to be contrary to the principles of authentic assessment. However, it may be necessary to use contrived contexts to elicit information about language abilities that are undermining a student's ability to function in authentic situations. Consequently, it might be useful to avoid considering these two approaches as mutually exclusive. Instead, using contrived situations can be helpful when additional probing of particular skills or eliciting the use of infrequently occurring language structures (e.g., adverbial connectives) is necessary, or when an adolescent's ability with language needs to be stressed. This approach can provide information about language behaviors that were not evidenced in what might be a less demanding conversational interaction and that reveal important information about an adolescent's language skills. Contrived situations might be particularly helpful for assessing language abilities involving aspects of figurative and literate language (e.g., proverbs, word definition skills, slang, idioms) and adverbial connectives.

Contrived situations may also be particularly helpful for examining adolescents' receptive language abilities when standardized testing for receptive language does not provide sufficient information for identification of language disorder or intervention planning. Receptive language ability is increasingly being recognized as an aspect of language performance that is often overlooked in terms of its impact on performance and outcomes from earlier language difficulties. For example, the evidence is mounting that children and adolescents who have receptive language impairments, with or without expressive language impairment, fare more poorly on measures of social adjustment and level of language abilities in adolescence (Asher & Gazelle, 1999; Beitchman, Wilson, Brownlie, Walters, & Lancee, 1996; Beitchman, Wilson, Brownlie, Walters, Inglis, et al., 1996). Careful assessment of an adolescent's receptive language abilities is important.

Portfolios.   In using portfolios as part of the assessment process, an adolescent and others who interact regularly with the adolescent (e.g., teachers, school counselors) add examples of the adolescent's work to a file. The file is intended to represent a collection of the adolescent's abilities in a variety of communication contexts and to reflect the adolescent's responses to different academic and communicative demands. The use of portfolios as a method of assessment is seen as a particularly ecologically valid approach. Wiig (1995) describes a 4×4 matrix that can be applied in a "structured, multidimensional assessment profile for focused holistic evaluation of portfolio samples across subject areas within a curriculum" (p.23). She refers to a profile resulting from such an assessment as an "S-MAP" (p. 23). Dimensions to be included in the assessment matrix vary by what are important dimensions for a particular communication task or context. Each dimension is then assessed on a rating scale of 1 (Good) to 4 (Unacceptable). For example, for a narrative sample, Wiig (1995) suggests that each of four dimensions (1. Organizational Structure; 2. Recall and Elaboration; 3. Coherence, Cohesion, and Conventions; 4. Evaluation, Monitoring, and Revision) be evaluated and assigned one of four ratings (1. Good; 2. Acceptable; 3. Marginal; 4. Unacceptable). Wiig (1995) provides descriptors to guide ratings within each dimension. For example, a description of "A recognizable narrative structure is followed; there is a clear beginning, middle sequence, and ending" for Organizational Structure is rated as "Good," whereas a description for Evaluation, Monitoring, and Revision of "There are many revisions or no revisions when appropriate; when there are revisions, they are abrupt and without transitions, become tangential and verbose" is rated as "Marginal" (p. 25). A matrix such as this has the potential to bring to analysis of adolescents' portfolios a more systematic approach than might otherwise occur.

Assessing the Educational System.   Success or failure in school significantly affects all aspects of life in adolescence, as well as adult life. When an adolescent suspected of having a language disorder has particular difficulty with certain subject areas, Larson and McKinley

(2003) believe that the student's educational environment, as well as his or her language skills, should be assessed. These authors suggest that such an assessment can help identify the source of the problem (either with the student or with the educational system), determine if the problem stems from the adolescent's lack of motivation or a lack of skill, and indicate whether or not an intervention plan needs to include curriculum modification as well as more direct language intervention. In completing a curriculum analysis, the language of instruction, the language of the textbooks, the student's attitude toward specific subjects, and the student's ability to comprehend the language used in the curriculum are assessed. A portfolio analysis of an adolescent's work from a number of different subjects and different types of communication tasks in these subjects might give us leads as to what and how to assess the educational system in which the adolescent is expected to use language to perform.

Larson and McKinley (1995) offer another strategy that can be used to facilitate completing such an assessment. These authors developed the Curriculum Analysis Form. The form is divided into three parts, all of which are completed for each course an adolescent is finding especially difficult. The first section analyzes the textbook used in the course, and the second focuses on the course's organization and the student's comprehension of classroom lectures/instructions and examinations. The last section of the form asks the adolescent to answer *yes* or *no* to a list of questions designed to probe the adolescent's attitude toward the course. When the analysis is completed, it helps clarify what strategies can be employed to assist the adolescent in dealing with educational language levels.

Lunday (1996) also developed a checklist to guide assessment of what communication skills are expected for postsecondary classroom and vocational success. This form consists of six aspects of language (Vocabulary, Use, Function, Organization, Form, Pragmatics), each of which is evaluated by answering a number of questions about expectations, for example, expected to participate in classroom discussions, expected to interpret and use nonverbal cues, required to understand figurative expressions. The teacher's expectation for each question is ascertained (i.e., yes it's an expectation, no it's not, or not applicable). For each question, the student's success in meeting each expectation is also evaluated as being positive, negative, or somewhere in the middle (+/–). The results provide a profile of what communication skills are important for the student from a teacher's perspective and the student's degree of ability to meet those expectations. This approach is quite consistent with the match/mismatch approach to assessment advocated by Larson and McKinley (1995), and the information obtained from such an analysis helps in determining intervention objectives.

The approach employed by Lunday (1996) to assessing classroom communication expectations recognized the importance of the perspectives of the teachers in influencing what communication skills adolescents need for success. What teachers perceive to be more and less important adolescent communication skills with them can set standards for adolescents' performances and influence their students' academic and personal success. To find out what high school teachers think are important communication skills for adolescents, Reed and Spicer (2003) asked grade 10 teachers to rank the importance of 14 communication skills. The skills represented a range of what would be considered primarily skills used for managing discourse (e.g., topic maintenance, conversational clarification and repair) and those related primarily to empathy and interpersonal relationships and considered to be addressee focused. Two metalinguistic/figurative language skills (verbal humor comprehension, appropriate slang usage) were also included among the 14 communication skills.

TABLE 5.8 High School Teachers' Ranking of the Importance of Communication Skills for Adolescents' Interactions with Their Teachers (in order from most to least important)

1. Relating narratives
2. Presenting differing points of view or thoughts logically
3. Employing conversational clarification and repair strategies
4. Taking a conversational partner's perspective
5. Turn-taking appropriately
6. Using appropriate vocal tone
7. Establishing and maintaining appropriate eye contact
8. Selecting conversational topics
9. Comprehending nonverbal communication
10. Comprehending vocal tone
11. Conveying messages tactfully
12. Maintaining topics
13. Comprehending verbal humor
14. Using appropriate adolescent slang

Source: Adapted from Reed & Spicer (2003).

Table 5.8 shows the teachers' ranking of the 14 communication skills from most to least important. The skills ranked as relatively high in importance were ones generally associated with discourse-management strategies, while the least important skills were the two metalinguistic/figurative language skills. To identify potential areas of mismatch and, therefore, potential intervention objectives, students' degrees of ability with each of these communication skills can be compared to the relative importance attached to them by their teachers, not unlike the approach used with Lunday's (1996) checklist.

Intervention

Unlike much of the intervention with language-disordered youngsters, who are often naive about the purposes and objectives of intervention, there is a general consensus among professionals working with adolescents with language disorders that these adolescents must participate in planning their own intervention (Bray, 1995; Ehren & Lenz, 1989; Larson & McKinley, 2003). As Larson and McKinley (1985) write, there can be "no 'hidden agenda' when providing services for adolescents" (p. 72). The principle of no hidden agenda means that

- Purposes of assessments are explained and results are shared with the adolescent.
- Responsibility for identifying, establishing, and prioritizing intervention plans and objectives is a task shared among the adolescent and relevant professionals (e.g., speech–language pathologist, classroom teachers, special educator).
- The reasons why particular skills are included in assessments and/or targeted in intervention are explained to and discussed with the adolescent.

Among the several reasons for adopting this approach are the following:

- Adolescents who recognize and accept that they have problems with communication and believe that intervention can help often begin to identify their own communicative behaviors that they wish to improve and that are important to them.
- Involvement in determining their own objectives leads the adolescents to accept responsibility for their problems, to take ownership of the problems, and to realize that they have the major role in modifying their language skills.
- Taking responsibility for their own problems and ways in which to address them means that adolescents are more likely to be motivated to improve.
- It begins to address what is a major objective of intervention with adolescents—improving their "meta" skills, that is, metalinguistics, metacognition, metapragmatics.

Principles in Determining Intervention Objectives

Emphasize Strategies and Regularities.   Objectives need to emphasize direct instruction that shows adolescents how to learn language and how to manage language demands of learning (Bray, 1995; Buttrill, Niizawa, Biemer, Takahashi, & Hearn, 1989; Comkowycz et al., 1987; Donahue, Szymanski, & Flores, 1999; Ehren, 2002; Larson & McKinley, 2003; Simon, 1998). That is, adolescents need to be taught strategies, rules, and techniques that will improve their communicative performances and their abilities to use their language to learn and function socially and vocationally. These are the skills that can be generalized to daily language use. The emphasis is, therefore, on using and improving metalinguistic, metacognitive, and metapragmatic abilities. Sometimes the terms *executive functioning* or *self-regulation* are used to describe the focus or processes related to this strategies approach, but as Singer and Bashir (1999) point out, "both are considered 'meta' constructs" (p. 265).

A number of different specific strategies approaches are described in the literature, for example, the Self-Regulated Strategy Development (SRSD) Model (Graham & Harris, 1999), the Strategic Process Model for Strategy Development (Wiig, 1990a), the Kansas University Strategies Intervention Model (Deshler & Schumaker, 1988), and Integrative Strategy Instruction (Ellis, 1993). What all of these have in common, according to Bray (1995), is that "students learn how to identify patterns in the information to be processed, select a plan of strategies to learn the information, implement the strategic plan, and later evaluate and monitor its effectiveness" (p. 67). This approach contrasts with intervention objectives focusing on tutoring in academic content areas. Intervention, then, includes teaching specific strategies and discussions about which of the strategies can be employed under what situations, including specific examples of other possible situations. Adolescents' conscious attempts to acquire strategies and to generate more examples of where else to apply the strategies can enhance, in very practical ways, the students' metalinguistic and metacognitive skills and facilitate generalization or bridging. Additionally, this approach stresses the pragmatic aspects of language and makes language functional for the adolescents, another guiding principle of intervention for adolescents with language impairments.

Authentic Intervention—but "Practice Makes Perfect."   Just as assessment processes with adolescents need to be authentic, so does intervention. Developing objectives that emphasize functional communication skills is another principle of language intervention for adolescents. Singer and Bashir (1999) advise to

> . . . avoid decontextualized interventions. Goals of intervention are not isolated from the day-to-day demands for communication and learning that students encounter. (pp. 271–272)

Authentic objectives include but are not limited to pragmatic language skills that promote positive human interactions, facilitate academic success, and allow people to operate on a day-to-day basis without recurring failures. Using information about what communication skills are more and less important to adolescents and their various communication partners in different situations, such as that shown in Table 5.9 as well as Table 5.8, can be helpful in selecting intervention objectives. As seen in Table 5.9, however, speech–language pathologists might not want to rely solely on what they believe would be important skills for adolescents because, as results of one of the studies shown in that table indicate, their opinions might differ substantially from those of adolescents, especially when adolescent peer interactions are being considered. When intervention centers on practical and relevant language abilities, adolescents are likely to recognize their importance and, therefore, be motivated to acquire them. This is especially true if the purposes of the objectives are explained and if real-life examples of effective and ineffective communication are provided.

It is unfortunate that for many adolescents with language impairments, their history of intervention will have been inconsistent, possibly with gaps in services, and objectives and directions of intervention may have suffered from a lack of coherence. This means that skills or strategies that might have been targets of intervention previously may have not been adequately learned in order to be stable or retained. Furthermore, these adolescents are typically inefficient learners who need additional time, repeated efforts, and more exposures than other students to learn and/or use a new skill or strategy. In contrast to their need for increased consistency and enhanced learning opportunities, their intervention has more than likely been inconsistent with inadequate opportunities and repetition of learning trials. This situation creates a wide gap between the learning opportunities that adolescents need to have provided for them to learn and achieve and what is often provided for them. Therefore, Simon (1998) advises that focused practice and overlearning of strategies and their implementation is essential and that "drill is not necessarily bad" (p. 263). She adds, however, that focused practice and drill need to be meaningful and to take place in context. That is, work on intervention objectives needs to be authentic, there needs to be a lot of it, and it needs to be consistent.

Different Intervention Emphases for Adolescents at Different Stages. The period of adolescence spans seven or more years. If thought of in terms of the changes that occur in a young child from infancy to 7 years of age, it should not be a surprising idea that the developmental stage known as adolescence needs to considered as consisting of substages, much in the same way that the 0- to 7-year period is thought of as several stages (infants, toddlers, preschoolers, primary-school age). When planning intervention, therefore, the adolescent's stage must be considered and the strategies, activities, and objectives need to correspond to his or her social-cognitive level (Larson & McKinley, 2003).

In the early years of adolescence, teenagers with language impairments have several years of school ahead of them, so there is still opportunity to improve academic performance.

TABLE 5.9 Rankings of the Importance of Fourteen Communication Skills for Adolescents in Different Communicative Contexts (in order from most to least important)

Whose Rankings:[1] Adolescents *Context:* In peers' communication for positive peer relationship	*Whose Rankings:*[2] Adolescents *Context:* In adolescent's own communication with peers for positive peer relationships	*Whose Rankings:*[2] Adolescents *Context:* In adolescent's own communication with teachers	*Whose Rankings:*[3] Speech–language pathologists *Context:* In adolescents' communication for positive peer relationships
1. Taking a conversational partner's perspective	1. Comprehending nonverbal communication	1. Turn-taking appropriately	1. Initiating topics of conversation appropriately*
2. Comprehending vocal tone	2. Taking a conversational partner's perspective	2. Taking a conversational partner's perspective	2. Selecting conversational topics
3. Conveying messages tactfully	3. Comprehending vocal tone	3. Presenting differing points of view or thoughts logically	3. Employing conversational clarification and repair strategies
4. Turn-taking appropriately	4. Using appropriate vocal tone	4. Employing conversational clarification and repair strategies	4. Presenting differing points of view or thoughts logically
5. Using appropriate vocal tone	5. Selecting conversational topics	5. Using appropriate vocal tone	5. Turn-taking appropriately
6. Establishing and maintaining appropriate eye contact	6. Conveying messages tactfully	6. Conveying messages tactfully	6. Comprehending verbal humor
7. Comprehending nonverbal communication	7. Presenting differing points of view or thoughts logically	7. Comprehending vocal tone	7. Comprehending nonverbal communication
8. Employing conversational clarification and repair strategies	8. Turn-taking appropriately	8. Relating narratives	8. Using appropriate adolescent slang
9. Selecting conversational topics	9. Employing conversational clarification and repair strategies	9. Establishing and maintaining appropriate eye contact	9. Relating narratives
10. Presenting differing points of view or thoughts logically	10. Establishing and maintaining appropriate eye contact	10. Selecting conversational topics	10. Establishing and maintaining appropriate eye contact
11. Relating narratives	11. Relating narratives	11. Comprehending nonverbal communication	11. Taking a conversational partner's perspective
12. Comprehending verbal humor	12. Comprehending verbal humor	12. Maintaining topics	12. Conveying messages tactfully
13. Maintaining topics	13. Maintaining topics	13. Comprehending verbal humor	13. Comprehending vocal tone
14. Using appropriate adolescent slang	14. Using appropriate adolescent slang	14. Using appropriate adolescent slang	14. Using appropriate vocal tone

* In this study, the item for topic initiation replaced the topic maintenance item in the other studies.

Sources: Adapted from: [1] Henry, Reed, & McAllister (1995); [2] Reed et al. (1999); [3] Reed, Bradfield, & McAllister (1998).

Relationships with peers are beginning to take on greater importance and there is greater expectation for appropriate interactions with a larger variety of people. For these reasons, intervention objectives with teenagers in the early years of adolescence that focus on language to improve both social and academic performance would likely be appropriate (Larson & McKinley, 2003). In contrast, teenagers in late adolescence, such as those between 16 and 18 years of age, are likely to have concerns about vocational options and employment, and peer relations are more important than in the early adolescent years. For these adolescents, objectives that emphasize improving language for vocational, as well as social, situations may be more important. For adolescents in the years between the early and later stages of adolescence (i.e., between about 13 and 15 years), peer relationships have considerable importance, and there is still some time to take advantage of academic input. However, vocational concerns may also emerge. For these reasons, there is considerable rationale for intervention objectives with these adolescents in the middle period of development to emphasize social, vocational, and academic language skills (Larson & McKinley, 2003).

Choosing Objectives for Success.   One maxim that we know well about human learning is that nothing succeeds like success; we know that success in learning leads to more success. This is a particularly important principle to consider in selecting intervention objectives for language-disordered adolescents, especially in the early stages of intervention. An adolescent with a language impairment likely has a history of academic and personal failure and may believe that he or she is not capable of learning when language is involved. It is not unusual for language-disordered adolescents to resist or avoid such learning situations. Therefore, as Bray (1995) writes, "it is important for a student to see results soon after learning and trying a strategy in order to 'buy into' the program" (p. 69). When adolescents see that they "can do it" and that it makes a difference in real ways for them, they are more apt to try to do more and to improve. Motivation problems are commonly ascribed to adolescents with language disorders. Choosing objectives that promote quick success, particularly in the early stages of intervention, can help overcome some of the problems related to motivation.

Factors in Implementing Intervention Objectives

Direct Teaching.   Intervention requires direct teaching of skills and specific strategies to adolescents (Ehren, 2002) so that they actually learn them and the analysis abilities needed to apply and evaluate them, to learn to recognize when the skills and strategies should be used and which should be tried, and to learn to self-initiate applying these. Other adolescents have learned a great deal of language, a great deal about how to learn, and a great deal about how to use their language to learn, usually without having been taught any of this directly; language-disordered adolescents have not, and there is little reason to believe that by the time these individuals reach adolescence they will learn these skills without being taught directly.

Considering Characteristics of Adolescents with Language Impairments.   Implementing intervention objectives, and in particular direct teaching that focuses on a strategies approach, can be trickier than it might seem. The things that these adolescents need to learn to do require them to use the very abilities and skills that are typically weak for them, and are actually considered to be characteristics of these teenagers. This is probably why the adolescents did not acquire the strategies and skills in the first place. Table 5.10 highlights what

TABLE 5.10 Discrepancies between Characteristics of Adolescents with Language Impairments and Requirements of Strategies Taught in Intervention

Some Characteristics of Adolescents with Language Impairments	Requirements Involved in Employing Language-Based Learning Strategies
An adolescent with a language impairment likely has weak metalinguistic and metacognitive skills.	A strategies approach requires an adolescent to analyze and think about communicative situations and language demands of a learning task, that is, metalinguisitc and metacognitive skills. In essence, what this does is ask the adolescent to use what are weak metalinguistic and metacognitive skills, rather than use what might be stronger skills, to learn new strategies and apply them in new situations that, in themselves, are "meta" skills.
Many adolescents with language impairments are quite poor and inefficient information processors. Inefficient information-processing abilities probably mean that an adolescent's problem-solving and task-analysis activities are slow. The educational system and interpersonal interactions expect quick responses; a language-disordered teenager may have learned over his or her many school years that adults and peers dislike incorrect responses less than delayed or no responses.	Using metalinguistic and metacognitive tasks can require that a considerable amount of information be stored in short-term or working memory long enough to be processed and mentally manipulated.
The adolescent might have figured out that if he or she guesses but is wrong, an adult will probably explain and fill in the missing parts or move on to something or somebody else so that the language-disordered adolescent is "let off the hook." To the adolescent, it may be better to respond quickly and be wrong than cause a delay or create a silence while trying to figure out a correct response. There is the possibility of a long history of a language-disordered adolescent having been provided with inadvertent positive reinforcement for quick, ill-considered responses. Adolescents with language disorders may have habituated a "guessing strategy." Response impulsivity is characteristic of many adolescents with language impairments.	A strategies approach requires that the adolescent take time to figure out an appropriate approach to a problem and arrive at a correct answer. Guessing is the exact opposite of what is necessary for the considered, analytical approach involved in using strategies
Adolescents with language impairments are often concrete thinkers. Many adolescents with language disorders are passive and dependent learners; "learned helplessness" is a term sometimes associated with adolescents with language impairments. Adolescents with language impairments often fail to self-activate or self-initiate the application of strategies even when they have learned the strategies and where to use them.	A strategies approach involves both situational analysis and performance evaluation, which are generally considered to be quite hypothetical and formal thought processes. Learning and using strategies requires that students initiate the process of analyzing a task, select one or more strategies from their repertoire, and then apply these and do so independently without needing to be prompted by another person.

might be incompatibilities and clashes between the requirements of learning and using language-related strategies and a number of the characteristics commonly seen in adolescents with language problems.

These adolescents have a long history—possibly as long as they are old—of "not quite having got it," "it" being whatever was in the environment to be learned at any point in time. These adolescents are also victims of the "Matthew effect" (Stanovich, 1986), explained as real-life examples of the second part of the proverb, "The rich get richer and the poor get poorer." Because adolescents with language disorders most likely started school with poor language skills when good language skills are required for becoming readers, they would not have learned to read fluently and well. And because reading is the greatest single source for further language acquisition and world knowledge, their poor reading skills mean that the gap between students with language problems and those able to take advantage of reading and formal education widens greatly through the early school years into adolescence. Because of the missed bits of information and the mislearning that have fed into these adolescents' concept formation and knowledge base for years, Simon (1998) suggests that "over time, a great deal of *misinformation can be acquired*" and that students' world knowledge can seem "quite weird" (p. 258). The misconceptions that adolescents with language impairment acquire means that they attempt to build new knowledge on top of flawed, distorted, and/or incomplete information. Wiig (1995) likens this to trying to build a house on a hole instead of a solid foundation. A somewhat different analogy is illustrated in Figure 5.6. In this illustration an adolescent's world knowledge is conceived of as

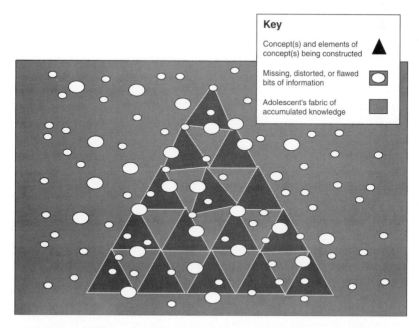

FIGURE 5.6 A Schematic Illustration of Adolescents' Constructions of Concepts on an Incomplete Fabric of Accumulated Knowledge Flawed over Time by Missing Bits of Information as a Result of Early and Ongoing Language Impairments

a piece of fabric into which pellets from a shotgun have been fired and which have left randomly sized and randomly located holes in information. Concepts and knowledge that underpin the formation of new, larger, and more complex concepts are flawed, distorted, and undermined in unpredictable ways by the holes in knowledge. In working with adolescents with language disorders, professionals cannot assume that the concepts these teenagers have formed are similar to those of their normally achieving peers.

Intervention Approaches to Accommodate Adolescents' Language and Learning Characteristics.   Although implementing intervention objectives for adolescents with language impairments might be tricky, a number of techniques and approaches can be helpful in getting around the barriers to learning raised by the language and learning characteristics exhibited by these adolescents. Among these are the following.

■ Teach, expect, and reward an adolescent's self-activation and self-initiation in applying strategies and skills; stress independent learning; identify self-activation and self-initiation as intervention objectives in their own right. This particular approach attempts to replace dependent, passive learning behaviors with those characteristic of active and independent learners and those more in line with learner expectations in the high school years.

■ Ensure overlearning and stabilization, plan for and build in redundancy, and incorporate repetition in many different situations; follow up; return regularly and frequently to previously targeted objectives to review performance and ensure the skills have been maintained; build in regular monitoring and checking of skills previously targeted that are no longer active intervention objectives. All of this is especially important in light of what has probably been an inconsistent intervention history for an adolescent and the evidence that skills and strategies often break down during periods of stress, typically when they are most needed, even when these appeared to have previously been learned quite well (Bray, 1995).

■ Because speed of response is the antithesis of what is trying to be achieved by a strategies approach for these adolescents, replace habituated guessing and response impulsivity with a strategy that allows them to delay responding and provides for processing time. Increasing wait time before making responses has been found to improve the quality of the responses of school-age children with language-learning disabilities to higher-level cognitive questions involving synthesis of information and to increase their verbal fluency (i.e., reduce maze behavior) in relating the information (Ellis Weismer & Schraeder, 1993). These findings are consistent with information from educational research involving both school-age and university students (Kaplan & Kies, 1994; Tobin, 1986, 1987). However, many of those with whom adolescents interact in the educational system and in peer relationships are likely to expect them to keep up in conversational turn exchanges and with responses in interactions. It is important, therefore, to help these individuals to employ an appropriate wait time as well assist the adolescents to adopt pragmatically appropriate ways to delay responding, such as making a statement that indicates an intentional delay ("Let me think about that," "Mmmm"). For school-age children with specific language impairment, Evans and her colleagues (1997) found that the use of verbal pauses (e.g., "ah," "um") at the beginning of the children's turns during conversational interchanges predicted their use of longer utterances. Such responses mark a turn, signal awareness of the previous utterance, indicate a need for a response, and fill the space while providing time to comprehend what was to be taken in and formulate a response. Such responses need to be well rehearsed and habituated, however, if they are to be of help to adolescents.

Although many adolescents with language disorders demonstrate a pattern of ill-considered, quick responses, there are some who do not respond at all or who exhibit long, silent pauses in their utterances (Dollaghan & Campbell, 1992), leaving silences to fill the spaces where others expect responses or disrupting the flow of conversation. If the reason for the silences is that an adolescent is using these "to buy" processing time, these inappropriate occurrences of unacknowledged silences, often misinterpreted by others as sullenness or obstinacy, can also be addressed by replacing the behavior with a more pragmatically appropriate delaying tactic involving a rehearsed statement or filler (Dollaghan & Campbell, 1992).

■ Employ concrete, hands-on activities to work on abstract "meta" tasks. The idea is to use activities consistent with concrete cognitive levels—for example, sorting cards or objects, creating models, using paper and pencil or a computer to map concepts—to facilitate development, use, and learning of various higher-level cognitive "meta"-level tasks associated with a strategies approach.

■ Reduce information-processing demands (e.g., how much information needs to be stored at a time in working memory, how much mental manipulation is involved in a task) by keeping needed information in the immediate environment. This can be accomplished by using intransient and stable stimuli (usually visual or graphic), such as lists and charts, to supplement or counter transient auditory stimuli. With this technique an adolescent can retrieve and consult bits of information in "permanent" (i.e., intransient) form that are needed to solve abstract or meta tasks or needed to implement a particular problem solving strategy.

Activities with an Authentic Focus That Integrate Aspects of Language. The suggested techniques above do not preclude the use of authentically based activities. In fact, the techniques can be ways to facilitate language-based strategies and to integrate work on several aspects of language. As an example, a functional activity might center around a very real life ability and, therefore, quite authentic objective, i.e., understanding a TV weather broadcast. A small-group setting might be used to address several functional aims: (1) to understand meanings of words, such as *precipitation, barometer,* and *prevailing,* as in *prevailing winds*; (2) to recognize cause–effect relationships based on the next day's forecast; (3) to identify specific differences between formal register as used in a TV broadcast and informal register inappropriate for such a communicative situation; (4) to select words, phrases, and sentences appropriate for use in a formal communicative context such as giving a weather broadcast; and (5) to adopt a formal communicative style appropriately. We see that these objectives encompass semantic, syntactic, morphological, and pragmatic aspects of language at both the receptive and expressive levels, yet they center on a functional survival skill while promoting metalinguistic and metacognitive skills.

Service Delivery

In Chapter 4, several different models of service delivery were discussed. What we know about intervention for adolescents with language impairments is that traditional service delivery models, such as the pull-out model, are not effective if used as the sole intervention approach (Buttrill et al., 1989; Comkowycz et al., 1987; Ehren, 2002; Larson & McKinley,

2003). Boyce and Larson (1983) give four reasons for the ineffectiveness of these traditional models:

1. When secondary students are removed from their classrooms for short periods of time twice a week, the usual daily schedules are disrupted.
2. Secondary students who need to walk in and out of classrooms during class periods are viewed as different from their peers during a developmental period when conformity to the peer norm is important to them.
3. Intervention can be viewed as punitive because, in addition to the first two reasons, the adolescents "receive no credit for work that may be very difficult for them" (p. 23).
4. Establishing and maintaining relationships with service providers is difficult when these professionals are removed from the usual routine of the schools. Additionally, the traditional one-to-one intervention fails to promote communicative interactions and provide opportunities to practice new language skills in varied communicative contexts.

The other thing we know about serving adolescents with language disorders is that an indirect intervention service delivery model, such as collaborative consultation, by itself is typically not sufficient to address to the academic and social needs of many of these students. However, it is important to integrate the principles of this service delivery approach into a more encompassing model of providing intervention for these adolescents. That is, close collaboration and consultation among all professionals who interact with an adolescent is essential for a unified and integrated intervention program. Not only is this good practice, it is also consistent with the legislation that guides and funds service delivery.

An alternative service delivery model for providing direct language intervention for language-disordered adolescents has been proposed (Larson & McKinley, 2003; Work, Cline, Ehren, Keiser, & Wujek, 1993). In this model, existing blocks of time in the school's daily schedule are frequently utilized for intervention. Students may be seen for an entire time period on a regularly scheduled basis, often five days a week corresponding with other academic class schedules. As with other classes, the students are generally seen in groups, although these groups are much smaller than the usual academic class. Small-group sessions facilitate interaction and communication practice. Furthermore, students can work on comprehension, production, and metalinguistic skills simultaneously. To describe such an intervention format, supportive titles, rather than punitive ones, are recommended, such as those of Larson and McKinley (1995), "Individualized Language Skills" or "Oral Communication Strategies" (p. 162). The Language Intervention Program for Secondary Students (LIPSS) (Comkowycz et al., 1987), implemented in Polk County Schools, Florida, selected the name Exceptional Student Education—Language Arts because the class "is taught under the rubric of a state-designed curriculum framework" (p. 204). A program in the Palo Alto Unified School District, California, chose the name Language/Study Skills Class (Buttrill et al., 1989).

Because the class schedule in this service delivery model is similar to that of other classes adolescents take, the intervention period can actually be added as a course in the school's curriculum. In some instances, credit may even be given. The adolescents can be awarded grades, or their performances can be evaluated on a pass–fail basis. With this intervention format, students' efforts are recognized, intervention is not viewed as penalizing or stigmatizing, and functional communication strategies can be learned and practiced in interactive situations. The model resolves the problems of traditional service delivery formats. Furthermore, because the format fits into the daily academic schedule, intervention becomes an integrated, accepted part of the school routine.

Summary

In this chapter we have seen that

- Important aspects of language continue to develop into adolescence as teenagers gain communicative competence.
- Many gaps remain in our knowledge of normal adolescent language development, and this group of individuals with language impairments continues to be relatively neglected professionally.
- Gaps make assessment of language-disordered adolescents an especially challenging process that must rely heavily on nonstandardized procedures.
- Fewer standardized language tests have been developed for adolescents than for youngsters, and the validity of several of these adolescent tests has been questioned.
- Intervention for language-disordered adolescents needs to
  - Involve the adolescents in helping to set their own intervention objectives.
  - Focus on functional communication skills and emphasize authentic objectives in authentic contexts.
  - Consider an adolescent's developmental stage and use a variety of intervention techniques to work around the barriers to learning that an adolescent with a language impairment can exhibit.
  - Emphasize communication strategies and improve metalinguistic, metapragmatic, and metacognitive skills.
  - Shift from traditional service delivery models to accommodate the needs of these adolescents.

If only one point is to emerge from the information in this chapter, it is that language disorders negatively impact on adolescents' academic and personal successes in junior and senior high schools and limit their social, vocational, and educational opportunities as adults. Neglecting these language-disordered adolescents would be a sad professional commentary.

6 Language and Children with Intellectual Disabilities

STEVEN H. LONG

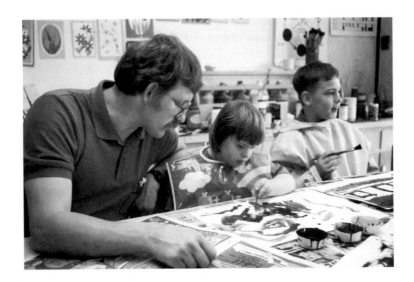

OBJECTIVES

After reading this chapter you should be able to discuss

- Definitions and etiological categories of intellectual disabilities
- How research on children with intellectual disabilities is conducted
- Differences between children with Down syndrome and children with intellectual disabilities due to other causes
- Characteristics of the language of children with intellectual disabilities
- Principles of language intervention for children with intellectual disabilities

In the study of language disorders, it is conventional to discuss children with intellectual disabilities as a group. This chapter will not break with that practice but will try to show how diverse these children really are. We find among children with intellectual disabilities a wide range of physical conditions and behaviors. Some children may show mild intellectual deficits but few other problems: they look like their peers, attend school and interact well with typically developing children, do not have seizures or other neurophysiological disorders, and speak intelligibly and effectively. Other children with intellectual disabilities may present a totally different picture. They have physical disabilities and attend a special school or special classroom with other severely disabled children. One child may occasionally scream and scratch himself; another may wear a helmet to protect her head when she falls during a seizure; and a third may not communicate with speech. When you read about research on children with intellectual disabilities, it is important to ask several questions: What kinds of children were studied? How old were they? What did they look like? How severe was their intellectual impairment? How severe were their physical, social, and educational problems? By challenging the information in this way, you will not fall into the trap of thinking about children with intellectual disabilities as all the same.

An Overview of Intellectual Disabilities

Definition

There is no official definition of intellectual disabilities, and not everyone is careful to say precisely what he or she means by the term. In fact, it is only recently that the term *intellectual disabilities* has been used. Previously, the commonly used term was *mental retardation.* As recently as 2002, a prominent association dealing with the area of intellectual disability was using the term *mental retardation* (American Association on Mental Retardation), although there was considerable debate within the organization about changing the association's name to the American Association on Intellectual Disabilities. For the most part in this chapter, the term *intellectual disabilities* will be used, unless it would be inappropriate to do so as in a quotation or a proper name.

　　The most influential definition of intellectual disability is that of the American Association on Mental Retardation (AAMR)[1] (American Association on Mental Retardation, 2002):

> Mental retardation is a disability characterized by significant limitations both in intellectual functioning and in adaptive behavior as expressed in conceptual, social, and practical adaptive skills. This disability originates before age 18.

What does this mean? An individual's "intellectual functioning" is determined from the results of an intelligence quotient (IQ) test, and "significant limitations" is quantified as "approximately IQ 70 or below." The AAMR deliberately uses the word *approximately* to allow for differences in the reliability of various IQ tests (Grossman, 1983). The range 70–75 is the cutoff recommended by the AAMR, but each state is allowed to set its own guidelines for identifying children with intellectual disabilities.

---

[1]Formerly called the American Association on Mental Deficiency (AAMD).

A number of tests are used to measure intelligence, depending on the age and verbal ability of the child:

- The Stanford-Binet Intelligence Scale—Fourth Edition (Thorndike, Hagen, & Sattler, 1996) has a long history and is still used with children of all ages.
- The Wechsler Intelligence Scale for Children—Third Edition (Wechsler, 1991) is another test used commonly with children of school age.
- As detection and intervention efforts focus increasingly on infants and preschoolers, the Bayley Scales of Infant Development—Second Edition (Bayley, 1993) has come into widespread use.
- For some individuals, tests that do not require verbal responses are needed, such as the Leiter International Performance Scale—Revised (Roid & Miller, 1997).

There are still other IQ tests with specific uses and advantages. What all IQ tests have in common, however, is that they yield a mental age (MA), an estimate of the individual's level of cognitive functioning. An IQ is derived by dividing the MA by the individual's chronological age (CA), that is, IQ = MA/CA.

Though the IQ scale is a continuous set of numbers, it is the practice of professionals in the field to describe levels of impairment for purposes of placement and research. Until 1992 the AAMR supported the use of descriptive labels based on IQ intervals. These labels paralleled an older set of terms that had traditionally been used in educational placement. In its last two documents on definition and classification (1992 and 2002), the AAMR has shifted to a concept that describes individuals with intellectual disabilities not in terms of their impairment but according to the intensity of support that they require to function across environments. These changes in labels and levels are shown in Table 6.1, which also includes the new levels. Because the concept of supports is such a radical departure from categorization based on IQ scores, it has not yet been fully embraced by governments and institutions. A recent survey of state agencies found that only four of them had updated their guidelines for definition and classification of intellectual disabilities to put them in line with the 1992 AAMR recommendations (Denning, Chamberlain, & Polloway, 2000).

Another term associated with definitions of intellectual disabilities is *adaptive behavior,* the ability to act as independently and responsibly as other people of the same age and cultural background. Adaptive behaviors are partitioned into the categories of conceptual skills (e.g., language, money concepts), social skills (e.g., following rules, self-esteem), and practical skills (e.g., eating, dressing, work skills). Examiners employ standardized tests that are normed on the general population to determine if an individual performs significantly below the mean in at least one of the three categories. It is important to note that most definitions of intellectual disabilities require evidence of lowered intelligence *and* adaptive behavior limitations. Also, the term *intellectual disabilities* is used only when these limitations appear during the *developmental period,* that is, up to 18 years of age.

In the literature on exceptional children, several other terms are used whose meanings are similar to intellectual disabilities. *Developmental disability* is one such term. This label is used in federal law to describe mental or physical disabilities, or both, that appear before age 22, are likely to continue indefinitely, and result in substantial functional limitations in self-care, language, learning, mobility, self-direction, capacity for independent living, and economic self-sufficiency. There is great, though not total, overlap between the categories of

TABLE 6.1   **Levels of Impairment of Individuals with Intellectual Disabilities**

	AAMR* Classification	**Traditional Label**	**IQ Range**	**Percentage of Persons with Intellectual Disabilities**
Previous labels	Mild	Educable	50–55 to 70	89
	Moderate	Trainable	35–40 to 50–55	7
	Severe	Custodial	20–25 to 35–40	3
	Profound	Life support	Below 20–25	1
Revised labels (adapted from AAMR, 2002)	Intermittent	Short-term supports, such as during an acute medical crisis		
	Limited	Supports needed regularly but briefly, such as employee assistance to remediate a job-related skill deficit		
	Extensive	Ongoing and regular assistance, such as long-term home living support		
	Pervasive	Potentially life-sustaining support, such as attendant care, skilled medical care, or help with taking medications		

*American Association on Mental Retardation.

intellectual disabilities and developmental disability. The differences occur at the upper end of the impaired range (e.g., an IQ of 65), at which an individual may receive a diagnosis of intellectual disabilities but *not* developmental disability (Grossman, 1983). There are, however, circumstances when the IQ of a child has not or cannot be determined. In these circumstances, it is common for the child to be identified by etiological category (e.g., fragile X syndrome) or simply labeled as *developmentally disabled* (Taylor & Kaufmann, 1991).

Autism is another term that has substantial overlap with intellectual disabilities. Around three-quarters of children with autism have IQ scores within the impaired range. Both researchers and practitioners, however, have tended to treat children with autism as a distinct group. Therefore a separate chapter in this text (Chapter 7) is devoted to them.

Learning disability is a category of impairment that is defined in federal law. Children with intellectual disabilities are specifically excluded from this category. In practice, though, there is a relationship between learning disability and intellectual disabilities. In just the 7 years following the enactment of P.L. 94-142, a 19 percent decrease was reported in the number of children receiving special education services who were identified as intellectually disabled. In actuality, however, this decrease may have reflected a shift in labeling practices, with many individuals with mild intellectual disabilities being reclassified as learning disabled (Frankenberger & Harper, 1988; MacMillan & Siperstein, 2001).

Causes of Intellectual Disabilities

In the preceding discussion, test performance was used to distinguish different levels of intellectual disability. Differentiation by level of performance is important to educators and administrators because it serves to place children with intellectual disabilities into programs and allocate funds to those programs. Other differences are frequently more important, however, to researchers who are interested in uncovering the causes of intellectual disabilities.

Research findings from many sources suggest that there are two broad categories of intellectual disability: *organic,* which results from major chromosomal, genetic, or traumatic causes; and *familial,* which has no known cause but tends to run in families. Table 6.2 summarizes the general characteristics of the two etiological categories.

The causes of organic intellectual disability are commonly identified by their period of occurrence: before the pregnancy (genetic), during the pregnancy (prenatal), or during delivery (perinatal). Several types of chromosomal or other genetic abnormality produce congenital syndromes associated with intellectual disabilities. Down syndrome and fragile X syndrome are the more common disorders of this type. Prenatal events, such as physical injury or substance abuse, may cause injury to the fetus and lead to an intellectual disability. Fetal alcohol syndrome (FAS), caused by excessive drinking during pregnancy, is one such condition (Coggins, Friet, & Morgan, 1998) and is estimated to occur in 0.3 to 2.2/1,000 births. During the actual delivery, there is a risk of hypoxia—inadequate oxygen going the brain of the baby—which may result in brain damage and intellectual disability.

Although organic intellectual disability is frequently studied and appears to have clear subtypes, it is less evident how familial intellectual disability should be viewed. One

TABLE 6.2   General Characteristics of Individuals with Organic and Familial Intellectual Disability

Organic Intellectual Disability	Familial Intellectual Disability
IQs most often below 50	IQs rarely below 50
Demonstrable organic etiology in 43–70% of cases	No demonstrable organic etiology in 76–80% of cases; parents may have this same type of intellectual disability
Found at all socioeconomic levels	More prevalent at lower socioeconomic levels
Siblings usually of normal intelligence	Siblings often have subnormal intelligence
Often accompanied by severe health problems	Health within normal range
Appearance often marred by physical stigmata	Normal appearance
Mortality rate higher (more likely to die at a younger age than the general population)	Normal mortality rate
Often dependent on care from others throughout life	With some support, can lead independent existence as adults
Unlikely to marry and often infertile	Likely to marry and produce children of low intelligence
Unlikely to experience neglect in their homes	More likely to experience neglect in their homes
High prevalence of associated physical disabilities (e.g., epilepsy, cerebral palsy)	Less likely to have other physical disabilities
Exhibit atypical patterns of development	Exhibit normal developmental patterns at a slower rate of growth

Sources: Adapted from Bennett-Gates & Zigler (1998); Murphy, Boyle, Schendel, Decoufle, & Yeargin-Allsopp (1998); and Zigler & Hodapp (1986).

proposal (Burack, 1990; Zigler & Balla, 1982; Zigler & Hodapp, 1986, 1991) is that there are three subtypes:

1. Either or both parents of a child with an intellectual disability are themselves intellectually disabled—about 35 percent of all individuals with intellectual disabilties.
2. The parents are not intellectually disabled but the intellectual disability is genetically inherited—another 35 percent of the total. In contrast to organic intellectual disabilities, which may also be genetic, inherited familial intellectual disability is not associated with a syndrome and produces less severe developmental disabilities.
3. Intellectual disability is due to extreme environmental deprivation—about 5 percent of the total.

Types and subtypes of intellectual disability are distinguished on the basis of what is presently known about genetic and environmental phenomena. As more becomes known, it is likely that our classifications will continue to shift.

Of all the known or suspected causes of intellectual disabilities, Down syndrome is unique because it can be identified relatively well at birth, and it has a clearly organic etiology. Consequently, children with Down syndrome have been the most intensively studied population of children with intellectual disabilities. This is especially true of early-developing behaviors. Because our information base is so much greater for Down syndrome, a separate section of this chapter will be devoted to a discussion of these children. Fragile X syndrome and FAS are two other conditions that are now being studied as biologically well-defined subgroups. Fragile X can now be identified prenatally, and it will therefore be possible in the future to study more thoroughly the developmental course of this group of children.

Associated Problems

Many children with intellectual disabilities show differences in appearance and have physical disabilities and health problems much more frequently than their non-intellectually disabled peers. As noted in Table 6.2, these problems are more frequent in children with organic intellectual disabilities. Few studies, however, have reported separate findings for the organic and familial populations. Table 6.3 summarizes information on associated problems as they have been reported for children with Down syndrome and for children with other intellectual disabilities syndromes or intellectual disability of unspecified cause.

The high prevalence of hearing loss is an important factor in understanding the language impairment of children with intellectual disabilities. Hearing impairment serves to multiply rather than just add to the disabilities of individuals with intellectual disabilities: learning is made more difficult, which delays cognitive development; and the delays in cognitive development diminish the use of auditory information and cause further intellectual impairment.

The causes of *sensorineural hearing loss* are often the same as the causes of intellectual disability—genetic factors, pre- and postnatal trauma, and diseases such as rubella and meningitis. *Conductive hearing loss,* on the other hand, is attributable to several organic and environmental factors. Congenital malformation of the middle ear is more common among children with intellectual disabilities. Estimates of abnormal middle ear function range from 30 to 63 percent, with the greatest problems found in individuals with severe intellectual disability (Givens & Seidemann, 1977; Lloyd & Fulton, 1972; Nolan, McCartney, McArthur, & Rowson, 1980). In addition, poor self-care habits may exacerbate hearing problems.

TABLE 6.3   Associated Problems of Appearance, Physical Disabilities, and Health Problems in Children with Intellectual Disabilities

Condition	All Children with Intellectual Disabilities	Children with Down Syndrome
Appearance		
Deviations in head size	Microcephaly and hydrocephaly	
Deviations in orofacial structure	Small eyes, poor head and mid-face growth are characteristic of children with FAS (Abel, 1998)	Upward-slanting eyes, prominent epicanthal folds, a small nose and chin, and a flattened bridge of the nose (Pueschel, 1992)
Physical Disabilities		
Epilepsy (seizures)	15–30% (McLaren & Bryson, 1987)	
Cerebral palsy and other motor impairments	20–30% (McLaren & Bryson, 1987)	
Sensory impairments (see also discussion in text)	20–60% require correction for refractive errors of vision (Maino, Rado, & Pizzi, 1996)	Visual: 40% show poor bilateral vision or amblyopia ("lazy eye") (Pueschel & Gieswein, 1993)
		Auditory: findings for conductive loss range from 21% to 58%, for sensorineural or mixed loss from 4% to 44% (Dahle & Baldwin, 1992)
Low muscle tone (hypotonia)		Causes gross motor delays, problems in feeding
Health Problems		
Congenital heart defects		40% to 60% (Martin, 1997; Pueschel, 1990)
Other problems	Obesity is more common than in the general population, with over-all prevalence estimates ranging from 29.5% to 50.5% (Rimmer, Braddock, & Fujiura, 1993; Rubin, Rimmer, Chicoine, Braddock, & McGuire, 1998)	Increased prevalence of leukemia (Hasle, Clemmensen, & Mikkelsen, 2000)
		Increased likelihood of diabetes (Kapell et al., 1998) and thyroid problems (Saenz, 1999) that may lead to obesity or decreased intellectual functioning
		Upper respiratory infections (Saenz, 1999)
		Abnormally high incidence of Alzheimer's disease in middle age (Janicki & Dalton, 2000)
		Sleep disorders, possibly due to upper airway obstruction (apnea) (Stores, 1993)
		Atlantoaxial instability, increased mobility between the first and second cervical vertebrae that increases the risk of spinal cord injury (Pueschel, 1998)

Hearing loss appears to be especially prevalent in the Down syndrome population (Saenz, 1999). The risk of hearing impairment is high in infancy and continues all the way into adulthood (Marcell, 1995). One reason children with Down syndrome are so prone to hearing loss is that they frequently have abnormally small outer ear canals, muscular hypotonia, and skull defects that inhibit middle ear drainage.

The Delay–Difference Controversy

A fundamental issue in intellectual disabilities research over the years has been the *delay–difference controversy*—that is, whether the cognitive and linguistic processes of individuals with and without intellectual disabilities are the same. No one disputes that the *achievements* of children with intellectual disabilities are lower. The debate focuses on the *explanation* for that lower achievement and whether it requires us to invoke the idea of specific qualitative differences in how these children develop. The argument is more intense for children with familial intellectual disabilities, about 75 percent of those identified as intellectually disabled, who show no evidence of central nervous system dysfunction. In those cases there are no "hard signs" to suggest that a qualitative difference does exist (Zigler & Balla, 1982).

To investigate the delay–difference controversy, researchers have applied the scientific method of making and testing predictions. These predictions have relied on the technique of matching subjects with and without intellectual disabilities according to their chronological age (CA), mental age (MA), or language age (LA). Examples of this matching are shown in Table 6.4. Only by comparing subjects matched according to one or another of these variables has it been possible to explore the issue of delay versus difference without misinterpretation.

Supporters of the difference position point to three findings, any or all of which may be areas of qualitative difference in individuals with intellectual disabilities:

1. They suffer from a deficit in verbal mediation ability due to the inactivity of the verbal system and its dissociation from the motor system (Luria, 1963).
2. They are inherently more rigid in their behavior (Dulaney & Ellis, 1997).
3. They have inadequate short-term memory (also called *working memory*) function, which is necessary to perform certain cognitive tasks (Bower & Hayes, 1994; Hulme & MacKenzie, 1992; Jarrold, Baddeley, & Hewes, 1999; Kay-Raining Bird & Chapman, 1994).

The notion of rigidity is hard to pin down, but it is most often illustrated by studies that show a deficit in abstract thinking. Children with Down syndrome, for example, have been found to classify objects by their common perceptual attributes (size, shape, color) rather than by abstract categories (fruit, clothing, furniture). They seem to have difficulty in hierarchical thinking, that is, recognizing that entities can be thought about at several levels. For example, the family pet has a proper name, *Rudy;* has a basic-level name, *dog;* has a subordinate name, *dachshund;* and has several superordinate names: *mammal, quadruped,* and *animal.* It may be hard for these children to accept that all of these names provide accurate descriptions of the same dog but at different levels of thinking.

TABLE 6.4   Examples of Subject Matching by CA, MA, and LA

	Typical Development				Intellectual Disabilities		
Subject	CA	MA	Language Test	Subject	CA	MA	Language Test
CA Matching[1]							
A	36	36	36	A	36	20	20
B	36	36	36	B	36	28	26
C	36	36	36	C	36	26	20
D	36	36	36	D	36	24	24
E	36	36	36	E	36	31	26
MA Matching[2]							
A	36	36	36	A	60	36	30
B	36	36	36	B	48	36	33
C	36	36	36	C	54	36	36
D	36	36	36	D	57	36	35
E	36	36	36	E	53	36	33
LA Matching[3]							
A	36	36	36	A	50	30	36
B	36	36	36	B	52	34	36
C	36	36	36	C	48	38	36
D	36	36	36	D	48	39	36
E	36	36	36	E	46	35	36

[1]Subjects are matched by chronological age (CA). Used to determine whether children with intellectual disabilities are delayed in specific language behaviors

[2]Subjects are matched by mental age (MA) as determined by an IQ test. Used to determine whether the language deficits of children with intellectual disabilities are attributable to their overall cognitive delay *mean length utterance*

[3]Subjects are matched by language age (LA) as determined by MLU or other language measure. Used to determine whether children with intellectual disabilities are delayed in specific domains of language (e.g., syntax) even though they show generally comparable communication abilities as the matched typically developing subjects.

Deficits in working memory have been offered as an explanation for a range of problems commonly seen in children with intellectual disabilities. It is generally believed that these children rarely employ strategies in situations that require active problem solving but can be taught to do so. However, the strategies taught for one task do not usually transfer spontaneously to other tasks. Most studies of problem solving, as well as most clinical descriptions, indicate that the performance of children with intellectual disabilities varies widely from one situation to the next. It has been suggested that this is due to limitations in functional working memory, which, in turn, may be the result of slowness in information processing (Ferretti & Cavalier, 1991). The problem should not be thought to extend to all memory functions. Research on long-term memory has been conducted on young children with mild intellectual disabilities. Though the database is still small, most studies suggest that there is no qualitative difference in the long-term memory functions of this population (Turnure, 1991).

In response to this evidence of differences, the delay position draws attention to the distinction between cognition and achievement. Some of the performance differences observed in familial intellectual disabilities may be simply due to lack of experience that results in deficits of knowledge. Other performance differences may be attributed to motivational differences in individuals with intellectual disabilities. Research has found persons with intellectual disabilities to be responsive to social reinforcement but at the same time wary of strange adults. They may be less likely to rely on their own cognitive resources and instead tend to problem-solve imitatively. They may have an expectancy of failure based on experience and therefore be more motivated to avoid failure than to achieve success. They respond better to tangible reinforcement and often exhibit *learned helplessness,* that is, not doing things even though they know how (Bybee & Zigler, 1999). Although intellectual disability is viewed primarily as a cognitive disorder, it may have associated with it the noncognitive characteristic of *passivity,* that is, not initiating the use of certain strategies known to be available. It has been noted that individuals with Down syndrome, who often possess reasonably good social skills, will often use those skills in order to sidestep difficult learning situations (Wishart, 1993).

Language Characteristics of Children with Intellectual Disabilities

It can be regarded as a truism that all children with intellectual disabilities exhibit some form of language impairment. The AAMR specifies that one component of the adaptive behavior deficits seen in all intellectual disabilities is communication disability. Consequently, professionals can expect that children with intellectual disabilities may need some form of language or communication intervention. It is important to note, however, that language impairment is caused by intellectual disabilities and not by a developmental syndrome in itself. One should be certain not to assume that developmental syndromes, such as De Lange syndrome, always result in communicative impairment.

Research Issues

One of the most consistent findings of research on the language of children with intellectual disabilities is that the findings are inconsistent. This inconsistency can be frustrating to professionals who want clear guidelines, but it is not surprising that research outcomes have differed, nor is it destined to always be the case. Some of the inconsistency may be attributed to the different methods of evaluation used by various investigators. For example, a study of comprehension that uses standardized tests may find that few children with severe or profound intellectual impairment respond appropriately to the structured format of the tests, but if comprehension were evaluated in these children using observational methods, there would likely be evidence of comprehension in certain familiar situations. It may also be that children with intellectual disabilities are especially likely to test poorly. In particular, some researchers have asserted that verbal performance in children with Down syndrome may be suppressed under the stress of testing (McCune, Kearney, & Checkoff, 1989).

　　An even greater impediment to language studies has been the tendency of researchers to treat all individuals with intellectual disabilities as a homogeneous group. In the future, we are likely to see the trend of more studies of subgroups (e.g., Down syndrome, fragile X syndrome, or FAS) as subjects continue. As we have noted, research with Down syndrome has already developed into a line of investigation distinct from other studies on children with intellectual disabilities. Following on this research, it is now believed that individuals with Down syndrome differ from individuals with other forms of intellectual disabilities in their more successful social and family functioning and level of peer acceptance (Kasari & Hodapp, 1996; Taylor, Bennie, & Buckley, 1996). For these reasons, in the following review we have frequently separated those studies in which the subjects were exclusively children with Down syndrome.

Pragmatics

The study of pragmatics in individuals with intellectual disabilities has examined behaviors in six areas: the development and use of speech acts, the ability to establish referents, the ability to repair conversational breakdowns, conversational turn taking, topic management, and generalization of language use from one setting to another.

Speech Acts.   As in other areas, much of the research in pragmatics has not carefully differentiated among types of children with intellectual disabilities. An exception has been the study of early speech act development, where identification of Down syndrome at or shortly after birth has resulted in the use of these children as subjects. Compared to nondisabled children matched for mean length of utterance (MLU), children with Down syndrome produce the same number and type of various speech acts but do so at a rate that is chronologically delayed (Coggins, Carpenter, & Owings, 1983; McCune et al., 1989; Owens & MacDonald, 1982; Sinson & Wetherick, 1982). The early stages of speech-act development have not been studied in other types of children with intellectual disabilities, but it appears that by adulthood, nearly all individuals with mild or moderate intellectual disabilities develop a full repertoire of speech acts (Owings & McManus, 1980; Rosenberg & Abbeduto, 1993).

Assertive communicative acts, such as requests for information, directives to perform an action, or unsolicited comments and statements, are the "icebreakers" we use to begin conversations. However, children with intellectual disabilities, especially those who are severely impaired, rarely use language to initiate social contact and tend to maintain responsive communicative roles (Bedrosian & Prutting, 1978; Beveridge, 1976; Calculator & Dollaghan, 1982; Eheart, 1982). As a result, unless they are in some way prodded, children with intellectual disabilities tend to show less peer interaction when placed in groups (Beveridge, 1976; Sinson & Wetherick, 1982). The distinction between the prompted and spontaneous pragmatic behaviors of children with intellectual disabilities can be clinically important. Unlike other children, they may show a considerable gap between the number of speech act types in their repertoire and the number of speech act tokens actually produced in conversation. When individuals with severe intellectual impairment do produce assertive speech acts, they are mainly imperatives that have the function of directing the listener to act. This is in contrast to the behavior of typically developing children of comparable mental age, who show greater balance between imperative and declarative types of utterances (McLean, Brady, McLean, & Behrens, 1999).

To get along socially and communicate information effectively, all individuals modify their style of speech in different situations. Studies of children and adolescents with mild to moderate intellectual impairment indicate that they learn to vary the linguistic form of their utterances in response to contextual cues but that they are delayed in this ability compared to nondisabled children of the same CA (Abbeduto, 1991). In one investigation, Guralnick and Paul-Brown (1986) compared children with mild intellectual impairment to typically developing children roughly matched in MA. They found that both groups made similar adjustments in language content, form, and use when talking to children with moderate and severe intellectual disability. That is, the children with mild intellectual impairment were sensitive to the fact that their conversational partners were even more impaired intellectually, and they adjusted their own language accordingly.

Referential Communication. Although studies of speech style suggest that children with intellectual disabilities do consider the comprehension abilities of their listeners, other research indicates that they frequently fail to take account of informational needs. This problem has been studied in terms of the children's abilities to establish referents, that is, to make it clear who or what they are talking about. The experimental task most often used to study this ability has been the barrier task. The barrier prevents the child from gesturing or from using deictic language while trying to get another person to select a picture identical to the one the child sees. The child must use specific vocabulary that provides an adequate amount of detail. Investigations using the barrier task to study adolescents with mild and moderate intellectual impairment have shown consistently that they fail to provide sufficient information (Longhurst, 1972, 1974; Rueda & Chan, 1980). The difficulties do not appear to be due entirely to cognitive delay, as the subjects with intellectual disabilities performed more poorly than typically developing younger children matched for MA (Longhurst, 1972). It was also clear from these studies that the problems in communication were the fault of the speaker, not the listener. The subjects with intellectual disabilities were able to select the correct pictures when the speaker was a nondisabled adult.

In other studies on referential communication, subjects were given commands that were ambiguous unless they made use of background information. For example, the experimenter would announce that he was looking for a gift for a child and then would ask the child to "Show me that cup." The correct response was to choose a child's small cup rather than an adult's cup. Children with mild-to-moderate intellectual impairment were found to perform these tasks as well as MA-matched, typically developing children (Abbeduto, Davies, Solesby, & Furman, 1991; Abbeduto, Short-Meyerson, Benson, Dolish, & Weissman, 1998). Taken together, studies of referential communication ability present a mixed picture. On some tasks, children with intellectual disabilities appear to function at a level consistent with their cognitive status; on others, they have more difficulty than would be predicted from intelligence alone.

Conversational Repair. One of the findings of experiments on referential communication is that children and adolescents with intellectual disabilities do a poor job of repairing breakdowns in communication. They rarely make requests for clarification when presented with an inadequate message, though, in this respect, they appear comparable to typical children of the same mental age (Abbeduto, Short-Meyerson, Benson, & Dolish, 1997). Additionally, when others make requests for clarification to children with intellectual disabilities, the children rarely respond (Abbeduto et al., 1991; Longhurst, 1972; Rueda & Chan, 1980). In natural communication settings as well, children with Down syndrome respond less frequently to requests for clarification than their nondisabled peers (Coggins & Stoel-Gammon, 1982). It is unclear whether the problem of making requests for clarification is due to inability or merely social reluctance, especially when the conversational partner is a nondisabled adult (Abbeduto, 1991). As for responding to such requests, it appears that persons with mild to moderate intellectual disabilities do develop this ability by the time they reach adulthood, though they may still fail to respond to subtle, especially nonverbal, requests for clarification (Abbeduto & Rosenberg, 1980; Longhurst & Berry, 1975; Paul & Cohen, 1984).

Turn Taking.   Normal conversations are characterized by finely tuned systems for taking turns and avoiding interruptions. It is thought that these behaviors have their origins in very early parent–child interactions involving feeding and reciprocal vocalization. Because infants with Down syndrome are identified early in life, it has been possible to study their early patterns of interaction. Some of these studies have found higher rates of *vocal clashing*—that is, simultaneous vocalization—than is the case with typically developing infants and their mothers (Berger & Cunningham, 1983; Jones, 1977). However, this difference does not seem to foreshadow later problems with turn taking. Young children with Down syndrome show no difference in the rate of turn-taking errors when they are compared to typically developing children (Tannock, 1988). A low rate of turn-taking errors has also been found in a heterogeneous group of preschoolers with intellectual disabilities (Davis, Stroud, & Green, 1988). Thus, turn-taking difficulties are not considered to be generally characteristic of children with intellectual disabilities, even though certain individuals may exhibit problems, especially in situations that suspend or vary the usual patterns of conversation (Abbeduto & Hesketh, 1997).

Topic Management.   It is one thing for children not to interrupt and to take their turn in a conversation. It is another for them to take a *good* turn. Research on what is called *discourse management* suggests that individuals with intellectual disabilities learn how to take a turn without adding significantly to a conversation (Abbeduto, 1991). They are able to maintain topics in conversations—that is, not change the subject—but they do so primarily with acknowledgments (e.g., *yeah, uh huh, okay*). They remain deficient in their ability to extend topics by providing new information or new shading on the current subject of discussion. There are several possible explanations for this deficit. Individuals with intellectual disabilities may simply lack the requisite knowledge for making topic extensions; they may not understand that topic maintenance is socially valued; or they may lack the cognitive ability to link information available to them to the current topic. Future research may help clarify which of these factors is most potent.

Generalization.   The quality of any language learning must be measured by how much the language is really used. An opinion commonly held is that children with intellectual disabilities do not generalize behaviors well outside the teaching environment. Two studies of nonverbal children with severe intellectual impairment illustrate the point. Calculator and Dollaghan (1982) observed the behavior of children at school and found that they used their communication boards in one-to-one sessions with a speech–language pathologist but used them much less frequently in classroom interactions. In another study, a child with severe intellectual impairment was taught to use iconic pictographs (Bliss symbols) by his classroom teacher and to sign by his speech–language pathologist. He reportedly used both systems effectively, but only in the settings in which they were taught (Nietupski, Scheutz, & Ockwood, 1980). These examples indicate that although children with intellectual disabilities can acquire new communication skills, the amount of functional improvement attained may be quite limited because of poor generalization of learning, to say nothing of poor interdisciplinary collaboration.

Comprehension

The language comprehension of children with intellectual disabilities has been studied from three vantage points: as a measure of information processing ability; as a component of linguistic competence; and as a test of contextual understanding.

Information Processing. Psychologists have long been interested in the efficiency with which individuals can derive knowledge from incoming stimuli. By varying the speed of different messages, they have found that individuals with intellectual disabilities require more time to encode incoming verbal information than nondisabled individuals of equal MA (Kail, 1992; Merrill & Mar, 1987). That is, it takes longer after hearing a sentence before it makes sense to children with intellectual disabilities so that they can answer questions about it or identify pictures that match it. Various experiments suggest that the problem occurs at the semantic–analytic rather than the phonological level. Words are heard as individual units of sound, but they do not quickly form a meaning in the mind of the listener.

Linguistic Competence. Language comprehension can also be considered in relation to the delay–difference controversy. Do children with intellectual disabilities understand language at a level that is consistent with their cognitive abilities, or are they selectively impaired in comprehension? In answer to this question, the evidence suggests that many (maybe 25–50 percent) (Abbeduto, Furman, & Davies, 1989; Miller & Chapman, 1984), but not all, children with intellectual disabilities may have language comprehension difficulties that exceed their cognitive delays.

Many different types of comprehension errors occur in children with intellectual disabilities, but it is not clear whether these errors signal a qualitative difference in language acquisition. Some studies suggest that children with intellectual disabilities learn to comprehend syntactic structures in approximately the same sequence as typically developing children (Berry, 1972; Dewart, 1979; Lamberts & Weener, 1976; Wheldall, 1976), but others suggest that sentence comprehension deficits are found even when subjects with and without intellectual disabilities are matched for LA (Dewart, 1979; Wheldall, 1976). It is therefore unwise to draw sweeping conclusions. Studies limited to children with Down syndrome (discussed later) are providing more detail about that population, and future research will probably concentrate on other biological subgroups. There is also some indication that children with intellectual disabilities show similar patterns of comprehension, learning up to, but not beyond, a certain developmental level. In children who have reached MAs of 7 and 9 years, for example, comprehension problems have been found to be concentrated in particular syntactic forms, such as passives and comparatives (Abbeduto et al., 1989).

Contextual Understanding. Formal evaluations of information processing or language comprehension may not accurately predict how well children with intellectual disabilities will comprehend in real situations, which provide redundancy and contextual cues to meaning (Abbeduto & Short, 1994). Both observational and experimental studies suggest that children with intellectual disabilities comprehend requests—even ones made indirectly—at a level comparable to MA- and LA-matched, typically developing children (Abbeduto et al., 1989; Hanzlik & Stevenson, 1986; Leifer & Lewis, 1984). What is more important, there is evidence that adolescents and adults with mild to moderate intellectual impairment learn to respond appropriately to speech acts produced within routine activities (Abbeduto, 1991). They appear to be aided by the predictability of these settings, which makes it unnecessary for them to analyze the content of a speaker's request fully. Thus, individuals with intellectual disabilities may often function more adequately in everyday activities than formal testing or performance in nonroutine situations would lead us to expect. This is especially true in interactions with their parents who, when studied, have demonstrated skill in scaffolding or structuring how they speak to their children so as to maximize their comprehension successes (Abbeduto, Weissman, & Short-Meyerson, 1999).

Semantics

Children with intellectual disabilities have long been characterized as having concreteness in their thinking and, consequently, in their learning and use of vocabulary. One of the clearest expressions of lexical concreteness is in the comprehension of idioms (e.g., "got cold feet," "broke her heart"), which rely on nonliteral interpretation. Idiom understanding is significantly poorer in 9-year-old children with mild intellectual disabilities than in typically developing children of the same age (Ezell & Goldstein, 1991a). Is this concreteness a unique feature of intellectual disabilities, or is it merely associated with younger MA? The consensus among researchers is that the learning of concrete words and semantic relations follows the same course as in typically developing children but moves at a slower pace in children with intellectual disabilities (Mervis, 1990; Rosenberg, 1982). When language samples produced by children with intellectual disabilties were compared with typically developing children matched for MA, no significant differences were found in the number of semantic relations produced (Kamhi & Johnston, 1982). Thus concreteness is probably best attributed to cognitive delay and can be expected to be greater in individuals with more severe intellectual impairment.

It should be noted that our picture of semantic development is far from complete. Although we believe that children with intellectual disabilities are delayed in their learning of concrete semantic categories, there is little evidence to indicate whether the acquisition of abstract semantic knowledge is similarly delayed. It is possible, though not yet demonstrated, that there is a level above which semantic development may not continue for these children.

Syntax

Any generalizations about the syntactic deficits of children with intellectual disabilities should be treated cautiously. Much of the recent research on children with Down syndrome has highlighted their syntactic difficulty, but similar conclusions do not yet appear warranted for other subgroups (Fowler, 1990; Stoel-Gammon, 1990). In addition, the majority of studies on syntactic development of non–Down syndrome children have been done with high-functioning individuals. Studies with low-functioning children suggest that patterns of syntactic learning may differ, depending on the severity of intellectual impairment (Bliss, Allen, & Walker, 1978). In all research in which syntactic abilities are judged from language samples, attention should be given to the type of sample obtained, as narrative samples are likely to be more complex than samples of conversation (Abbeduto, Benson, Short, & Dolish, 1995; Chapman, Seung, Schwartz, & Kay-Raining Bird, 1998).

The general conclusion drawn in the past was that syntactic functioning in children with intellectual disabilities shows a developmental lag and that MA is therefore a better predictor of syntactic performance than CA (Rosenberg, 1982). For example, language samples gathered from adolescents with mild to severe intellectual disabilities showed a high correlation between MA and the length and syntactic complexity of their sentences (Graham & Graham, 1971).

The interpretation of delay appears to hold regardless of the level of syntax that is measured. Compared to typically developing children, children with mild intellectual disabilities master bound morphemes in approximately the same order but at a slower rate (Newfield & Schlanger, 1968). The number of inflectional errors occurring in language samples is about the same in children with mild intellectual disabilities and in typically developing children (Kamhi & Johnston, 1982). A finding inconsistent with the delay position was reported by Lovell and Bradbury (1967), who studied the inflections produced by 14- and 15-year-old English children with mild intellectual impairment. When the results were compared to those from typically developing American first graders, the English children's scores were significantly lower, despite their higher MAs. However, this finding may have been due to cultural differences or to the test that was used, which employs nonsense words and has been found to overestimate morphological errors (Berko, 1958; Dever, 1972).

The acquisition of phrase structures appears to follow a similar developmental pattern in children with and without intellectual impairment, even though the rate of learning is significantly different. On a sentence-imitation task, children with intellectual disabilities who had an MA of 5 years performed like typically developing children who were 3 years of age (McLeavey, Toomey, & Dempsey, 1982). This suggests that phrasal learning follows the typical developmental sequence but is even more delayed than MA would predict. On the other hand, Kamhi and Johnston (1982) measured spontaneous production of pronouns, noun phrases, verb phrases, and negatives and found differences between children with and without intellectual disabilities that were consistent with their MA differences. It may be that the discrepancy in results is attributable to differences between imitative and spontaneous language production.

The area of syntactic development that does provide some evidence of a difference rather than a delay is the acquisition of clause structures. The same two studies described in the preceding paragraph (Kamhi & Johnston, 1982; McLeavey et al., 1982) both found significant differences in the production of subordinating conjunctions, for example, *who* introducing a relative clause or *because*. In spontaneous speech, children with intellectual disabilities relied on *and* as the only form of clausal linkage. They also produced significantly fewer question forms (interrogative reversals and *wh-* questions) and used only developmentally simple question forms, such as copula reversal and *what* questions. As a whole, these findings indicate that a difference in clausal syntax development may exist among children with intellectual disabilities but that it may emerge only in the later stages of language acquisition.

Speech Production

Among all subgroups of children with intellectual disabilities, there is evidence that speech production problems are more prevalent than among typically developing children. Some of the factors that contribute to speech difficulties are the high prevalence of hearing impairment and the neuromotor deficits and orofacial anomalies that are associated with certain developmental syndromes. These factors do not explain, however, why speech production problems are common among children with nonorganic intellectual disability. In one study on the issue, words produced by 5-year-old children with mild intellectual impairment were compared to those of preschool groups of communicatively disabled and typically developing children (Klink, Gerstman, Raphael, Schlanger, & Newsome, 1986). All subjects were roughly matched for MLU. It was discovered that problems occurring as a result of phonological processes were significantly more frequent in the children with intellectual disabilities and communicative disability but that the profile of process usage (types of processes used) was comparable across all three groups. The only characteristic that distinguished the children with intellectual disabilities was the presence of the final-consonant devoicing process (e.g., *cap* for *cab*). This evidence, though limited, suggests that at least some children with intellectual disabilities should be considered to have specific phonological delays that are inconsistent with their general level of language development.

Language Characteristics of Children with Down Syndrome

Because Down syndrome is the most common chromosomal cause of intellectual disabilities and because it can usually be identified from birth, this subgroup is the best studied of all subgroups of children with intellectual disabilities (Gerber, 1990). Many studies also indicate that children with Down syndrome are especially impaired in their development of language compared with other groups of children with intellectual disabilities (Abbeduto et al., 2001; Fowler, 1990). There is evidence that this language deficit manifests itself even before spoken language begins, in that children with Down syndrome make fewer nonverbal requests than typically developing children (Mundy, Kasari, Sigman, & Ruskin, 1995). Once spoken language emerges, children with Down syndrome are consistently below CA expectations and frequently show deficits that are incommensurate with other areas of development. To be sure, a major issue in research on children with Down syndrome has become the extent to which some language domains (e.g., phonology, syntax, vocabulary) may be specifically impaired, that is, lower than MA would predict.

Comprehension

Although the comprehension of children with Down syndrome is clearly delayed, research has not yet indicated conclusively whether it is specifically impaired. Some reviewers have claimed that specific language deficits observed in Down syndrome affect production but not comprehension (Lynch & Eilers, 1991; Stoel-Gammon, 1990). Others see the impairment affecting both aspects of language development (Fowler, 1990). Still others confine themselves to the statement that comprehension abilities often exceed production abilities (Mahoney, Glover, & Finger, 1981; Miller, 1988).

Another question that can be asked about comprehension is whether children with Down syndrome are equally competent at all levels of language. To find an answer, Chapman, Schwartz, and Kay-Raining Bird (1991) compared the lexical and syntactic comprehension test scores of children and adolescents with Down syndrome with those of an MA-matched group of typically developing children. They found that what distinguished the two groups was the difference between lexical and syntactic test scores. The subjects with Down syndrome achieved age-equivalence scores on the vocabulary test that were nearly a year better than their syntax scores. Moreover, this gap steadily widened with age. During the period from 5 to 8 years the scores were nearly equal, but by 16 to 20 years they were over 2 years apart. Consistent with this finding, children and adolescents with Down syndrome have been found to have fast-mapping ability comparable to that of typically developing children matched for MA (Chapman, Kay-Raining Bird, & Schwartz, 1990). Together these studies suggest that comprehension should not be regarded as a singular ability in these children. The evidence indicates that syntactic comprehension is most likely to be specifically impaired compared to vocabulary comprehension.

Semantics

We have just reviewed the relationship between vocabulary and syntax for comprehension. From the perspective of production, a similar pattern can be seen. When children with Down syndrome and typically developing children are matched for MA, language samples obtained from the children with Down syndrome are found to contain a smaller number of different words. However, when the children are matched for MLU, the result is reversed and the samples from children with Down syndrome show more diverse vocabulary (Miller, 1988; Miller, Budde, Bashir, & LaFollette, 1987). Parent reports reveal that children with Down syndrome show spurts of vocabulary growth but fall steadily behind their typically developing peers (Miller, 1992). These comparisons suggest that vocabulary development lags behind what would be predicted from MA but is superior to syntactic development.

In the area of relational semantics, very limited research suggests that the behavior of children with Down syndrome should be described as delayed but not different. Longitudinal studies reported on five children with Down syndrome and mild-to-moderate intellectual impairment have found that the frequency and distribution of semantic relations were comparable to those reported for typically developing children at the same level of language development (Coggins, 1979; Fowler, Gelman, & Gleitman, 1994). Language samples gathered from adolescents with Down syndrome and an MA of 6 to 7 years also showed no significant differences in thematic relations when compared to typical children at the same language level (Fowler et al., 1994).

Syntax

The notion of a specific language impairment in children with Down syndrome is best supported in the domain of syntax. Researchers followed the development of cognition, language comprehension, and language production in a group of young (11 to 58 months) children with Down syndrome (Miller, 1988). Over a 2-year period, unlike typically developing children, the language production skills of children with Down syndrome gradually fell behind both their cognitive and comprehension abilities. The discrepancy has been found to persist into adolescence and early adulthood (Chapman et al., 1998; Jenkins, 1993). Because of this specific impairment in expressive syntax, children with Down syndrome produce narratives in which their content matches their MA but their linguistic structure does not (Boudreau &

Chapman, 2000; Miles & Chapman, 2002). It has been suggested that, once the number of informational items becomes great, these children are unable to use mental representations to coordinate their ideas with the syntax necessary to express them. As a result, they fail to use successfully various syntactic devices (pronouns, adverbs of time, connective adverbs, etc.) that help listeners keep track of more complex narratives (Moore, Clibbens, & Dennis, 1998)

Speech Production

Research on the phonetic and phonological development of children with Down syndrome has produced a set of inconsistent findings. The early phonetic behaviors of infants with Down syndrome seem to unfold in a pattern similar to that of typically developing children. In general, they produce similar vocalizations, have a similar age of onset for reduplicated babbling, and show a comparable repertoire of vowels and consonants in their babbling (Smith & Oller, 1981; Smith & Stoel-Gammon, 1996; Steffens, Oller, Lynch, & Urbano, 1992). However, a study of infants with Down syndrome not receiving intervention found that the onset of babbling was slightly later than that of typically developing children and that mature syllable production was less consistent through the end of the first year (Lynch et al., 1995). This inconsistency in production may be attributable to hypotonicity and delays in motor development commonly found among infants with Down syndrome (Stoel-Gammon, 2001). Early intervention may help to reduce the impact of those delays on early speech production.

As meaningful speech begins, the order of phoneme acquisition has been found to be very similar between children with Down syndrome and mild intellectual impairment and typically developing children matched for MLU (Stoel-Gammon, 1980). The phonetic inventories of the children with Down syndrome included nearly all the sounds that were simplified in spontaneous production, showing that their problems are due to phonological delay rather than phonetic impairment resulting from anatomical or physiological differences. Furthermore, the specific patterns of sound omission and substitution produced by children with Down syndrome are comparable to those found in typically developing children (Bleile & Schwarz, 1984; Smith & Stoel-Gammon, 1983; Stoel-Gammon, 1980).

Not all the research, however, has been consistent with the interpretation of phonological delay. Dodd (1975) compared children with Down syndrome and an average age of 9 years to a CA- and MA-matched group of children with intellectual disabilities but not Down syndrome. She found that while the children with Down syndrome were better at recognizing real and nonsense words, they were poorer at repeating them after delays of 15 and 30 seconds. This was interpreted as evidence of a specific motor disability that impeded correct articulation. In other studies, Dodd (1976; Thompson & Dodd, 2001) has found a higher frequency of phonological errors and greater inconsistency in word production in children with Down syndrome. This finding is inconsistent with other studies of the same population (Bleile & Schwarz, 1984; Stoel-Gammon, 1980). Dodd's data were taken from older children and were elicited through picture naming rather than spontaneous speech, but a final explanation of the discrepancy awaits further research.

Phonological Awareness and Literacy

Children with Down syndrome span a wide range of intellectual abilities. For those at the lower end of this range, the likelihood of learning to read is very low (Carr, 1995). However, many do acquire literacy skills at varying levels (Buckley & Bird, 1993). In contrast to typically developing children, the phonological awareness skills of children with Down syndrome begin to slow in development earlier than their word-recognition abilities. The result is that they will likely reach a stage in learning to read where new words must be recognized from their visual appearance rather than through an analysis of letter–sound relationships (Kay-Raining Bird, Cleave, & McConnell, 2000). At this point, their rate of learning will decline unless instruction can stimulate further growth in phonological awareness (Kennedy & Flynn, 2003).

Rate of Language Learning

One of the most interesting findings to emerge from studies of children with Down syndrome is that they do not appear to learn language at a constant rate. The broad pattern revealed by research (Cardoso-Martins, Mervis, & Mervis, 1985; Chapman & Hesketh, 2001; Fowler, 1988; Jenkins, 1993; Oliver & Buckley, 1994; Rondal, 1988; Rutter & Buckley, 1994) is that children with Down syndrome show strong development during the infant and toddler years, especially when facilitated by early-intervention programs. In many cases these children perform at levels comparable to those of their typically developing peers. Thereafter, language development continues at a slightly slower pace into the early school years. During these years, comparisons with typically developing children begin to reveal more gaps in language ability. From roughly 8 years of age until the middle or end of adolescence, many children with Down syndrome appear to reach a plateau in development. What little language change occurs tends to be growth in vocabulary, so the discrepancy between lexical and syntactic abilities becomes greater during this time. In early adulthood there appears to be some slight additional growth in language.

Not all scholars agree that individuals with Down syndrome show a developmental ceiling, beyond which it is difficult or impossible for their language to advance. Though some evidence exists in support of this notion, it is unclear whether the ceiling is attributable to physical changes associated with aging or to some type of cognitive limitation. One interpretation of the available information is that individuals with Down syndrome do not progress further than the language level associated with a mental age of 5 years (Fowler, 1988).

Use of Imitation

It sometimes seems that children with Down syndrome use gesture and verbal imitation more often than typically developing children, especially during the early stages of language development. However, a carefully controlled study of 12- to 26-month-old typically developing children and MA-matched children with Down syndrome found the groups to be highly similar, using equal amounts of speech and gesture (McCune et al., 1989).

As for verbal imitation, some studies have found it to be delayed in children with Down syndrome but others have found no difference in its frequency (Coggins & Morrison, 1981; Mahoney et al., 1981; McCune et al., 1989; Owens & MacDonald, 1982). Conclusions are made even more difficult by the fact that subjects in these studies have often been enrolled in language therapy. Thus, the findings may be contaminated by changes in imitative behavior caused by intervention (McCune et al., 1989). When Tager-Flusberg and Calkins (1990) compared the spontaneous and imitative utterances of children with Down syndrome, they found them to be comparable in length and complexity. This suggests that imitation is not a crucial language-learning mechanism for these children.

Explanations for Specific Language Deficit in Children with Down Syndrome

It is now well established that children with Down syndrome are delayed in language acquisition. It also appears likely that they are specifically impaired in syntactic development, and perhaps in other language domains, even when compared to MA. How do we account for the special language problems of this subgroup? Table 6.5 provides a short account of some possible explanations and some of the flaws of those explanations. As the table suggests, none of these explanations provides a completely satisfactory answer to the question. Certain accounts are logically flawed, and others must await further research before they can be stated in precise terms.

Implications for Intervention

Each child with intellectual disabilities presents a unique pattern of communicative abilities and difficulties, which must be identified as a result of a thorough individual assessment. There is, therefore, no one intervention prescription for children with intellectual disabilities. There is, however, a set of general principles and considerations that apply to all intervention efforts.

In this chapter we will discuss intervention that focuses on enhancing language and communication via speech as the output modality. There are, however, children with intellectual disabilities who have significant difficulties using speech for communication. For these children, *augmentative and alternative communication* (AAC) approaches may be viable options. There are also other children with intellectual disabilities whose language development can be promoted by employing some forms of AAC. AAC in relation to children with intellectual disabilities is discussed in Chapter 12.

Social and Legislative Influences

Recall that federal legislation has mandated equal educational opportunity for the disabled. This has led to the end of institutionalization for all but the most severely impaired children with intellectual disabilities and to the mainstreaming of disabled children into regular classrooms. To help these children and their teachers, specialists are increasingly being asked to serve as classroom consultants as part of their role as interventionists. This consultant role involves skills in assessing communicative needs, developing intervention strategies, training personnel who will administer programs, and developing methods of reviewing and improving the treatment programs (ASHA, 1997; Kumin, 2001). The shift to community integration of children with intellectual disabilities also means that an increasing number of intervention strategies are designed to promote interaction with peers (Goldstein, English, Shafer, & Kaczmarek, 1997; Goldstein & Ferrell, 1987; Goldstein & Mousetis, 1989; McGee, Almeida, & Sulzer-Azaroff, 1992) and to increase the communicative experiences of the children in public places such as shopping malls, museums, and sports arenas (ASHA, 1996).

TABLE 6.5 Explanations for Specific Language Impairment in Children with Down Syndrome

Explanation	Critique
They are less motivated than other children to perform linguistically. In institutions, and even at home, their needs are met without requiring them to use language.	This argument ignores the fact that motivation does not explain normal language development, which requires children to learn forms that do not necessarily improve their ability to express needs and wants. We would also expect that there would have been some "motivational" improvement as institutionalization has decreased. Yet studies have shown no differences in syntactic development between home-reared and institutionalized children with Down syndrome (Fowler, 1990).
Parents of children with Down syndrome do not provide a good language-learning environment.	Most studies of interaction between parents and children with Down syndrome show behaviors that are comparable to parental interactions with nondisabled children. Even where differences exist, they have not been shown to cause delays in language learning (Rosenberg & Abbeduto, 1993).
There are neurological differences in children with Down syndrome that are responsible for the observed language deficits. Dichotic listening tests have found that many children with Down syndrome do not show a right-ear advantage as normal children do (Fowler, 1990). Also, infants and children with Down syndrome may show difficulty in processing some of the acoustic cues that signal the difference between consonants (Lynch & Eilers, 1991).	These studies are methodologically complicated and hard to interpret. The findings from dichotic listening tasks may be the result of language delays rather than the cause of them (Buckley, 1993).
There is a maturational plateau, either an MA or a linguistic stage, beyond which language learning, and syntactic learning in particular, become much more difficult (Fowler, 1990; Fowler et al., 1994; Grela, 2003).	The neurological mechanisms responsible for such a plateau are not understood.
Hearing loss produces impairment of both language and nonverbal cognition (Lynch & Eilers, 1991; Stoel-Gammon, 1990).	Does not suffice as an explanation. The level of hearing loss observed among individuals with Down syndrome does not produce marked impairment when it occurs in individuals without intellectual disability. Hearing loss is therefore best thought of as a contributory factor.
Structural differences in the speech mechanism, such as a small maxilla, missing teeth, small oral cavity, high palate, or tongue hypertrophy (Stoel-Gammon, 1981, 1990) are responsible for a speech–specific motor difficulty.	Difficult to understand why this would produce a specific syntactic deficit. It is best thought of as a contributory factor.

Intelligibility

Because a high percentage of children with intellectual disabilities have a speech production problem, it is important to consider whether articulatory and phonological impairments will hinder efforts to change other aspects of language and whether improving intelligibility might allow children to display more linguistic abilities, enhance conversational interaction, and promote faster language learning. In addition, we should always recall that language production teaching requires us to judge children's attempts at target forms. If those attempts are unintelligible, we cannot reinforce or even respond appropriately; under these circumstances, treatment will languish.

In some instances, attempts have been made to improve intelligibility through surgery rather than therapy. Children with Down syndrome often exhibit tongue hypertrophy, which has been thought to contribute to their articulatory difficulties. However, pre- and postsurgical evaluation of a tongue reduction procedure performed on eighteen children with Down syndrome found no significant differences in the number of consonant errors produced on a single-word articulation test (Parsons, Iacono, & Rozner, 1987). This suggests that surgery alone will not produce an improvement in intelligibility. Intervention should instead be based on a child's phonetic repertoire, phonological profile, and cognitive level, as is generally recommended in cases of poor intelligibility.

Facilitating versus Compensatory Intervention

Scholars who view children with intellectual disabilities as delayed rather than as different also believe that these children reach a developmental plateau beyond which they show relatively few gains. We also know that language learning of children with Down syndrome is most rapid during the early years of life and that the rate and extent of learning appears to slow dramatically in later childhood and thereafter. Considering these findings, we may need to distinguish between early and late developmental periods and develop different intervention strategies for the two stages. In the early years, the professional role may be to facilitate language by providing and fostering greater cognitive and language stimulation. In the later years, the role may be to teach compensatory strategies that will help both the children and those who interact with them to communicate more functionally. For example, a program for infants and toddlers with intellectual disabilities may provide intensive general stimulation. As the children grow older, increasingly specific language forms and functions may be targeted so that ultimately, in the adolescent and adult years, communicative intervention is designed to teach abilities that will improve performance in a particular school or job setting.

Developmental versus Remedial Logic

One of the clearest areas of disagreement regarding intervention is found in response to the question, "Should children with intellectual disabilities be taught like typically developing children?" This dispute has been described as a contrast between developmental and remedial logic (Fey, 1986). In simple terms, *developmental logic* argues that language targets should be presented to children with intellectual disabilities in the same order that they are acquired by typically developing children. This is consistent with a delay view of intellectual disabilities, which emphasizes that the developmental processes of these children show far more similarities to than differences from those of typically developing children. On the other hand, *remedial logic* makes the straightforward point that children with intellectual disabilities are by definition not developing typically; therefore, nondevelopmental approaches are required to assist them. There is, moreover, some research evidence to suggest that children with intellectual disabilities learn language differently. In particular, they do not show the same kinds of interrelationships between language comprehension and production processes as typically developing children. In the case of children with Down syndrome, syntactic skills may be especially problematic compared to other language abilities (Fowler, 1990).

In intervention, it is likely unnecessary to choose one rationale over the other. The heterogeneity of children with intellectual disabilities makes it impossible to generalize, and the critical point is to select approaches that help the individual children most effectively. It is apparent, however, that most programs that employ remedial logic are used with severely and profoundly impaired individuals. In contrast, developmental logic is more likely to be the basis of treatment regimens for children with mild to moderate intellectual impairment. Miller (1984) points out that all instructional approaches—behavior modification, cognitive learning strategies, and naturalistic ecological models—should be used with children who are intellectually disabled. Naturalistic methods may be preferred if there is evidence that the child is doing a lot of incidental learning, that is, acquiring language forms that are not specifically trained. On the other hand, if incidental learning stops, new behaviors might be introduced behaviorally and then generalized through more naturalistic strategies.

Language–Cognition Relationships

To those who regard intellectual disabilities from the delay perspective and who accept the cognitive hypothesis, the presence of a gap between a child's MA and LA is regarded as a positive prognostic sign for intervention. The reason is simple. From this perspective, the ceiling for a child's language development is set by the child's cognitive development: if MA exceeds LA, then a child has room to grow. Another similar interpretation would be that when a child's LA approaches or matches MA, language development can be expected to plateau. At that point, as noted in the preceding section, a change in intervention tactics may be warranted.

These interpretations of the language–cognition relationship are speculative, and not everyone who intervenes with children with intellectual disabilities will want to accept them. There is little doubt, however, that to teach language to children with intellectual disabilities, the cognitive requirements for learning must be evaluated. Generally, for example, children with intellectual disabilities will require more redundancy in instruction and are likely to need model or physical guidance accompanied by verbal instruction to learn as effectively as possible.

The suggestion has been made that, if cognitive development is prerequisite to language acquisition, a good intervention strategy would be to train cognition before attempting to introduce language targets. For example, at least one researcher has found that training in *object permanence* and *means–end behaviors* enhanced the learning of referential speech by children with profound intellectual impairment (Kahn, 1984). With more cognitively mature individuals in whom language is well established, cognitive training is more likely to focus on developing *strategies* for accomplishing particular language tasks.

For example, rehearsal strategies have been taught successfully to adolescents with mild intellectual impairment. It may be, then, that cognition training can facilitate language learning and language performance in children with intellectual disabilities. As Finch-Williams (1984) has noted, however, there is a sticky issue attached to cognition training, namely, who should do the training—a speech–language pathologist, a school psychologist, a special education teacher, or another professional? At present there are no guidelines to refer to, so each decision is made on an individual basis, hopefully with consultation of the various professionals involved in assisting a child.

Pragmatics and Pragmatic Relevance

Practically minded professionals have long recognized that language intervention for children with intellectual disabilities must result in functional gains. There is little point in teaching a child to produce a new set of words, a new bound morpheme, or a new grammatical operation if these forms do not help everyday communication in the short or long term. Fey (1986) suggests that the basic goal of language intervention should be to achieve a balance in the child's ability to respond and to produce assertive communicative acts. Yet, as we saw earlier, children with intellectual disabilities may be passive communicators. Intervention for these children may require procedures that will increase the range and frequency of assertive communicative behavior. Table 6.6 gives examples of specific goals that might be pursued and some procedures that might be used to implement those goals.

Another important consideration in achieving pragmatic success is that we must achieve a reasonable fit between a child's communicative behavior and the typical conditions of everyday life. If the fit is poor, a behavior tends not to be used. Cipani (1989) suggests that in order to be maintained, a communicative behavior must meet three criteria: (1) it must be fluent, that is, occur within an acceptable time after the stimulus; (2) it must be used neither too little nor too much; and (3) it must occur in response to a variety of natural stimuli. In short, the language behaviors we teach must be sufficiently fine-tuned that they do not give the impression of having been learned as a result of intervention.

A logical approach to pragmatics intervention is to concentrate in areas where individuals with intellectual disabilities would be expected to show little development on their own (Abbeduto, 1991). Research to date suggests that conversational turn taking is the most easily acquired pragmatic behavior. Therefore, intervention might have more impact if it is targeted toward one of the five other areas discussed earlier: speech acts, referential communication, conversational repair, topic management, and generalization of use.

What kinds of techniques can be used to promote pragmatic development? There are no pat methods for stimulating change in this area. However, research on problem solving indicates that children with intellectual disabilities will improve their performance when they are prompted to apply a particular strategy (Ferretti & Cavalier, 1991). It is easy to see that many of the behaviors we consider pragmatic involve a type of interpersonal problem solving, for example, judging what a listener needs to know. Therefore, prompting to apply pragmatic knowledge in certain situations may improve performance, just as it has been shown to improve performance in cognitive tasks (Abbeduto, 1991). The simple reminder may be one of the most powerful techniques.

The use of a reminder, of course, assumes that a particular behavior is already within a child's repertoire. If this is not the case, then the behavior must be established. For exam-

TABLE 6.6   Goals and Procedures for Children with Intellectual disabilities Who Are Inactive Communicators or Passive Conversationalists

Basic Goals (after Fey, 1986)	Example of Specific Goal	Example of the Procedure
Increase the child's frequency of social bids (verbal *and* nonverbal) in a variety of social contexts	Increase the number of spontaneous vocalizations	Allow periods of silence during interactions with children who are severely intellectually impaired so that they have more opportunity to initiate vocalization.
Increase the frequency of use of available assertive conversational acts in a variety of social contexts	Increase the number of verbal requests	Wait 5 seconds after approaching a child who is in need of help and is capable of requesting it. If no request is produced, provide an imitative prompt.
Increase the child's repertoire of requestive conversational acts, using existing forms, when possible	Increase the number of requests for action	Use interactive routines to create both need and opportunity for adults with severe or profound intellectual impairment to communicate. For example, an individual with intellectual impairment can be shown how to operate a radio by using a special stick to turn it on. After repeating the demonstration several times, give the radio to the individual with intellectual disability but without the stick needed to operate it (McLean, McLean, Brady, & Etter, 1991).
Train new linguistic forms that are useful in performing available assertive acts	Increase the number of verbal forms for requesting action	Use a combination of focused stimulation and incidental teaching to train the forms "Pass me the —, please" and "Help me, please."

ple, to address a problem of conversational repair, Ezell and Goldstein (1991b) trained five children with mild or moderate intellectual impairment to request clarification when they were presented with instructions that were obscured by noise, contained an unfamiliar word, or were too lengthy to be comprehended. The experimenters deliberately created the communication breakdowns and then taught the children how to respond to them. The barrier game, modified to suit the cognitive level of the child, is a commonly used approach to increase awareness of referential difficulties such as deictic language and provide practice in overcoming them.

Goal Attack Strategy

Deciding how many and in what sequence target behaviors will be introduced to a child is an important intervention consideration. As with any children, the number of goals worked on at one time is determined by factors such as attention span, motivation, cooperation, and rate of learning. Compared with their typically developing peers, children with intellectual disabilities generally have problems in all of these areas. This suggests that the number of goals should be limited, possibly even to one at a time for some children.

Caretaker Interaction

The relationship between adult caretakers and children with intellectual disabilities has important implications for the development of these children and for intervention efforts. Consequently, this relationship has been frequently studied to determine whether and how parents act differently toward children with intellectual disabilities, to uncover the causes of any differences, and to see if parents' behavior can be changed with positive effects. Table 6.7 summarizes the results from various studies on this topic. Collectively, this research suggests that parents and teachers act and talk somewhat differently to children with intellectual disabilities. Many of the adults' behaviors, however, appear to be in reaction to the conduct of the children. Regardless of how the interaction begins, it appears possible to help parents to modify their behavior toward children with intellectual disabilities and, by so doing, to achieve developmental gains.

Materials Selection

One of the foremost practical considerations in planning an intervention procedure is selecting materials that will engage children's attention and motivate them to participate in the designed activity. In this regard, we should remember that children with intellectual disabilities are often delayed in other areas of development. Delays in sensory and motor development and social skills, combined with cognitive impairment, make it very difficult to predict a child's level of interest with a particular toy or activity. Neither MA nor CA can be expected to provide an unerring guide, although a child's level of intellectual disability may provide a guide to materials selection. There may be an advantage in using materials that are relatively concrete and as realistic as possible

Comprehension

Promoting comprehension can take many forms, depending on the intellectual level of the child and on whether there is a significant hearing impairment. In all cases it is important to continue to monitor hearing status in order to ensure the success of comprehension training.

It is clear that operant conditioning procedures can be effective in training comprehension of specific language forms, particularly if rehearsal strategies are also employed. Operant techniques may be the method of choice for children with severe or profound intellectual disabilities. The use of operant procedures, however, does not mean that language teaching must occur in sterile surroundings or that it cannot take advantage of certain natural tendencies toward learning. In one study, operant methods were used in two forms to enhance comprehension of agent–action–object and action–object–locative sentences by preschool children with moderate intellectual disabilities (Kim & Lombardino, 1991). In one form, the methods were script based, that is, the sentence stimuli were presented in the context of a meaningful story. In the other form, they were not. The researchers found that the script-based technique resulted in more rapid learning and better generalization to nontraining contexts.

A much different set of methods for facilitating comprehension is found in child-oriented intervention approaches. Here the clinician follows the child's lead while enriching the verbal environment through self-talk, parallel talk, repetition, or recasting, techniques that are often used with other children with language disorders. Fey (1986) asserts that these

TABLE 6.7   Questions Raised and Answers Given by Research on Interaction between Adult Caretakers and Children with Intellectual Disabilities

Question	Research Indicates That . . .
Do parents talk differently to children with intellectual disabilities?	Some say no. Marshall, Hegrenes, and Goldstein (1973) compared the language of mothers of children with intellectual disabilities to that of mothers of typically developing children. The children were matched for CA. Despite the clear developmental differences between the two groups of children, they found few differences in the language used by the mothers when talking to their children.
	Others say yes. Mothers were found to produce more frequent but shorter utterances in conversation with children with Down syndrome than with their nondisabled siblings (Buium, Rynders, & Turnure, 1974). Mothers of children with Down syndrome often use larger numbers of imperatives than mothers of typically developing children (Cardoso-Martins & Mervis, 1985).
	Even if parents *do* talk differently to children with intellectual disabilities, there is little evidence that such behavior causes the language acquisition of those children to be different (Rosenberg & Abbeduto, 1993)
Do parents act differently with children with intellectual disabilities?	There is evidence that parents of children with intellectual disabilities (Stoneman, Brody, & Abbott, 1983) and mothers of children with Down syndrome (Cardoso-Martins & Mervis, 1985; Eheart, 1982; Smith, 1989) are more likely than parents of typically developing children to take a dominant managerial role in interactions with their children.
Why do parents of children with intellectual disabilities tend to take a dominant role?	One factor contributing to this tendency may be that children with intellectual disabilities have been found to be less responsive to their parents than typically developing children. It may also be that the parents of children with Down syndrome, being aware of their disability, feel the need to provide additional stimulation or draw their children's attention in certain directions (Lynch & Eilers, 1991; Smith, 1989). Parents of children with Down syndrome are especially concerned with the social acceptability of their children's behavior and tend to be more directive when, for example, the children exhibit nonstandard play with toys (Maurer & Sherrod, 1987).
Can parental behavior be changed?	Girolametto (1988) found that an 11-week parent education course was effective in reducing the directiveness and increasing the responsiveness of mothers of children with developmental delays. The children showed significant gains in both assertive and responsive conversational acts, number of verbal turns, and diversity of vocabulary.
Do changes in parental behavior lead to developmental gains in children with intellectual disabilities?	Some say no. Girolametto (1988) found that parent education produced no language gains, as measured by the Sequenced Inventory of Communication Development.
	Others say yes. A number of studies (Bidder, Bryant, & Gray, 1975; Ludlow & Allen, 1979; MacDonald et al., 1974) have found that early parent training improves the language development of children with Down syndrome.
What methods of parent training work best?	Researchers have not yet undertaken studies comparing different instructional methods, so we must use the suggestions made from studies of language development in children with Down syndrome (Pruess, Vadasy, & Fewell, 1987).
Do teachers talk differently to children with intellectual disabilities?	Teachers have been found to modify their speech to children with intellectual disabilities in accord with their perceived communicative level (Hodapp, Evans, & Ward, 1989). The changes are largely functional: they request different kinds of responses (attend, identification or yes/no, labeling, topic comment) based on each child's immediate linguistic performance. Syntax and vocabulary are not altered.

techniques "may be especially useful when general gains in language comprehension are the focus of the intervention program" (p. 203). Training parents to stimulate their children in one of these ways may result in gains not only in comprehension but in production as well.

Lexicon

Because of the deficits in syntax shown by children with intellectual disabilities—especially those with Down syndrome—professionals may target vocabulary as a way of teaching to a strength. But lexical teaching should not be carried out without regard to impairments in other areas of language. It should be integrated with syntactic teaching so that children are able to express a variety of ideas.. Vocabulary teaching is too often limited to nominals. A child who already knows a set of nouns (*bike, ball, rope, car*) must learn other words that function syntactically with those nouns: verbs (*ride, throw, jump, drive*), modifiers (*big, little, thick, nice, blue*), adverbs (*fast, far, hard, safely*), and so on.

Attention should also be paid to the semantic field structure of a vocabulary. For example, a child may possess a vocabulary that is full of words and idiomatic phrases to express semantic fields such as man (*daddy, sister, team*), clothing (*shoes, zipper, take off*), food (*eat, sandwich, stir*), and animals (*dog, meow, walk the dog*). These are both common to experience and for the most part physically tangible. The vocabulary may be weak, however, in semantic fields such as sight (*look, blind, invisible*), smell (*nostril, whiff, odor*), and flowers (*petal, thorn, rose*). These words are either less common or more abstract or both. Professionals should consider whether their aim is to work within existing semantic fields and merely increase the number of functional words that are available to the child, or whether they want to try to stretch the child cognitively and semantically by introducing areas of the lexicon in which the child has not ventured previously. The aim is likely to be different for various children with intellectual disabilities.

Syntax

Two major types of syntax teaching programs, which will be discussed more fully in Chapter 14, have been described as hybrid and trainer-oriented approaches (Fey, 1986). These two types are distinguished primarily by the role of the child. In *hybrid intervention,* situations are structured to encourage a child to make a specific communicative attempt, which then serves as the focus for a teaching interaction between the child and an adult. Table 6.8 shows examples of two hybrid procedures, the mand-model and incidental teaching techniques (Warren & Bambara, 1989).

Although these approaches have been used successfully to train syntax in several experiments with disadvantaged and specifically language-impaired children, there are few studies of the procedure with children who are intellectually disabled (Warren & Kaiser, 1986). Warren and Bambara (1989) reported on one milieu teaching program (see Chapter 14) carried out with three children with borderline to moderate intellectual impairment. Using a combination of mand-model, incidental teaching, and systematic commenting (similar to focused stimulation, discussed later) techniques, they were able to train action–object forms. Training was conducted three or four times per week for 15 minutes. The authors observed varying amounts of generalization to other communicative acts but very little generalization to other settings or persons.

TABLE 6.8   Examples of Two Hybrid Intervention Procedures

Mand-Model

Context: Child is scooping beans with a ladle and pouring them into a pot.

Trainer: "What are you doing?" (target probe question)

Child: No response

Trainer: "Tell me." (mand)

Child: "Beans"

Trainer: "Say, pour beans." (model)

Child: "Pour beans."

Trainer: "That's right, you're pouring beans into the pot." (verbal acknowledgment + expansion)

Incidental Teaching

Context: Making pudding activity. Trainer gives peer a turn at stirring the pudding as the subject looks on.

Child: "Me!" (Child initiates) and reaches for ladle.

Trainer: "Stir pudding." (model)

Child: "Stir pudding."

Trainer: "Alright. You stir the pudding, too." (verbal acknowledgment + expansion + activity participation)

In *trainer-oriented intervention,* as the name implies, the procedure is more fully under the control of the professional. Operant procedures are one form of trainer-oriented intervention. Although different in their details, all operant procedures are based on a teaching strategy that introduces new language behaviors in a series of small steps. Following is an example of the steps followed in teaching a child to respond to an open-ended question with an action–object sentence.

Goal: Train Action–Object Sentence

(Trainer shows car to child)

TRAINER: What's that?

CHILD: Car.

TRAINER: (Reinforecement) Point to car.

(Child points to car)

TRAINER: (Reinforcement) Is that a car?

CHILD: Yes.

TRAINER: (Reinforcement) What do you want?

CHILD: Want car.

TRAINER: (Reinforcement)

(Trainer shows spoon to child)

TRAINER: What's that? Is that a car?

CHILD: No.

TRAINER: (Reinforcement)

(Trainer shows spoon and car to child)

TRAINER: What's that? (points to car)

CHILD: Car.

TRAINER: (Reinforcement) What's that? (points to spoon)

CHILD: Spoon

TRAINER: (Reinforcement) What do you want?

CHILD: Want car.

The behaviorist principles of prompting, shaping, and reinforcing are used to elicit a high rate of correct responses from the child. These procedures have been used successfully to teach noun and verb inflections (Baer & Guess, 1973; Schumaker & Sherman, 1970), simple clauses (Lutzker & Sherman, 1974), and elements of noun-phrase structure (Smeets & Streifel, 1976). There is no doubt that operant procedures can be used successfully to train behaviors that resemble language. Successful outcomes have been achieved with children at all levels of intellectual impairment, though the behaviors taught to children with severe and profound intellectual impairment are basic communicative functions such as pointing, vocalizing, or crude signing.

The primary criticism of operant procedures to teach language has been that they are not ecologically valid, that is, the behaviors learned lack the flexibility and context sensitivity of normal communicative functions. The result is that language taught by operant techniques tends not to generalize to situations outside those in which it was taught. In response, it may be said that for some children with intellectual disabilities, the ability to use language in a limited number of situations is a satisfactory result. Furthermore, the failure of certain language behaviors to generalize may merely reflect incomplete teaching—inadequate stimulus generalization, to use behaviorist terms—rather than any fundamental flaw in operant procedures.

An alternative trainer-oriented approach is modeling (see Chapter 14). In the techniques known as *focused stimulation* or *systematic commenting,* the professional bombards the child with contextually relevant models of a target form, but the child is not asked to respond (Fey, 1986). Modeling is often used in a modified form with children with intellectual disabilities. The following procedure (Warren & Bambara, 1989) illustrates how a model might be presented with additional repetition, prosodic emphasis, and direct prompts for response.

Trainer makes frequent comments describing the child's and trainer's activity, placing emphasis on the target form:

TRAINER: I'm *making cookies.* See? *Make cookies.*

Also used as an antecedent to a direct prompt for a target response:

(Trainer shakes baby powder on a doll.)

TRAINER: "Let's *shake powder* on the baby."

(Child attempts to grab the powder away from the adult.)

TRAINER: What do you want to do?

These modifications are intended to overcome problems of poor attention and verbal passivity, which are often presented by children with intellectual disabilities. In the Environmental Language Intervention Program (ELIP) (MacDonald, Blott, Gordon, Spiegel, & Hartmann, 1974; MacDonald & Horstmeier, 1978), a program used successfully with preschool children with Down syndrome, a model is presented but the children are then also prompted to use certain language targets and are reinforced when they do. The program promotes generalization by using the parents as trainers and requiring responses in conversational and play situations (MacDonald et al., 1974).

Another modeling program, Interactive Language Development Teaching (ILDT) (Lee, Koenigsknecht, & Mulhern, 1975), which is described more fully in Chapter 14, has been similarly modified for use with children with moderate intellectual impairment (McGivern, Rieff, & Vender, 1978). In its modified form, children were provided reinforcement for attending behavior and correct grammatical responses. Only one new language story was introduced each week, and additional time was spent on vocabulary instruction. To assess the success of the program, children in an experimental group received instruction for 30 minutes per day, 4 days a week, for 7 months. Children in a control group received an equal amount of "stimulation" but without a consistent focus on syntactic targets. Investigators found significant improvement in the children's ability to repeat modeled structures, as well as improvement in syntax scores obtained from spontaneous language samples. As used with children with intellectual disabilities, the ILDT program requires the following entrance abilities: (1) spontaneous production of phrases with more than two words and subject–verb clauses; (2) ability to repeat at least two words from a modeled sentence; and (3) ability to attend auditorily for at least 10 minutes when reinforcement is provided.

Some children with Down syndrome have been found to present cognitive profiles in which reading skills are relatively advanced compared to their overall mental age (Byrne, Buckley, MacDonald, & Bird, 1995). Perhaps owing to this, teenagers with Down syndrome have been shown to benefit from a syntax instruction program in which target structures were modeled through reading (Buckley, 1995). The long-term effect of these gains is not presently known.

Speech Production

In most respects, intervention for speech production difficulties is the same for children with and without intellectual disabilities. As noted earlier, accommodation is made in materials and instructions to suit the cognitive level of the child. Also, because of the oral and facial differences they present, oral motor stimulation and exercises are often recommended for children with Down syndrome to improve sucking, oral awareness, and tone of the lips and tongue, as well as to decrease drooling (Swift & Rosin, 1990). With children who show variability in how they produce the same word, parents can be enlisted to accept only renditions that are consistent and do not contain nondevelopmental errors (Dodd, McCormack, & Woodyatt, 1994).

Summary

In this chapter we have seen that

- Intellectual disabilities is a category of disability defined by testing of intelligence and adaptive behavior.
- The major etiological categories of intellectual disabilities are organic and familial. Individuals in the two categories show distinct profiles.
- Children with intellectual disabilities frequently show differences in appearance and have more physical disabilities and health problems than typically developing children.
- Research has yet to resolve the delay–difference controversy over the nature of cognitive and linguistic systems in children with intellectual disabilities. At least part of the controversy can be attributed to inadequate research methods. Future refinements in research techniques should help to advance our knowledge.
- Compared to their CA peers, children with intellectual disabilities show impairments at all levels of language: pragmatics, comprehension, semantics, syntax, and speech production.
- Compared to children equivalent in MA, children with Down syndrome appear to show a specific impairment of syntax. These children also show a decline in rate of language development as they grow older. The causes of these phenomena are presently unknown.
- Intervention for children with intellectual disabilities should be planned with consideration of legal, cognitive, linguistic, logical, environmental, and motivational factors.
- Trainer-oriented, child-oriented, and hybrid approaches to language intervention can all be implemented successfully with children who are intellectually disabled.

Children with intellectual disabilities, though discussed as a group, must be treated as individuals. The problems of each child are uniquely complex and require us to consider broad issues of personal development and quality of life. The professional challenge is to find resourceful solutions that extend each individual's capacity for communication and social participation.

7 Language and Children with Autism

STEVEN H. LONG

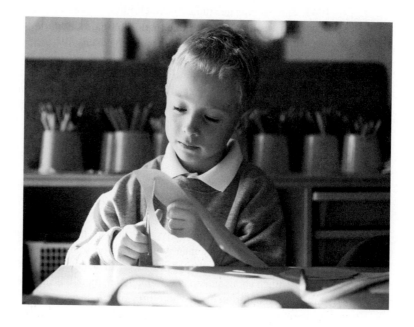

OBJECTIVES

After reading this chapter you should be able to discuss

- Definitions and description of autism
- Other etiological categories with which it overlaps
- General characteristics of the language of children with autism
- Principles of language intervention for children with autism

Professionals who serve children with language disorders are prone to change their minds. Usually these changes are relatively small: a theory might be updated to take account of new research information, or a new intervention tactic might be adopted that refines previous practice. The disorder of autism, however, has been associated with wide swings in thinking. Such large changes cause many reactions among professionals. There is fascination with the enigmatic nature of autism, frustration that many previous beliefs about it are eventually proven wrong, and optimism that the new ideas will improve the efficacy of treatment.

An Overview of Children with Autism

Autism was first described as a syndrome, or unique collection of behaviors, by Kanner in 1943. The patients he studied were children of normal or near-normal intelligence. Therefore, the focus of his description was on their unusual social and communicative impairments. He characterized the children as aloof and withdrawn, able to communicate only in repetitive utterances, fascinated by inanimate objects, and intolerant of changes in routine (Kanner, 1943). The cause of autism was, and still is, unknown, but for the next three decades following Kanner's published observations it was generally considered to be a type of emotional disturbance. As such, it was sometimes interpreted as resulting from environmental influences during the early years of life (Bettelheim, 1967). Because of this belief, the parents of children with autism were often—and, we now know, unfairly—held responsible for the condition. Treatment efforts were as likely to be concerned with changing the family as with changing the child.

Since the 1970s three major shifts in thinking about autism have occurred. The first has been in the conception of the disorder. Autism is now clearly viewed as a *developmental* rather than an *emotional* or *psychiatric* disorder (American Psychiatric Association, 2000). Hence, it is more closely aligned with intellectual disabilities and other forms of developmental disability than with childhood schizophrenia and other types of psychotic disorders. The second change has been in our beliefs about the origin of the disorder. Though much about autism is still not understood, it is now generally accepted that the condition is present from birth. Therefore, autism does not stem from the actions of the parents in rearing their children but, in all likelihood, results from the genes they contributed in making their children. The third shift in thinking has been a subject of some controversy. It has resulted from an innovative—some would say illegitimate—method of intervention known as *facilitated communication*. Although this method is a form of augmentative and alternative communication (AAC), which will be discussed more fully in Chapter 12, it must be mentioned at the outset because of its prominence in the literature on autism.

Diagnostic Criteria

Despite the relatively short history of autism as a clinical category, it has become one of the most complicated areas of medical and educational diagnosis. The number of terms used to describe children with autism and related disorders has grown quickly, especially in recent years. A group of these terms is listed and defined in Table 7.1. The proliferation of labels

TABLE 7.1 Terminology Used to Describe Children with Autism and Related Psychotic and Developmental Disorders

Term	Description/Comment
Asperger's disorder	A diagnostic label first appearing in DSM-IV in 1994 but often used prior to that in the literature on pervasive developmental disorder (PDD). Individuals with this condition, primarily boys, exhibit social and communicative deficits, but typically at a higher level than individuals with autism. For example, an individual with Asperger syndrome may interact socially but display numerous behavioral oddities such as social unawareness, lack of common sense, repetitive interests, and pedantic speech (Gillberg, 1991). The condition overlaps with mild forms of autism but has a better prognosis (Bishop, 1989).
Autistic disorder	The most severe form of PDD recognized in DSM-IV-TR (American Psychiatric Association, 2000). See Table 7.2 for a description of diagnostic criteria.
Autistic spectrum (disorder)	Originally, a term introduced to describe a group of conditions broader than PDD that share impairments in social interaction, verbal and non-verbal communication, and imagination (Wing, 1997). The term has since come to be used as a synonym for PDD or to refer to (a) a continuum of intellectual ability among children with PDD; or (b) a range of symptom severity among children with autism; or (c) the developmental changes that may occur in children with autism, such as the improvement of language ability (Tonge, 2002).
Childhood disintegrative disorder	Also known as Heller syndrome, this is a rare condition in which a child's social, communicative, and cognitive development is normal at least until age 2 but then suddenly disintegrates, and behaviors characteristic of pervasive development disorder emerge (Rutter & Schopler, 1987). In DSM-IV, the American Psychiatric Association (2000) recognized this as a form of pervasive developmental disorder separate from autistic disorder.
Infantile autism	Older diagnostic category used in DSM-III (American Psychiatric Association, 1980). It was merged into the category of autistic disorder when DSM-III was revised in 1983.
Kanner's syndrome or "classic" autism	A term used by some professionals to designate children with autism who resemble the patients originally described by Kanner (1943). Specifically, these are children who show the social, communication, and behavioral aberrations associated with autism but do not show intellectual impairment.
Pervasive development disorder (PDD)	The broader category of mental disorders in DSM-IV-TR that includes autistic disorder.
Pervasive development disorder not otherwise specified (PDDNOS)	A diagnostic category described in DSM-IV-TR which is used for children who exhibit behaviors characteristic of pervasive developmental disorder but do not meet the criteria for a specific disorder (autistic disorder, Asperger's disorder, Rett's disorder, or Childhood disintegrative disorder (American Psychiatric Association, 2000). Clinically, these children typically appear to be less impaired than children diagnosed with autistic disorder.
Residual autism	A term used to describe individuals who once met the criteria for autistic disorder but, because of developmental changes and improvements, no longer do.
Rett's disorder	A progressive neurological disorder occurring in girls. It is associated with worsening dementia, loss of facial expression and purposeful hand use, ataxia, diminished interpersonal contact, and stereotyped hand movements (Rutter & Schopler, 1987). Rett's disorder must be specifically excluded as part of the diagnosis of autistic disorder (American Psychiatric Association, 2000).
Schizoid and schizotypal personality disorder	Two types of personality disorders, in contrast to developmental disorders, described in DSM-IV-TR. The chief feature of schizoid personality disorder is detachment from social relationships and a restricted range of emotional expression (American Psychiatric Association, 2000). Individuals with these characteristics might be diagnosed by some professionals as having Asperger syndrome (Rutter & Schopler, 1987). Schizotypal personality disorder is associated with social deficits but also shows distortions of thinking and behavioral eccentricities (American Psychiatric Association, 2000).
Schizophrenia	A condition in which social and communicative behaviors are affected in ways similar to those seen in autism. Schizophrenia, however, is classified as a *psychosis* in contrast to a *pervasive developmental disorder*. It contrasts with autism in several ways (see Table 7.4)

has resulted from research on what constitutes the core of autism and distinguishes it from other similar disorders. To many professionals, the distinctions among these terms are subtle and may even seem irrelevant in matters of clinical practice. After all, if several children are labeled differently but receive the same treatment, what purpose does the label serve? It is a fair question, and the framers of diagnostic categories may in the future need to consider "response to treatment" as one of the characteristics that define subgroups of children with autism and related disorders.

Nevertheless, professionals rely on diagnostic categories to do their work, so we must address the issue of how syndromes are defined and distinguished. To begin with, we should note a simple linguistic and clinical distinction. The word *autism,* a noun, should refer always to a clinical syndrome that is defined by a unique set of behavioral criteria. Those criteria have changed at various points over the last half-century, but the notion of autism as a syndrome has remained unchanged (Wetherby, 1989). In contrast, the word *autistic,* an adjective, has frequently been used by clinicians to describe individual behaviors in children who may or may not meet the criteria for the syndrome of autism. For example, many children with profound intellectual disabilities exhibit self-injurious (head banging, biting) or stereotypic (arm flapping, grimacing) behaviors that are also observed in children with autism. Perhaps because these actions are so dramatically bizarre and are associated with autism, they are often called *autistic* or *autistic-like behaviors.* This practice is regrettable for two reasons. First, it gives a sloppy description of the behaviors themselves. To say that a child has "autistic-like behaviors" is akin to saying that someone "acts depressed." Second, the term *autistic-like* suggests to the uninformed listener or reader that a child has been diagnosed with autism, when this may not be the case.

As noted previously, the category of autism has been revised over the years. Several well-recognized scholars have had substantial influence in shaping professional opinion about the diagnostic boundaries of the disorder (Rutter, 1978; Wing, 1981). Since 1980, however, the major arbiter in the matter of definition has been a group of professionals assembled by the American Psychiatric Association, whose work is published in the *Diagnostic and Statistical Manual of Mental Disorders.* The fourth edition of this manual (DSM-IV) was published in 1994; a revision (DSM-IV-TR) was published in 2000. The definition of Autistic Disorder contained in DSM-IV-TR is cited in Table 7.2. This definition now serves as the standard for scholars in the field and for many professionals involved in the diagnosis of autism. Although the DSM-IV-TR definition carries the weight of scholarly authority, the legal definition of autism is determined by each state. A survey conducted in 1985 indicated that the two state agencies most commonly providing diagnostic services for autism—the departments of mental health and of public instruction—often utilize different diagnostic criteria and permit different professionals (e.g., psychiatrist, school psychologist, special education teacher) to make the diagnosis (Vicker & Monahan, 1988). Without some investigation of a child's individual case history, therefore, the criteria that were applied in a diagnosis of autism may not be clearly known.

The DSM-IV-TR diagnostic criteria for autism are designed to deal with the inherent heterogeneity of the disorder. That is, they recognize that children with autism present a wide range of aberrant behaviors. Stereotyped descriptions of children with autism nearly always include behaviors such as echolalia, idiosyncratic language (e.g., repeating television commercials), fascination with mechanical objects, and unusual motor behavior (e.g., toe walking). But these behaviors, though they may be common, are not found in all cases of autism.

TABLE 7.2 DSM-IV-TR Diagnostic Criteria for Autistic Disorder

Prior to age 3, the child must show six or more behaviors characteristic of the disorder. Of these, there must be at least . . .

Two behaviors that demonstrate qualitative impairment of social interaction:

	Example Typical of Younger or More Handicapped Child	Example Typical of Older or Less Handicapped Child
1. Marked impairment in the use of multiple nonverbal behaviors such as eye-to-eye gaze, facial expression, body postures, and gestures to regulate social interaction	Does not wave bye-bye	Mechanically imitates others' actions out of context
2. Failure to develop peer relationships appropriate to developmental level	No interest in making peer friendships	Shows interest in friendship but does not understand conventions of social interaction, for example, reads phone book to uninterested peer
3. Lack of spontaneous seeking to share enjoyment, interests, or achievements with other people	Does now show or point out objects of interest to others	Does not talk about his own or others' interests
4. Lack of social or emotional reciprocity	Does not seek comfort even when ill, hurt, or tired	Seeks comfort in a stereotyped way; for example, says *cheese, cheese, cheese* whenever hurt
5. No or abnormal play	Does not actively participate in simple games	Involves other children in play only as "mechanical aids"

One behavior that demonstrates qualitative impairment in communication:

1. Delay in, or total lack of, the development of spoken language (not accompanied by an attempt to compensate through alternative modes of communication such as gesture or mime)	No communicative babbling, facial expression, gesture, mime, or spoken language
2. In individuals with adequate speech, marked impairment in the ability to initiate or sustain a conversation with others	Monologues are produced without allowing others opportunity to speak
3. Stereotyped and repetitive use of language or idiosyncratic language	Monotonous or question-like intonation, high pitch, immediate echolalia, use of *you* for *I*, invented words, irrelevant remarks
4. Lack of varied, spontaneous make-believe play or social imitative play appropriate to developmental level	No playacting of adult roles, fantasy characters, or animals

One behavior indicative of restricted, repetitive, and stereotyped patterns of behavior, interests, and activities:

1. Encompassing preoccupation with one or more stereotyped and restricted patterns of interest that is abnormal either in intensity or focus	Interested only in lining up objects, amassing facts about meteorology, or in pretending to be a fantasy character
2. Apparently inflexible adherence to specific, nonfunctional routines or rituals	Insists that the same route be followed when shopping
3. Stereotyped and repetitive motor mannerisms	Hand flicking or twisting, spinning, head banging, complex whole-body movements
4. Persistent preoccupation with parts of objects	Sniffs objects, repetitive feeling of texture of materials, attachment to unusual objects (e.g., carrying around a piece of string)

Source: Adapted from American Psychiatric Association (2000).

Is there a behavior or behaviors that unambiguously identify autism in a child? If the question is asked this way, the answer has to be no. However, researchers have asked another related question: do certain behaviors found in autism more reliably distinguish it from other disorders? Two studies have examined the records of children with autism and similar disorders and have used statistical analyses to determine the distinctive characteristics of autism (Dahl, Cohen, & Provence, 1986; Siegel, Vukicevic, Elliott, & Kraemer, 1989). The studies agree that social impairment is the hallmark characteristic. Specifically, of the behaviors cited in the DSM-III-R definition and maintained in DSM-IV-TR, the most predictive characteristic was a marked lack of awareness of the existence or feelings of others, followed by a persistent preoccupation with parts of objects.

Prevalence

Current estimates from the National Institute of Child Health and Human Development (2001) are that autism occurs in approximately one to two children in every 1,000. This represents a sizable increase from rates reported in the 1970s (3.5–4.5 per 10,000 children), but most of this change can be accounted for by differences in how autism is now defined and studied (Tonge, 2002).

All forms of pervasive developmental disorder occur more frequently in males than females, with different studies suggesting ratios from 2:1 to 5:1 (American Psychiatric Association, 2000). The ratio for autistic disorder, in particular, has been estimated at 3:1 or 4:1. The more frequent impairment of males has no ready explanation, but it is one of the features of autism that distinguish it from intellectual disabilities. Although females with autism are diagnosed less frequently, they may be skewed toward the low end in IQ distribution (Bryson, 1997). Inasmuch as IQ is the best-known predictor of outcome in individuals with autism, it can be inferred that females tend to present as more difficult clinical cases (Gillberg, 1991). Females have also been found to develop seizure disorders in higher proportions than males, which may contribute further to their poorer observed outcomes (Volkmar & Nelson, 1990).

Associated Problems

The core features of autism, which are outlined in the DSM-IV-TR diagnostic criteria, are social impairment, communicative impairment, and repetitive or highly restricted (stereotyped) behavior that replaces more imaginative forms of action. These features most accurately distinguish autism from other developmental disabilities, but they do not describe all the aberrant behaviors one is likely to find in children with autism. Table 7.3 summarizes some of the other significant conditions that are associated with autism. Of particular note, especially because of impacts on intervention, is the high co-occurrence of intellectual disability with autism. Largely as a result of these associated problems, individuals with autism have a reduced life expectancy (Shavelle, Strauss, & Pickett, 2001).

What Causes Autism?

The short answer to this question is, simply, that we do not know. There are a number of methodological problems that make the search for the cause difficult:

TABLE 7.3 Associated Problems in Children with Autism

Intellectual disabilities	Over three-quarters of all children with autism have intellectual disabilities, based on IQ test scores. In most cases the tests indicate a moderate level of intellectual impairment (IQ 35–49) (American Psychiatric Association, 2000; Rutter & Schopler, 1987).
Motor behavior deficits	Along with their propensity for repetitive movements (see Table 7.1), many children with autism are poorly coordinated and display odd hand and body postures (American Psychiatric Association, 2000). Their performance on copying tasks suggests that deficits in visual monitoring of motor performance are responsible for some of their motor difficulties (Fulkerson & Freeman, 1980). Proponents of facilitated communication have suggested that one of the primary impairments of autism is an inability to *initiate* voluntary movements, a motor apraxia (Biklen, 1990). This claim has been strongly disputed (Calculator, 1999).
Unusual sensory behavior	Children with autism may show either hyposensitivity or hypersensitivity to certain stimuli. They may be oblivious to heat, cold, or pain but show extreme distress when they hear certain sounds or are touched unexpectedly. In one survey, 18% of children with autism showed hyperacusis, a collapsed tolerance to normal environmental sounds (Rosenhall, Nordin, Sandstroem, Ahlsen, & Gillberg, 1999).
Hearing loss	Fluctuating, negative middle-ear pressure is more common in children with autism than in unimpaired children. This results in more frequent middle ear infections (Konstantareas & Homatidis, 1987), though it is not necessary for an infection to develop in order for a child's hearing to be affected. Pronounced or profound bilateral hearing loss occurs in 3.5% of cases (Rosenhall et al., 1999).
Seizures	Approximately one-third of all patients develop epilepsy during early childhood or adolescence (Gillberg, 1991; Volkmar & Nelson, 1990). The onset of seizures tends not to occur during *middle* childhood, for reasons that are not understood (Volkmar & Nelson, 1990).
Fragile X syndrome	Children with autism show a higher than normal prevalence of fragile X syndrome, a genetic condition associated with intellectual disability and certain behavioral abnormalities. Fragile X syndrome has been found at rates varying from 0% to 20%, depending on the identification criteria employed. When stringent criteria were followed, it appeared in only 2.7% of cases (Piven, Gayle, Landa, Wzorek, & Folstein, 1991). The reason for the association, even though it may be small, is unknown.

1. Autism is not a discrete disorder but represents the most severe form of pervasive developmental disorder. Therefore, the cause of autism must also account for the problems of children who have related disorders.
2. There is significant variation in the types and severity of problems manifested by children with autism. Whatever is causing the disorder must be interacting with other developmental factors to produce such a diverse array of behavioral profiles.
3. In most children with autism, the disorder is first manifested as an impairment in social skills observed around 18 months (Johnson, Siddons, Frith, & Morton, 1992). Even then, however, it may not be possible to make a confident diagnosis. Consequently, researchers are unable to study the disorder until the children have become

toddlers or preschoolers. This serves to keep certain information about the origins of the problem hidden from investigators.

4. The social and communicative impairments of children with autism have always made developmental testing extremely difficult, especially when the children are young (Lord, 1997). When the accuracy of measurements is doubted, it is hard to find support for causal theories. After all, the data they are based upon may be wrong.

In spite of these obstacles, research on autism has assembled an impressive amount of information and has brought many issues into focus. For many years, there has been a consensus that the underlying problem in autism is neurophysiological rather than environmental. Acknowledgment of this fact has led researchers to compare autism with other childhood disorders known to have a neurophysiological cause, such as intellectual disabilities and schizophrenia. The reasoning is that if autism can be linked to any of these other disorders, then it may be possible to develop an explanation of autism based on what is known about the other disorders. The evidence has indicated, however, that autism is distinctive. Table 7.4 summarizes some of the findings that differentiate autism from other neurophysiological disorders of childhood.

Some scientists have taken the position that the behaviors evidenced in autism can be traced to specific neurophysiological mechanisms and that these mechanisms must, therefore, be dysfunctional. Thus, it has been suggested that the primary deficit is in

1. Areas of the limbic system that are responsible for arousal, attention, and motor responsiveness (Bauman & Kemper, 1994), *or*

2. Areas of the cerebellum that facilitate arousal and attention (Townsend, Courchesne, & Egaas, 1996), *or*

3. A combination of cortical and subcortical areas that are responsible for attachment and social behavior (Ozonoff, Pennington, & Rogers, 1991), *or*

4. Neuromotor systems underlying voluntary or intentional movement (Biklen, 1990). This last suggestion is linked with the therapeutic approach of facilitated communication.

Where brain abnormalities are implicated in autism, these most likely occur before birth as a result of a number of possible causes (e.g., infection, metabolic imbalance, immune response, neurophysiological disturbance, or environmental insult). These many causes may all lead to similar patterns of brain development, which result in autism (Bristol et al., 1996).

A further factor related to causation relates to baby and childhood vaccinations. Beginning in the late 1990s, reports began to circulate of a possible link between the measles–mumps–rubella (MMR) vaccine and autism. Scientific investigation to date has not shown any causal relationship between the two, and thus no recommendation has been made for changes in either the use or timing of the MMR vaccine (Immunization Safety Review Committee–Institute of Medicine, 2001). Research on this topic continues, however.

Heredity

As with all serious developmental disorders, investigators have been intrigued with the role of heredity in causing autism. Although research in this area is ongoing, the current body of opinion may be summarized as follows.

TABLE 7.4   Evidence Distinguishing Autism from Other Neurophysiological Disorders

Autism versus . . .	Intellectual Disabilities
Onset of seizures (in about 25% of children) occurs during adolescence	Onset of seizures occurs during early childhood
Occurs infrequently in Down syndrome (about 10% of children) or cerebral palsy	Usually occurs in Down Syndrome and cerebral palsy
Occurs much more frequently in males (approximately a 4:1 ratio)	Occurs only slightly more frequently in males
Children have difficulty discriminating socioemotional cues (e.g., facial expressions)	Children can read such cues at a level commensurate with MA
Autism versus . . .	**Schizophrenia**
Onset typically occurs before 30 months of age	Onset typically occurs during adolescence
Family history of schizophrenia is rare	Family history of schizophrenia is greater than chance
Delusions and hallucinations are rare	Delusions and hallucinations are hallmark behaviors
Abnormal behaviors are persistent	Abnormal behaviors are episodic
Seizures occur in about 25% of cases	Seizures are rare
Autism versus . . .	**Developmental Disorder of Receptive Language**
Occurs much more frequently in males (approximately a 4:1 ratio)	Approximately equal in sex distribution (males are predominant in *expressive* language disorder)
Prognosis for improvement is generally poor	Prognosis is generally good
Wider and more severe cognitive handicaps	Milder cognitive handicaps
Persisting socioemotional and behavioral problems	Emotional and behavioral problems appear secondary to language impairment and tend to improve as language does

Source: Adapted from Folstein & Rutter (1988), Howlin, Wing, & Gould (1995), Rutter & Schopler (1987), and Yirmiya, Erel, Shaked, & Solomonika (1998).

■ There is a slight tendency for autism to aggregate (occur more than once) in the same family. This occurs in approximately 1 to 3 percent of families who have one child with autism. Although this is a small percentage, it is 50 to 100 times greater than the chance probability (Folstein & Rutter, 1988). Thus, for a subgroup of individuals there may be a genetic susceptibility to the disorder (Bristol et al., 1996). In cases that can be linked to specific genetic disorders such as fragile X syndrome, the role of heredity is better understood and more accurate genetic predictions can be made

■ There is a greater likelihood of other cognitive, social, or psychological disorders within the families of children with autism. This increased risk is not due solely to the stress of raising a child with autism (Bolton, Pickles, Murphy, & Rutter, 1998). The parents of children with autism indicate that they may have subtle communication problems of their own and that, compared to the parents of children with Down syndrome, they show a higher rate of anxiety and manic–depressive disorder (Landa, Folstein, & Isaacs, 1991; Piven, Chase et al., 1991). It is important to note that these findings do not support the earlier—and now discredited—theory that autism results from insensitive parenting practices.

■ The precise mode of genetic transmission is not yet understood. It appears, from examination of family histories, that autism results not from a single gene but from multiple interacting genes. Research in this area is complicated by the fact that autism is manifested in many different forms and is part of a spectrum of social–cognitive disorders. Results can therefore vary as a consequence of how the disorder is defined and identified in each study (Rutter, Bailey, Simonoff, & Pickles, 1997).

Natural History of Autism

One of the many mysteries about autism is that the condition is not generally recognizable until around 18 months. At that age, some but not all children who will eventually be diagnosed show a noticeable difference in social behaviors such as smiling, pointing, or responding to people (Johnson et al., 1992). In most cases, the onset of autism occurs between 18 and 36 months of age but, studies of home videos of infants have revealed that as early as 8- to 12-month-old children with autism can be identified by deficits in several areas: decreased eye contact, orienting to name, pointing, and showing (Baranek, 1999; Mars, Mauk, & Dowrick, 1998; Osterling & Dawson, 1994). Children who later present more severe symptoms tend to have an earlier age of onset. This probably reflects the behavior of the parents more than that of the child: severe symptoms are more likely to be recognized at an early age than mild ones. Thus, the term *age of onset,* as it is commonly used, is more accurately described as *age of recognition* (Short & Schopler, 1988).

Many of the early signs of autism are deficiencies in a child's communicative behaviors prior to the emergence of speech. Whereas both typically developing children and nonautistic children with intellectual disabilities show a strong attraction to the sound of their mother's voice, children with autism show no such interest or even prefer to listen to environmental sounds such as restaurant noise (Klin, 1991). When they are engaged in interactions with other people, children with autism show deficiencies in gestural joint attention skills (Kasari, Freeman, & Paparella, 2001). That is, they rarely point to or show objects to their partners. These behaviors are frequent among preverbal typically developing children, as is the use of eye contact to attract and then direct a partner's attention. Yet compared to MA- and LA-matched groups of children with intellectual disabilities, children with autism rarely show these behaviors (Mundy, Sigman, & Kasari, 1990).

In later childhood, children with autism begin to display the wide range of impairments in social interaction, communication, and imaginative play that characterize the disorder (see Table 7.2 for summary). Recently a number of scholars have suggested that these diverse problems may have a single underlying cause, namely, an inability to attribute mental states to themselves or to others, or as it is sometimes referred to, "theory of mind" (Baron-Cohen, 1991; Frith, 1989; Silliman et al., 2003; Tager-Flusberg, 1992; Yirmiya, Sigman, Kasari, & Mundy, 1992). This inability to engage in metarepresentational thinking means that children do not understand or relate to the thought processes of people with whom they interact. Obviously this problem would significantly limit their capacity to initiate and sustain social relationships, which rely on the ability to "read" the mood, desires, and intentions of social partners. Similarly, communication requires an ability to evaluate messages according to the context in which they are produced. Part of that context is the thinking and emotional state of the speaker. We routinely relate the two in statements such as "Mommy is sad because she thought you were lost." Children with metarepresentational problems are likely to be confused by this kind of sentence because they cannot imagine the emotions of the mother that would result in sadness. A further consequence of a metarepresentational problem is that children do not observe the subtle cues issued by their conversational partners that signal when they are expected to talk, when they should yield their turn, when they should clarify a statement they have made, and so on. Hence, the marked deficiencies in the pragmatics of communication they often exhibit may result from metarepresentational problems. These are some of the reasons social deficits are viewed as significant features of autism.

Most imaginative activity also depends on representations of what others are thinking. This is apparent in role-playing games, which demand that children be able to think like the individual they are impersonating, whether it is a parent, a policeman, a store owner, or a doctor. Imaginative activity is closely aligned to symbolic thought processes, another problematic area characteristic of autism.

The social and communicative impairments observed in young children with autism often improve in later childhood. Treatment, of course, is one of the factors influencing this improvement. Long-term studies of individuals with autism have indicated, however, that many of them suffer an aggravation of symptoms during adolescence. Most commonly there is an increase in hyperactivity, aggressiveness, self-destructiveness, and insistence on routine. The reason for this deterioration, and the reason it strikes some individuals but not others, is unknown. Some of the causes that have been suggested are the adolescent onset of epilepsy in some individuals, the hormonal changes of puberty and their influence on the nervous system, and the physical growth of the child, which exacerbates the effect of any behavioral problems (Gillberg, 1991).

Communication in Children with Autism

Recall that many studies of language impairment in children with intellectual disabilities have relied on the technique of matching subjects by CA, MA, or LA. A similar procedure has been used to study language impairments of children with autism. In principle, this method should yield comparisons between groups of children (e.g., children with autism, children with intellectual disabilities, and children who are developing typically) that are unconfounded by differences in age, intelligence, or general language level. However, children with autism are frequently difficult to match with others. Because of their tendencies to echo speech addressed to them and to produce stereotyped phrases and sentences, MLU counts are likely to be less stable and less representative than for other children. Similarly, IQ matching is difficult for children with autism because their performances are highly variable at different ages and with different types of intelligence tests (Sparrow et al., 1997).

The verbal abilities of children with autism range from the total absence of speech to communication that is fully adequate in phonological and grammatical form but is remarkable for its semantic or pragmatic irregularities. At both ends of this severity continuum, the behaviors evidenced by children with autism overlap with those shown by children with other developmental disorders. Obviously, a child with no speech may have one of several disorders: autism, intellectual disability, selective/elective mutism, hearing impairment, and others. On the other hand, a child whose problems are exclusively semantic and pragmatic may have a history of autism, learning disability, intellectual disability, or head injury. Thus, neither the degree of severity nor the level(s) of language impairment will unambiguously identify a child with autism. Nevertheless, various studies have suggested a profile of language skills that is generally characteristic of the disorder. In this profile certain abilities are relatively *preserved,* that is, they appear to be commensurate or nearly commensurate with a child's intellectual level. It is important to note that these components of the child's language typically will not be age appropriate and, therefore, may be a focus of clinical intervention. It is generally believed, however, that these language difficulties are secondary to intellectual impairment and, therefore, can be expected to improve as general developmental gains are made. In contrast is a set of abilities that appear to be relatively *impaired* in children with autism. These are the communication behaviors that are most distinctive of autism and are frequently cited as diagnostic criteria (see Table 7.2).

Preserved Abilities

Segmental Phonology and Syntax.   One of the most important generalizations that can be made about the language abilities of children with autism is that they typically do not show specific developmental impairment at the levels of segmental phonology (consonant and vowel production) or syntax (Mundy & Markus, 1997; Tager-Flusberg, 1981). As with all generalizations, however, exceptional cases can be found (Wolk & Giesen, 2000). Nevertheless, one can usually expect the following:

1. The speech the children produce will be generally intelligible, in the same way that the speech of a typically developing child can be understood at any age, even though it is not yet adultlike. There is some evidence that distortion errors may tend to persist into adulthood (Shriberg, Paul, McSweeny, Klin, & Cohen, 2001).
2. Utterances will be free of glaring syntactic problems and will show a balance in structural growth, meaning that they will not have a telegraphic quality caused by limited development of phrase structures and bound morphemes.

The presence of these abilities is a major linguistic difference between children with autism and children with language handicaps due to other causes such as intellectual disabilities, deafness, or specific language impairment.

Lexical and Syntactic Comprehension.   Many factors influence a child's understanding of language, among them the familiarity of the grammar and vocabulary, the familiarity of the topic, and the familiarity of the interactants. Under controlled conditions, it appears that children with autism are able to comprehend the linguistic *code* at a level consistent with MA. That is, they can decode word meanings and semantic contrasts signified by changes in word order or by inflectional morphemes (Beisler, Tsai, & Vonk, 1987; Eskes, Bryson, & McCormick, 1990). This does not mean that a child with autism will understand language as would a typically developing child of the same age. For instance, a 5-year-old child with autism who has an MA of 2 years will doubtless present with comprehension difficulties because of limited vocabulary and immature cognitive development. Moreover, the child is very likely to exhibit deficits in those social interactional behaviors (eye contact, joint attention) that are crucial to speech comprehension in the early years of life (Baron-Cohen, 1988; Watson, 2001).

Imitation.   Imitation is often considered an area of impairment for children with autism because of their tendency to imitate excessively and inappropriately, which we will discuss later. However, we should also observe that, unlike many children with other forms of language impairment, children with autism *can* imitate verbal stimuli. Thus, the ability to decode, store, and encode verbal messages is present, even though the use of this ability can seem strange and sometimes even bizarre.

Impaired Abilities

Nonsegmental Phonology.   In contrast to their ability to master individual sound segments (consonants and vowels), children with autism commonly display significant impairment in nonsegmental speech production, also referred to as *prosody*. Problems of this type take many forms and can vary considerably among children. Some of the most frequently reported aberrations are as follows (Baltaxe & Simmons, 1985; Goldfarb, Braunstein, & Lorge, 1956; Shriberg et al., 2001):

1. A stereotyped rhythmic pattern, described as "singsong," that is characterized by excessive sound prolongation
2. Overly frequent and contextually inappropriate whispering
3. Unusual fluctuations in loudness
4. Limited pitch range, resulting in monotonous speech
5. Inappropriate or disfluent phrasing, akin to stuttering
6. Excessive nasal resonance
7. Tonal contrasts that are inconsistent with the meanings expressed verbally, for example, sentences produced with rising intonation that clearly are not requests

Explanation of these problems is complex because appropriate prosody has so many necessary components: perceptual–motor skill, grammatical organization, and awareness of what is socially acceptable in different circumstances (Shriberg et al., 2001). A simple explanation that children with autism do not perceive prosodic contrasts is not supported by the available research (Baltaxe & Guthrie, 1987; Frankel, Simmons, & Richey, 1987).

Idiosyncratic Language.   Children with autism display several unusual verbal behaviors that, as a group, are referred to as idiosyncratic language. This term draws attention to the fact that, although there are similarities in how idiosyncratic language is learned or used, each child is unique in the specific words or phrases that are produced and the contexts in which they occur.

All forms of idiosyncratic language appear to reflect either peculiarities of semantic processing or deficits in pragmatic competence. Children with autism have a proclivity to recall certain words or phrases only in the context in which they were first learned. Thus, a child may learn a word initially (e.g., *shoe*) as a result of experiences with a particular object (sneaker) but will never generalize use of the word to other stimuli (other shoes, other people's shoes, pictures of shoes). Similarly, a word or phrase may seem to be triggered by the recurrence of the original conditions of learning, as in this example:

Alex, when he was about 3 years old, was riding home at dusk with his mother, who told him that for supper they would have "sea scallops to eat." Just as she said this, the car ahead

(Mercury-Comet, 1960 vintage) with peculiar slanting tail lights stopped and the tail lights lit up. For three or four years afterward, Alex would recite "sea scallops to eat" whenever he saw this type of tail-light on a car. (Simon, 1975, p. 1442)

A distinction is sometimes made between idiosyncratic language, in which conventional words or phrases are used with unconventional meanings, and neologisms, in which a new word or words are coined. Examples of the two behaviors are given in Table 7.5. Children with autism produce both forms, though neologisms are far less frequent and usually consist of incorrect combinations of morphemes (e.g., *glassable* for *breakable*) rather than wholly invented strings of phonemes (e.g., *glufer*). Neither idiosyncratic language nor neologisms are unique to children with autism. They are found less frequently in the spontaneous speech of children with intellectual disabilities, as well as that of young children who are developing typically. In children with autism, however, they are more likely to draw attention. This is because they are more frequent and because they occur in older children who are no longer given license to use language in these ways (Volden & Lord, 1991).

TABLE 7.5   Examples of Neologisms and Idiosyncratic Language in Children with Autism

Utterance	Interpretation
Idiosyncratic Language	
"It makes me want to as deep as economical with it" (Volden & Lord, 1991, p. 118)	"withdraw as much as possible"
"They're having a meal and then they're finishing and *siding the table"* (Volden & Lord, 1991, p. 118)	"clearing the table"
"go get pizza" (Mayes, Calhoun, & Crites, 2001, p. 268)	"I am hungry"
"And *wave their things* on the floor in the bathroom" (Volden & Lord, 1991, p. 118)	"leave their things"
"look what you hear downstairs" (Mayes et al., 2001, p. 268)	"I hear something downstairs"
"If they *even take it true enough"* (Volden & Lord, 1991, p. 118)	"If they take it seriously enough"
"But in the car, *it's some"* (Volden & Lord, 1991, p. 118)	"But in the car, there's something different"
"Q: and what was inside the paper, when you took the paper off? A: that's my cousin" (Preece, 2002, p. 100)	Uninterpretable
Neologisms	
"And he's seriously wounded *like cutes and bloosers"* (Volden & Lord, 1991, p. 118)	"cuts and bruises"
"She's *bawcet"* (Volden & Lord, 1991, p. 118)	"She's bossy"

Source: Mayes et al., (2001); Preece (2002); Volden & Lord (1991).

Idiosyncratic language varies in frequency and character among different children with autism. In some children the process is highly creative, so that idiosyncratic forms will appear at one time and may not reappear in other conversations. In contrast, other children make repeated use of the same word or phrase, often in contexts in which it seems meaningless. It appears unlikely that this behavior has the same function for all children that produce it. The suggestion has been made, however, that highly repeated utterances serve some form of communicative function. For example, Coggins and Frederickson (1988) studied a 9-year-old boy with autism who frequently repeated the phrase "can I talk." By analyzing where the utterance occurred in conversational sequences, they were able to determine that it did not occur randomly but nearly always was directed to the conversational partner, the child's father. Furthermore, the utterance tended to occur in the middle of speaking exchanges and often followed adult attempts to direct activities or introduce new topics. The conclusion was that the utterance was used to force a change in speaker turn and thereby help the child to cope with conversational demands.

Pronoun Difficulties.   Confusion and substitution of pronominal forms occur frequently in the speech of children with autism. Some of their errors, such as confusion of gender (*he* for *she* or *it*) or case substitution (*him* for *he*), are also commonly found in young typically developing children and in children with other forms of language impairment. To some extent, therefore, the pronoun difficulties observed in autism are merely a predictable component of the total language impairment. The problem that appears distinct to autism is the persistent confusion of the first- and second-person singular forms. Children with autism often use *you* to refer to themselves and *I* or *me* to refer to others. They do not appear to have difficulty in comprehending these pronouns (Lee, Hobson, & Chiat, 1994). A number of explanations for this phenomenon have been proposed. In years past the problem was viewed as a failure of ego differentiation, but this idea has been abandoned along with other psychopathological accounts of autism. Among the current explanations are the following.

1. Children with autism are specifically impaired in their ability to understand and use certain deictic forms, that is, words whose meaning is determined by the communicative context. Because the interpretation of *I, you,* and *me* changes along with the speaker, they find it difficult to grasp the underlying meaning of these words.

2. The problem with pronominal reference is another aspect of the difficulty children with autism have with metarepresentation, or theory of mind deficits. That is, they do not clearly differentiate between their own and others' mental states and, therefore, struggle with the language forms that explicitly mark this difference. If this explanation is correct, one would expect pronoun use to improve as gains are made in nonverbal behaviors that direct others' attention (e.g., eye contact, gesturing).

3. Children with autism may have attention deficits that interfere with their ability to observe pronoun use in speech between other individuals (Oshima-Takane & Benaroya, 1989). Because they do not attend to conversation when others are speaking, they do not witness the normal shift in pronoun use. This means that they will not master pronouns as a result of incidental exposure to conversational models. Additional focused exposure to pronoun shifting, as might be provided in a language intervention program, should be helpful, according to this explanation.

There is currently no resolution, however, as to which, if any of these accounts is accurate.

Echolalia.   One of the most salient characteristics of children with autism is the frequency with which they repeat utterances addressed to them. This behavior is described as echolalia when it seems to occur in an automatic and apparently unthinking way. This tendency to imitate speech too much has been described as occurring in children who frequently fail to show "social imitation" of gesture and facial expression early in development (Malvy et al., 1999). Descriptions of echolalia frequently distinguish between two types: immediate echolalia, the exact repetition of a word or words directly after they are spoken, and delayed echolalia, which occurs some time after the original utterance is produced. A third type sometimes mentioned, mitigated echolalia, refers to immediate repetitions that contain some change to the utterance. In both research and clinical practice, the distinctions among these types of echolalia are often difficult to make. For example, there is no standard for judging how much of a time delay must occur before echolalia is considered delayed rather than immediate (5 seconds? 1 minute? half an hour?). Similarly, there is no agreement on the quantity or quality of changes that must be present in a mitigated echolalic response (one word changed? one inflection? change in intonation?). All in all, one must be careful not to assume that these terms are used with identical meanings by all professionals.

In the past it was often assumed that the repetitions of children with autism were without intention and therefore should be regarded as pathological signs of their language disorder. At the same time, however, it has always been recognized that echolalia is not limited to children with autism but also occurs in children with intellectual disabilities, as well as in typically developing children. A distinction between normal and pathological echolalia has been maintained on the basis of three pieces of evidence. First, the frequency of echolalia is higher in children with autism than in those who have intellectual disabilities or who are developing typically. Second, echolalia continues to occur at later ages in children with autism, while it usually disappears by the age of 2½ to 3 years in typically developing children. Third, some research has suggested that imitation serves a role in facilitating the grammatical development of typically developing children. It is also sometimes said that the repetitions of children with autism are qualitatively different, being almost exact copies of what is said to them, whereas those of other children more frequently contain changes in certain words or inflections or to the prosodic features of the utterance. Support for this belief comes largely from published clinical observations rather than experimental measurements and comparisons.

In recent years, echolalia has come to be viewed as less of a pathological behavior in individuals with autism, mostly because of research demonstrating that their repetition does have communicative intent. That intent is not found in the words themselves—these are borrowed from the conversational partner—but rather in the combined effect of the repetition, its prosody, any simultaneous nonverbal cues, and the context in which it is produced. Studies have confirmed that not all echolalia is interactive, that is, intended to be communicative. However, careful videotape analysis has revealed that echolalia can often serve a range of interactive communicative functions. For example, echolalia might begin when the listener's attention is diverted and persist until attention is gained; in this instance it appears to serve a "calling" function. In another case, echolalia might be used merely to fill a conversational turn. The child is facing the listener and it is the child's turn to talk, but there is no overt indication of communicative intent, such as heightened prosody, in the echolalic utterance. Different types of echolalia, immediate or delayed, might occur in response to directive or facilitate utterances addressed to the child (Rydell & Mirenda, 1994).

It also has been speculated that the poor comprehension skills of children with autism may be a primary variable in causing echolalia. There is limited empirical support for this position. One study of ten children with autism found a striking relationship between the frequency of echolalia in speech samples and scores on a standardized comprehension test (Roberts, 1989). It is possible, then, that echolalia is an adaptive response to breakdowns in comprehension. If this is the case, as understanding improves and other means become available for solving specific comprehension problems (e.g., requests for repetition or clarification), echolalia would no longer be needed and should, therefore, decrease in frequency.

Interestingly, as evidence has accumulated showing that echolalia serves various pragmatic purposes for children with autism, other research indicates that it does not seem to help in the acquisition of grammar. Studies comparing the spontaneous and immediately imitated utterances of children with autism have found that their echolalic utterances are less grammatically complex, with the possible exception of the early stages of acquisition Thus, imitation does not appear to be the primary means by which new grammatical forms are learned, though it may play a more significant role in phonological or lexical acquisition.

Communicative Functions.   Even though echolalia is frequent in many individuals with autism, it does not make up their total communication system. If echolalia is put to one side, what sort of speech acts are most commonly performed by these children? Results from different studies on this question are not easily compared because of differences in the way verbal and nonverbal behaviors are classified. However, it appears reasonably clear that children with autism are most competent in performing instrumental communicative acts. These acts serve either to regulate the behavior of a conversational partner (e.g., by asking for an action to be performed or an object to be retrieved) or to comply with requests (e.g., by giving the partner a requested object). Children with autism are much less competent at gaining and directing the attention of the conversational partner, as might be achieved by making eye contact, pointing, or showing objects (Kasari et al., 2001). Compared to children with developmental language delay and typically developing children matched for language level, children with autism initiate communicative acts much less frequently (Koegel, 2000; Taylor & Harris, 1995). They prefer, as a rule, to follow rather than lead in a conversation and to engage their partners at a level that requires little sharing of interest and attention.

The Concept of Asynchronous Development

Studies of the communicative functions used by children with autism have indicated that the frequency of those functions across categories is significantly different from that of other children. Those studies do not show, however, that the functions themselves are aberrant. Children with autism display the same communicative behaviors as typically developing children, but the profile of pragmatic functions they use is likely to be significantly different. It has been suggested that the essential problem is one of timing and sequence. Normal communicative functions are acquired in an abnormal order, so that at any one time, a child with autism may exhibit a set of behaviors that is developmentally scattered (VanMeter, Fein, Morris, Waterhouse, & Allen, 1997). For example, children with autism commonly lack many of the joint attention functions seen in preverbal typically developing children, but they may possess other, more developmentally advanced functions such as requests for information. This asynchrony in the emergence of pragmatic communication functions may be the result of underlying social and cognitive deficits in autism. As with typically developing children, the emergence of more advanced pragmatic behaviors appears to be correlated with the use of more symbolically advanced forms of communication (Stone & Caro-Martinez, 1990). As higher-level functions increase, so does the frequency of speech and gesture, replacing motoric acts and vocalization as the primary means of communication. Asynchrony in development is also seen, for example, when pragmatic development is compared to syntactic development or prosodic development is compared to phonological development.

Implications for Intervention

All language disorders are complex and require careful assessment to sort out different levels of impairment. In children with autism, this complexity is raised one or more notches because of the intricate interactions between language, cognition, and social behavior, all of which are impaired at the same time, although not always in the same degrees. Faced with the enormity of the problems in this population, professionals have struggled to find effective intervention approaches. The lack of success many have experienced has resulted in an understandable tendency to abandon older methods whenever a recognizably new treatment comes along (McLean, 1992). Consequently, the swings in clinical practice have been wider in the area of autism than with other types of childhood language impairment. Regardless of the specific treatment approach a professional employs, it is important to understand and observe certain general principles of clinical practice. These principles should be consistent with the core information about autism reviewed to this point in the chapter.

Assessment

Assessment of children with autism is difficult and may not be appropriately done by the nonspecialist. Depending on the type of population they serve most frequently, many professionals may routinely use some norm-referenced tests to evaluate their clients. However, the nature of the social impairment in children with autism makes most standardized testing unreliable. Many of these children lack the ability to attend to stimuli presented in a fixed manner; they may have no consistent verbal or nonverbal means of responding; and the responses they produce may be contaminated by the intrusion of echolalia or idiosyncratic language. The best results may therefore be obtained from a standardized observation protocol such as the Autism Diagnostic Observation Schedule (ADOS) (Lord, Rutter, DiLavore, & Risi, 1999) or the Childhood Autism Rating Scale (CARS) (Schopler, Reichler, & Renner, 1988). In these procedures a child's behavior is rated across those categories that identify and distinguish the disorder of autism. The CARS can be used with any sample of behavior, whereas the ADOS uses a series of games and activities in which the child is subtly invited, i.e., "pressed," to participate. Both instruments are flexible enough to meet the challenges presented by individuals with autism.

Service Model

As we have seen elsewhere in this text, a traditional model for providing intervention in the schools has been to remove a child from the classroom and provide brief therapy sessions at another location. This pull-out model makes several assumptions about the entry-level skills and motivation of the child that are not tenable for children with autism. It is designed to supplement, not replace, an academic curriculum and therefore presupposes a minimum level of language development, an ability to learn and generalize, and a motivation to acquire language that may not be present in a child with autism. When the traditional model fails, creative approaches must be tried that balance structure and flexibility. Because many children with autism insist that routines be observed and will become highly distressed if they are not, it is important that intervention approaches cater adequately to this need. On the other hand, programs that are too structured may not allow children to develop skills in the use of natural language (Prizant & Wetherby, 1998). The result may be language that appears unnatural to others and does not generalize well outside of the school setting. Efforts at developing a collaborative service model to address the needs of all handicapped children in school are especially important for individuals with autism.

The timing of services is another issue pertinent to intervention with autism. As noted earlier in this chapter, autism is rarely identified by infant screenings conducted during the first 18 months but is recognized in nearly all cases before 36 months of age. The implication, of course, is that one does not find infant stimulation programs for children with autism of the type that exist for other conditions (e.g., Down syndrome). On the other hand, it is not necessary—and indeed, would be ill-advised—to wait until a child with autism is of school age before initiating services. Evaluation of one early intervention program for high-functioning preschool children with autism found that they made significant developmental gains, as measured by IQ scores and standardized language test scores (Harris, Handleman, Gordon, Kristoff, & Fuentes, 1991). Some of the children were mainstreamed with typically developing preschoolers, while others were enrolled in a class consisting solely of individuals with autism. Interestingly, both groups showed equivalent gains in language ability (Harris, Handleman, Kristoff, Bass, & Gordon, 1990).

Special Considerations

Children with autism are known to have a number of associated problems (see Table 7.3) that may require special management during intervention. It is plain that all children must be evaluated and, if appropriate, treated for hearing loss and seizure, two conditions that appear to have elevated risk in autism. The hypersensitivity of certain children may also dictate a change in teaching methods. Touch can be used to guide or reinforce—it is, for example, used systematically in some forms of AAC—but a period of adjustment may be needed. Because of the auditory sensitivity of many children with autism, behavioral problems may be reduced and comprehension improved by avoiding excessive speech, speaking in a clear and unexaggerated manner, and supplementing speech, when necessary, with gesture and physical direction (Prizant, Schuler, Wetherby, & Rydell, 1997). In a school setting, the technique of *priming* or exposing students with autism to school assignments before their presentation in class has been found to reduce episodes of disruptive behavior (Koegel, Koegel, Frea, & Green-Hopkins, 2003).

As we have seen, studies of the communicative functions used by children with autism indicate that they emerge in a different sequence than in typically developing children. One may argue, therefore, that language intervention should be structured to reflect this different order of acquisition. Specifically, it should be expected that a child with autism will establish instrumental functions before ones that attract or direct attention. This means that in the first stage of intervention the goal may be to facilitate requests or protests. Procedures that often induce a communicative need for requests and protests, such as placing objects out of reach, withholding an important part of a toy, or sabotaging a play activity, are described elsewhere in this text and in other therapy texts. It is not certain, however, whether such techniques are effective for children with autism. One study has found that neither adult direction (e.g., looking at and tapping an object) nor procedures designed to motivate communication (e.g., not sharing a desired food) increased joint attention behaviors (Landry & Loveland, 1989).

At a second stage of intervention, children with autism can be encouraged to use communications that attract attention to themselves. The inherent tendency toward ritualistic behavior might be used to establish behaviors such as greeting or requesting a social routine (e.g., playing patty-cake or peekaboo). At the third stage, children may be taught functions that direct another person's attention. The earliest of these are labeling an object or commenting on an environmental event. The behaviors themselves can be introduced through various modeling approaches, discussed in Chapter 14. Clinicians should be mindful, however, that children with autism often begin to direct others' attention by means of echolalia. Hence, it is important to monitor children's contextual use of echolalia and evaluate whether changes in that behavior indicate the emergence of more sophisticated communicative functions.

Intervention Models

Three theoretical approaches are apparent in the different methods used in the treatment of autism. Though many current intervention approaches borrow elements from all of these models, the distinction remains useful for sorting among various methods.

Behaviorism.   In the 1960s and 1970s the elements of behavior modification were applied with great enthusiasm to the treatment of autism (Lovaas, 1977). Behavioral methods begin by analyzing language behaviors into a detailed series of steps. For example, to teach a child to name might require training the following behaviors in sequence: sitting, attending to the trainer's face, nonverbal imitation, verbal imitation, labeling in response to questions, and labeling in response to other stimuli. Behavior modification was also used to decrease self-injurious behavior and promote social interaction.

During this early period of investigation, both rewards and aversive stimuli were employed to establish operant control over a behavior. In one notorious experiment, electric shock was used as a negative reinforcer (Lovaas, Schaeffer, & Simmons, 1965). Most recent behaviorist proposals, however, are strictly nonaversive. Desirable behaviors, such as the acquisition of specific gesturing and signing skills, the asking of questions, more appropriate play, and greater social interaction with peers, have been taught through a sequence of prompting, fading, stimulus rotation (the systematic introduction of new targets), and reinforcement (Buffington, Krantz, Poulson, & McClannahan, 1998; Carr, Kolo-ginsky, & Leff-Simon, 1987; Gonzalez-Lopez & Kamps, 1997; Stahmer, 1999; Williams, Donley, & Keller, 2000). Undesirable behaviors have also been reduced by teaching a replacement behavior (Buschbacher & Fox, 2003). For example, autistic leading—a request made by grasping an adult's wrist and leading him or her to the desired object—was diminished by teaching children to point to what they wanted (Carr & Kemp, 1989). Delayed echolalia was reduced in one child by observing the behavior and discovering that it served the communicative function of requesting help. The child was then taught an appropriate substitute behavior, the request "Help me" (Durand & Crimmins, 1987).

Psycholinguistic Theory. Early behavior modification programs to teach language were characterized by massed practice, a specialized treatment setting, and instructional episodes initiated by an adult (Carr et al., 1987). These techniques were effective in training new forms, but they often failed to produce results that generalized outside the training sessions and yielded true communication. To meet this problem, many current intervention programs now emphasize *incidental teaching,* a technique in which teaching interactions occur in a child's typical environment (home or classroom) and are allowed to arise naturally out of the situation that transpires (see Chapter 14). Comparisons of incidental teaching with traditional behaviorist methods have indicated that the more natural method is just as efficient in establishing new language behaviors in individuals with autism and is more effective in promoting generalization to everyday settings and producing positive affect between parents and children (Elliott, Hall, & Soper, 1991; Koegel, O'Dell, & Koegel, 1987; Shreibman, Kaneko, & Koegel, 1991; Woods & Wetherby, 2003). The method lends itself to classroom use and can be taught effectively to classroom teachers (Dyer, Williams, & Luce, 1991).

Social Interaction Theory. In contrast to the methods that grow out of behavioral and psycholinguistic theory, social interaction theory does not recommend a specific intervention strategy. Instead, it offers a perspective on communicative interactions and suggests that some of the pragmatic deficits associated with autism may arise when adults do not make good conversational adjustments. For example, children with autism tend to produce more adequate responses when adults ask them yes/no questions, questions that are conceptually simple, and questions that are related to the child's topic (Curcio & Paccia, 1987; Prizant et al., 1997). In an effort to help, adults often rely on a teaching mode of conversation. They consistently set the topic and use directive communication acts to elicit specific responses from the child. This, in turn, leads the child to produce a very narrow range of communicative behaviors. There is no simple solution to this problem. Attempts to be nurturing are generally ineffective with children with autism, because they tend to remain socially withdrawn (Holmes, 1998). When a child does not act spontaneously, adults are thwarted from using nurturing behaviors such as utterance expansions and responses related to the child's topic. The solution may be to (1) modify directive behaviors so that they allow more flexibility of response, for example, asking questions that have several correct answers, and (2) show nurturance by construing abnormal behaviors as normal, for example, responding to the intent of an echolalic utterance rather than its content (Duchan, 1983).

These insights from social interaction theory can be applied to intervention in three areas.

1. Professionals can observe or record conversations between children and their parents or teachers. By coding the type of utterances produced by the adult(s) and the adequacy of the child's responses, it is possible to determine any relationships between the two. This may lead to recommendations to the adults that they increase certain behaviors and decrease others to promote more adequate language use by the child.

2. Professionals should observe themselves and carry out the same type of analysis on their own interaction with the child. Many clinical conversations contain stimuli that are intended to be facilitating (e.g., requests for repetition or clarification) but that may have undesirable effects on a child with autism.

3. If a child with autism is enrolled in a classroom with typically developing children, then social interaction analysis can be used to improve the effectiveness of peer-mediated intervention. In *peer-mediated programs,* typically developing children are shown how to initiate social interactions with children with autism, for example, by commenting on what an impaired child is doing or offering to share a toy. Once the typically developing children have been shown how to make initiations, they are verbally prompted to do so. Then, gradually, prompts are eliminated so that the behavior becomes spontaneous (Odom & Watts, 1991). Early analysis of how children with autism interact with adults or with their unimpaired peers may indicate what types of gambits are most successful at stimulating social interactions. These gambits would then become the ones taught to all the typically developing children involved in the intervention program.

Augmentative and Alternative Communication (AAC).   Facilitated communication, as one AAC option for intervention, has been mentioned earlier, and we have raised the issue that there are concerns arising from the literature regarding the empirical validity of the approach. Other forms of AAC, including the use of manual signing, have also been used with children with autism, and these are becoming increasingly popular (Mirenda, 2003). Because AAC as an intervention approach is used with children whose communication impairments cross a number of "diagnostic" categories, it is discussed separately later in this text.

Summary

In this chapter we have seen that

- Autism is a developmental rather than an emotional or psychiatric disorder. Evidence suggests that it has a genetic basis, though a single cause has yet to be identified.
- Autism is one of several pervasive developmental disorders, all of which are characterized by social, communicative, and cognitive deficits.
- Children with autism are heterogeneous. Consequently, the diagnostic criteria established in DSM-IV-TR specify a wide range of behaviors as signs of the disorder. All children diagnosed with autism must exhibit some impairment in each of the categories of social interaction, communication, and repertoire of activities and interests.

- Autism is associated with a number of sensory and motor handicaps. These handicaps are not found in all individuals with autism, however, and they are not included among the diagnostic criteria for the disorder.
- In nearly all cases, autism is identified between 18 and 36 months of age, with more severe cases usually identified earlier.
- Certain language abilities tend to be relatively preserved in autism, that is, they are commensurate with the MA of the child. Segmental phonology and syntax, lexical and syntactic comprehension, and imitation are the abilities in this category.
- Language abilities that appear to be specifically impaired in children with autism are nonsegmental phonology (prosody) and pronoun use. These children produce language that is frequently idiosyncratic or echolalic. Pragmatically, they may be especially impaired in their use of language to share or direct attention, and they infrequently produce communicative acts considered to be initiating.
- Asynchrony in the development of different parameters of language is characteristic of children with autism (e.g., syntax versus pragmatics).
- An underlying cognitive deficit in children with autism may be their inability to think about and compare their own and others' mental states, that is, "theory of mind."
- Intervention for children with autism requires special skills in assessment and a nontraditional service delivery model. Treatment methods based on principles of behaviorism, psycholinguistic theory, and social interaction theory have all been used successfully to promote verbal language learning and reduce aberrant communication behaviors.
- AAC can be an intervention option, but not all forms of AAC (i.e., facilitated communication) are equally supported empirically.

Autism is often described as an enigmatic disorder because of its mysterious origin and the unusual behaviors that characterize it. Recent research has added to our understanding of autism but, at the same time, raised new questions about the causes and attributes of the disorder. Our views of what autism is and how it can be remediated seem destined to change—perhaps fundamentally—in the coming years.

8 Language and Children with Auditory Impairments

KERRIE LEE

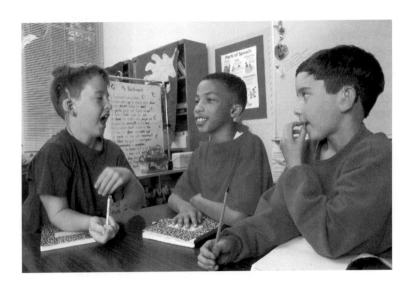

OBJECTIVES

After reading this chapter you should be able to discuss

- Different types of auditory impairments, including peripheral hearing loss, central auditory processing disorder, and auditory neuropathy

- The impact of sensorineural hearing impairment and conductive hearing impairment has on receptive and expressive speech and language

- Language skills of children with auditory impairments in relation to intervention implications, academic achievement, and communication choices

- Different technology options for hearing-impaired children, including hearing aids, cochlear implants, and FM aids

Some children are born with little, if any, hearing, or they lose it before they acquire speech and language (i.e., prelinguistically hearing impaired). These children will have communicative, academic, and social difficulties that arise as consequences of their hearing loss. While outcomes are difficult to predict for an individual child, improvements in technology, including digital hearing aids and cochlear implants, and more effective approaches to therapy have led to better outcomes for many children born with a profound or total hearing loss or who lose their hearing before the acquisition of language. Other children are born with some hearing. For these children, there tends to be an inverse relation between language and speech outcomes and amount of hearing; that is, as hearing loss increases; outcomes tend to be poorer.

This chapter describes current knowledge and understanding about the relationship between hearing loss and language disorder. The relationship will be explored on the basis of severity of the loss, which is partially related to *sites of lesion* (where in the auditory system the problems leading to the hearing impairments occur) and *etiologies* (the causes of the problems in the auditory system). There is a relationship between the site of lesion underlying the hearing loss, the etiology, and the severity of the loss. Although most of our discussion about hearing losses will focus on problems located in the peripheral auditory mechanism or system, which we know from Chapter 1 consists of the outer, middle, and inner ear, this chapter will also discuss two other dysfunctions in the central auditory system: *central auditory processing disorders* (CAPD) and the less well known and understood *auditory neuropathy*. We have seen elsewhere in this book references to some children with language problems possibly related to inefficient processing of incoming auditory stimuli associated with speech. The topic of CAPD is related to these references. CAPD is assumed to be the result of auditory input dysfunction in functional areas of the auditory system not associated with peripheral hearing loss affecting the middle ear or the cochlea. Auditory neuropathy arises from dysfunction in the central auditory system at the level of the brain cortex.

Overview of Hearing Loss

Because hearing loss underlies most of the language problems exhibited by deaf and hearing-impaired children, audiological assessment to measure the hearing loss helps provide a broad framework for estimating the impact of the hearing loss on children's language.

Types and Degrees of Hearing Loss

Hearing loss is typically described in terms of type of loss (sensorineural, conductive, and mixed) and degree of loss. *Sensorineural hearing loss* occurs when there is damage to the hair cells located in the cochlea or in the auditory neurological pathways to the brain. Sensorineural hearing loss is usually considered irreversible and is characterized by reduced sensitivity to sound and distortion of incoming speech sounds because of limitations in the coding of frequency and intensity information in the signal. The severity of the loss depends on the extent of the damage (from having no hair cells to minimal damage to outer hair cells for a limited frequency range). As a result, sensorineural losses all have the same site of lesion (the hair cells in the cochlea or auditory nerve) but due to differences in etiology can be differentiated in terms of their severity. Severity can range from mild to total loss.

Hearing loss is measured in *decibels* (dB) a logarithmic metric, in which 0 dB HL is close to the softest sound a normally hearing person can hear, whereas a sound of about 120 dB HL produces a pain sensation in people with normal hearing. The hearing-level range for sensorineural hearing losses can be from 10 db (mild loss) to more than 120 db (total loss). A hearing loss up to 60 dB HL typically involves only damage to the outer hair cells and results in loss of sensitivity to sound and abnormal loudness perception. Losses greater than 60 dB HL must also involve the inner hair cells, and in addition to sensitivity and loudness there are also problems with distortion. Although amplification devices can boost the level of intensity of sound to counteract loss sensitivity, they are not as good at countering the distortion effects of sensorineural hearing losses.

Conductive hearing loss occurs when the cause of the loss lies in the external or middle ear, changing the normal operation of these areas and reducing sound transmission through them to the cochlea. The primary consequence of conductive loss is a loss of sensitivity without associated distortion. This means that the effects of conductive loss can be compensated effectively with amplification. In general, conductive losses are also responsive to medical treatment, which can often restore hearing to normal levels. Various pathologies in the middle ear cause conductive hearing losses, including a buildup of fluid in the middle ear itself (*otitis media*) which reduces the efficiency of the mechanical and resonant subsystems. The hearing problems associated with conductive losses result from impedance of the transduction system of the middle ear, and the degree of loss can range from 10 to 60 dB HL, keeping in mind that the average speaking level measured at about a yard away is approximately 40 dB HL. However, conductive losses are typically around 30 dB HL.

In addition to types of hearing loss, the other important way of characterizing hearing loss is by degree of loss. Besides the term *normal*, the five terms used to identify degree of loss are *mild, moderate, severe, profound,* and *total.* Children with profound and total hearing losses previously were labeled as *deaf,* and those with mild to severe losses were labeled *hard of hearing,* but this division has been challenged recently. Now, the term *hearing impaired* is more typically used to cover all degrees of hearing loss for children who use some form of oral communication, and *deaf* is used for children who use a sign language system.

Total hearing loss results in the most severe communication disruption. In this case there is no auditory receptive capability as a result of significant damage to or absence of cochlear structures and damage to the auditory nerve. Next in severity, but with some auditory input capability, is profound hearing loss, followed by severe hearing loss. Children with severe, profound, or total hearing losses are incapable of hearing speech, even shouted speech, unless they are fitted with appropriate amplification devices. A hearing loss that is severe or greater must involve the cochlea and/or auditory nerve as the site of lesion. Mild or moderate hearing loss may be due to dysfunction in the cochlea (sensorineural hearing loss), or in the middle ear or outer ear (conductive hearing loss), or a mixture of both (mixed hearing loss). With moderate hearing loss, speech can be detected, but many of the information-bearing components of the speech signal are missing (e.g., the high-frequency "hiss" of /s/, some of the less intense but essentially distinguishing formats of vowels). With mild hearing loss most of the speech signal is audible, provided a child is listening in good acoustic conditions, such as being close to the speaker and having minimal background noise.

One complication in discussing degree and type of hearing loss and its effect on receptive communication is that hearing losses can affect different frequencies of sounds, resulting in different configurations of hearing loss. Most sensorineural hearing losses are more severe in the high frequencies, so hearing levels can drop off from near normal levels (10–20 dB HL) for low-frequency sounds to moderate and severe losses (60–80 dB HL) at higher frequencies. The configuration of a hearing loss can add to the effects of the degree and type of loss on receptive communication function and require different amplification characteristics to aid communication. Similarly, conductive hearing losses in the middle ear can be predominantly at low or high frequencies, depending on the middle ear components that are affected.

It might be expected that the relationship between hearing loss and speech-receptive communication function would be reasonably deterministic. That is, if you know the severity of the hearing loss, you could predict the auditory input dysfunction for speech reception. In general, this is true, and Boothroyd (1982) has shown that, based on overall speech-reception capacities, it is possible to divide degree of loss on an audiogram into six categories, five categories corresponding to the terms presented earlier (mild, moderate, severe, profound, total), and normal hearing. These are shown in Figure 8.1, which is laid out like an audiogram. An audiogram is a chart for plotting hearing levels in decibels. A person's responses to the presentation of tones at various frequencies are recorded according to the softest level at which he or she hears each of the tones, that is the person's hearing threshold for the tone.

Hearing Loss and Speech–Language Reception

The deterministic relationship between tone thresholds and speech–language reception is statistical and not predictive of an individual child's abilities to understand speech and language. It is therefore important to measure speech–language reception capacity in individual children to understand their specific capacities. As an example, consider the results for two adolescent boys with severe hearing impairments. These two listeners are the same age and have very similar hearing losses. Figure 8.2 shows their performances on a measure of receptive language capability, the Token Test (De Renzi & Vignolo, 1962). The Token Test uses oral directions for the listener to manipulate colored squares and circles. Parts 1 to 4 of

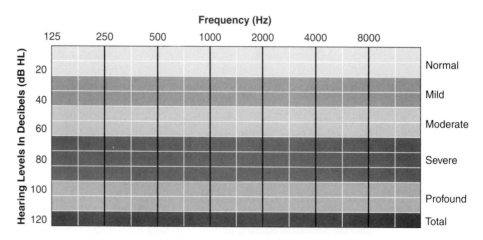

FIGURE 8.1   Audiogram Showing the Classification of Degree of Loss

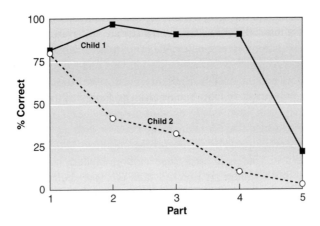

FIGURE 8.2   Examples of Results for Two Children with Severe Bilateral Sensorineural Hearing Loss on Parts 1 to 5 of the Token Test Items

the test rely more on working memory capability, while Part 5 introduces some linguistic complexity into the instructions to manipulate the tokens. The results show that, despite similar severe bilateral hearing losses, their two Token Test results are very dissimilar. The reasons for these differences can be due to several possible developmental factors, among these cognitive capacity and social development. The important issue is that hearing loss alone should not be used to determine potential language outcomes. Similar differential results can be found across a range of even simpler speech–language reception measures. Children with the same hearing losses do not handle speech reception in qualitatively similar ways, and each child needs to be assessed to determine that child's individual capacity.

We need to keep these large individual differences associated with hearing loss in mind. A number of factors interact to make generalizations difficult. Among these are family demographics (e.g., socioeconomic status, presence of other family members who are/are not hearing impaired or deaf), age of identification of hearing loss, age of receipt and success of amplification devices, and the modality for language learning, that is, sign language (signed English or a language of a Deaf culture such as American Sign Language), auditory–oral (audition plus visual cues from speech reading), auditory–verbal (using primarily auditory cues), or total communication (TC) (a combination of sign and auditory cues), along with the related educational/habilitation approaches associated with the language-learning modality. Nevertheless, for the sake of achieving a coherent view, the following sections will present average data and generalizations for the groups that are described.

Language of Children with Differing Degrees of Hearing Loss and Intervention Implications

Children born with hearing impairments will have communicative, academic, and social difficulties that develop as a direct consequence of their hearing impairment. Interventions to ameliorate the impact of their hearing impairment include technology devices, such as hearing aids and cochlear implants, and intensive speech and language therapy. Although outcomes for an individual child are difficult to predict, technological and intervention advances have meant improved outcomes for many children with prelinqual hearing impairment. This chapter describes current knowledge and understanding about the impact that hearing loss has on children's language and speech.

Children with Greater Degrees of Hearing Loss (61–121+ dB HL)

Total Hearing Loss (121+ dB HL).   Although the situation of many children with total hearing loss has improved recently as the result of increased resources for education and improved technology (including cochlear implants and tactile aids), the challenge for many is still considerable. In a qualitative research study, Sainsbury (1986) provided a graphic report of the difficulties faced in society by those with practically no intelligible speech or useful hearing. Her subjects were 171 hearing-impaired adults, including those who were born with a total hearing loss, those who had acquired their loss before 2 years of age, and those who were completely dependent on manual sign language (British Sign Language, BSL). Sainsbury noted that the problems these adults faced in making themselves understood and in being able to make hearing family and friends understand their difficulties were almost insurmountable. This group typically had low literacy levels, reducing even further their communication and integration options. Television with teletext[1] was, at that time, either unaffordable (because of the considerably lower education levels achieved by many adults with total hearing loss, with resulting lower earning potential), or the message was often misunderstood because of their slow reading and poor language comprehension, resulting in only partial information understanding at best. Sainsbury also found that while a family member who could act as an intermediary between the person with total hearing loss and society is a critical source of information about the wider world, such an intermediary often had limited time and might not be as sympathetic as necessary.

These findings have significant bearing on issues related to integration of children with total hearing loss within normal hearing environments and the role of a Deaf culture within society. Children with little or no hearing in their childhood as well as in adulthood experience markedly fewer problematic communications and interactions within the Deaf community compared to their interactions with normally hearing individuals in the hearing world. While informal communication networks may be well developed, the person with little or no hearing remains highly dependent on the communicative functions of the formal network of both government and voluntary service providers, who must provide the necessary intermediary communicative function to overcome the significant language barrier.

Although studies of both expressive and receptive language capabilities have been conducted with adults with total hearing loss, the results are highly individual. Generally, however, results do not show well-developed language skills unless successful management of a technology aid has been available to the person. Cochlear implants can produce results

---

[1]Teletext or closed captions is a system of subtitling developed for TV or movie viewers who cannot follow the spoken dialogue.

for some individuals with total hearing loss equivalent to those achieved for profound- or severe-hearing-loss groups, but there is substantial variability in the results. It is important to remember that the fitting of a cochlear implant does not, in itself, guarantee easy transition to the hearing world if that is the desired goal for the family of a child with a total hearing loss.

Profound Hearing Loss (91–120 dB HL).   Profound hearing loss has a significant impact on speech, language, communication, and psychosocial adjustment. However, with early and intensive therapy, as well as an appropriate hearing device and educational placement, children can learn language, establish intelligible speech, develop easy communication with family and peers, and have good psychosocial adjustment.

Psychosocial and Cognitive Considerations.   Frequently throughout this book, the association between language ability and psychosocial issues has been raised. We are about to raise it again because there is consistent evidence that more children with hearing loss end up with a range of psychosocial complications than their normal-hearing peers (Ridgeway, 1998). The percentage of children with severe and profound hearing loss who experience psychosocial adjustment problems is significant, suggesting some relationship between degree of hearing loss and psychosocial development. For more significant psychosocial difficulties, the incidence of psychotic illness in the hearing-impaired population seems not to differ from that of the hearing population (de Feu, 1997; Kitson & Fry, 1990). However, with regard to less significant psychosocial difficulties, Ridgeway (1998) found that 38 percent of the group with hearing impairments in her study reported psychological difficulties, a proportion considerably higher than the 17 percent found in the hearing population. Ridgeway also found that 40–50 percent of children with hearing impairments have emotional or behavioral problems, compared to around 25 percent for the general child population. However, as Ridgeway (1998) indicates, the 40–50 percent of individuals with identified mental health problems in the hearing-impaired population do not need specialist intervention, suggesting that it is their hearing loss combined with the environment in which the individuals find themselves that causes their difficulties and not any biological or innate characteristic. Given that both identity and psychosocial adjustment in a verbal world are highly dependent on language, it can be hypothesized that difficulties with language are a primary determiner of social and psychological adjustment for this population.

The relationship between language development and cognition in children with significant sensorineural hearing loss also needs consideration. In terms of cognitive abilities, differences between children with hearing loss and children with normal hearing on measures of IQ, for instance, can depend on what aspect of IQ is tested. Tests of verbal IQ showed depressed scores (e.g., 85.54 compared to 100) in a meta-analysis of studies completed by Braden (1994). In contrast, there was no difference in performance tests (in which the child can be shown what was required), with scores of 99.95 compared to 100. This result is, however, not as simple as it seems, because there was a difference in "nonverbal" IQ tests that did not involve motor skills and therefore relied more on verbal explanations of the tasks to the children. In the case of nonmotor "nonverbal" IQ tests, the mean performance for those with hearing loss was 94.57, compared to 100 for those with normal hearing. It is important to note that although the scores for the children with hearing impairment were within normal limits, they were still significantly lower than the scores of individuals without hearing loss, findings not unlike those that we have seen for children with specific language impairment. Differences noted for children with hearing loss on a range of cognitive and IQ tests need to be carefully evaluated to understand the contribution of their auditory isolation and language disorder on the test results. We address this again in Chapter 13.

Speech and Expressive Language.   Speech and language will not develop spontaneously in children with profound hearing loss without technology aids and special education assistance. The child with a profound hearing loss will need help with all aspects of language, grammar, vocabulary, reading, and writing. The developing child will have reduced speech intelligibility and, depending on the age of fitting and type of technology aid, the child may have varying problems with voice and resonance quality.

A complete description of speech characteristics of a child with a profound hearing impairment needs to include assessment of overall intelligibility, segmental errors (sounds of speech), and suprasegmental errors (errors in speech rhythm and prosody). In the past, children with profound hearing impairments have been difficult to understand (only about 20 percent of their speech may be understandable). Cole and Paterson (1984) reported that over half of all school-aged children in the United States and Canada with significant hearing loss had speech that was rated as unintelligible. However, emerging patterns of results, as a result of cochlear implant technology, are modifying these descriptions. With cochlear implants there can be significant improvements in speech outcomes, but it is important to note that unintelligible speech is also found in children with implants (Serry & Blamey, 1999; Tobey, Geers, & Brenner, 1994; Tye-Murray & Kirk, 1993). While the cochlear implant may improve the production of individual speech sounds and aid their acquisition in the same developmental order as normally hearing children, the development process is slower for the children with implants, and the evidence to date suggests that only some children attain speech that is fully intelligible (Serry & Blamey, 1999).

In a review of the data on segmental speech production of hearing-impaired infants with profound losses, McCaffrey (1999) concluded that these infants show differences in the normal pattern of development from a very early age. In babbling, separate consonants and vowels are produced more than consonant–vowel syllables, and multisyllabic utterances are minimal (Oller & Eilers, 1988; Stoel-Gammon, 1988). Canonical babbling emerges later, and infants with profound hearing loss may not achieve this stage or can be delayed for this production by between 15 and 18 months (Oller & Eilers, 1988). Overall there are fewer consonants produced by infants who are hearing impaired, as well as qualitative differences including more labial than alveolar production (Stoel-Gammon, 1988). This difference, the opposite of the production patterns in children with normal hearing, is more pronounced as the severity of the loss increases (Yoshinaga-Itano, Stredler-Brown, & Jancosek, 1992). This may arise because even though alveolars are more frequent in English, they are less visible and therefore are not as accessible as labial production to children with hearing impairment (Osberger & McGarr, 1982; Stoel-Gammon & Kehoe, 1994). Another effect of hearing loss is greater production of nasal consonants. McCaffrey (1999) suggests this may be because audition is required to "motivate changing from the basic resting position of an open velopharyngeal port characteristic of quiet breathing to elevating the soft palate in order to achieve closure of the velopharyngeal airway for production of non-nasal" (p. 151). Finally, vowel production is more neutralized in the speech of children with profound hearing loss (Kent, Osberger, Netsell, & Hustedde, 1987; Yoshinaga-Itano, 1998) and has more schwa /ə/ qualities (Tye-Murray & Kirk, 1993). This reduced and neutralized vowel space of speakers with hearing loss contributes to the poor intelligibility of their speech. These findings make clear how important it is to manage early-intervention programs effectively for children with a hearing loss, both in terms of early identification as well as technology aids and speech–language intervention.

Children with profound hearing loss also tend to have a distinctive voice quality. Their speech is often characterized as being breathy, labored, staccato, and arrhythmic. Errors in suprasegmental speech patterns are correlated with these qualities, including errors in stress, speaking rate, coarticulation, breath control, pitch, and intensity (Tye-Murray, 1998).

In general, children with profound hearing loss do not learn language very well. These problems can be categorized as problems of form (syntax and morphology), content (semantics and vocabulary), and use (pragmatics) (Tye-Murray, 1998). Seyfried and Kricos (1996) identified a number of problems of form as the result of hearing impairment, including overuse of nouns and verbs and exclusive use of simple sentence structure with reduced word content. These children exhibit poor use of normal syntax. Some show only delayed patterns of development, whereas others end up with quite deviant language use.

Although hearing impairment, regardless of severity, results in use of a restricted vocabulary, profound hearing loss produces the most significant and evident consequences for vocabulary development and usage. For example, White and White (1987) conducted a 3-year longitudinal study of infants with profound hearing loss aged 8–30 months. By the third year of their study they found that the children had acquired vocabulary levels equivalent to 12-month-old children with normal hearing.

Pragmatics are also disrupted. Children with profound hearing loss may not follow social rules of conversation in turn taking or understand how to develop interactions (e.g., asking inappropriate questions at the wrong time). The child with a hearing loss may not be able to initiate or maintain a conversation. Most obvious is the problem of being able to repair communication breakdowns, leading to the behaviors of "bluffing" and "passing," in which the child may simply nod to misunderstood questions and statements.

Levels of writing skills are typically depressed, with written patterns often following spoken expression deficits (e.g., omission of function words, poor vocabulary, use of very simple sentences). In addition, extended, discursive writing will often lack clear organization. While many children will progress in narrative skills between the ages of 7 and 18 years, they will rarely achieve the same levels of performance as normally hearing peers (Yoshinaga & Downey, 1996).

Speech and Language Reception.   What children with profound hearing loss perceive in terms of their speech and language reception may be reflected in their expressive language and speech. Even when they have received appropriate amplification, they may not be able to detect all speech sounds and, because of damage to the ear, will also have problems with discrimination of speech sounds that they can detect. In general, vowels, because of their longer duration and lower frequency characteristics, are easier to detect and discriminate than consonants. Children with profound hearing loss will hear very little if they are unaided by a technology device and, depending on type of device, may have access only to vowel sounds, with little differentiation of consonant sounds. As a result, they have traditionally demonstrated poor performance in the areas of receptive vocabulary, morphological markers, and function words such as prepositions and articles which are characterized by lower sound levels and limited visual cues. Children with hearing loss will also have trouble understanding verbs and verb tenses, especially those that take auxiliaries (Davis & Hardick, 1981). They will often have problems understanding word order, because of emphasis on content, not function words.

The relationship of literacy to oral language development in children with normal hearing leads to the prediction that children with profound hearing loss will have poor literacy outcomes. Typically, results show that these children are at least 3 years or more behind in reading level than their peers with normal hearing. Paul (1998) claims there has been little improvement in reading levels in over 80 years. Poor literacy can be due to a number of problems related to the degree of hearing loss, including limited access to auditory–verbal information in language acquisition, less acquired experience and world knowledge, and the type of instruction received, which may be based on a phonics approach using a sound system to which the child with hearing impairment has limited access (Tye-Murray, 1998).

Severe Hearing Loss (61–90 dB HL). Children with severe hearing loss demonstrate the greatest variation in speech and language skills. In general, as their hearing loss approaches 90 dB HL, the characteristics of the group are more like the profound-hearing-loss group. In contrast, children with hearing loss around 60 dB HL show characteristics similar to moderate- and even mild-hearing-loss groups if they have been appropriately fitted with hearing aids, language development delays have been identified early, and consistent intervention has been provided. In most cases, however, some depression of the children's speech and language skills exists (Smith, 1975).

Every hearing loss, even those in the mild range, produces significant barriers to easy communication in environments with background noise, and that includes almost all environments including school classrooms (Northern & Downs, 2002). The communication skills of children who have a severe hearing impairment particularly need to be understood in terms of the extra concentration and attention required to communicate. These difficulties are exacerbated by the effects that even mild expressive and receptive communication problems can have, not only on academic achievement, but also on self-identity. This can become a particular issue in adolescence for teenagers already differentiated by having to wear a technology aid.

Counseling about these issues is, however, often made more difficult by the actual language skills developed by the child. In particular, limited vocabulary and its subsequent effect on concept development means that special programs need to provide both information and emotional counseling that takes into account the language problems that are present for individual children. In this sense, speech and language evaluations of children with severe hearing impairments can be critical in providing a clear basis on which to base other intervention support that will be required, which can range from education training to counseling support.

Intervention

Technology Aids. There are two main options available for providing auditory input to children with significant degrees of hearing loss. These are *hearing aids* and *cochlear implants*. Children with severe hearing loss are typically fitted with high-power hearing aids, although some are fitted with cochlear implants. Modern hearing aids provide not only amplification to make sounds loud enough to be heard, but also offer sophisticated signal processing using programmable digital technology. This means the aids can be better "tuned" and adapted to hearing needs related to more specific listening environments. Current clinical practice includes monitoring the speech and language development of children fitted with hearing aids. Changeover to cochlear implant technology is considered if children plateau in their development. Cochlear implants are more likely for children with hearing loss in the profound to total loss ranges. A third option, the tactile aid, which converts sound into vibrations on the skin, is also available for children with no response to sound with hearing aids and for whom a cochlear implant is not possible.

Cochlear implants became a viable aid for hearing-impaired children in the 1980s and today are fitted to a significant percentage of children with profound and total hearing loss. While some children may not be able to be fitted with cochlear implants (for reasons ranging from having no cochlea to other medical or psychological contraindications or because they do not want an implant) and may therefore be fitted with a tactile aid, the preferred technology aid now is a cochlear implant. The cochlear implant will often provide the same functionality for a child with total or profound hearing impairment as that of a child with at least a severe hearing loss with hearing aids (Blamey et al., 2001). That is, many of the results discussed for language development of children with hearing impairments are currently changing, at least for a proportion of these children who are fitted with cochlear implants. This means that some of the generalizations about language, speech, and literacy that we have just reported may not apply in the next several years as outcomes data on children with cochlear implants become more available.

Some outcomes data are already available (e.g., Geers, 2003; Geers & Brenner, 2003; Geers, Brenner, & Davidson, 2003; Geers, Nicholas, & Sedey, 2003; Nicholas & Geers, 2003; Rattigan, Reed, & Lee, 2002; Rubinstein, 2002; Tomblin, Spencer, Flock, Tyler, & Gantz, 1999). A snapshot of some of these results is presented here. For example, Rubenstein (2002) has reported that for children who acquire hearing loss after they have acquired language, there is usually a rapid improvement in speech-reception ability as measured by speech discrimination scores after fitting a cochlear implant (from 0 to 45 percent). Rubenstein (2002) also presented data showing that these children fitted with cochlear implants began to parallel the results of children with normal hearing. That is, their rate of growth matched that of children with normal hearing. Tomblin and colleagues (1999) looked at children with cochlear implants who had prelingual hearing impairment and compared their performance to children with hearing impairment not using implants. These researchers showed that, as a group, the implant group, with at least 3 years of implant experience, showed greater progress gains compared to the nonimplant group, and that these gains continued to increase for 5 years postimplant.

Geers and Moog (1994a) reported results for a range of language domains for 13 children with cochlear implants. The children showed an advantage for cochlear implants compared to other devices including hearing aids and tactile aids. The children with implants showed greater linguistic complexity in their spontaneous language and larger expressive and receptive vocabularies and, overall, demonstrated expressive and receptive language skills above the 60th percentile relative to normally hearing children after 36 months with the implant and intensive auditory–oral instruction. Geers and Moog also found that the language abilities of the children with the implants, whose hearing losses averaged 118 dB HL, closely resembled the abilities of children with hearing losses of 90–100 dB HL using hearing aids. Rattigan and colleagues (2002) have also reported data for children with prelinguistic, severe–profound hearing losses that indicate that, for the majority of these children, aspects of their language, literacy, and phonological processing abilities can move into the normal range on standardized tests after several years of using cochlear implants. Like the children in the Geers and Moog study (1994a), the children in the work of Rattigan et al. (2002) had received considerable auditory–verbal intervention.

With regard to vocabulary abilities, Waltzman and colleagues (1997) reported the results of a study involving 38 children who were profoundly hearing impaired, had been implanted prior to age 5 years, and had used their implant for a minimum of 1 year. All the children had experience with only auditory–verbal input (except one child who was using total communication). The results indicated significant increases in vocabulary development relative to preimplantation baselines. Over a 36-month period, expressive vocabulary increased by 48 months and receptive vocabulary by 33 months. A slightly mixed finding arises from the work of Dawson, Blamey, Dettman, Barker, and Clark (1995), who examined thirteen adolescents who had been using cochlear implants for a number of years. Although these researchers found that vocabulary scores increased significantly for the entire sample, only three of the children reached age-appropriate vocabulary levels 5 years after receiving their implant.

Protocols that enabled babies under 12 months of age with significant hearing losses to be implanted have only been introduced in the past 5 years, and as a result outcomes data are more limited for this group. However, in a longitudinal study providing a preliminary look at the language and speech development of these very young children with profound hearing impairment and cochlear implants, Wright, Purcell, and Reed (2001a, 2001b, 2002) have reported that, although the infants used a range of nonverbal communicative intents between the ages of 8 and 15 months of age prior to implantation, they used no verbal communicative intents until implantation. After implantation, verbal communicative intents emerged about 3 to 4 months later regardless of the children's chronological ages, which then ranged between 11 to 12 months and 14 to 15 months of age. Patterns with regard to types of communicative intents used by the children basically corresponded to patterns seen in children without hearing loss. These infants, like other children for whom results have been reported here, received considerable intervention in addition to having received cochlear implants, and in a number of cases the intervention was mostly auditory–verbal in nature.

Another important aspect is that while children who are implanted may perform similarly whether their deafness was pre-, peri- or postlingual (although children who acquire their hearing loss postlingually may catch up more quickly), the degree of hearing impairment may have some impact on the outcome of language development, with children with greater hearing impairment performing less well than children with more hearing. Boothroyd (1993) disputes that degree of residual hearing loss actually impacts on outcome, but Dowell and Cowan (1997) have reported that over 85 percent of 192 children who had residual hearing at the time of implantation were able to complete an open-set speech-reception test, which contrasted with the results when these authors pooled the data for children with and without residual hearing. The pooled data indicated a drop to 65 percent of the children who could complete the test. Because the functioning of a cochlear implant is not dependent on the performance of hair cells in the cochlea, and in fact destroys these as part of the surgical implantation process, the benefits of residual hearing are due to more intact neuronal connections from the cochlea to transmit the information produced by the cochlear implant.

Cochlear implants represent the single greatest advance in technology for profound hearing impairment, but while this technology has produced quite remarkable results, it is necessary to ensure that parents develop realistic expectations about the range of possible outcomes in terms of expressive and receptive speech and language abilities and in terms of their children's social inclusion. Tooher (2002) and her colleagues (Tooher, Hogan, & Reed, 2002a, 2002b) have reported on the psychosocial and language abilities of adolescents who had used cochlear implants for a number of years. A theme that emerged as a result of interviews with the adolescents was that some of the language, educational, and psychosocial issues associated with hearing loss do not simply disappear because of the implant, even with extensive intervention and mainstream education. It is important to recognize that the technology is only part of the support the children need. These children will need to engage successfully with intensive speech and language stimulation that is essential for them if they are to acquire good oral communication skills. For example, the adolescents noted above performed broadly within the ranges expected of teenagers without hearing impairments on measures of language, as well on psychosocial measures.

For children who, for whatever reason, cannot take advantage of cochlear implants, the other main alternative is a tactile aid (Osberger, Robbins, Todd, & Riley, 1996). Although cochlear implants remain the preferred option, it is encouraging to note that a prospective study of speech-perception capabilities in children using tactile aids over a 3-year period approximated the skills in groups who had used cochlear implants over a similar period (Eilers, Cobo-Lewis, Vergara, & Oller, 1997). In addition, the language development of children using tactile aids has shown improvement over not using auditory input stimulation, at least in early school years (Geers & Moog, 1994b; Osberger, Robbins, et al., 1991; Osberger, Chute, et al., 1991).

Intervention and Education Approaches.   About 90 percent of children who are born with significant hearing impairment have parents with normal hearing. One result of this is that the dominant mode of communication that the children are exposed to is auditory–oral. For children who cannot acquire language by the auditory–oral channel, the options are sign language alone or total communication. However, for sign-alone or total communication, hearing parents rarely develop their sign communication skills to the level required so that they can interact with their child at levels equivalent to their auditory–oral skills (Moeller & Luetke-Stahlman, 1990). In employing sign to communicate, hearing parents may omit function words and use only three- to four-word sentences, and their sign vocabulary may be limited and presented in a less consistent manner than for auditory–oral presentation. These conditions lead to slower language development in home environments than if the children could take advantage of their parents' language presented in the auditory–oral channel. Children of hearing parents who are exposed to alternative environments where there are fluent signers (such as in bilingual programs) in their first 5 years develop fluent sign language, whereas later acquisition of sign language results in incomplete mastery, especially of grammar (Mayberry & Eichen, 1991).

The selection of a communication approach to intervention for hearing-impaired children remains controversial. Traditionally, the choices have been a manual approach using Deaf sign language, a total communication approach in which auditory–oral input is supplemented by signed language, an auditory–visual approach in which hearing is supplemented by visual speech-reading cues, or an auditory–verbal approach in which the child has to rely on auditory input. In addition, there are several variations, ranging from cued speech (Cornett, 1985), in which a hand cue supplements speech sounds, to an approach that favors the initial use of a manual signed approach to kick-start language development, followed by more emphasis on auditory–oral input at a later age (Johnson, Liddell, & Erting, 1989).

With improved technology available for hearing-impaired children, the auditory–verbal approach aims to provide a systematic program for providing auditory-only stimulation for the language channel. Auditory–verbal therapy (AVT) (Estabrooks, 1994) emphasizes early detection of hearing loss, early fitting with an appropriate technology aid (hearing aid or cochlear implant), ongoing diagnostic therapy, and a strong support system across the family and the professionals involved in the intervention process. AVT is focused on providing support for hearing-impaired children to learn to listen, process spoken language, and talk in regular learning and living environments. In some settings, AVT is an integrated part of children receiving their academic instruction in mainstreamed environments. It is important to realize, however, that AVT, too, is not without controversy.

While auditory–verbal stimulation provides a direct path toward "normality" of speech and language function, this goal can be unrealistic for some children and it is important to monitor a child's speech and language development closely. Nevins and Chute (1996) reviewed academic achievement of hearing-impaired children in mainstream schools and noted higher achievement in this group than in nonmainstreamed peers. This effect also carries across to improved speech intelligibility for the mainstreamed group. However, this result may simply be because those children who can cope with mainstream education do so because of better auditory input ability in the first place. Technology aids also play a role here. In the Nevins and Chute review, about 75 percent of children with 5 years experience with a cochlear implant tended to shift their educational placement from a special school or unit to a mainstream class. Similarly, children receiving a cochlear implant at a young age tended to proceed to a mainstream setting, although all children needed varying forms of follow-up to maintain success. These trends are consistent with the findings of Geers, Spehar, and Sedey (2002), in which the children with cochlear implants in a total communication setting achieved better speech perception, speech intelligibility, and language scores if they used speech as their primary communication mode, instead of primarily using sign or total communication. And compared to their signing or total communication peers, these children were also more likely to move into mainstream educational settings.

Within educational and home environments using exclusively auditory–oral only, total communication, or manual sign–only approaches there are also different options for intervention that range from very structured approaches to very naturalistic approaches. Traditional structured approaches, for example, Fitzgerald (1949), have been criticized for not including the full developmental patterns necessary to facilitate flexible language acquisition and lacking connection to concept expansion methods to utilize new vocabulary. Naturalistic conversational approaches (Horstmeier & MacDonald, 1978) try to provide daily input through a range of communication experiences. However, these might be introduced before the child is able to utilize them properly, thereby leading to failure. Most current methods offer a combination of both approaches but still tend toward one or the other.

Regardless of the educational environment or intervention methods, it has long been recognized that as much language input as possible in any communication mode will improve the language development outcomes for children with hearing impairment. For instance,

Calderon and Greenberg (1997) reviewed literature concerning a variety of early-intervention programs and found that, when children who have a profound hearing loss are enrolled in such programs and receive early exposure to sign language as well as auditory–verbal input, they demonstrate more competent language development than children who do not receive those interventions.

Geers (2002) investigated auditory, speech, language, and reading outcomes in a reasonably large sample (130) of children with prelingual profound hearing loss after they had been fitted with a multichannel cochlear implant for 4 to 6 years. Approximately 20 percent of the variance in level of performance for the variables measured was accounted for by family factors. About 24 percent of the variance was accounted for by implant results, and 12 percent by educational variables. These results indicate that professional and family intervention and support for the children are major factors in success for children with significant hearing impairment, and that educational approaches have a significant but lesser effect on outcome.

Because all hearing loss creates problems for children's communication in environments where there is ambient noise in the background, part of assisting children with significant hearing losses involves trying to encourage optimal listening contexts for listening to learn. This approach needs to involve parents, teachers, clinicians, and as the children mature, the children themselves, in learning about how to minimize background noise and optimize listening conditions. Other considerations related to improving the listening environment are discussed later in this chapter.

Children with Lesser Degrees of Hearing Loss (15–60 dB HL)

Moderate Hearing Loss (31–60 dB HL).   Davis and colleagues (1986) investigated the relationship between hearing loss, educational achievement, language development, and personality development in a group of forty children, aged 5 to 18 years of age, with mild and moderate sensorineural hearing losses, as well as children with severe hearing losses. These researchers found that language development and academic success could not be predicted by hearing loss or age, again reminding us that degree of hearing loss by itself is not a good simple predictor of behavioral functioning. Many of the children, however, did demonstrate aggressive tendencies and expressed more somatic complaints than their hearing peers. Parents reported experiencing more behavioral difficulties in social and school situations. These findings underscore the importance of considering all aspects of the development of children with hearing loss, regardless of the severity of the losses.

Provided that children with mild-to-moderate hearing losses have been provided with use of appropriate amplifications (usually hearing aids) and speech and language delays are addressed in early intervention, their difficulties with speech and language are likely to be limited to mild-to-moderate problems (Elfenbein, Hardin-Jones, & Davis, 1994). When these positive conditions have not occurred, their difficulties can be more serious. As with all hearing-impaired children, it is important to evaluate each child to determine the degree of intervention required and understand that moderate hearing impairment can result in significant language problems for some children (Davis, 1990). Children with mild and moderate hearing impairment may have difficulties with poor vocabulary development (probably as the result of more limited exposure to different alternatives for expressing concepts and difficulties dealing with figurative and metalinguistic features of vocabulary), delays and difficulties in the use of morphological markers requiring high-frequency sounds, such as plurals, third-person present tense, and regular past tense for English, and delays in the development of functional words, such as prepositions and articles (Davis & Hardick, 1981).

Mild Hearing Loss (15–31 dB HL).   Some of the characteristics associated with mild hearing loss were raised in the previous section on moderate hearing losses. It is important to realize that mild hearing loss is problematic for language development, not so much because of the extent of the effects it produces on receptive communication, but because the mild effects are often not identified until a child is older, by which time mild disruptions in language have turned into significant effects on academic achievement. Children with mild hearing loss are less likely to be identified in early screening programs, and their apparent inattentive behavior is often not associated with hearing loss until their poor academic achievement is investigated with routine vision and hearing tests (Yoshinaga, 2000). The other problem at issue for mild hearing losses is that children, and particularly adolescents, resist wearing hearing aids because the advantage they get from personal amplification does not balance the disadvantage of being stigmatized by the wearing of a technology aid, thereby associating them with a group that in most communication circumstances they do not resemble.

As a result, a main developmental problem this group experiences is academic under-achievement. Subtle expressive and receptive language problems will be present in the child with mild hearing loss, and as the loss reaches the borderline between mild and moderate loss, the more the receptive capacity and behavior of children will demonstrate the same problems as the moderate-loss group (particularly for spoken language elements requiring more high-frequency sound information, such as morphology, tenses, etc.). This continuum of deficit is also not discrete in that some children with a mild loss will also show quite poor receptive communication skills, again emphasizing the need both to identify and profile communication capacity in all children with hearing loss.

Unilateral Hearing Loss.   Unilateral hearing loss (hearing loss in one ear only) has a reasonably large prevalence, with estimates ranging from 3 to 13 per 1,000 (Northern & Downs, 2002).   Total unilateral deafness is most commonly due to mumps developed in very early childhood. As with mild hearing loss, the child and parents may be unaware of the problem until it begins to affect specialized communication requirements (e.g., telephone use).

The traditional wisdom was that children with a unilateral loss but normal hearing in the other ear will develop normally. This view was, however, questioned in the 1980s by Bess and his associates (Bess & Tharpe, 1988; Bess, Klee, & Culbertson, 1986). They showed that at least one-third of a group of children with unilateral hearing loss had delayed academic progress, and that 50 percent of the group needed special resource support in their educational programs. This has similarities to the effects of mild bilateral hearing loss. Oyler, Oyler, and Matkin (1987, 1988) found similar results.

These data indicate that children with unilateral hearing loss are at risk for academic difficulties, but not all children with unilateral loss will have these problems if early intervention is provided. A study by Kiese-Himmel (2002) reported that children who were identified early and managed appropriately (fitted with hearing aids when appropriate, monitored educationally) performed similarly to normally hearing children on standardized linguistic tasks.

This argues that if children are identified early and managed appropriately, unilateral hearing loss does not necessarily lead to language and associated academic problems.

Amplification in the Classroom.   Children with a hearing loss may have persistent speech-perception problems in many listening environments even with a hearing aid fitted and can benefit from management strategies including appropriate classroom seating, FM aids, and management of the listening environment. The problems associated with poor listening environment are evident for all levels of hearing loss discussed above, including unilateral loss. These problems are particularly evident in the classroom environment, where noise, reverberation, and distance from the speaker are usually present together. For children with hearing loss who are educated in a mainstream classroom, options such as acoustic treatment of the classroom are usually not practical and FM amplification represents the best means of overcoming the effects of poor classroom acoustics. An FM aid consists of a microphone and transmitter worn by the teacher and a receiver worn by the child. The receiver can be coupled to a child's hearing aid so the sound through the FM is appropriate to the child's hearing. The main advantage of the FM aid is that it produces an improvement in signal-to-noise ratio of 6 to 10 dB. FM aids should offer options that permit listening with FM alone, cutting out all sounds except those transmitted through the microphone, or using both the microphone from the hearing aid and from the FM device together. This latter condition provides less advantage in terms of signal-to-noise ratio but allows the listeners to hear others speaking in the classroom and to monitor their own voices.

Conductive Hearing Loss.   In many ways, conductive hearing loss could be considered along with mild-to-moderate sensorineural hearing loss, but there are a number of complicating factors that indicate that it should be considered in its own right. First, conductive hearing loss can co-occur with sensorineural loss, thereby adding to the impact of that loss on speech reception. Second, conductive hearing loss is most prevalent in young children as a result of otitis media. Otitis media typically causes a fluctuating conductive hearing loss. That is, because its site of lesion and etiology are the result of the fluid in the middle ear, it does not always remain constant. Children suffering long-term middle-ear disease can have either a sustained hearing loss or one that fluctuates over time, even returning to normal hearing for extended periods of time. Third, a special literature has developed around middle-ear problems because of the hypothesized relationship between the occurrence of otitis media (middle-ear disease) in early childhood and language disorders.

Conductive hearing losses are the most common type of hearing loss found in children and can be caused by impacted wax in the external ear canal (easily observed and remedied) or infection (otitis media) in the middle ear with a residual of fluid (effusion) in the middle-ear cavity. Most children will have at least one episode of otitis media before the age of 5 years. Most of these will repair spontaneously, but a substantial proportion may require some form of medical intervention. The average hearing loss in children with middle-ear effusion is about 27 dB HL (for frequencies typically averaged at 500, 1,000 and 4,000 Hz) (Fria, Cantekin, & Eichler, 1985). In certain populations (including Native Americans, Aboriginal Australians), the prevalence and effects are much greater.

As with most of the lesser hearing problems (including mild bilateral sensorineural hearing loss and unilateral loss), the effects of conductive hearing loss were traditionally thought to relate mostly to the need for medical intervention. This intervention consists of either antibiotics or surgery to drain the infected ear and insert ventilation tubes to aerate the middle ear. Medical intervention is undertaken to alleviate the pain caused by the acute otitis media, to ensure that infection does not spread to brain areas (meninges), and to restore normal hearing. However, this tradition was questioned in a study by Holm and Kunze (1969), who showed that a group of children with a history of otitis media (reported retrospectively) had minor performance differences on a range of educational achievement and language measures. Although this report has since been criticized for its flawed methodology, it had a significant impact on the beliefs held by professionals about conductive hearing loss and on later research. The Holm and Kunze study was followed by a range of either retrospective studies of children with otitis media or with testing for the effects of otitis media carried out during active otitis media episodes. Both sorts of studies suggested a strong association between almost any otitis media event and a later language disorder (Howie, 1975; Needleman, 1977).

There are several issues that need to be considered in determining the relationship between otitis media/middle-ear effusion and language development in children. The first is that in special populations in which otitis media with middle-ear effusion is highly prevalent, persistent, and produces maximum effects on hearing levels over a long time, the problem needs to be managed in the same way as mild-to-moderate sensorineural hearing loss. In the absence of reinstatement of near-normal hearing (either by medical or technology intervention), the child with protracted middle-ear problems is likely to develop significant language disorders. These can impact dramatically on academic performance. The same would be true if we left bilateral sensorineural hearing loss unaided for an extended length of time during language development. The relationship between actual hearing loss in otitis media with effusion (OME) and effects on language was stressed by Friel-Patti and Finitzo (1990).

The contribution of mild, fluctuating loss during language development is more controversial. If middle-ear infections are common in individual children and remain untreated for substantial periods of time, then they clearly will have an effect. However, it is the actual extent and duration of hearing loss that is probably the main determinant of language development effects. The simple occurrence of a bout of otitis media (given its very prevalent nature) is unlikely to cause problems in itself. Haggard, Birkin, and Pringle (1994) reviewed 13 major studies that had investigated the effects of otitis media with effusion (OME) on language outcomes. These authors were very critical of the design of most of the studies, and even when effects were statistically significant they were very small. However, 9 of the 13 studies did report adverse effects of OME on language development. The effects occurred only between the ages of 2 and 4 years and were not consistent across different language skills. Overall, Haggard, et al. (1994) concluded that there is an effect of OME on language development but it varied depending on age of onset, length of duration of episodes, and number of bouts of OME. This is consistent with the previous analysis indicating that, if the OME affects hearing loss during critical language-development periods, then it may have the same effects as unmanaged mild/moderate sensorineural hearing loss. Because average hearing levels in OME are rarely poorer than 30 dB HL, there should be only subtle effects on speech input. However, young children require louder levels to perceive speech with the same performance as older children (e.g., Mackie & Dermody, 1986), so it is possible that speech perception scores might be poorer in young children with even mild hearing losses.

There is evidence for the effects of OME on speech perception. For instance, Clarkson, Eimas, and Marean (1989) reported results showing children with a history of OME and matched controls. Two OME groups were included, one with OME history and language delay and one with OME history and no language delay. The children in the OME without language delay group performed more poorly than those in the control group, while the children in the OME with language delay group, in turn, performed more poorly than those in the OME without language delay group. Other studies that indicate that speech perception in noise, which more closely approximates normal environment listening conditions, is also impaired in OME groups relative to controls (Gravel & Wallace, 1992; Jerger & Jerger, 1983).

The role of either the hearing loss due to transient OME or its effect on speech perception as the basis for later language disorders remains controversial. The first to point out the methodological issues related to studies in this area was Ventry (1983). Despite the early availability of a set of criteria, most subsequent studies have failed to provide prospective designs, standardized measures for evaluation of language effects, appropriate statistical analysis of differences, and most critically, have used OME itself for prediction of effect on language rather than the presence of a hearing loss associated with the OME. As a result, there remains some uncertainty in the actual effects on language development that can be attributed to OME during early language-development years. Strong recommendations both about early identification and the most effective treatment cannot be made at this time.

Early Identification of Hearing Loss

Early identification of hearing loss is a major key to intervention. The prevalence of hearing loss in newborns has been estimated in a number of studies to range from 1.5 to 6 per 1,000 live births (Mauk, White, & Mortensen, 1991; Mehl & Thomson, 1998; Northern & Hayes, 1994). These figures are higher than the historical figure of 1 per 1,000 live births. The increase is based on the ability of new technologies such as otoacoustic emissions (OAEs) and automated auditory brainstem response (AABR) to identify mild and moderate losses and unilateral hearing loss, as well as severe and profound hearing loss. Hearing loss in infants results in a serious, life-long disability (Northern & Hayes, 1994), which can be ameliorated with early identification and intervention.

Early identification has traditionally relied on the use of high-risk registers, whereby a child with risk factors for hearing loss is screened before discharge from hospital after birth or within the first 3 months (JCIHS, 1995). Although these risk factors enable the identification of high-risk infants, a number of studies (Mauk et al., 1991; Mehl & Thomson, 1998) has reported that only 50 percent of children with hearing loss have any high-risk indicators. Programs that target only high-risk infants are therefore limited to identifying at most 50 percent of the children with hearing loss.

The JCIHS (1995) argued that while high-risk registers provide important help in the early identification of hearing loss, the goal is really universal hearing screening. In 2000 the JCIHS released a paper advocating the introduction of universal hearing screening using a physiological measure, such as OAE or AABR, with full diagnostic testing and referral for intervention by 6 months of age (JCIHS, 2000). Universal hearing screening programs are becoming more widespread, with Northern and Downs (2002) reporting that more than twenty states in the USA had passed legislation for statewide universal infant hearing screening programs. More states and countries are expected to follow suit.

Central Auditory Processing Disorders (CAPD)

The role of transient middle-ear disorders in language disorders remains conjectural but, to the extent that defined OME is present, it is likely that a child is also experiencing hearing loss that could produce adverse effects on language development. However, another group of children show no evidence of hearing loss but have language disorders that some purport are because of clinical evidence of poor auditory processing. These children demonstrate poor performance compared to their peers in hearing tests that are more complex than the pure-tone hearing test. Descriptions of children that are compatible with auditory processing problems can be found in clinical reports going back to the turn of the last century, although the actual diagnoses vary depending on the fashion of the time (Aram & Nation, 1982). Among the diagnostic terms that have been used are *childhood aphasia, central auditory processing disorders* (CAPD), and *auditory processing disorders.* The term *central* refers to the distinction between peripheral hearing and the perceiving and "deciphering" of auditory stimuli (i.e., processing) more centrally in the auditory systems of the brain.

The argument about the role of auditory processing in the absence of hearing loss as a cause of language problems is made by the following logical progression. The children have language disorders, which is why they have been referred for testing. The children have normal hearing (typically), but when tested on a range of complex auditory perception or speech processing tasks show poorer performance than age-related peers. Therefore, the auditory processing disorder could be the cause of the language disorder in the same way that hearing loss can cause language disorders. This idea had begun to gain considerable momentum (Eisenson, 1972; Myklebust, 1954) when Rees (1973) published an influential paper suggesting that despite the evidence showing poor auditory/speech task processing performance in clinical groups of children with language disorders, the evidence for demonstrating that auditory processing disorders caused language disorders was weak. Although these arguments occurred over 30 years ago, they remain relevant today. Despite Rees's early significant criticisms, the area of CAPD continued to grow, and batteries of tests based on those criticized by Rees were still developed and used. Noting these developments, Rees (1973, 1982) wrote another analysis of CAPD, and this provided further guidelines about the major difficulties with the CAPD approach.

Rees (1973, 1982) pointed out that the notion of auditory processing is used in two quite different ways. One use is by persons interested in providing intervention for language disorders, while the other is by neuro-audiologists who are interested in using behavioral and electrophysiological tests to diagnose central auditory dysfunction. Despite a range of studies from the 1960s, there was little evidence of central auditory dysfunction of auditory brain structures underlying language disorders in otherwise healthy children. Other professionals promoting CAPD but interested more in intervention adopted the notion that complex language behavior, as Rees (1982) wrote, "is composed of a finite number of sub-skills that can be reduced even further to fundamental perceptual-motor abilities" (p. 94). The inventory of basic skills can include auditory discrimination, auditory sequencing, and auditory memory. However, other skills can be included, such as identifying speech in noise (figure–ground perception). A major motivation for this approach is that if children demonstrate poor performance on these types of auditory skills, then these could be remediated and this process could be correlated with improvements in their language development.

Rees (1982) suggested that there are several weaknesses with this basic hypothesis. The first is that there is no coherent or unified theory of basic auditory skills. As a result, each test battery includes a different range of tasks, response requirements, and suppositions about their relation to intervention. At one extreme, the tasks can include a simple digit span task (requiring a child to repeat back spoken digits with increasing string length, say from three to seven spoken digits depending on age, because memory span increases with age). At another extreme, there are tasks requiring acoustic treatment of stimuli that degrades the signal in some way (filtered, time compressed, or with noise added at different signal-to-noise ratios). Response requirements in degraded-speech tests can range from requiring the child to respond to syllables, words, or sentences. The evidence is overwhelming that many children with language disorders have trouble on these tasks. However, the question remains as to whether they have trouble because they have auditory processing problems producing language disorders, or whether language disorders produce poor performance on the tasks, or whether poor language performance and poor performance are both the result of some other condition. The failure to engage the speech processor in these children with stimuli, for instance, lacking in redundancy could be just as much evidence for a poorly established language processing system as for an auditory processing disorder. Similarly, failure to deal with distorted or unexpected versions of stimuli again could point to poorly developed language skills, not auditory processing disorders.

In support of Rees' analysis, Leonard (1979) emphasized the problems of interpreting poorer auditory skills as causally related to language disorders and suggested that the auditory processing tasks, themselves, frequently confounded aspects of the disordered language performance (for which the child had already been identified). Furthermore, at about the same time, a review of thirty-four studies that attempted to determine whether intervention to improve auditory processing skills produced positive results on language showed that there was little success with such intervention approaches in actually remediating the language disorders (Hammill & Larsen, 1974). These theoretical issues have endured, but so has the development of auditory skills test batteries (Flowers, Costello, & Small, 1970; Katz, Curtiss, & Tallal, 1992; Keith, 1986, 2000; Willeford, 1977), and a number of clinics administers them on a regular basis.

At about the same time as these criticisms of the auditory processing skills approaches to children's language disorders were occurring, the issue of auditory processing problems as underlying factors in language disorders received a significant boost by a series of studies by Tallal and her colleagues (Tallal, 1975, 1976, 1980; Tallal & Piercy, 1973a, 1973b, 1974, 1975; Tallal, Stark, & Curtis, 1976). These researchers tested a group of well-defined children with language disorders on a series of different speech-processing tasks. Using controlled, synthetic speech, Tallal and her colleagues altered the critical perceptual elements of the speech, in particular the speed of transition between consecutive speech sounds. She found that the group of children with language disorders who had trouble identifying the sounds when presented with normal transition times between speech sounds improved when the transition was lengthened. Similarly, the children could only identify the order of two sounds when the duration between them was extended. These results appeared to demonstrate the presence of a specific auditory processing problem in the children with language disorders. The findings of specific auditory processing problems can be found in other studies as well. For example, using a dichotic listening task (in which spoken stop consonants are presented in simultaneous pairs to listeners for them to recognize), a group of children with well-defined reading problems, many of whom would be expected to have language impairments, had significantly poorer performance relative to their typically developing peers when the stimuli were presented dichotically (that is, one to each ear simultaneously), but not when the same stimuli were presented monotically (both stimuli to the same ear) (Dermody, Katsch, & Mackie, 1983; Dermody, Mackie, & Katsch, 1983).

Arguing in favor of a CAPD approach, Jerger (1998) suggests that there is converging evidence in support of auditory perceptual disorders. There exist a considerable amount of data showing that both children and adults with identified brain dysfunctions have disrupted auditory processing on tasks similar to those used in CAPD batteries to identify children with language disorders. This raises an index of suspicion that children with language disorders may also have subtle, at present unidentified, dysfunctions of the central auditory system. Independent of this, there is also clear evidence of significant disruption of language development from peripheral hearing loss, so results showing at least poor auditory processing might also act in the same way but at a central processing level.

Because of the debate surrounding CAPD, the American Speech–Language–Hearing Association (ASHA) convened a task force a number of years ago to develop a consensus statement for the profession (ASHA, 1976). The Task Force defined central auditory processes as the auditory system mechanisms and functions responsible for a range of behavioral responses in tasks such as auditory discrimination, sound localization, temporal aspects of hearing such as judging the order of tones presented in rapid succession, and speech perception under degraded conditions such as presenting speech in noise. CAPD is demonstrated by failure on tests of these functions related to norm-related performance, but this failure may be due to specific dysfunction of the auditory system mechanisms or to more general cognitive processes such as attention problems or even language disorders. As a result, there remained significant problems with the consensus viewpoint, as pointed out by Jerger (1998). The consensus simply listed the kinds of performance deficits reported in the literature. Jerger again raised the lack of a conceptual framework for describing the results obtained.

A second attempt at some consensus was formulated by a group from the American Academy of Audiology (Jerger & Musiek, 2000). They proposed a name change from CAPD to auditory processing disorders (APD) and defined the condition as a deficit in the processing of information that is specific to the auditory system. As pointed out above, there is some evidence for reasonably specific auditory processing disorders in children with associated language disorders but no direct evidence to prove a causal link between these and specific language disorders.

In terms of intervention based on auditory processing testing, a range of approaches has been developed for CAPD. More recently there are also approaches that are based on the evidence of specific auditory processing problems. This latter approach was discredited initially (Rees, 1973) but has recently produced data leading to the development of commercial programs for intervention. The most known of these programs is the Fast ForWord program (Scientific Learning Corporation, 1997). It uses computer games and computer-generated synthetic speech in adaptive training to improve children's abilities to identify rapidly presented sounds and temporally altered speech. Tasks include discrimination of sounds, analysis of order of presentation, and identification of speech sounds. After children have mastered 90 percent of the games they have completed the program. Trials with around 500 children suggest significant gains in language skills after completing the training program (Tallal et al., 1996). Several of the unanswered questions about the effects resulting from the training have included whether the changes in language can be attributed to the systematic and incremental nature of the practice associated with completing the tasks, the amount of practice provided in the program, or fundamental improvements in processing auditory information.

Fast ForWord has developed further to gradually incorporate a wider range of tasks, including phonemic awareness, language structures, and story comprehension. These changes reduce the emphasis of the program on auditory processing and increase the emphasis on language intervention. The Fast ForWord program remains an expensive, proprietary program that now combines auditory processing training tasks and language therapy and therefore does not provide good evidence for the specific effectiveness of auditory training to improve language function.

Other programs based on similar principles are appearing, such as a UK computer game system called *Phonomena,* by MindWeavers (MindWeavers, 1996), that has been developing since 1996. This program is based on training in auditory discrimination skills. Unpublished field trials also show effects similar to Fast ForWord in improving some aspects of language skills (word listening abilities). However, as with the Fast ForWord program, there remain limited peer-reviewed independent data and no real conceptual framework for indicating why simple auditory discrimination would lead to improvements in complex language skills.

Differing and unresolved conceptual and clinical issues hamper the quest for consensus on CAPD assessment and indeed CAPD, although Keith (1999) purports that there is a general consensus surrounding the actual existence of CAPD. The confusion surrounding CAPD can be partially attributed to disciplines coming from different conceptual viewpoints. For example, according to Friel-Patti and Finitzo (1990), speech–language pathologists work within a network model that assumes that sound, meaning, and the intention of a message are all integrated, distributed, and processed at multiple levels throughout the nervous system, not just the central auditory nervous system. These professionals, then, are interested in the relationships that occur at different levels of processing. Audiologists, on the other hand, adopt a model based around the central auditory nervous system (Cacace & McFarland, 1998) that assesses the integrity of various sections within that pathway and do not encompass the full language system. There are also two other main theoretical issues that frustrate consensus. These are:

- Whether an auditory-specific perceptual deficit exists alone (Cacace & McFarland, 1998; McFarland & Cacace, 1997), or whether it is actually a broader information-processing deficit that affects processing more generally and other sensory modalities as well
- Whether there is a general auditory processing difficulty (Tallal et al., 1996), or whether it is actually a deficit specific to speech perception (Mody, Studdert-Kennedy, & Brady, 1997)

We can see in these points a number of issues related to information processing accounts of specific language impairment in children and the surface account of the grammatical deficits of children with specific language impairment that were presented in Chapter 3.

Just to make it more interesting, there is also a myriad of clinical issues with regard to CAPD assessment, including the lack of diagnostic criteria, lack of appropriate norms, and confounding with language and memory factors. As a response to some of these, a test-battery approach for CAPD has been advocated as the main method of choice for assessment (Musiek, 1999), although it, too, has been questioned as to whether it actually is diagnostically superior to individual tests (Turner, Robinette, & Bauch, 1999).

It is clear, then, that the quest for consensus needs to be twofold—consensus on the conceptualization of CAPD and consensus on current assessment approaches. Of course, the latter is strongly determined by the former, as we will only make advances if we integrate theoretical and clinical perspectives. Already, there have been suggestions in the literature related to widening our diagnostic lens to encompass phonological working memory issues in an attempt to identify the underlying, fundamental nature of processing deficits (Friel-Patti & Finitzo, 1990). We need to tackle these conceptual and clinical issues from a multidisciplinary, if not transdisciplinary, perspective as well as from a holistic approach in which children's auditory, language, literacy, and cognitive abilities are analyzed and reported upon. We need to critically evaluate current assessment tools by examining the underlying processes that are required in order to carry out such tasks.

The evidence to date indicates that professionals should maintain a reasonably high index of suspicion about the role of auditory processing problems in children with language disorders, but the possibility of auditory processing problems in children with language disorders should not be dismissed out of hand. Approaches that assess aspects of processing auditory information essential for language learning might provide good ways for early identification of children at risk for language disorders, including reading problems.

Auditory Neuropathy

Studies during the 1990s reported on a new clinical entity called *auditory neuropathy* (Berlin et al., 1998; Hood, 1998). Diagnosis of auditory neuropathy is dependent on a range of complex audiological tests, which can be used to demonstrate the characteristics of the condition: normal middle-ear function (based on tympanometry) but absent acoustic reflexes; normal outer hair cell function in the cochlea (based on normal otoacoustic emissions) but poor neural synchrony (based on an abnormal or missing auditory brainstem response, ABR).

Hood (1998) speculates that there is more than a single etiology for auditory neuropathy despite the fact that all patients display this common pattern of test results. Individuals with auditory neuropathy have audiograms ranging from normal hearing to profound hearing losses, and when there is measured response to pure tones, their speech perception abilities are much poorer than would be expected (Berlin, 2000). Hood (1998) also points out that

> while any disorder of the auditory neural pathways from the VIIIth nerve to the cortex might be defined as an auditory neuropathy, the current use of the term relates specifically to more peripheral portions of the auditory pathways in the area between the outer hair cells and brainstem. Auditory neuropathy differs from other disorders affecting the VIIIth nerve, such as a vestibular Schwannoma, in that there is no space occupying lesion and radiological findings are normal. (Section 15)

The consequences of auditory neuropathy for communication vary, depending on age of onset and amount of residual hearing. Generally these individuals are aware of sound around them, but cannot discriminate speech. Hood (1998) reports that individuals with auditory neuropathy with residual hearing ability or those with a postlingual onset and progressive neuropathy must use lip reading (speech reading) to follow speech. Their own speech, however, is usually intelligible, with normal vocal quality. For infants and young children identified with auditory neuropathy, the lack of clear auditory information results in problems in the development of speech and language, and active intervention is necessary. Berlin and his colleagues (Berlin et al., 1998) recommend introducing a sign system that follows the grammatical structure of English, such as signed English or cued speech. These authors point out that auditory function may improve, and if this happens, spoken language can be assimilated into a language system that already follows English language structure.

Summary

In this chapter, we have seen that

- Hearing loss may be peripheral or central.
- Peripheral hearing loss may be either conductive (located in the external or middle ear) or sensorineural (located in the cochlear or 8th nerve).
- Peripheral hearing loss is categorized by degree of loss and, while all hearing loss affects speech and language development, in general the more severe the hearing loss, the greater the potential impact on speech and language development.
- Hearing loss affects written, spoken, and receptive communication skills, academic achievement, and social development.
- Cochlear implants provide significant input stimulation for children with total or profound hearing loss, which may produce results that are superior to those with hearing aids in this group of children.
- There is no single best communication choice for a child with a significant hearing loss. Outcomes are affected by the language environment of the child and the type of technology aid being used, as well as individual variables, such as cognitive abilities.
- Children with mild hearing loss and unilateral loss are at risk for language and academic problems unless identified early and managed appropriately.
- Conductive hearing loss due to OME affects a child's ability to hear and understand speech, but the impact of OME itself on speech and language development is uncertain.
- Universal newborn hearing screening is recommended for early identification of hearing loss.
- There is ongoing debate about the role of central auditory processing disorders in language disorders.
- New assessment procedures have enabled us to identify children with auditory neuropathies, and more research is needed to determine the most appropriate management options for these children.

Any degree of hearing impairment puts a child at risk for language learning and academic achievement. Early identification followed by early intervention are key in helping these children.

9 Language and Linguistically-Culturally Diverse Children

STEVEN H. LONG

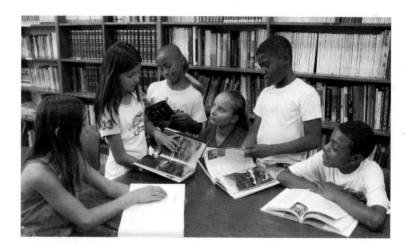

OBJECTIVES

After reading this chapter, you should be able to discuss

- Concepts of multiculturalism, linguistic variation, and second language learning and their relevance to assessment and intervention of language disorders in children

- General linguistic characteristics of the language of children from linguistically-culturally diverse backgrounds, specifically those from some African American, Hispanic American, Asian American, and Native American homes

- Discuss principles of language assessment and intervention for linguistically-culturally diverse children

The linguistic and cultural character of the United States is rapidly changing, nowhere more than in its schools. From 1986 to 1999, nonwhite children enrolled in public elementary and secondary schools increased from 30 to 38 percent (U.S. Department of Education, 2001a). Many children are raised in homes in which languages other than English are spoken at least some of the time. For the 2000–2001 school year, it is estimated that more than 4.5 million students learning English as a second language were enrolled in U.S. public schools, approximately 9.6 percent of total public school enrollment (Kindler, 2002). Other children, both nonwhite and white, learn a form of spoken English that differs from that used in most U.S. schools and workplaces. As a result, many students are at risk for educational failure because of their language background and not because of a language impairment. At the same time, children who grow up in linguistically and/or culturally diverse households that are ethnic, bilingual, or both, are not immune from specific disabilities in language learning. Consequently, professionals must be able to distinguish between language differences, which are the result of a child's linguistic and/or cultural environment, and language disorders, which are due to an impairment of language-learning mechanisms.

Concepts of Cultural Diversity

Cultural diversity is commonly also referred to *as multiculturalism,* which is a cover term for the racial, linguistic, and cultural variation in society. Although there is much overlapping and interaction among the factors of race, language, and culture, they are, in principle, separate concepts:

■ *Race* is a statement about an individual's biological attributes. By itself, race is of little importance to discussions of language acquisition and language disorders. The few exceptions occur when there are physical differences among races, which in turn can be related to variations in language learning. For example, African American children have a lower incidence of middle-ear infection because the size and angle of their eustachian tubes permits better drainage. Insofar as otitis media may be a source of language difficulties in children, this racial difference may be of some significance.

■ Most broadly, *language* refers to all the behaviors by which individuals communicate with one another. In the context of multiculturalism, however, we attend primarily to the differences in form (phonology, grammar) and lexicon that distinguish one language (e.g., English, Spanish, Japanese) from another and one variety of the same language (e.g., standard, nonstandard, American English, New Zealand English) from another variety. Differences in pragmatics are viewed as a communication aspect of culture rather than language *per se.* For example, Hispanic American speakers tend to have a small distance between them during conversation (Pajewski & Enriquez, 1996; Taylor, 1987). This appears to be true whether the speakers are monolingual (having only one language) or bilingual (sharing aspects of two languages) and, if they are bilingual, whether they are speaking Spanish, English, or a mixture of the two. Thus, the language behavior (Spanish) and the cultural behavior (standing close during conversation) are separable components of the communication of many but not all Hispanic American speakers. When we speak of language as a multicultural variable, the meaning should be restricted to those formal elements that will be learned and used by speakers.

■ *Culture* is a statement about behaviors that are shared by a group of individuals. Many of these behaviors can influence communication. Members of an ethnic group share many cultural elements as a result of ancestral links. Four large ethnic groups in the United States—African Americans, Hispanic Americans, Native Americans, and Asian Americans—are commonly contrasted with one another and with white Americans of mostly European descent. As shown in Table 9.1, this comparison of behaviors across cultural groups reveals several differences with the potential to cause miscommunication and misinterpretation of behavior. It is important to recognize, however, that even though ethnicity cannot be changed, it does not compel an individual to follow certain cultural standards. To expect that all members of an ethnic group will behave in the same way is prejudicial. On the other hand, to be unaware of cultural differences and their potential effect on communication is unprofessional. Balance is, therefore, a key factor in serving children with linguistically-culturally diverse backgrounds.

TABLE 9.1 Some Differences in Communicative Behavior across American Cultural Groups

White Americans	African Americans	Hispanic Americans	Asian Americans	Native Americans
Touching of hair is considered a sign of affection, especially between adults and children	Touching of hair may be considered offensive	Touching occurs commonly during conversation	Touching is more acceptable between members of the same sex than between men and women	Learning through quiet observation is valued; group teaching activities that encourage each child to speak may be disfavored
Uninvited touching between men and women may be considered harassing	Direct eye contact is avoided during listening but maintained during speaking	Direct eye contact may be considered disrespectful	Backslapping is considered offensive	"Wait time"—the amount of time speakers are given to speak and respond—is substantially longer
Direct eye contact is maintained during listening but avoided during speaking	Public behavior may be emotionally intense and demonstrative	A small distance is maintained between speakers during conversation	Men and women do not customarily shake hands	
Public behavior should be emotionally restrained	Interruption of another speaker during conversation is acceptable	Parent–child conversation is usually directive, not collaborative	Children tend to wait to participate, unless otherwise requested by the teacher	Individual humility and group harmony are valued; displaying knowledge in front of others may be uncomfortable
			Being singled out can cause distress	
			Many children are socialized to listen more than speak and to speak in a soft voice	

Sources: Adapted from Espinosa (1995); Feng (1994); Fung & Roseberry-McKibbin (1999); Madding (2002); Swisher (1991); Taylor (1987); and Tharp & Yamauchi (1994).

Concepts of Linguistic Variation

Around the world, no two individuals communicate in exactly the same manner. The differences among people can be described in several ways. At the broadest level, we can identify nearly 1,000 different languages, each produced by 10,000 or more speakers (Crystal, 1997). Many of these languages are produced in several different forms or dialects, which vary from one another in grammar, vocabulary, and phonology. A language is distinguished from a dialect in two ways:

■ A dialect is assumed to be a subset of a language and therefore should share a common core of grammatical and other characteristics with all other dialects of that language.
■ Speakers of different dialects should be able to understand one another, whereas speakers of different languages should not.

The common core of a language is more evident in its written form than in its spoken form. Thus, an individual who knows English will be able to read a newspaper published in Canada, the United States, England, Australia, or any other English-speaking nation. However, the same individual, if he or she is from Kansas, may be unable to understand the English spoken in some parts of Scotland, Jamaica, New Zealand, or even Los Angeles. This calls attention to the fact that differences in pronunciation, or accent, are conspicuous features of a dialect and cause difficulty in spoken communication between two individuals using the same language.

There is nothing inherently better about one dialect than another. Within a society, however, factors of history, economics, and education can combine to favor a particular dialect and establish it as the standard. *Standard American English* (SAE) is the phrase used to refer to what is considered characteristic of "mainstream" speakers of American English. All English-speaking nations are considered to have their own standard dialects, so it is customary to use the terms *American English, South African English,* and so on, to refer to various standard dialects.

The concept of a standard dialect is strongly associated with the educational level of the speaker. Individuals with considerable formal education tend to speak the standard dialect of the nation in which they live. They may also speak other dialects, depending on their personal backgrounds and experiences. The most invariant feature of a standard dialect is grammar. Whereas differences in vocabulary and pronunciation are identifiable features of regional dialects, these dialects are not usually considered nonstandard unless they include grammatical variation. Thus, we would expect that educated speakers in Mississippi, New Hampshire, and Minnesota will show discernible differences in their speech, but these will be primarily at the levels of phonology and vocabulary.

Because the standard dialect of a nation is generally the dialect of its more educated inhabitants, it is usually preferred in the classroom. Historically, this has led many speakers to identify standard dialectal forms as correct and nonstandard dialectal forms as wrong or substandard. At one time it was believed that nonstandard dialects were immature forms of Standard English and that speakers who produced them were less developed in their linguistic abilities. However, research by sociolinguists has shown convincingly that nonstandard forms of English are equally complex and have the same cognitive and linguistic requirements as the standard dialect.

Table 9.2 summarizes four of the factors contributing to communication differences among speakers of English. Geography and membership in an ethnic group are often considered together as comprising an individual's speech community. For example, speakers who are reared in Texas may produce speech that has phonological, lexical, and grammatical characteristics distinctive of that region. Collectively, these features are sometimes described as a *twang* or *drawl* (though some might restrict those terms to descriptions of the differences in pronunciation). The features of Texan speech are sufficiently distinctive to constitute a regional dialect of English. However, this regional dialect is altered to varying degrees by the ethnic background of each speaker. We are likely to find the prototypical Texas dialect among white speakers, but some African American speakers from that state might also produce African American Vernacular English (AAVE), an ethnic dialect used across the United States. Regional and ethnic influences can interact, so that the AAVE spoken by some African Americans living in Dallas is likely to differ in some respects from the AAVE produced by some African Americans living in Seattle or Cleveland.

The influence of an ethnic dialect is sometimes difficult to separate from the effect of a native language other than English. Many characteristics of the dialect spoken by some Hispanic Americans are the result of linguistic borrowing from Spanish. English words may be pronounced with a Spanish accent, Spanish vocabulary may be substituted for English words in some contexts, and English syntax may be modified in ways that make it more consistent with Spanish syntax. Some individuals speak only English but nevertheless maintain an influence from Spanish in their dialect. Others speak both English and Spanish, though their English will likely reveal characteristics of Spanish, and vice versa. All immigrant groups from non-English-speaking countries can be expected to show a similar pattern.

TABLE 9.2   Factors Contributing to Communication Differences among Speakers

Regional Dialect	Ethnic Dialect	Register	Idiolect
Examples: Southern, Brooklyn	Examples: Black English Vernacular, Spanish-influenced English	Examples: formal, informal, caretaker	Examples: every individual speaker
Produces variation in: ■ Phonology (e.g., use of vocalic /r/) ■ Rate of speech ■ Syntax (e.g., use of *y'all*) ■ Use of gestures ■ Use of specific words or idioms ■ Vocal intensity ■ Vocal quality (e.g., nasality)	Produces variation in: ■ Distance between speaker and listener ■ Morphology (e.g., use of plural marker) ■ Phonology (e.g., use of theta) ■ Rate of speech ■ Stress and intonation ■ Syntax (e.g., use of copula) ■ Use of specific words or idioms	Produces variation in: ■ Distance between speaker and listener ■ Eye contact ■ Lexical specificity ■ Rate of speech ■ Stress and intonation ■ Syntax (e.g., simple/complex) ■ Use of gestures ■ Use of specific words or idioms (e.g., formal/informal, common/uncommon) ■ Vocal intensity	Produces variation in: ■ Rate of speech ■ Stress and intonation ■ Use of gestures ■ Use of specific words or idioms ■ Vocal quality

However, we tend to focus on particular ethnic dialects for social and demographic reasons. When the number of immigrants from a particular country or region becomes large, the language differences of those individuals can become a social issue, especially in education. This has occurred in the United States with both Hispanic Americans and Asian Americans; consequently, we tend to identify dialectal issues with those two groups. The large Asian and Hispanic immigration to the United States has also resulted in the formation of ethnic enclaves, especially in the bigger cities (Council of Economic Advisers, 1998). The insulation of these subcommunities helps to maintain ethnic dialects by keeping native languages in use and by mitigating the influence of English-speaking culture.

Beyond the effects of geography and ethnic background, we all vary our speech to suit the requirements of specific social communicative events. That is, we *code* switch, a concept we first encountered in this text in Chapter 1. Speakers of nonstandard ethnic dialects who are also competent users of standard English often adjust their use of nonstandard features to meet the expectations of a conversational partner. In a work or educational setting, the standard dialect might be used; in an ethnic social setting, the nonstandard dialect.

Of course, not all the features of an individual's communication are determined by region, ethnicity, or social situation. If they were, then many of us would sound far more alike than we do. What keeps us different is our uniqueness as individuals. Variation in everything from vocal tract anatomy to personal experiences provides everyone with an *idiolect,* that is, a distinctive combination of language characteristics.

Each person's idiolect can be compared to those of other individuals within a speech community. When we evaluate children for language disorders, this is what is done. Typically, a child's idiolect is first compared to the standard dialect of the nation in which the child lives. If the child's language is found to be different, then the following possibilities must be explored:

- The child is learning the standard dialect but is language disordered.
- The child is learning a nonstandard dialect.
- The child is learning a nonstandard dialect *and* is language disordered.

To evaluate either of the last two possibilities requires a knowledge of the child's nonstandard dialect or other language. Features of the child's language that differ from the standard dialect must be evaluated to determine whether they are disordered or merely dialectal variations.

Concepts of Second Language Learning

In theory, the perfect bilingual speaker is one who can comprehend and use two languages with equal facility. However, apart from professional translators, such competence is rarely attained. Far more common are individuals who

- Are fluent with both written and spoken forms of their first (native) language and have less proficiency with a second language; or
- Have equivalent but different areas of competence in two languages and therefore prefer to use one or the other in particular circumstances (e.g., at school, during play) or while engaged in certain tasks (speaking, reading, writing).

Many factors affect the process and result of second language learning. The model environment for children is to learn two languages from birth. They would hear the two languages being spoken by both of their parents, as well as by their peers, other adults, and speakers on radio and television. The children would be able to speak, read, and write both languages at school and in all other social experiences such as church, sports teams, and clubs. Of course, such an environment does not exist, even in the most linguistically diverse nations. Bilingual acquisition is influenced by every variation from the model situation we have described. For example, a daughter is born to a German university professor. Although the father speaks English, he does not use it at home. When the girl is 4, the father accepts a position at a U.S. university and the family moves. The daughter is exposed to English through her American friends and their families, through television, and through her father, who now begins to speak it to her at home. The mother has limited knowledge of English and, therefore, speaks mostly German with the girl and with her father. In this scenario, the girl's language learning is affected by (1) the ages at which she was first exposed to German and English; (2) the switch in the language used by her father; (3) the difference in the languages used by her mother and father; and (4) the language used by her American peers and teachers. Because she learned German and English in sequence rather than simultaneously, the girl is less likely to mix the two languages. There will likely be differences in the speed and accuracy with which she names items in German or English (Kohnert, Bates, & Hernandez, 1999). At age 4 and beyond, she will be aware of the difference in language skills of her two parents. Not only will she expect her mother to speak German, she may object if her mother attempts to use English with her (Volterra & Taeschner, 1978). On the other hand, the girl and her father may develop an elaborate system for code switching between German and English (Juan-Garau & Perez-Vidal, 2001). For instance, they may use German when speaking affectionately but switch to English for an instructional purpose. Discipline may be meted out in English unless the child resists or disobeys in some way. In that case, the father may switch to German to emphasize his determination.

Children who learn two languages simultaneously appear to go through a sorting-out process during the preschool years. How this sorting occurs has been a controversial subject in recent decades (De Houwer, 1995). Under the "single system" or "fusion" hypothesis, children are supposed to traverse three stages, beginning with a system that mixes vocabulary and grammatical features from the two languages and ending with a system in which the two are clearly differentiated (Volterra & Taeschner, 1978). The fusion hypothesis gives attention to the phenomenon of code mixing, a developmental stage in which bilingual children may for a time mix vocabulary from the two languages or, at a slightly later stage, mix the grammatical systems of the two languages. For example, a child learning Spanish and English may vary the order of nouns and adjectives, thereby creating ungrammatical or unusual sentences in both languages (e.g., "It's a clown silly" or "Es un tonto payaso"). Clinically, there has been concern that such code mixing indicates a confused stage of language learning. Thus, speech–language pathologists and others have sometimes advised parents of a bilingual child who is slow to acquire language that it would be best to limit the child to a single language input (De Houwer, 1999). Recent research indicates, however, that bilingual children can differentiate their languages from very early in development and that code mixing represents an adaptation to other linguistic influences. In particular, there is evidence that most code mixing can be explained as the result of lexical gaps in one language, imperfect attempts on the part of the child to develop pragmatic skill in code switching, or the prominence of particular aspects of the culture in which the child is exposed to the two languages (Brice & Anderson, 1999; Koeppe, 1996; Nicoladis & Secco, 2000; Peña, Bedore, & Zlatic-Giunta, 2002).

Language Characteristics of Linguistically-Culturally Diverse Children

Although it is convenient at times to consider linguistically-culturally diverse children as a group, there are important linguistic and cultural differences among various ethnic populations. Analysis of language and culture can be done along a continuum of detail. At a broad level, we can identify four major ethnic groups in the United States: African Americans, Hispanic Americans, Asian Americans, and Native Americans. Together, these groups are expected to comprise almost 34 percent of the U.S. population by 2015 (U.S. Bureau of the Census, 2000). At a fine level of analysis, every major ethnic group can be seen to consist of many subgroups, which often vary greatly from one another in language and culture. Thus we could distinguish among African Americans living in different regions of the country; among Hispanic Americans based on their country of origin (Cuba, Mexico, El Salvador); among Asian Americans who have immigrated from different nations (Korea, Cambodia, Vietnam); and among Native Americans with different tribal ancestries (Arapaho, Navajo). Detailed knowledge of such subgroups may be crucial in certain educational settings. For the purposes of this chapter, however, we will examine only those broad linguistic and cultural differences that exist among these four groups.

Hispanic American Children

A major factor in the English produced by Hispanic American bilingual-bicultural children is the Spanish language. A unique dialect is formed as a result of the influence of and borrowing from Spanish phonology, grammar, and vocabulary.

Varieties of Spanish-Influenced English.   Spanish, like English, has many national standard forms as well as nonstandard forms. Individuals from Mexico, Puerto Rico, and Cuba form the predominant groups in the Hispanic population of the United States. Consequently, those national varieties of Spanish are the most influential. The last two censuses, however, have shown a significant increase in Central and South American immigration, so that groups from El Salvador, Guatemala, Colombia, and Honduras are now more numerous and will have a greater impact on dialectal learning (U.S. Bureau of the Census, 2001). Clearly, many varieties of Spanish are spoken in America, which means that a wide range of effects on children are possible.

Language Profiles of Hispanic American Bilingual-Bicultural Children.   Several variables interact to produce different language profiles among Hispanic American children. First, and most important, children's relative proficiency in English and Spanish can vary greatly, depending on such factors as the following:

- The age at which they were introduced to English and its effect on simultaneous or sequential acquisition

- The bilingual fluency of the parents and other significant language models
- The bilingual requirements or opportunities of the environment in which the children live

Table 9.3 shows the different ways in which two languages may be mixed or kept separate. Some Hispanic American children may be truly bilingual, highly competent in both their comprehension and production of Spanish and English. Others may have a dominant language that they are able to speak and understand well. They will naturally prefer to use this language in all situations that allow it. Another possibility is for children to know elements of both Spanish and English but lack competence and confidence in either one. These children may be able to communicate effectively only by switching back and forth between the languages and by mixing Spanish and English vocabularies. Children with such low mixed dominance are not necessarily language disordered. Those who are language impaired probably mix languages as a compensatory strategy but may not do it well, while those who are not, mix languages as a result of environmental influences and probably do so with relative ease.

A final group of Hispanic American children may be monolingual, communicating only in English or Spanish. Obviously, children who are ethnic Hispanics and may have Spanish surnames are not obligated to know the Spanish language. This situation will occur more frequently in second- and later-generation families. Because of cultural traditions the children may know a considerable number of Spanish words and idioms, but they are functionally monolingual. In contrast, children who have recently arrived in the United States or have been raised in tightly knit Hispanic American communities may speak only Spanish.

TABLE 9.3   Profiles of Language Mixing and Separation

Monolingual English	Comprehends and produces English only.
Low mixed English/other language	Comprehends and produces both languages imperfectly, though English is slightly stronger. Mixes the languages in speaking.
English dominant	Comprehends and produces English well. Uses other language when required but has less proficiency with it.
Bilingual	Comprehends and produces both languages equally well. Code-switches easily.
Other language dominant	Comprehends and produces other language well. Uses English when required but has less proficiency with it.
Low mixed other language/English	Comprehends and produces both languages imperfectly, though other language is slightly stronger. Mixes the languages in speaking.
Monolingual other language	Comprehends and produces other language only.

Like other monolingual children, they may have acquired some vocabulary, but otherwise they are incompetent in English.

A second variable affecting Hispanic American children's language profiles is the dialect or dialects to which they are exposed. One child might learn a Puerto Rican standard form of Spanish and an AAVE nonstandard form of English. Another child might combine a nonstandard form of Mexican Spanish with SAE. The possible combinations are potentially as great as the number of varieties of Spanish and English. In actuality, however, common combinations will be determined by patterns of immigration and settlement in the United States.

Individual variation in Hispanic American children's pragmatic language profiles will be largely influenced by variables such as family expectations, ethnic pride, and cultural beliefs (Brice, 2001; Salas-Provance, Erickson, & Reed, 2002). We have noted that the Hispanic community in the United States is now quite diverse, which makes it increasingly difficult to generalize about "Hispanic culture" or "Hispanic value systems." It remains fair to say, however, that Hispanic American children often display pragmatic communicative behaviors that are different from those of white middle-class children. They may, for instance, show more reluctance to extend topics—providing more information than is requested—in conversations with adults (Pajewski & Enriquez, 1996). Extending topics, which is valued as a sign of creativity and social skill among most whites, may be considered disrespectful among certain Hispanic American groups.

Phonological Differences.   Spanish has slightly fewer consonants than American English, about eighteen versus about twenty-four. Table 9.4 compares the two consonant systems in terms of three groups. There are several sounds that are produced identically or very nearly so. The pronunciation of these sounds presents little difficulty to bilingual or second language learners of English. There is a smaller group of sounds that occur only in English. Speakers of Spanish will typically substitute phonetically similar Spanish sounds. For example, /s/ or /t/ will be substituted for "th," /s/ for /z/, and "ch" for "sh." Sounds in the sec-

TABLE 9.4   Consonants of Spanish and English

1. Consonants pronounced alike: f, s, h, m, n, l, w, j, "ng"

2. English consonants that do not exist in Spanish: z "sh," "zh" (except in Argentina),
   /dʒ/ "th" (except in central Spain)

3. Consonants pronounced differently	Explanation of Spanish pronunciation
b, v	Pronounced the same, as a voiced bilabial fricative, a sound that does not exist in English.
p, k, "ch"	Produced without the following aspiration.
t, d	Produced as dental rather than alveolar stops. In intervocalic position, /d/ is produced as a voiced interdental fricative /ð/.
g	Produced as /g/ only when it follows /n/, e.g., in *tango*. Otherwise, it is produced as a voiced velar fricative, a sound that does not exist in English.
r	Produced either as a flap or an alveolar trill, depending on phonetic context.

Sources: Adapted from Butt & Benjamin (2000) and Goldstein (2001).

ond group in the table are ones that are sometimes or always produced differently in Spanish than in English. To the ear of a native English speaker, these consonants sound slightly distorted when native speakers of Spanish pronounce English words.

The Spanish vowel system also contains fewer sounds than its English counterpart, five as compared to twelve. Table 9.5 summarizes the points of contrast. All the Spanish vowels and diphthongs also exist in English, but there are seven vowels unique to English. Speakers of Spanish tend to substitute for these English vowels phonetically similar vowels, for example, /i/ for /ɪ/ and /a/ for /ʌ/.

Another major influence on vowel production in the two languages is the difference in prosodic features. In English, the duration of vowels varies, depending on whether they occur in stressed or unstressed syllables. Thus, in the word *elephant,* the vowel in the first, stressed, syllable is /ɛ/; the vowel in the second, unstressed, syllable is /ə/. In Spanish, vowel length is nearly constant. Therefore, in the word *elefante,* the vowels in the first, second, and fourth syllables are all /ɛ/. There is a natural tendency for native speakers of Spanish to retain their habit of producing equal vowel duration when they speak English. This habit, along with the vowel substitutions mentioned earlier, yields pronunciations such as /presiden/ for *president,* /telefon/ for *telephone,* and /mekani/ for *mechanic.*

The contrasts we have drawn thus far are between the phonetic features of English and Spanish, that is, differences in which sounds are produced and how they are produced. There are also a number of phonological differences that can affect the pronunciation of bilingual children. Some of the most important ones are as follows.

- The fricative /ð/ occurs only in intervocalic position in Spanish. Thus, in speaking English, it is typically substituted for by /d/ in prevocalic (e.g., *this*) or postvocalic (e.g., *smooth*) positions.
- In several dialects of Spanish (e.g., Cuban), /s/ is omitted in postvocalic position.
- Consonant clusters containing /s/ as the first sound such as /sp/, /st/, and /sk/ do not occur in the word-initial position in Spanish. Consequently, native speakers will often insert a vowel before the cluster so that it conforms to the Spanish phonological rule, for example, /eskul/ for *school.*
- Consonant clusters containing /s/ as the last sound, such as /ps/, /ts/, and /ks/, do not occur in word-final position in Spanish. These clusters are commonly reduced in English words, for example, /βak/ for *box* or /kot/ for *coats.*
- The only word-final consonants in Spanish are /s, n, r, l, d/. All other words end in vowels. Therefore, the tendency is to omit consonants (e.g., /kæn/ for *can't*) or add vowels to the ends of words, especially when the English and Spanish words are cognates (e.g., /fruta/ for *fruit*).

TABLE 9.5 Vowels and Diphthongs of Spanish and English

Vowels pronounced alike: a, e, i, o, u (though they are not lengthened as in English)

Diphthongs pronounced alike: aɪ, aʊ, iu, ɔɪ

English vowels and diphthongs that do not exist in Spanish: ɪ, ɛ, æ, ʌ, ə, ɔ, ʊ, oʊ

Sources: Adapted from Butt & Benjamin (2000) and Goldstein (2001).

It is important to be aware of phonological differences such as these because they frequently contain the key to understanding what seem to be inconsistencies in pronunciation. For example, a Hispanic American child may correctly pronounce the consonants in the words /feðo/ *feather,* /soni/ *sunny,* and /mostod/ *mustard* but have difficulty with some of the same sounds in the words /do/ *those,* /leto/ *lettuce,* and /estó/ *stove.* It is also important to remember that the different dialects of Spanish can influence pronunciation differentially and that this, too, can be a key in understanding a child's phonological characteristics (Goldstein & Iglesias, 2001).

Grammatical Differences.   Comparison of English and Spanish grammar is considerably more complex than comparison of phonology because of the number of features involved. Many differences are relevant only to the language of adults and need not concern us in our discussion of children's grammatical learning. Some of the distinctions that are most pertinent to children are these:

■ The position of adjectives in the noun phrase is more flexible in Spanish. The rules determining which adjectives precede and which follow a noun are difficult to formulate (Butt & Benjamin, 2000). However, the fact that Spanish allows postmodifying adjectives makes it more likely that bilingual children will attempt to use this structure in English, for example, *car green* instead of *green car.*

■ Nearly all Spanish adjectives can function as nouns if preceded by an article or demonstrative. English requires an indefinite pronoun to express the same meaning; for example *los rojos* (literally, *the reds*) has the same meaning as *the red ones* in English.

■ Indefinite articles are omitted following certain uses of the copula, certain common verbs (*have, buy, take, look for, wear*), and certain prepositions.

■ In referring to parts of the body, clothing, or other personal belongings, the possessive pronoun is replaced by the definite article; for example, "Me quité los calcetines" is translated literally as "I took off the (i.e., my) socks."

■ Spanish does not require the auxiliary verb *do* to support the transformation of statements into questions ("He did it"→ "Did he do it?") or statements into negative commands ("Do it!"→ "Don't do it!"). Questions are instead marked by rising intonation and negative commands by the insertion of *no* at the beginning of the sentence.

■ Plurality is marked more redundantly in Spanish than in English. For instance, in the sentence, "Han llegado los dos niños colombianos"/"The two Colombian boys have arrived," plurality is marked five times: on the auxiliary verb, the article, the quantifier, the noun, and the adjective. Such redundancy permits Spanish speakers to omit some of the markers without loss of information. Omission of plural markers is especially common in dialects that delete the postvocalic /s/ (Iglesias & Anderson, 1993).

■ Negation is marked on all constituents of a negative sentence; for example "Nunca veía a nadie en ninguna de las habitaciones" translates literally as "I never saw nobody in none of the rooms." *No* is used for all negation in the verb phrase, for example, "No puedo" ("I can't") or "No está aquí" ("He isn't here"). There is no equivalent to *not.*

Characteristics of Spanish-Influenced English.   The basic framework for identifying and understanding characteristics of Spanish-influenced English is knowledge of the two languages and the differences between them. We should recall, however, that the interaction between the languages is influenced by dialectal variation within Spanish and English. Moreover, it is not clear that interference from Spanish is the major cause of errors in Hispanic American children's learning of English. Recent research on bilingual language learning suggests that grammatical forms are used in a language-specific manner (De Houwer, 1995). That is, children tend to maintain separation between the syntactic rules and morphological forms relevant to different languages they are acquiring.

Interference effects appear to be more potent in explaining the phonological characteristics of Spanish-influenced English. Table 9.6 provides examples of both grammatical and phonological interference errors that may be observed in Hispanic American children. The frequency and consistency of such errors is likely to vary depending on when and how the children begin to learn English, as well as the degree of balance in their competence with the two languages.

African American Children

Many African American children learn a nonstandard dialect of American English. At one time this dialect was commonly described as "Black English." However, that term implied that the dialect was used by all African Americans, which is not the case. Consequently, it was replaced by the description "Black English *Vernacular*" and then, more recently, *African American Vernacular English* (AAVE), to emphasize that it is the dialect of a particular speech community and not of an entire race. Sociolinguistic studies suggest that AAVE is used to some extent by most African Americans, but that the degree of usage

TABLE 9.6   Phonological and Grammatical Interference Errors Found in Spanish-Influenced English

Example	Errors	Explanation
She /tʃ i/ no can help	■ Substitution of /tʃ/ "ch" for /ʃ/ "sh" ■ Incorrect negative in the verb phrase	■ /tʃ/ "ch" not used in Spanish; /ʃ/ "sh" is the closest form ■ *no* is the only negative form in the verb phrase and always precedes the verb it modifies
I want /wan/ *the* /di/ *big*	■ Reduction of cluster /nt/→ /n/ ■ Substitution of /d/ for /ð/ ■ Omission of indefinite pronoun *one*	■ Spanish words do not end in /t/; cluster is reduced to conform with this rule ■ /ð/ not used in word-initial position; /d/ is the closest form ■ Article + adjective is the Spanish equivalent of the English phrase article + adjective + *one*
He wearing /weɾin/ *shirt* /tʃut/, *no?*	■ Substitution of flap for /r/; substitution of /n/ for "ng"; substitution of "ch" for "sh" ■ Omission of auxiliary verb *is* ■ Omission of indefinite article *a* ■ Use of *no* and rising intonation to form tag question	■ Sounds do not exist in Spanish or are not allowed in certain phonetic contexts; closest forms are substituted ■ Immature verb form (*not* an interference error) ■ Indefinite articles not used following verb *wear* ■ *No* + rising intonation is the Spanish tag form when seeking agreement from listener

varies by socioeconomic group. African Americans of lower socioeconomic groups are more likely to use a higher percentage of AAVE linguistic features, whereas those of upper and middle socioeconomic groups tend to use fewer features (Wolfram & Schilling-Estes, 1998). Although AAVE is socially stratified, its use does not necessarily indicate a difference in the social background or education of the speaker. However, because the dialect can be difficult for SAE speakers to understand, even listeners who are professionals can mistakenly form impressions about intelligence from speech characteristics alone (Bleile, McGowan, & Bernthal, 1997).

Historical Issues.   The origin of AAVE has in the past been a disputed and controversial subject. Language is a major source of ethnic identity, and the origin of a language can become an issue of ethnic pride as well as a topic of academic study. One early view of AAVE was that it was merely a *restricted code,* that is, a variety of language used by lower social classes that is characterized by, among other things, reduced syntax and a reliance on context for the interpretation of meaning (Crystal, 1997). This opinion of AAVE has been largely abandoned, though the issue of a restricted code among lower social classes continues to be argued.

Scholars agree that AAVE had its origins among the slave communities of the U.S. South and then spread to northern urban centers as African Americans migrated to those regions. There has been disagreement, however, about how the dialect first became established among the slaves. For example, some of the linguistic features of AAVE are also found in British dialects that were spoken in the early periods of southern U.S. history. The best-supported and most widely accepted view is that AAVE began in Africa as a *pidgin,* or very limited trade language, used to facilitate commerce between Europeans and Africans. When a slave trade developed during the 1600s, this pidgin language came with the Africans to southeastern America. There it gradually merged with English to form a language of its own, known as a *creole* language, which has a systematic and elaborated grammar and vocabulary (Rickford, 1998). This creole language gradually evolved into what we recognize today as AAVE. What is apparent from historical study is that AAVE is a systematic and rule-governed variety of English that has evolved through processes that are well known to linguists. It should be viewed, therefore, as an independent linguistic system that is related to SAE but that has many of its own formal and functional characteristics.

Characteristics of AAVE.   AAVE may be contrasted with SAE at each level of linguistic structure: pragmatics, semantics, phonology, and grammar. To a speaker of SAE, the interaction of AAVE speakers may appear to be highly assertive and perhaps even excessively demonstrative. Loud talking, heated public arguments, and frequent interruptions of one's conversational partners are considered acceptable pragmatic behaviors in AAVE. On the other hand, certain behaviors that SAE speakers may consider acceptable or only mildly rude are intolerable to AAVE speakers—for example, asking personal questions of a new acquaintance or trying to break in on a conversation (Taylor, 1990). Thus, neither dialect should be considered more polite than the other.

AAVE has been a fertile ground for the development of slang, especially among inner-city populations. This is hardly surprising, because slang's most consistent function is to mark social or linguistic identity (Crystal, 1997). Some of the slang generated by AAVE, such as the adjective *cool,* the verb *diss,* or the noun *props,* have crossed over and become part of SAE. Other words and idiomatic phrases have remained unique to AAVE and are not understandable to individuals who do not know the dialect (Smitherman, 2000).

The major phonological features of AAVE affecting vowels and consonants are summarized in Table 9.7. Other phonological differences exist in the prosody of AAVE, such as greater vowel prolongation and varied intonation contours (Hyter, 1998). As indicated earlier, these features are characteristic of the dialect as a whole but are found to varying degrees in individual speakers. Many features common to AAVE phonology, such as weak-syllable deletion and final cluster reduction also occur in other English vernaculars, spoken by other ethnic groups (Pollock, 2001). There is also overlap between AAVE and the phonological features common to young children, regardless of whether they are learning a standard or nonstandard dialect of English (Bleile & Wallach, 1992; Seymour & Seymour, 1981). It appears, therefore, that the phonological systems of AAVE and SAE speakers do not become fully differentiated until later in childhood.

Table 9.8 shows some of the principal features of AAVE grammar. Some grammatical markers that are obligatory in SAE are deleted in AAVE in contexts where they are redundant. For example, the possessive noun marker will be absent in the sentence "That be Rhonda purse" but present in the sentence "That be Rhonda's." Interactions can occur between phonological and grammatical features of AAVE (Stockman, 1996a). For instance, the singular form of *desk* would be pronounced in AAVE as /dɛs/. To form the plural and yet still avoid a consonant cluster, AAVE speakers will produce /dɛsəz/ unless the word follows a numerical quantifier. In that case, the plural marker will be omitted: "My school got a hundred desk /dɛs/." Thus, the dialect's variations from SAE are both consistent and logical.

TABLE 9.7   Phonological Features of AAVE

Phonological Variation	Example
Deletion of nasal at the end of a word and nasalization of the preceding vowel	comb → co/ko/ (with vowel nasalized) man → ma/mæ/ (with vowel nasalized)
Deletion of semivowels /r/ and /l/	store → sto/sto/ fool → foo/fu/ help → hep/hɛp/
Devoicing and weakening of final stops	hat → ha/hæ/ mad → mat/mæt/ or ma/mæ/ cake → ca/k/ big → bid/bɪd/ or bi/bɪ/
Simplification of consonant clusters at the end of a word	last → lass/læs/ soft → sof/sɔf/
Substitution of f/th"th" in the middle and at the end of a word; substitution of /v/θ/ in the middle of a word	tooth → toof/tuf/ brother → brover/brʌvə /
Substitution of stop for interdental fricative at the beginning of a word	that → dat/dæt/ thin → tin/tɪn/

Sources: Craig, Thompson, Washington, & Potter (2003) and Pollock (2001).

TABLE 9.8   Grammatical Features of AAVE

Grammatical Variation	Example
Deletion of possessive marker with adjacent nouns	That Bobby bike (= Bobby's bike)
Deletion of plural marker when a numerical quantifier is used	I got two card
Different formation of indirect questions	I asked him did he know her name
No final -s in the third-person singular present tense	That dog bark all the time
Use of double negatives involving the auxiliary verb at the beginning of a sentence	Can't nobody fix that thing
Use of *be* to mark habitual action	I be goin' to school every day
Use of the copula is not obligatory	He mad
	My brother real big

Sources: Adapted from Nelson (1998); Nelson & Hyter (1990); and Wolfram & Schilling-Estes (1998).

Asian American Children

Asian Americans are the most culturally and linguistically diverse of the major ethnic groups in the United States. There is no agreement on which nationalities should be included in the category of *Asian,* as it is not clear whether this term refers to a racial sub-type, a geographic area, or a linguistic grouping. For our purposes, it will refer to a particular group of languages. Some languages, such as those spoken in India and the Philippines, will be excluded from our discussion, even though these might also be considered Asian.

Varieties of Asian Languages.   The classification of languages raises some problems for which there are no clear solutions. Languages are usually compared in terms of their structural characteristics (grammar, vocabulary, and phonology) and historical origins. However, the weighting given to different structural levels is purely arbitrary. Thus, two languages that are grammatically distinct might be placed in different families, even though they share many phonological features. Historical information can assist in resolving some structural issues, but there are problems even here. Two languages that are historically distinct may be used by ethnic groups that, through migration and resettlement, come to live in the same area. Over time the two languages that were once distinct will begin to influence and borrow from one another.

Asian languages that are widely spoken by immigrants to the United States are listed in Table 9.9, along with some of the phonological features of those languages that contrast with English. As can be seen, the phonological structure of Asian languages is markedly different from that of English. They tend to have a simpler segmental structure, with fewer vowels and consonants and with word shapes that are largely monosyllabic and contain few consonant clusters. However, the suprasegmental structure of Asian languages, most of which are tonal languages, is generally richer, with variation in tone and vowel length used

TABLE 9.9   Examples of Languages Widely Spoken among Asian Immigrant Populations and Their Contrasting Phonological Features

Language	Where Spoken	Contrasting Phonological Features
Japanese	Japan	No word-final consonants, only five vowels, contrastive vowel length
Korean	North and South Korea, parts of China, Japan, and Russia	Contrastive vowel length
Mon-Khmer family		
Khmer	Kampuchea (Cambodia)	Large repertoire of consonant clusters
Vietnamese	Kampuchea (Cambodia), Laos, Vietnam	Tone language, no consonant clusters, essentially monosyllabic, only six final consonants
Sino-Tibetan family		
Chinese (Cantonese and Mandarin)	China	Tone language, no consonant clusters, essentially monosyllabic, few final consonants
Hmong	Northern Laos, Thailand, Vietnam	Tone language, only word-initial consonant clusters, only one final consonant
Tai family		
Lao (Laotian)	Laos, Thailand	Tone language, essentially monosyllabic

Sources: Adapted from Cheng (1987a, 1987b); Crystal (1997); and Hwa-Froelich et al. (2002).

to signal differences in word meaning. In fact, intonation patterns are often identified as among the major contributors to linguistic differences between some Asian languages and English.

Characteristics of Asian-Influenced English.   The English spoken by Asian American children may show the effect of interference from their native Asian language. The extent of this interference depends on the bilingual profile presented by each child. Recall that Table 9.3 shows a range of profiles that may be demonstrated by different children learning two languages. The precise nature of the interference will depend on the cultural and linguistic experiences of each child. For example, the language and behavior of a Hmong child may show little resemblance to that of a Korean child. Table 9.10 summarizes some of the phonological and grammatical interference errors that are likely to occur in native speakers of Chinese or Vietnamese. Similar errors may be found among speakers of other Asian languages.

Besides their differences in language form, Asian American children may vary in their pragmatic behavior. Because Asian cultural mores generally discourage children from interrupting or asserting themselves with adults, they may appear passive when observed alongside other American children. They may seem to avoid eye contact in dyadic conversation and yet stare openly in other situations (Cheng, 1998). While pragmatic differences of this kind are subtle and may not interfere at all with peer interaction, they can interfere with assessment efforts and might be wrongly taken as an indication of limited language competence.

TABLE 9.10   Phonological and Grammatical Interference Errors Found in the English of Native Chinese and Vietnamese Speakers

Example	Errors
We go you house /haʊ/ yesterday /jɛtuʼde/ (= We went to your house yesterday)	■ Omission of word-final /s/ (*house*) ■ Reduction of cluster /st/→/t/ (*yesterday*) ■ Incorrect syllable stress (*yesterday*) ■ Use of unmarked verb form (*go*) for irregular past-tense form (*sent*) ■ Substitution of pronominal forms (*you/your*) ■ Omission of preposition *to*
Him no buy book /bʊ/? (= Didn't he buy the book?)	■ Omission of word-final /k/ (*book*) ■ Omission of article *the* ■ Simplified interrogative: auxiliary verb *did* omitted; question marked only by rising intonation ■ Use of unmarked verb form (*buy*) for expanded verb phrase (*did buy*) ■ Substitution of pronominal forms (*him/he*) ■ Simplified negation: marked only by use of *no*
That /dæ/ man two dollar /daral/ me (= That man gave me two dollars or That man gave two dollars to me)	■ Omission of word-final /t/ (*that*) ■ Substitution of /ð/→/d/ (*that*) ■ Substitution of liquid consonants /r/ and /l/ (*dollar*) ■ Omission of plural marker when preceded by numerical quantifier (*two dollar*) ■ Reversed ordering of direct and indirect objects (*two dollar me*) or omission of preposition *to*

Sources: Adapted from Cheng (1987a, b) and Hwa-Froelich et al. (2002).

Native American Children

Roughly half a million American Indian and Alaska Native students attend elementary and secondary schools in the United States. About 90 percent of these students attend public schools, while 10 percent attend schools operated or funded by the Bureau of Indian Affairs and tribes. Although Native American students represent less than 1 percent of the school-age population, they make up 1.3 percent of the special education population (U.S. Department of Education, 2001b). Native American students in special education are most often identified as having a specific learning disability, intellectual disability, emotional disturbance, or a speech–language impairment.

Language Preservation.   A unique consideration in discussing the language skills of Native American children is the growing efforts to preserve tribal languages. The issues surrounding these efforts are a complex mixture of history, linguistics, culture, and politics. Among the more pertinent considerations are these:

■ Only 2.5 percent of limited-English-proficient students in the United States are Native American (Fleischman & Hopstock, 1993). This means that the vast majority of Native American children learn English as their first language.

■ The impetus to maintain tribal languages is to prevent the demise of culture, though there is disagreement on this point within the Native American community.

■ Few curriculum materials exist for the teaching of Native American languages.

■ Some Native American students are under peer pressure not to learn or use their tribal language.

■ Dialectic differences and the absence of an acceptable orthography (spelling of the language) impede language maintenance in some communities.

■ Native American students living in cities may find access to tribal language instruction hindered by the fact that many different tribes and languages are represented in their schools and the community (Peacock & Day, 1999).

Cultural-Linguistic Differences.   The assessment of language skills in Native American children is complicated by differences in parenting practices and overall cultural expectations for language use (Harris, 1985; Robinson-Zañartu, 1996). Because of these differences, children from Native American homes may appear delayed in language and other developmental traits compared to children from the cultural mainstream. Robinson-Zañartu (1996) alerts us to the possibility that

> . . . direct and timed question and answer sequences common in psychometric testing and in classroom discourse are experienced as culturally inappropriate in many Native American groups. Such questioning may elicit silence, an "I don't know" response, or a reply that may seem unrelated. (p. 376)

Children may also struggle with the task of dealing with the materials used in many norm-referenced, standardized tests, such as pictures and booklets, particularly if their background is a more traditional one characterized by learning without books (Robinson-Zañartu, 1996). Cultural influences reflecting story traditions in Native American societies may also be seen in many of the narratives produced by these children, influences that potentially lead to content and structures of narratives that differ from those of mainstream narratives (John-Steiner & Panofsky, 1992; Kay-Raining Bird & Vetter, 1994; Westby & Roman, 1995). In particular, narratives may not progress in the linear, cause–effect fashion expected in most classrooms. It is also possible that some children will not have had practice in telling stories or communicating events in narrative form because only adults have the privilege of being designated storytellers (Paul, 2001). Results from parent questionnaires and standardized language tests, as well as narrative assessment, must therefore be interpreted with great care and an awareness of cultural influences (Long, 1998; Long & Christensen, 1998).

Characteristics of English Spoken by Native Americans.   Although most Native Americans learn English as their first language, the dialect that many of them speak differs from SAE in terms of its grammar, phonology, semantics, and rules of discourse. Table 9.11 lists some of the most commonly observed linguistic differences in what has been termed Indian English (Leap, 1993). Even among individuals who speak their ancestral language, standard English, or both, Indian English fluency is a way of reinforcing one's cultural identity for many Native Americans, especially where it is the only Indian-related language tradition that has been maintained in a community. Under such circumstances, Indian English fluency

TABLE 9.11   **Linguistic Features of English Spoken by Native Americans**

Variation	Example
Phonology Vowel shifting	Among Navajo English speakers, exchange of /ɪ/ and /ɛ/, /i/ and /ɪ/, /e/ and /ɛ/
Morphology Frequent deletion of plural and possessive marker	I read Diane['s] book Many of my relative[s] live in Shiprock
Use of base form or overregularized form for past tense verbs	I hear him sing yesterday I eated some
Syntax Left-branching dependent clauses	They ride bikes is what I see them do From the family is where we learn to be good
Deletion of articles and demonstratives	They find [a] bone in [that] deep yard He asked [the] shopkeeper for [that] sheep
Deletion of *be, have,* and *get* as auxiliary or copular verbs	She [is] Red Corn people Then they would tell them what law he [has] broken

Sources: Leap (1993) and Thurston (1998).

becomes a highly valued social skill, and the nonstandard features of the dialect take on an even greater cultural significance (St. Charles & Costantino, 2000).

The Influence of Poverty

To this point, we have examined the language development and language differences of ethnic American children from a purely cultural and linguistic perspective. In an ideal world, this would be the only viewpoint we would need to consider. It is apparent, however, that in a disproportionate number of cases, ethnic children are also children of poverty. While 9 percent of white children are poor, 30 percent of African American children and 28 percent of Hispanic American children are so classified (National Center for Children in Poverty, 2002). The effects of poverty on the general health and development of children are well known. Work (1991) writes:

> Children of poverty lack food, clothing, housing, medicine, and early learning assistance. These children face sickness, psychological stress, malnutrition, and underdevelopment. . . . As poor children progress through the school system, they face school failure, pregnancy, substance abuse, and economic stress. Illiteracy in the poor is endemic and cyclic as poor children become poor parents of more poor children. (p. 61)

Each of the problems identified in the preceding paragraph can increase the risk of disabling conditions, including language disorders. Poor mothers may not have received prenatal care during their pregnancies, and malnutrition and substance abuse can lead to premature delivery of babies with low birth weight. These babies have a substantially greater risk of incurring developmental problems, among them fetal alcohol syndrome (FAS), which is associated with conditions such as language-learning disabilities and intellectual disability. Even when poor children are born healthy, they can be raised in an environment that can be less stimulating and more dangerous than that of other children. As a result, they are likely to be delayed in certain areas of language learning compared to middle-class children. Poverty is also not disassociated with what might be familial transmission of specific language impairment, given the resultant literacy and consequent academic difficulties with the related vocational and economic limitations. This means that some children of poor parents may have an inherited language impairment because one or both of their parents has a language impairment.

All professionals should differentiate between environmental conditions that result from cultural differences and those that are due to poverty. Nutritional choices, methods of discipline, and styles of verbal interaction all vary across cultural groups. Though differences in these behaviors may have short-term effects on language learning, they are not associated with a greater prevalence of language disorders. In contrast, the consequences of poverty can harm a child's nervous system, either from birth or during the early formative years. Such damage can lead to long-term language deficits from which a child is unlikely to recover.

Issues in Assessment

It is estimated that 10 percent of the members of all racial/ethnic minority groups have disorders of speech, language, or hearing, the same percentage as the U.S. population as a whole (Deal-Williams, 2002). The unique issue in the case of linguistically-culturally diverse children is that their language can be evaluated and categorized in any of four different ways:

1. Typically developing and speaking SAE
2. Typically developing and speaking a nonstandard dialect or form influenced by another language
3. Atypically developing and speaking SAE
4. Atypically developing and speaking a nonstandard dialect or form influenced by another language

The key to fair assessment is to determine each child's dialectal status and not allow a language variation to interfere with the judgments made about language learning-ability. This requires an awareness of the structural differences found in the particular linguistic influences and a critical attitude toward assessment instruments, which may ignore the possibility of linguistic variation (Seymour, Roeper, & de Villiers, 2003).

Testing Bias

Standardized testing is based on the premise of peer comparison. Stimuli are presented in an invariant manner to children of the same age so that their responses can be compared and each child's performance ranked. In order to determine a valid ranking, no child can be put at a disadvantage in responding to the test items. Thus, a child who is ill would not be tested, and special assistance must be provided if tests are to be used with children who have sensory or motor handicaps. It is sometimes more difficult to recognize the disadvantages faced by linguistically-culturally diverse children who undergo standardized testing. There are obstacles to be overcome in nearly every aspect of the evaluation process (Sattler, 2001). Some of the most common are as follows.

1. *Cultural bias.* Many standardized tests reflect white, middle-class backgrounds. This is typically seen in the choice of tasks and stimulus items. For example, it is routinely assumed that children will enjoy the activities of listening to stories, pointing to pictures, and answering requests for information. Such activities are common in middle-class households, and children from these homes have usually been reinforced extensively for taking part. But linguistically-culturally diverse children may lack these experiences. Hence, these children may arrive at a testing session unprepared and unmotivated for the kinds of activities that will be presented to them.

2. *Examiner sensitivity bias.* Professionals who administer standardized tests may not be familiar with the linguistic and cultural characteristics of the linguistically-culturally diverse children they are asked to evaluate. This condition opens up the possibility of several types of misinterpretation. The speech of the linguistically-culturally diverse children may be only marginally intelligible to the examiner, who then must frequently ask for repetition or clarification. Such frequent requests can be interpreted by children as an indication that they are performing poorly, which may make them reluctant to participate in the assessment. Another source of misinterpretation may be the pragmatic behavior of a child. As we have seen, linguistically-culturally diverse children may differ in their pattern of eye contact and in their willingness to respond to requests for information. An examiner who is unaware of these differences may construe these behaviors as nervousness, uncertainty, ignorance, defiance, or disorder.

3. *Examiner expectations bias.* The experiences of certain examiners may lead them to anticipate a particular pattern of behavior from linguistically-culturally diverse children. Although standardized tests try to reduce variation in examiner procedures, some discretion is always allowed. For example, most tests do not specify how long an examiner must wait for a child to respond to an item. Most examiners rely on their intuition in deciding whether a child is still thinking or does not know an answer. This intuition is formed from previous experiences with children. If those experiences suggest that a child will perform poorly, then the examiner is less likely to believe that additional time will enable a correct response.

4. *Overinterpretation bias.* A danger attached to all standardized assessment is that the examiner will draw broad conclusions from limited test data. For instance, it is inappropriate to conclude that a child's language comprehension is generally impaired when the only data to support this statement is a low score on a test of receptive vocabulary. With monolingual, middle-class children without issues of linguistic and cultural variation, such bias is avoided by administering more than one test and by combining information from standardized and nonstandardized assessment procedures. The same practice should be followed with linguistically-culturally diverse children. However, fewer tests are available that have been standardized on this population, and nonstandardized assessment can be difficult without the assistance of someone knowledgeable about a child's linguistic and cultural background.

5. *Linguistic bias.* Some tests may contain English words or idioms that are unfamiliar to linguistically-culturally diverse children. This may reduce the number of items to which a child responds or may change the demands of a task. For example, a child from a linguistically-culturally diverse background may not know some of the English words for common household items, which are frequently used in tests because they are assumed to be familiar. Language bias may also occur inadvertently in the idiomatic prompts and reinforcers used by the examiner, such as "Don't take your eyes off it" or "That's the way."

The problem of bias is not limited to tests or examiners. Linguistically-culturally diverse children are likely to vary their performance, depending on how they perceive a communicative situation. For example, African American children may not use AAVE in settings that are perceived as formal (Hester, 1996). If children try to communicate in SAE and they do not know this dialect as well as AAVE, the results of the assessment will be misleadingly low. On the other hand, children who are able to code-switch effectively from AAVE to SAE may leave the impression that they speak only the standard dialect.

The concern over test bias applies to all instruments used to evaluate children's developmental abilities. Federal education law (IDEA) mandates that all students be evaluated using nondiscriminatory evaluations and multiple forms of assessment. IDEA also requires that students be assessed in their native language or other mode of communication. If tests are not available in the student's native language, interpreters should be used. For students identified as limited English proficient, tests should focus on assessing the impact of the child's disability on his or her educational performance rather than assessing the child's English language skills.

Standardized intelligence tests have long been criticized for underestimating the competence of linguistically-culturally diverse children (Sattler, 2001). To reduce the bias inherent in intelligence instruments, it has been proposed that they be administered to linguistically-culturally diverse children only in a translated form. Translation of test items is difficult, however, without affecting the sensitivity of the test. An alternative approach is to develop norms for specific ethnic groups, as has been done for the Wechsler Intelligence Scale for Children—Third Edition (WISC-III) administered to Navajo children (Tempest, 1998).

For many years, standardized language tests have also been analyzed for evidence of bias. Examples of findings from the literature over three decades are the following.

■ From kindergarten to fourth grade, African American students obtained increasingly lower scores than white students on the Grammatic Closure subtest of the Illinois Test of Psycholinguistic Abilities (Kirk, McCarthy, & Kirk, 1968). This appears to be due to the appearance of more AAVE grammatical features in older African American students (Arnold & Reed, 1976).

■ African American children in Head Start programs in a rural area of Alabama scored significantly lower on the Preschool Language Assessment Instrument (Blank, Rose, & Berlin, 1978) than white children from the same programs (Haynes, Haak, Moran, Rice, & Johnson, 1995). On components of the same tool that tap higher level, decentralized, and metalinguistic tasks (Levels III and IV), African American children in Georgia again performed significantly lower than their white peers (Fagundes, Haynes, Haak, & Moran, 1998).

■ On another preschool language test, the Preschool Language Scale—3 (Zimmerman, Steiner, & Pond, 1992), African American preschoolers from low-income families scored an average of one standard deviation below the expected mean for their age, primarily because of their poor performance on items containing language features not part of their dialect (Qi, Kaiser, Milan, Yzquierdo, & Hancock, 2003).

- Both white and African American children from a rural area of northeastern Georgia obtained scores on the Wepman Auditory Discrimination Test (Wepman, 1958) that were lower than those predicted by the test's norms (Hirshoren & Ambrose, 1976).

- African American children matched for age and grade level with white children obtained statistically lower scores on the Peabody Picture Vocabulary Test (Dunn, 1965) (Kreschek & Nicolosi, 1973).

- The scores of bilingual Hispanic children were almost two standard deviations below the mean for monolingual children on both the Expressive One-Word Picture Vocabulary Test (Gardner, 1979, 1983) and the Peabody Picture Vocabulary Test—Revised (Dunn & Dunn, 1981; Teuber & Furlong, 1985).

- Hispanic American and African American preschool children were more successful at imitating sentences containing AAVE features, while their white counterparts performed better with SAE stimuli (Stephens, 1976).

- The Test of Language Development (Newcomer & Hammill, 1977), when administered to young AAVE-speaking children, yielded scores significantly lower than those reported in the norms (Wiener, Lewnau, & Erway, 1983).

- A wide range of scores has been obtained when the Spanish version of the Test for Auditory Comprehension of Language (Carrow, 1973) has been administered to different groups of Hispanic American children (Linares-Orama & Sanders, 1977; Rueda & Perozzi, 1977; Wilcox & Aasby, 1988). This variation appears to be due to differences in the socioeconomic status and educational experiences of the different subject groups. Similarly, Spanish-speaking bilingual children with normal language skills performed notably below the norms on the Spanish Version of the Preschool Language Scale—3 (Zimmerman, Steiner, & Pond, 1993), further indicating potential bias even in tests designed to be appropriate for bilingual children (Restrepo & Silverman, 2001).

It is apparent, therefore, that many standardized language tests are significantly biased against linguistically-culturally diverse children. This issue is of enormous concern to professional organizations involved in debates over assessment practices. Several organizations and task forces have called for a moratorium on the administration of tests in translation or the use of tests that do not take account of nonstandard language forms or include ethnic minority populations in their standardization group (Figueroa & Hernandez, 2000; Vaughn-Cooke, 1983). Such dramatic action, along with other efforts to increase professional awareness of multiculturalism, has prompted publishers to revise existing tests and develop new instruments that better meet the needs of linguistically-culturally diverse children. One such example is the Diagnostic Evaluation of Language Variance (DELV)—Criterion Referenced (Seymour et al., 2003), a language test described as attempting to neutralize the impact of a child's use of nonmainstream American English on results. While these efforts to revise tests and develop new ones are positive steps in addressing the issues of test bias and producing valuable and useful assessment instruments, it is not always a strategy as successful or valid as it might appear (Anderson, 1996; Restrepo, 1998; Restrepo & Silverman, 2001).

We know that children's production of narratives can especially reflect cultural differences (John-Steiner & Panofsky, 1992; Kay-Raining Bird & Vetter, 1994; Robinson-Zañartu, 1996; Westby & Roman, 1995). It is essential, therefore, that professionals attempt to consider the ways in which storytelling activities are reflected in children's particular cultures so that these can be analyzed in ways that do not lead to biased interpretations and misidentify different narrative structures, content, or sequences as evidence of impairment when these may be quite appropriate and consistent with expectations in the children's home and cultures. It is possible, however, that differences identified as culturally based can become a bridge to helping children learn other ways of conveying narratives that are more consistent with the mainstream classroom in which they are needing to function (Westby & Roman, 1995).

Differential Diagnosis of Communicative Behaviors

Professionals who work with linguistically-culturally diverse children face the challenge of distinguishing between language differences and language disorders. The principles and requirements of this task were stated succinctly in a 1983 position paper and have remained the same since:

> . . . no dialectal variety of English is a disorder or a pathological form of speech or language. Each social dialect is adequate as a functional and effective variety of English.
> . . . It is indeed possible for dialect speakers to have linguistic disorders within the dialect. An essential step toward making accurate assessments of communicative disorders is to distinguish between those aspects of linguistic variation that represent the diversity of the English language from those that represent speech, language, and hearing disorders. The speech-language pathologist must have certain competencies to distinguish between dialectal differences and communicative disorders. These competencies include knowledge of the particular dialect as a rule-governed linguistic system, knowledge of the phonological and grammatical features of the dialect, and knowledge of nondiscriminatory testing procedures. (ASHA Committee on the Status of Racial Minorities, 1983)

The process of language evaluation for linguistically-culturally diverse children follows the usual steps of screening, assessment, and intervention. Figure 9.1 illustrates the progression of a language evaluation for such a child. Because not all minority children are bilingual or use a nonstandard dialect, Step 1 is to screen the child with an instrument that is based on and standardized for SAE. If the child passes this screening, an optional second screening may be carried out to determine whether the child is also competent in a second language or in a nonstandard dialect. Children who fail the initial SAE screening should then be tested, if possible, in their native or dominant language or nonstandard dialect (Peña, Bedore, & Rappazzo, 2003). A passing score on this screening would then tend to establish that a child is not language impaired but rather language different.

Children who fail both language screenings arrive at Step 2, along with children who fail the SAE screening and cannot be tested in their native language or dialect. These children should now be evaluated more fully to determine whether they are actually language impaired. If nonbiased, norm-referenced tests are available, they can be administered. If a child receives passing scores on these tests, the result of the screenings would be discarded and the child would be assessed as a competent speaker of a second language or nonstandard dialect. If appropriate norm-referenced instruments do not exist to suit a particular

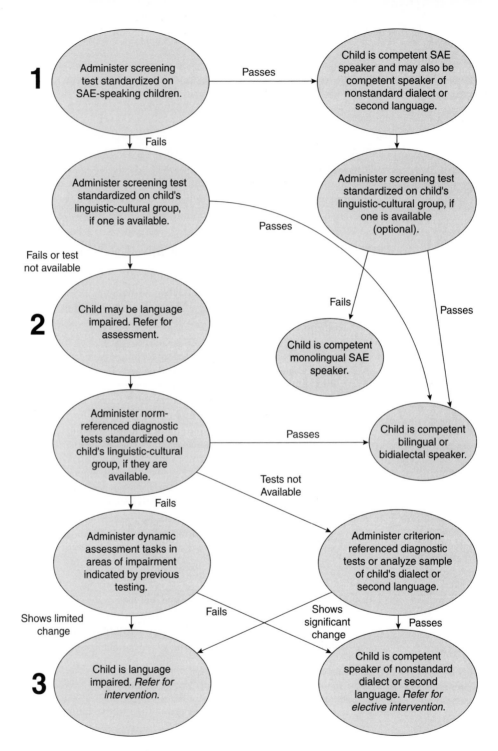

FIGURE 9.1   Model of Differential Diagnosis for Linguistically-Culturally Diverse Children

child, then criterion-referenced tests or language sampling can be used to evaluate competence (Hernandez, 1994). Language samples can be obtained by recording conversation that occurs during play. During this interaction, however, care should be taken to avoid the kinds of interactions (e.g., interview) that are uncommon among members of certain racial/ethnic groups. Samples gathered in settings familiar to the children or while interacting with family members may increase the ecological validity of the samples. The samples that are gathered should be evaluated using developmental criteria that have been well referenced for the speech community to which a child belongs. For example, Black English Sentence Scoring (BESS) (Nelson & Hyter, 1990), an adaptation of Developmental Sentence Scoring (Lee, 1974), represents an attempt to honor the grammatical features of AAVE, as well as to compare young African American children to their linguistic peers.

A child who fails a norm-referenced assessment using culturally and linguistically fair test instruments should then undergo dynamic assessment trials in those areas of language that appear deficient. If the child shows significant behavioral change during these trials, the poor test score can be attributed to cultural differences rather than an underlying language impairment (Peña, Iglesias, & Lidz, 2001; Ukrainetz, Harpell, Walsh, & Coyle, 2000). Intervention in that case should focus on the elective goal of helping the child adjust to the mainstream culture and its methods of evaluation. However, if the child responds poorly to dynamic assessment— fails to attend or generalize new learning—then intervention for language impairment should proceed (Step 3), still with consideration of the child's multicultural needs.

The protocol just described and shown in Figure 9.1 is truly workable only if more nondiscriminatory assessment instruments become available. As a first step, some tests written in SAE and originally normed on mostly mainstream populations have been renormed on minority populations. Such an approach is inadequate, however, because it only serves to verify that a child is incompetent as a speaker of SAE. What is needed are measures that can establish children's competencies in their native languages or nonstandard dialects. To serve this purpose, the tests must be conceived and developed specifically to evaluate a minority population. For example, in the case of AAVE speakers, test tasks and stimulus items should be developed and field tested with African American children to ensure that they are both motivating and familiar. The standardization population for the test must be representative of AAVE speakers nationwide. At a minimum, it should be reflective of the social class distribution of African Americans. In line with these requirements is Stockman's (1996b) Minimal Competency Core, which seeks to identify the linguistic components that differentiate typically developing and language-impaired children learning AAVE. Investigations of the phonological and grammatical systems of AAVE-speaking children have found that the features that best identify those with language impairments are ones shared between AAVE and SAE (Bleile & Wallach, 1992; Seymour, Bland-Stewart, & Green, 1998). Thus, traditional measures of language performance, such as the number of different words or complex syntactic constructions used in a language sample, can be used to identify children with language impairment, even when they speak a nonstandard dialect (Craig & Washington, 2000). The task of differentiation is made easier as normative data on the performance of minority populations become widely available (Craig & Washington, 2002).

The problems of nonbiased assessment are equally great for children who speak languages other than English. Currently, more tests and other assessment materials exist in Spanish than in any other foreign language. These include global language tests such as the

Preschool Language Scale—3: Spanish Edition (Zimmerman et al., 1993), parent report measures such as the Fundación MacArthur Inventario del Desarrollo de Habilidades Comunicativas (Jackson-Maldonado, Bates, & Thal, 1992), and procedures for the analysis of language samples such as the Developmental Assessment of Spanish Grammar (Toronto, 1976). Most of these instruments were originally developed in English and then translated into Spanish. As a result, they may or may not demonstrate good validity in their translated form (Gutierrez-Clellen, Restrepo, Bedore, Peña, & Anderson, 2000; Restrepo & Silverman, 2001; Thal, Jackson-Maldonado, & Acosta, 2000). Moreover, these instruments are based on different dialects of Spanish. What may be appropriate vocabulary and cultural assumptions for a Mexican American child may not be suitable for a child from El Salvador. In all cases of assessment involving children who speak limited English, the assessment should be carried out in the child's native language. To do this, the examiner must possess "native or near native fluency in both the minority language and the English language" (ASHA Committee on the Status of Racial Minorities, 1985). If the examiner is not trained in language assessment—for example, if a parent or relative or even a professional translator serves this role—then time must be allowed for adequate instruction regarding the purposes, procedures, and goals of the assessment. Working with translators, whether family members or professional translators, is far from straightforward and not an easily implemented alternative.

Implications for Intervention

Language assessment of linguistically-culturally diverse children can have three different outcomes:

1. Intervention is not recommended for children who are competent users of SAE and who may also be competent users of another language or English dialect.
2. *Therapeutic language intervention* is recommended for children who fail to show competence in *any* language or dialect.
3. *Elective language intervention* is recommended for children who are not competent users of SAE but who are competent in a nonstandard dialect or a language other than English.

The distinction between therapeutic and elective language intervention is based on the view that the traditional role of a language professional is to provide services to the communicatively disordered individuals, whereas children who do not use SAE may not be impaired in their ability to communicate; they merely communicate through another language form. Hence, following the traditional model, intervention would not be recommended for them. Nevertheless, professionals recognize that individuals who do not use SAE may be penalized educationally, socially, or vocationally. Many children, or their parents, may, therefore, request intervention to develop skills in the use of SAE.

Intervention for Language Differences and Language Disorders

Children recommended for therapeutic language intervention need to develop competence with some language form, whether it is standard English, nonstandard English, or a language other than English. It is likely that many of the linguistically-culturally diverse children in this category have a *low mixed language dominance,* that is, they combine elements of English and another language to form a mixture that is inadequate by the standards of both languages. Children whose language is influenced by a nonstandard dialect of English may also show signs of mixing. Among typically developing children, the acquisition of more than one language or dialect does not seriously slow the rate of acquisition for extended periods. However, the commonsense assumption of most professionals is that a language-disordered child is hindered by bilingual instruction. The different rules for phonology and grammar, the greater vocabulary load, and the need to master the subtleties of code switching all place demands on the child without necessarily improving the child's communicative effectiveness. The routine practice, therefore, is for professionals to begin by determining which language form will serve as the target of intervention.

There is no single formula by which to select the language form for instruction. Among the factors that must be weighed are the following.

- *Dominant language or dialect.* Although children receiving therapeutic intervention are not competent in any language form, they may show greater strength in one than another. For example, a 4-year-old Asian American child from Korea may respond to simple commands in both Korean and English but display a larger receptive vocabulary in English. The child may speak in both languages but produce only minor or formulaic utterances in Korean, in contrast to two- and three-word combinations in English. In both languages, then, the competence is less than would be expected of a typically developing child of this age, yet English appears clearly to be the dominant language. The possibility should also be considered that a child will have "domain-specific" competencies in different languages, for example, better speaking ability in one language but better reading ability in another (American Educational Research Association, American Psychological Association, & National Council on Measurement and Education, 1999).

- *Availability of service provider.* If intervention is to be provided in a language form other than SAE, it must be conducted by a professional or by a hired translator who is fully proficient in that other form. There are presently large discrepancies between the number of linguistically-culturally diverse children who qualify for therapeutic language intervention and the number of professionals able to work in language forms other than SAE. For example, as of 2002 only 2.1 percent of the membership of the American Speech–Language–Hearing Association (ASHA) was African American, and only 2.5 percent was Hispanic American (ASHA, 2002a). Because speech–language pathologists play an essential role in working with linguistically and culturally diverse children, data for that professional group are concerning. Fewer than 2 percent of members identify themselves as having bilingual skills, including American Sign Language (Deal-Williams, 2002). In many instances, therefore, professionals will need to rely on a hired translator or substantially improve their knowledge of a nonstandard dialect such as AAVE. Regrettably, a recent report indicates that, of a number of actions that could be taken to improve service to linguistically-culturally diverse children, ASHA members are unlikely to learn another language or train interpreters/translators for use in clinical practice (ASHA, 2002c).

- *Parental preference.* In all language intervention, the support and assistance of a child's parents is essential (Westby, Stevens, Dominguez, & Oetter, 1996). This will obviously be difficult if (1) the parents are opposed to the language form selected for instruction, (2) they themselves are not proficient in that language form, and/or (3) they have different culturally based beliefs about adult–child communication patterns, education and health services for children and their families, and child-rearing practices (Chao, 1996; Crago, 1990; Johnston & Wong, 2002; van Kleeck, 1994b). Some parents want their children to become SAE speakers, even though they themselves may not be. Immigrant families may insist that their children learn SAE, as it is viewed as crucial to their economic improvement and cultural assimilation.

■ *Speech community.* The most important insight that sociolinguistic study affords us is that language develops within a cultural context. We learn to speak and understand the variety of language used by those with whom we live and interact. For children, this means that peers and adult supervisors (parents, teachers, day-care providers, relatives, etc.) will be the most important linguistic influences. A child will have difficulty learning SAE when a nonstandard dialect is routinely heard at home, on the street, on the playground, and in the classroom. Conversely, it makes little sense to avoid SAE when that form dominates the child's environment.

Once a language form is chosen as the target for intervention, goals should be formulated that will increase the linguistically-culturally diverse child's language competence. In the main, the process of goal selection should observe the same principles as with mainstream language-impaired children. Some multicultural materials are available that may enhance a child's progress by providing stimuli that are more personally relevant (Deal & Rodriquez, 1987). The major differences in the intervention procedure will be to (1) identify instances when a child's performance in the target language form appears to be influenced by the other language or dialect; (2) use assistants as models when necessary; and (3) clearly identify what is an acceptable target behavior. An example of the first point is that Hispanic American children being taught SAE syntax may be slow to learn interrogative reversals because of interference from Spanish syntax. This does not affect the manner in which the form is introduced (operant learning, modeling, etc.), but it does lead to a different expectation for how quickly the children will progress with that form. A case can be made for initially avoiding certain target forms when interference can be anticipated.

If instruction is provided in a language form other than SAE, professionals must be very careful to ensure that correct models are presented. This may require the use of an assistant who can present stimuli under the guidance of the professional. The intervention task and the stimuli to be presented should be worked out in advance, so that the interaction with the child is as natural and uninterrupted as possible. Similarly, professionals must identify, perhaps with the assistant's or parents' help, what are acceptable responses to certain tasks. Once these are distinguished, the professional and the assistant may share the job of reinforcing the behaviors when they are produced by the child. The parents or assistants can also help to select what are culturally, as well as linguistically, appropriate intervention objectives and even intervention materials.

Intervention for Language Differences

Elective language intervention can occur under the following circumstances:

- A child is a proficient speaker of a nonstandard dialect or language other than English.
- The child or his parents request intervention to facilitate the acquisition of SAE.

- Resources are available to support elective intervention for children with language differences, as well as therapeutic intervention for children with language impairment.

The proficiency of these linguistically-culturally diverse children in a language form other than SAE means that they are competent language learners and should respond well to instruction. This conclusion, in turn, provides a rationale for working with the children in larger groups and using teacher aides and peer instructors to maximize resources. The role of the professional may vary from providing direct, individualized instruction to conducting inservice training and oversight of classroom activities.

The practice of elective language intervention is controversial and raises issues of ethnic identity, nationalism, economics, and professional training. To some extent, the issues are different for speakers of nonstandard dialects and speakers of languages other than English. In 1977 a lawsuit was brought in Ann Arbor, Michigan, by African American elementary school children because they were faring poorly as a result of disadvantage because they were required to speak and read SAE in school even though they were speakers of AAVE (*Martin Luther King Jr. Elementary School Children v. Ann Arbor School District Board,* 1977). The interpretation of the problem was not the use of SAE in the classroom but the fact that teachers were insensitive to the African American children's problems in learning that dialect. The solution devised by the Ann Arbor School Board, under court order, was to organize inservice programs to increase teachers' awareness of AAVE and improve their ability to teach SAE to the African American children.

The issue of ethnic sensitivity involves a different response in the case of children who speak little or no English. Politically, it has been more difficult to make the case that these children should receive special instruction to help them make the transition to the use of SAE. As of 2003, twenty-six states had declared by statute, resolution, or constitutional amendment that English was the official language of the state (Crawford, 2003). The effect of these laws has been mixed, and they have been challenged in court. However, they speak to the concern many citizens feel over the increasing linguistic diversity of the United States. They also reflect an apprehension that programs to accommodate non-English-speaking children will take resources away from other aspects of public education.

There is disagreement over which group of professionals should be responsible for elective language intervention. Some within the field of speech–language pathology are highly supportive of the practice and feel competent to serve as teachers. Others argue that elective intervention, especially with non-English speakers, requires skills not possessed by speech–language pathologists. The position of ASHA is that speech–language pathologists may, by virtue of their individual experiences and education, be qualified to provide English as a Second Language (ESL) instruction. Without such qualification, however, they should limit their role to collaboration with ESL instructors in providing assessment and/or intervention services in school settings (ASHA, 1998).

At least three distinct purposes for elective language intervention can be identified. It may be that some but not all of these objectives are relevant to professionals in different settings.

1. *Cultural assimilation.* Especially in conditions where linguistically-culturally diverse children are a small minority, the mastery of SAE may help the development of peer relationships and facilitate interactions with adults at school and in the community.

2. *Vocational opportunity.* Difficulty in obtaining work is a problem that many children will face in the future if they do not speak SAE. It is futile to prepare children in other areas if they will be denied opportunities because of their language differences.

3. *Literacy instruction.* This was the basis of the Ann Arbor trial, and it remains a significant issue. The only form of English that is written—apart from creative works—is the standard dialect. To become literate, therefore, a child must learn that dialect. In the case of AAVE, it remains unclear whether use of that dialect, as opposed to other socioeconomic or cultural factors, is the cause of reading difficulty (Rickford & Rickford, 1995). Experience with Hispanic American children suggests that their reading success correlates with their oral language proficiency (Gottardo, 2002; Quiroga, Lemos-Britton, Mostafapour, Abbott, & Berninger, 2002). However, it is also clear that lack of English proficiency is not the sole cause of poor reading skill. Other factors that must be considered are cultural differences in family attitudes toward literacy as well as low motivation and low educational aspirations that are the result of discrimination (Snow, Burns, & Griffin, 1998).

If the decision is made to support elective language intervention for linguistically-culturally diverse children, instructional procedures should be tailored to match their age, environment, and language needs. Young children who speak languages other than English are often mainstreamed successfully in classes of predominantly SAE-speaking peers. They may require some initial support in making their needs known, and some of them will be silent for an extended period before they begin speaking in English (Saville-Troike, 1988). In circumstances where bilingual children form a sizable percentage of a class, mainstreaming may need to be supplemented with special programs to introduce English as a second language.

Children who use a nonstandard dialect should receive instruction targeted at contrasting structures in SAE. For example, speakers of AAVE may benefit from SAE practice in the use of the copula, the formation of indirect questions, and the use of negation (see Table 9.8). It may assist children to practice switching from nonstandard to standard dialectal forms within the same communication task.

A child's age must be considered in relation to interference effects and to the amount of time available for instruction. In general, older non-native speakers of English will have more difficulty with interference from their native languages. The same might be presumed to be true for speakers of nonstandard dialects. In both cases, however, a child's age may be offset by a high motivation to learn SAE (Taylor, 1990). The linguistic needs of older children are more immediate, as they have fewer remaining years of school. In this case, professionals may opt for a more intense and selective approach to instruction, emphasizing those features of SAE that will most improve the intelligibility and public acceptability of an individual's communication.

Intervention for Linguistically-Culturally Diverse Children with Other Disabilities

As we have seen in many of the chapters in this book, the underlying deficits of intellectual disabilities, autism, specific language impairment, and other developmental disorders have particular negative effects on language-acquisition mechanisms. Linguistically-culturally diverse children with these deficits are especially at risk. Furthermore, the association between language impairment and emotional or behavioral disorder is high in linguistically-culturally diverse children (Toppelberg, Medrano, Pena Morgens, & Nieto-Castanon, 2002). Decisions regarding language input to these children are especially important because they are generally more dependent on that input and their pragmatic deficits make them less likely to engage speakers in conversation on their own. Increasingly, a case is being made to maintain bilingual input to children with language impairment (Gutiérrez-Clellen, 1999). Given the number of linguistic and social variables at issue, however, it is difficult to justfiy a single approach. Instead, professionals should follow a set of guidelines such as these (Toppelberg, Snow, & Tager-Flusberg, 1999):

1. Determine the critical communicative needs of the child and the language(s) with which the child absolutely must be familiar.
2. Determine the child's relative ability in the first and second languages, the willingness and ability of family members and school personnel to function in the various possible languages, and the child's attitude toward and aptitude for language in general and learning a second language in particular.
3. Discuss with the family the risks, benefits, and availability of a particular language given the child's abilities and needs. Weigh the value of maintaining the home language (for emotional and behavioral regulation and for family and cultural relatedness) against competing needs (such as learning the language of instruction, society, and occupations) and limitations (such as the child's inability to handle several languages).
4. Do not ask the child to learn languages that will not be central to communicative needs, e.g., by studying a foreign language in middle childhood.
5. Provide optimal, intense, well-structured, native input in the language(s) it is determined the child absolutely must learn.

Summary

In this chapter we have seen that

■ Changes in the population of the United States are resulting in increased multiculturalism, that is, variation in race, language, and culture.
■ Language variation exists on many levels: in different nations, in different regions of the same nation, among different ethnic groups, in different social situations, and among different individual speakers.
■ Children learning more than one language can show varying degrees of competence with the different languages. Bilingual learning is affected by many factors. Patterns of acquisition appear to be different in children who learn the languages sequentially rather than simultaneously.
■ A major influence on the English produced by Hispanic American bilingual-bicultural children is the Spanish language. Most of the phonological variation and some of the grammatical differences they show from SAE can be explained as interference from a dialect of Spanish.
■ Some African American children learn a nonstandard dialect, known as African American Vernacular English, that evolved from the interaction of English and

African languages. The dialect is systematic, with rule-governed features of phonology, grammar, semantics, and pragmatics.

- The English of Asian American children may be influenced by the phonological and grammatical features of their native Asian languages, as well as suprasegmental characteristics. Some general contrasts exist between English and several Asian languages. However, there is considerable variation in the linguistic and cultural behaviors of Asian American children.

- The majority of Native American children learn English as their first language, but many of those learning a nonstandard dialect. However, growing efforts to maintain tribal languages could place more of these children in the position of being bilingual language learners. Differences between Native American and mainstream culture increase the threat of bias in standard language assessment.

- A high percentage of linguistically-culturally diverse children live in conditions of poverty. This may be responsible for a higher prevalence of certain language disorders in this population.

- Professionals who assess linguistically-culturally diverse children must distinguish between language differences and language disorders, either or both of which can occur in an individual.

- Many current tests of language contain significant sources of bias when they are used with linguistically-culturally diverse children. They must be administered with caution. In the future, they should be replaced by new instruments developed for and standardized on racial/ethnic minority populations.

- Screening and assessment procedures for linguistically-culturally diverse children lead to a recommendation of no intervention, therapeutic intervention, or elective intervention. Therapeutic language intervention is for children who do not show proficiency in any language or dialect. Several factors must be considered by professionals in selecting the language or dialect for use in instruction. Assistance in interpreting a child's language or culture may be necessary, but working with translators, even professional translators, is challenging and not a perfect solution.

- Elective language intervention is for children who are competent in a nonstandard dialect or another language but not in SAE. It may not be supported by all professionals or political factions. The form of intervention will vary, depending on the identified purposes of instruction, the number and ages of the children to be seen, and the resources that are provided.

The communication needs of linguistically-culturally diverse children have been highlighted by demographic changes, linguistic research, and legal action. Professionals are still in the process of responding to these needs, which require many changes in traditional methods of assessment and intervention. Much work remains to be done.

10 Children with Acquired Language Disorders

STEVEN H. LONG

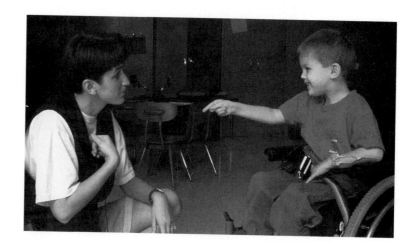

OBJECTIVES

After reading this chapter you should be able to discuss

- Definitions and etiologies of acquired aphasia in children
- Basic concepts of language recovery in children as a function of physiological restitution and normal language development
- General characteristics of the language of children with acquired aphasia
- Principles of language assessment and intervention for children with acquired aphasia

Most children learn to talk, read, and write only once and then use those abilities for the rest of their lives. For a special group of children, however, the experience of language acquisition is at least partially repeated. These children sustain some type of brain injury that pushes them down the ladder of language development and forces them to climb it again. Fortunately, nature is able to heal or compensate for much of the damage that occurs. But recovery is not complete, and the changes children undergo create enormous stress on them and their families (Hawley, Ward, Magnay, & Long, 2003). Professionals must be available to help interpret and explain these changes as well as to provide intervention that complements the natural recuperation process.

An Overview of Acquired Childhood Aphasia

Definition

Historically, the term *aphasia* has been used to describe two different conditions in children. From Chapter 3 we know that the terms *developmental* or *congenital aphasia* have sometimes been used to describe children who show language impairment without sensory dysfunction, intellectual disability, or other neurological damage. These are, however, older labels. In more recent clinical and research literature these terms have commonly been replaced by *developmental language disorder* or *specific language impairment.* In contrast, the terms *acquired aphasia* or *childhood aphasia* refer to children who have a language disorder stemming from a disease or accident that alters neurological functioning. Children with acquired aphasia had begun to develop language normally but then lost all or part of their communicative abilities as a result of neurological damage they sustained.

Types of Brain Injury

Brain injuries occur in localized and diffuse forms. *Localized* or *focal lesions* are confined to specific areas of the brain and result from penetrating injuries (such as gunshot wounds), vascular lesions (strokes or hemorrhages), or tumors. *Diffuse lesions* are spread out over many brain regions and usually result from traumatic head injuries or poisoning. In all types of brain injury, nerve cells are killed in one of three ways:

1. Directly, as a result of mechanical shearing or lack of oxygen carried by blood
2. Indirectly, as a result of the degeneration of their connections with other nerve cells
3. Inadvertently, as a result of electrical overstimulation associated with the interruption of blood flow

Nerve cell death caused by overstimulation has been discovered relatively recently and appears to be amenable to early drug treatment (Almli & Finger, 1992; Felberg, Burgin, & Grotta, 2000). Thus, in the future, it may be possible to reduce the amount of permanent damage caused by certain kinds of brain injuries.

Traumatic Brain Injury.   Every year U.S. children 14 years and younger sustain traumatic brain injuries that result in an estimated 3,000 deaths, 29,000 hospitalizations, and 400,000 emergency department visits (Langlois, 2000). Different terms are used to describe the neurological damage that results from accidents involving the head. *Closed-head injury* (CHI) indicates that a child has suffered diffuse rather than focal brain injury as a result of a blow to the head. Drawing on information from the National Head Injury Foundation, the other frequently used term, *traumatic brain injury* (TBI) can be defined as (Savage, 1991)

> . . . an insult to the brain, not of a degenerative or congenital nature but caused by an external physical force, that may produce a diminished or altered state of consciousness, which results in impairment of cognitive abilities or physical functioning. It can also result in the disturbance of behavioral or emotional functioning. These impairments may be either temporary or permanent and cause partial or total functional disability or psychosocial maladjustment. (p. 3)

TBI should not be confused with minimal brain dysfunction (MBD), an older term for children with behavioral evidence of neurological dysfunction but no history of injury (see Chapters 3 and 4). Professionals often use the terms *head injury* and *traumatic brain injury* interchangeably. The latter is more specific and leaves no doubt that a child's problems are the result of injury to the brain, not the head.

TBI results from several causes, which are more likely among particular age groups. Infants and toddlers are generally hurt through falls or abuse. Older preschoolers suffer falls, while young school-aged children suffer injuries through sports and accidents involving them as pedestrians, bike or skateboard riders, or passengers. Adolescents sustain the most accidents, primarily as the result of motor vehicles accidents. Beginning in the preschool years, boys become two to four times more likely than girls to suffer a TBI. Children and adolescents with TBI are a much higher-incidence population than is generally realized. Estimates are that approximately 4 percent of all children kindergarten through twelfth grade have experienced some type of head trauma. Among children enrolled in special education, this figure jumps to somewhere between 8 and 20 percent (Savage, 1991). Automobile accidents causing head injury in children are more likely to be at low speeds. The rotational acceleration to which their brains are subjected is therefore likely to be less than that of adolescents and adults involved in high-speed crashes. Damage may be confined to the cortex of the brain, whereas in adolescents and adults it can extend into the deeper white matter. In addition, children are less likely to develop contusions and hematomas. On the other hand, infants often have a poorer outcome in head injury cases. They are more susceptible to hematomas, may have white matter damage because their brains have little myelination, and in cases where the trauma is caused by abuse, may be delayed in receiving medical attention (Duhaime, Christian, Rorke, & Zimmerman, 1998).

Classification of brain injury is based on scores from the *Glasgow Coma Scale* (GCS), shown in Table 10.1, which measures eye opening, motor responses, and verbal responses. Scores from the three categories are summed and then a severity rating is assigned from this scale:

13–15	mild brain injury
9–12	moderate brain injury
3–8	severe brain injury

Although initial GCS scores are generally predictive of which children will die or have a poor outcome from an accident, the ratings do not necessarily correlate with the level of

TABLE 10.1   The Glasgow Coma Scale

Best Eye Opening	Best Motor Response	Best Verbal Response
4 Opens eyes on own	6 Follows simple commands	5 Carries on a conversation correctly and tells examiner where he is, who he is, and the month and year
3 Opens eyes when asked to in a loud voice	5 Pulls examiner's hand away when pinched	
2 Opens eyes when pinched	4 Pulls part of body away when examiner pinches patient	4 Seems confused or disoriented
1 Does not open eyes	3 Flexes body inappropriately to pain	3 Talks so examiner can understand victim but makes no sense
	2 Body becomes rigid in an extended position when examiner pinches victim	2 Makes sounds that examiner can't understand
	1 Has no motor response to pinch	1 Makes no noise

Source: Teasdale & Jennett (1974).

difficulty surviving children will experience in motor performance, education, and socialization (Haley, Cioffi, Lewin, & Baryza, 1990; Savage, 1991). The GCS was originally developed for use with adults, but it is also the most commonly used scoring tool for children. However, it is less appropriate for very young children whose motor and verbal skills are not yet fully developed, and for this reason alternative scales have been developed (Durham et al., 2000; Simpson, Cockington, Hanieh, Raftos, & Reilly, 1991). The *Pediatric Glasgow Coma Scale* uses age-adjusted maximal scores but is based on a 14-point GCS instead of the 15-point one (Reilly & Simpson, 1988).

Strokes and Tumors.   The most common causes of aphasia in adults are relatively uncommon in children. For example, in 2000, the death rate for cerebrovascular disease in the United States was 0.5 per 100,000 for children under 15 years of age. The comparable figure for adults age 65 and older was 422. Similarly, the death rate for cancerous tumors of all kinds was 5.2 per 100,000 for children, while for adults it was 1,127 (Minino & Smith, 2001). Obviously, in comparison to the incidence of traumatic injuries, vascular lesions and malignant tumors are rarely seen conditions. Yet, when they do occur and produce unilateral damage to the left hemisphere, they result in aphasic symptoms that are comparable to those seen in adults.

More than a third of childhood strokes occur during the first two years of life. The usual causes of stroke in children are cardiac disease, vascular occlusion, sickle cell disease, vascular malformation, and hemorrhage. Blockage of a cerebral artery may result from trauma, infection, cellular changes, or for no discernible reason. It frequently causes a sudden hemiplegia in a child and may be accompanied by seizures. In sickle cell anemia, deformed red cells cause vascular obstruction, leading to a crisis in which coma and seizures occur. Cerebral hemorrhage is often produced by the rupture of malformed blood vessels. Children with this condition are at risk for recurrence throughout their lives.

Landau-Kleffner Syndrome.   The least frequent cause of acquired aphasia in children is a distinctive syndrome in which convulsive disorder, indicated by abnormal electroencephalogram (EEG) tracings, occurs at about the same time as a breakdown in language. The condition has been profiled as follows:

- It has a low incidence. As of 1992, at least 198 cases had been reported in the literature (Beaumanoir, 1992).
- Age of onset ranges from 1½ to 13 years.
- Language regression may be gradual or sudden.
- All children show abnormal EEG results, and over two-thirds experience some type of seizure before, simultaneous with, or after the language regression.
- Affected children show such a severe disturbance in auditory comprehension that they appear to be deaf, but there is typically no loss of hearing sensitivity for pure tones.
- Males are affected twice as often as females.
- Changes in aphasia, seizures, and EEG findings do not correlate well. Some children stop having seizures and show normal EEG tracings but continue to exhibit aphasia. Others show an opposite pattern.

Associated Problems

Children with acquired aphasia are certain to have other problems as a result of their brain injuries. The number and extent of these difficulties will vary widely from one injured child to the next. However, studies suggest some general characteristics of children in three etiological categories: those with TBI, those with Landau-Kleffner syndrome, and those with vascular lesions. Findings for these three groups are shown in Table 10.2. The impairments associated with acquired aphasia can have a significant impact on the procedures used for evaluating and treating the language disorder. For example, perceptual and motor difficulties may make it necessary to adapt test materials and procedures. Behavioral disturbances may interfere with attempts to include a child in group instruction or recreation.

Language Development and Language Recovery

The same kinds of brain injuries can affect both children and adults, yet it is commonly believed that the effects of these injuries on language are different for the two age groups. The prevailing view has been that brain-injured children differ in at least three respects:

1. They have a lower risk of aphasia.
2. They present different language symptoms.
3. They recover faster and more fully than adults.

These assertions have been tempered as research has progressed. A key issue has been the validity of the progressive laterality or equipotentiality hypothesis, which maintains that cerebral dominance is not present at birth but develops slowly over the course of childhood (Lenneberg, 1967). If it is true that language has not yet fully lateralized in preadolescents, then it is understandable that damage to the dominant hemisphere (usually the left one) would not produce aphasia or would produce only mild symptoms. Moreover, the absence of cerebral dominance suggests that higher-level functions, including language, are less localized in a

TABLE 10.2   Associated Physical, Cognitive, Perceptual Motor, Behavioral, and Social Problems in Children with Acquired Aphasia

Etiology	Traumatic Brain Injury (TBI)	Landau-Kleffner Syndrome	Vascular Lesion
Gross and fine motor	Severe TBI: spasticity, ataxia, delayed motor milestones Mild TBI: fine motor and visuomotor deficits, reduction in age-appropriate play and physical activity	Gross and fine motor skills are usually good, sometimes superior	Hemiparesis on side opposite to brain injury
Cognitive	Problems with long- and short-term memory, conceptual skills, problem solving Reduced speed of information processing Reduced attending skills	Normal performance intelligence in most cases	Lower scores on standardized intelligence tests with performance scores higher than verbal scores
Perceptual motor	Visual neglect, visual field cuts Motor apraxia, reduced motor speed, poor motor sequencing	Normal hearing sensitivity to pure tones but may not respond to speech stimuli Long-term effects: difficulty understanding speech in competing noise situations; difficulty with tasks that challenge visual perception and visual memory	Visual neglect, motor apraxia Visual discrimination problems in cases of crossed aphasia (right hemisphere lesion)
Behavioral	Impulsivity, poor judgment, disinhibition, dependency, anger outbursts, denial, depression, emotional ability, apathy, lethargy, poor motivation	Inattention, withdrawal, aggressiveness, temper outbursts, nightmares, refusal to respond, hyperactivity	Inattention, distractibility
Social	Does not learn from peers, does not generalize from social situations Behaves like a much younger child, withdraws Becomes distracted in noisy surroundings and becomes lost even in familiar surroundings	May have periods of social withdrawal	May have periods of social withdrawal (elective mutism reported in one case)

Sources: Burd et al. (1990); Catroppa & Anderson (2003); DePompei & Blosser (1987); Haley et al. (1990); Martins, Ferro, & Trindade (1987); McNaughton (1991); Miller et al. (1984); Raybarman (2002); White & Sreenivasan (1987); and Ylvisaker (1989).

child's brain. This means that uninjured parts of the brain might be able to assume the functions previously handled by injured regions because of neurological plasticity, a concept introduced in Chapter 1. However, not all the evidence supports the notion of progressive laterality. Certain anatomical and electrophysiological studies indicate that some features of lateralization, such as dichotic ear preference, are present very early in life. Other research, however, suggests a great deal of neuronal plasticity in young children's brains (Dapretto, Woods, & Bookheimer, 2000; Mills, Coffey-Corina, & Neville, 1993). Studies of children's recovery from unilateral damage to the left hemisphere of the brain are difficult to interpret because of differences in methods of investigation. Taken as a whole, the evidence to date does not support the notion that a child's chances of recovery decline consistently (monotonically) with age. We must therefore await further studies to determine exactly how plasticity varies with age and affects the chances for recovery from brain injury (Bates & Roe, 2001). It is possible that language representation in children is like that of adults, but this similarity is masked by the greater neural interconnections that characterize the young brain (de Bode & Curtiss, 2001).

The language symptoms of children with aphasia have traditionally been thought to be different from those of adults. Aphasia in adults is broadly categorized into two groups: *nonfluent,* in which speech is halting, speech comprehension is relatively good, and the site of injury is in the frontal lobe of the brain; and *fluent,* in which speech contains errors but is produced without effort, speech comprehension is poor, and the site of injury is in the parietal and temporal lobes. Most cases of acquired aphasia in children have been traditionally described as presenting as nonfluent, regardless of the location of the brain injury (Satz & Bullard-Bates, 1981). As more studies are conducted, however, it appears that, as with adults, children with aphasia demonstrate either nonfluent or fluent speech (van Dongen, Paquier, Creten, van Borsel, & Catsman-Berrevoets, 2001), although descriptions of the nonfluent form still predominate in the literature. In other respects, children also appear to show the same language disturbances found among adults with aphasia. They have disorders of auditory comprehension, writing, reading, and naming (Aram, 1998; Jordan & Ashton, 1996; Jordan, Murdoch, Buttsworth, & Hudson-Tennent, 1995).

Although the symptoms of children with aphasia are similar to those of adults, the prognosis for the two groups is considerably different. When all cases of acquired aphasia are taken together, the great majority of children—estimated at about 75 percent—show a dramatic recovery of language that is unrelated to their recovery of motor function (Aram, 1988; Eisele & Aram, 1995; Satz & Bullard-Bates, 1981). The rate of recovery is considerably lower for children who suffer from seizures (Bates & Roe, 2001). However, recovery is rarely complete. One-fourth or more of children with brain injuries show residual aphasia more than a year postonset and, even in cases where they appear to be clinically recovered from the aphasia, they continue to show deficits on tests of intelligence and academic achievement (Jordan & Murdoch, 1994). The strong recovery of some children with aphasia raises two questions:

1. Why do other children not recover as well?
2. Why do children recover so much better than adults?

Recovery in adults with aphasia has been related to several factors such as age, type of aphasia, etiology, and severity of injury. These factors also have been presumed to affect recovery in children. For adults who suffer strokes, younger age is regarded as a positive prognostic factor (Sarno, 1998). Among children who suffer traumatic brain injuries, age interacts with factors such as anatomical development, type of injury, and state of language development to determine the prognosis (Anderson et al., 1997). Toddlers and young children generally appear to recover best because: (1) their brains withstand injury better than those of infants, (2) they have established certain spoken language skills and sometimes written language skills prior to injury, and (3) they still have enough plasticity for functional reorganization of the brain to occur. After age 5, however, children's patterns of recovery from TBI become increasingly like those of adults (Chapman, Levin, Wanek, Weyrauch, & Kufera, 1998). In contrast, children who acquire aphasia secondary to convulsive disorder (Landau-Kleffner syndrome) generally recover better when onset occurs at older ages. This has been attributed to the syndrome's disruption of further language development (Bishop, 1985).

The type and location of a brain injury may also affect a child's recovery. In the smaller number of instances where brain-injured children present the symptoms of fluent aphasia immediately after the injury, the prognosis for recovery is generally worse (Martins & Ferro, 1992). Also affecting the prognosis for recovery is the cause of brain injury. The pattern most often observed is that recovery is best with traumatic injuries, not as good with vascular lesions, and poorest with infectious etiologies (Dennis, 1992; Martins & Ferro, 1992).

Language Characteristics of
Children with Acquired Aphasia

Because children with acquired aphasia often recover much of their premorbid communicative ability, we cannot give a single description of their language characteristics. Aphasiologists characterize the first 3 months to a year following brain injury as a period of "spontaneous recovery," during which the nervous system is able to recover a number of functions even without any type of intervention (Sarno, 1998). Language impairment is most pronounced during this acute period. After the phase of spontaneous recovery, children with acquired aphasia will likely be left with residual language difficulties that affect interpersonal communication to some degree but, in most cases, have their greatest impact on academic performance. In the following sections we will delineate the common language characteristics during the acute recovery period and afterwards. Distinctions will be drawn between the behaviors of children with TBI, vascular lesion, and Landau-Kleffner syndrome.

Acute Recovery Period

Comprehension.   A wide range of comprehension impairments are found among children with acute aphasia. In general, the severity of the comprehension disorder corresponds to the severity of the injury. For example, a child with a severe TBI will usually show more difficulty at first than a child with a mild TBI. Complexity of what is to be comprehended is also a factor. A study of 57 children and adolescents with mild to moderate-severe closed-head injury found that more than 18 percent had poor auditory comprehension of syntactically complex sentences but only 2 percent had trouble understanding single words (Ewing-Cobbs, Fletcher, Landry, & Levin, 1985).

Children with vascular lesions also show individual variability in their comprehension problems. Dennis (1980) described a 9-year-old girl who, immediately following a left-sided stroke, was impaired in her auditory comprehension of words and simple commands. Her reading comprehension of the same content was better but suffered interference if she read aloud. In a larger investigation, two of eight children with left-sided nontraumatic brain injuries exhibited problems of auditory comprehension (Hécaen, 1976).

The most serious comprehension impairments are found in children with Landau-Kleffner syndrome. The impairment ranges from a limited ability to understand commands to a complete obliviousness to speech (Baynes, Kegl, Brentari, Kussmaul, & Poizner, 1998; Mantovani & Landau, 1980; Miller, Campbell, Chapman, & Ellis Weismer, 1984; Pearce & Darwish, 1984; Sieratzki, Calvert, Brammer, David, & Woll, 2001). These children may not even respond appropriately to nonspeech auditory stimuli, which has led some investigators to label the condition as an "auditory agnosia," an inability to make sense of sound (Baynes et al., 1998).

Word Retrieval.   Difficulties with word retrieval are frequently observed in children with acquired aphasia. They may appear as an inability to name pictures and objects or as excessive hesitation and nonspecific word use in spontaneous speech. One study found that a relatively small percentage (9 percent) of children and adolescents with mild-to-moderate to severe head injuries were hampered in confrontation naming; a larger number (more than 18 percent) had trouble retrieving words in a specific category (Ewing-Cobbs et al., 1985). In their spontaneous speech, children and adolescents with TBI produce significantly fewer words and fewer different words than control subjects when first evaluated after their injury. Significant improvement in vocabulary usage occurs for most children during the first year following injury, but some continue at a lower level (Campbell & Dollaghan, 1990). In general, some word-finding difficulty can be expected in closed-head-injury cases, regardless of the severity of the injury or the age of the child (Dennis, 1992; Jordan, Murdoch, Hudson-Tennent, & Boon, 1996).

Few studies have documented lexical difficulties in children with left-sided vascular lesions. The 9-year-old girl described previously (Dennis, 1980) had a number of word-finding impairments 2 weeks after a stroke, including semantic paraphasias (*bottle* for *cup*) and random misnamings. Perseverative responses were common. Her ability to write names was better than her ability to speak them. Lexical problems have been reported in other children with nontraumatic brain injuries, though these may appear more on word association rather than naming tasks (Jordan et al., 1996).

Children with Landau-Kleffner syndrome show word substitutions and word-retrieval problems in spontaneous speech. These problems are similar to those of children with language-learning disabilities. The most common signs of word-finding difficulty are filled pauses (*uh, um*), word and phrase revisions, substitution of semantically or phonologically related words for the intended word, and overuse of indefinite reference terms (*this, that, thing, stuff*) (Miller et al., 1984).

Syntax.   When evaluated soon after sustaining TBI, children and adolescents show significant differences on a number of global measures of spontaneous speech: a smaller number of utterances produced, a shorter mean length of utterance (MLU), a smaller percentage of complex utterances, and a larger percentage of utterances with mazes and disruptions (filled pauses, false starts, revisions, etc.) (Campbell & Dollaghan, 1990). Performance is also impaired on various structured communication tasks such as object description, sentence repetition, and formulation of sentences containing target words. Writing tends to be even more impaired than speaking.

Case studies of children who suffer strokes suggest a similar pattern of syntactic deficits. A child who suffered a massive left-sided stroke was impaired, 2 weeks postonset, in describing the use of common objects, repeating sentences, and formulating sentences with target words. Much of the difficulty was still present at 3 months postonset (Dennis, 1980). Another child, a 5-year-old who exhibited a crossed aphasia (resulting from a right-hemisphere lesion), was initially mute. Over the next 3 months, syntax progressed to single words, then two- and three-word combinations with lengthy delays between words, then short phrases, and finally, short sentences (Burd, Gascon, Swenson, & Hankey, 1990).

Children with Landau-Kleffner syndrome may become mute or show speech limited to grunts, gestures, and production of isolated vowels and consonants (Miller et al., 1984; Soprano, Garcia, Caraballo, & Fejerman, 1994). Shoumaker et al. (1974) described three children whose speech fluctuated over the course of the disorder but, at its worst, was limited to a few words. McNaughton (1991) reported about a 6-year-old boy who inconsistently produced about 30 word approximations that could be understood only by familiar listening partners. He also developed a repertoire of 15 idiosyncratic gestures such as drawing the letter "M" in the air to signify "McDonalds" or drawing a grid in the air to request a game of tic-tac-toe. A Dutch girl has been described who experienced seizures and aphasia from 5 to 8 years. Measurements of MLU and number of words spoken fluctuated as she experienced language breakdown, recovery, another breakdown, and another recovery (van de Sandt-Koenderman, Smit, van Dongen, & van Hest, 1984).

Speech Production.   Problems of speech intelligibility are found in many children with acquired aphasia. Damage to motor-planning regions of the brain or to cranial nerve pathways may produce sound substitutions and omissions or slurred speech, the symptoms of apraxia of speech or dysarthria. Problems may also emerge in speech prosody. Following TBI many children may recover a lot of their articulation skills during the first year, and improvement in articulation may be the earliest and strongest of all gains in expressive language (Campbell & Dollaghan, 1990). Articulation problems have also been observed in children with left-sided nontraumatic brain injuries (Dennis, 1980; Hécaen, 1976). For children with Landau-Kleffner syndrome, a variety of misarticulations may occur, and prosody may resemble that of deaf children, that is, a high fundamental frequency used with little variation in intonation.

Later Recovery and Residual Language Impairment

Though it is plain that children with aphasia recover more fully than adults, recent findings also indicate that children experience some persistent language impairment. This appears to be true regardless of the etiology of the aphasia. Following TBI, the difficulties that persist are often subtle and may be associated with higher-level language skills. For example, in spontaneous conversation or when giving narrative accounts, there may be residual problems in word retrieval, recall and organization of information, syntactic formulation, and use of cohesion devices that help the listener follow the events and characters of a story (Brookshire, Chapman, Song, & Levin, 2000; Campbell & Dollaghan, 1990; Chapman et al., 1998; Dollaghan & Campbell, 1992). Verbal explanations may be disorganized, confusing, and ineffective because of unnecessary repetition or the inclusion of irrelevant detail (McDonald, 1993). In reading or listening, children with brain injury may understand facts that are stated directly but fail to comprehend information that must be inferred (Barnes & Dennis, 2001; Dennis & Barnes, 2001). The superficial emotions of characters in a story may be understood, but not the more deceptive emotions that motivate certain behaviors (Dennis, Barnes, Wilkinson, & Humphreys, 1998). In any type of language task involving nonliteral meanings—the understanding of humor, sarcasm, and so forth—children recovering from head injury are more prone to misunderstanding than their peers (Dennis, Purvis, Barnes, Wilkinson, & Winner, 2001; Docking, Jordan, & Murdoch, 1999; Docking, Murdoch, & Jordan, 2000; Jordan, Cremona-Meteyard, & King, 1996). Higher-level language abilities are perhaps among the most debilitating communication problems these children can experience, because they have the potential to negatively impact on their academic and social success. These are also the language functions that are often overlooked in the children and hardest to document. Professionals need to be particularly alert for difficulties in these areas.

Children's recovery from vascular lesions shows a similar pattern. There appears to be a strong initial recovery of language functions, but despite their early progress, most children remain impaired to some degree well after the original injury. For example, an evaluation of 11 children and adolescents with nontraumatic brain injuries more than a year postonset found that they were able to communicate verbally and engage in conversation but still exhibited residual language and academic difficulties (Cooper & Flowers, 1987). The spontaneous spoken language of these children is less elaborated syntactically and contains more errors in the complex sentences that are produced (Aram, Ekelman, & Whitaker, 1986). Naming is slower than in normal subjects, but the pattern of errors produced is generally similar to that of normal children and does not resemble the dysnomia of adults with aphasia (Aram, Ekelman, & Whitaker, 1987). Unfortunately, time alone does not heal these problems. Follow-up of young adults who experienced strokes as children has shown a wide range of language impairments, with resulting effects on not only their academic performance but also their social lives (Watamori, Sasanuma, & Ueda, 1990).

Children with Landau-Kleffner syndrome also show long-term language disability. Review of the literature shows that language difficulties either recur or persist beyond 6 months in 94 percent of the reported cases (Miller et al., 1984).

It is clear, then, that children with acquired aphasia can be expected to exhibit some measure of language difficulty well after the time of their brain damage and probably into adulthood. These problems can be expected to impact academic achievement.

Academic Achievement

Despite the previous discussion, there can be a tendency to view many children with acquired aphasia as "fully recovered," given the amount of recovery that children with acquired aphasia often achieve. It is apparent, however, that the effects of brain damage are widespread and can influence a child's performance, particularly at school. Even intelligence testing may not be sensitive to certain deficits incurred by children with head injury and consequently may not be predictive of academic success (Ewing-Cobbs, Levin, & Fletcher, 1998).

Classroom performance can be affected in many different ways. Table 10.3 shows the results of one follow-up study of children with acquired aphasia. As can be seen, deficits were detected on several formal language tests as well as on measures of academic achievement. Though most of these children are able to continue in regular school, the research clearly indicates that academic difficulties can be expected.

Writing skills appear to be especially susceptible to impairment as a result of brain injury. These skills seem to be more affected in younger children with closed-head injury than in adolescents. This may be due to the effect of the injury on acquiring new skills or to the greater writing experience of adolescents, which makes their writing more resistant to disruption (Ewing-Cobbs et al., 1985). Regardless of age, the prognosis for recovery of writing skills is worse for individuals who sustain more severe head injuries (Yorkston, Jaffe, Liao, & Polissar, 1999).

Much of the research that has documented academic difficulties among children with acquired aphasia has relied on standardized language or achievement tests to measure their abilities. However, these tests do not reflect the full extent of the problems these children experience in the classroom (Ewing-Cobbs et al., 1998). A survey of the teachers of severely head-injured students indicated an even wider range of academic difficulties, especially with more complex tasks requiring processing and integration of information (Ylvisaker, 1989). The results of this survey are summarized in Table 10.4. Clearly, the problems these children can face in school are extensive and cut across all academic areas.

TABLE 10.3   Residual Language and Academic Problems of Children with Acquired Aphasia

Language Ability Tested	Number of Children Scoring More than 2 SD below the Mean
Comprehension of single words	9/15
Comprehension of spoken sentences	7/15
Comprehension of contextual spoken language	4/15
Oral production of sentences of varying grammatical complexity	9/15
Recall of vocabulary within a semantic category (word fluency)	4/15
Single word picture labeling	8/15

Achievement Test	Number of Children Scoring More than 1 SD below the Mean
Reading recognition	3/15
Reading comprehension	5/15
Spelling	8/15
Arithmetic	12/14

Source: Cooper & Flowers (1987).

TABLE 10.4 Academic Difficulties Reported by Teachers of Children with Severe Head Injuries

Reading	25% of the children had difficulty with reading vocabulary
	50% had difficulty with rate of reading
	70% had difficulty with higher levels of comprehension
	90% had trouble comprehending reading passages of substantial length
Auditory comprehension	70% showed deterioration in auditory comprehension when the amount of language was increased
	25% performed more poorly on a standardized comprehension test when stimuli were presented at a rapid rate
Expressive language	14% had difficulty expressing simple ideas
	75% had difficulty expressing complex ideas, in both spoken and written form
	Recall of vocabulary within a semantic category (word fluency) was below normal limits
Writing	75% scored below the 15th percentile on a timed writing test
Memory	77% showed deficits in long-term recall of verbal material
Attention	60% were distracted by auditory and visual stimuli in the classroom

Source: Ylvisaker (1989).

The academic problems created by brain damage are not limited to deficits in specific skills. It is not uncommon to find a disturbance of metacognitive and metalinguistic functions. Ylvisaker and Szekeres (1989) have identified seven problems:

1. *Limited self-awareness* of communication problems, which leads to a reluctance or unwillingness to work on them
2. *Poor planning* of language responses, resulting in disorganized, haphazard narratives
3. *Difficulty in initiating* conversation
4. *Problems in inhibiting* inappropriate remarks
5. *Failure to self-monitor* situations and conversations, resulting in inappropriate behavior or poor comprehension
6. *General self-evaluations* ("it's okay" or "it's all wrong") that do not lead to constructive responses
7. *Lack of flexibility* in considering various solutions to problems

Thus far, metacognitive/metalinguistic problems have been described in detail only for children with closed-head injury. However, children with vascular lesions and

Landau-Kleffner syndrome have also been depicted as having difficulties with narrative organization, self-awareness of their impairments, and timely initiation of speech. Future studies may reveal more about the metacognitive/metalinguistic deficits in these populations.

Differences between Developmental and Acquired Language Disorders in Children

Throughout this chapter we have noted that children with acquired aphasia are a unique population because they have developed and then lost a competence with language. The evidence of rapid recovery of some skills makes it apparent that children do not actually relearn language following a brain injury. They appear instead to reaccess some of the abilities that existed premorbidly, to compensate for some of the abilities that are lost, and to resume acquiring new skills.

Compared to children with developmental language disorders, children with acquired aphasia differ in attitude, in profile of abilities, and in pattern of improvement. Among the characteristics commonly noted in children with closed-head injury are the following (Catroppa & Anderson, 1999, 2003; DePompei & Blosser, 1987; Tucker & Colson, 1992; Ylvisaker & Gioia, 1998):

- They have previous successful experiences in social and academic settings.
- Before their injury, they had a self-concept of being normal.
- They have many discrepancies in ability levels.
- They show inconsistent patterns of performance.
- During recovery they are likely to show great variability and fluctuation.
- They have greater problems in generalizing, structuring, and integrating new information.

The differences in the experiences of these children and in our expectations for their rate of progress should lead us to organize intervention programs that cater to their special needs and yet still recognize their commonality with other children. Intervention for children with acquired aphasia cannot rely on the same strategies that are used for developmental language disorders. Many professionals have reported that they feel ill prepared to provide services to students with TBI. Although increased training in this domain has improved the overall quality of service, there remain significant gaps in knowledge and uncertainties about professional competence (Hux, Walker, & Sanger, 1996). To assist professionals in knowing what approaches to intervention have been shown to be effective with individuals with TBI, Tate, Perdices, McDonald, Togher, and Mosely, an interdisciplinary group of Australian researchers, have been developing a database that evaluates the available evidence about interventions, including language interventions, that have been used with people with TBI 5 years of age and older (Tate & Douglas, 2002). The database, known as PsycBITE, is to be available free of charge on the World Wide Web in early 2004.

Implications for Assessment and Intervention

Assessment

The incidence of acquired aphasia in children is significantly lower than either the incidence of developmental language disorders or the incidence of aphasia in adults. As a result, few tests have been developed specifically to evaluate childhood aphasia. It is possible to administer norm-referenced tests that are used to identify developmental language disorders. These will at least establish how children with acquired aphasia compare to their typically developing peers. However, these tests cannot be used to answer questions about rate or pattern of recovery, as can tests constructed for adults with aphasia. In any language test administered to children with acquired aphasia, it is crucial to differentiate effects that are due to language impairment (e.g., language comprehension deficits) from effects due to the method of testing (e.g., sustained attention, speed of information processing) (Turkstra & Holland, 1998).

It is tempting to administer a battery of tests to compare a child's performance across different modalities (e.g., speaking, listening, writing). However, in most instances the tests have been standardized on different populations, and any conclusions about patterns of impairment must therefore be severely limited (Swisher, 1985). Even tests such as the Clinical Evaluation of Language Fundamentals—Third Edition (CELF—3) (Semel et al., 1996b), which assess both receptive and expressive language abilities and are standardized on a single population, must be used with caution. Tests like various versions of the CELF are intended to identify linguistic impairment but do not necessarily identify problems of verbal memory, learning, and fluency that can significantly affect a student's academic performance (Turkstra, 1999).

Two tests are available that are adaptations of instruments originally devised for use with adults. The child adaptation of the Neurosensory Center Comprehensive Examination for Aphasia (Gaddes & Crockett, 1975) provides norms for children from 6 to 13 years of age. The Porch Index of Communicative Ability in Children (Porch, 1979) has norms from 3 to 12 years. These tests cannot be interpreted in the same fashion as their adult counterparts, and questions remain about whether the aphasia models on which they are based can be validly applied to children. Nevertheless, they may prove useful in assessment, if only as a criterion-referenced measure of a child's behavior during the period of spontaneous recovery.

A much better alternative for assessment will come with the development of tests that are standardized on children and adolescents with acquired aphasia. One such instrument, the Pediatric Test of Traumatic Brain Injury, is designed for use with school-aged children and adolescents in acute care and rehabilitation settings after TBI (Hotz, Helm-Estabrooks, & Nelson, 2001). It allows for the evaluation of cognitive and linguistic skills immediately following injury and during the period of recovery. Eventually, this will enable researchers to develop psychometric profiles for recovery based on a child's age and type and severity of injury. Other instruments will assist in the detection of subtle deficits in pragmatic skills such as the ability to negotiate, hint, describe a simple procedure, or understand sarcasm (McDonald & Turkstra, 1998; Turkstra, McDonald, & Kaufmann, 1996).

The assessment process for children with acquired aphasia needs to be multidisciplinary. Among the professionals who may be involved are a classroom teacher, nurse, occupational therapist, special educator, parent, pediatrician, physical therapist, psychologist, recreational therapist, and speech–language pathologist. To synthesize information from a variety of sources (tests, interviews, observations) and facilitate team decision making, a common rating scale may be used to track a child's progress (Bagnato et al., 1988).

Social and Legislative Influences

Children with TBI are now included in the federal laws on education for children with disabilities and thus are eligible for services from public school systems. However, the cost of such services is prohibitive for many smaller schools. Consequently, many children with mild and moderate TBI are not served. In the past, children with nontraumatic brain injuries resulting from stroke, infection, poisoning, and other causes were not included in the definition of TBI and therefore did not receive services. Several states have recently changed their statutes in this regard.

Interestingly, these laws do not define what "education" is, with the result that education and rehabilitation professionals may disagree on what are appropriate services for a child. A plan for therapy that is deemed necessary by rehabilitation personnel may be rejected or severely reduced by public schools on the grounds that it is not strictly necessary for educational purposes (Savage, 1991). Economy may be a factor in the acceptance, rejection, or modification of these plans.

Nonspeech Options

Later in this text is a discussion of augmentative and alternative communication (AAC) and relevance to children with acquired aphasia. In early stages of recovery following TBI, AAC may be necessary to establish a way for the children to communicate if their speech is unintelligible or they are unable to speak. AAC may also be part of their intervention, as we shall see in Chapter 12.

Behavior Disorders

Professionals working with children with acquired language disorders need to be prepared for the possibility that these children may demonstrate behavior problems. These can be described as aggressive, impulsive, disinhibited, or antisocial behaviors or the opposite, such as lack of drive and motivation or depression. The behavioral outcome in each child is the result of an interaction among the effects of the brain injury, the adjustment made to the new situation created by the accident (e.g., new living quarters, parent–child relationships, school, peer group), and the behavior predispositions of the individual (e.g., tendencies toward aggressiveness, depression). This latter factor relates to issues of preinjury behaviors that the children may have demonstrated (e.g., impulsivity, aggressiveness, risk taking) and that, in some cases, might have been associated with reasons for their injury. All these factors must be considered in understanding a child's behavior and developing an intervention plan to deal with it. In addition, certain types of behavior problems may be driven by neurological damage and may therefore require drug treatment along with behavioral intervention.

Intelligibility

Children with acquired aphasia who also present some kind of speech-production problem may require intervention so that efforts to promote language recovery are not hindered by poor intelligibility. Improvements in intelligibility will allow children to display linguistic abilities without frustration. Gains in intelligibility will also benefit any other intervention strategies that require judgments about the correctness of children's attempts at target forms.

Problems of aphasia, dysarthria, and apraxia of speech can coexist in children with TBI. During the early stages of recovery, treatment is limited to facial and oral stimulation and feeding therapy. If a child is alert but unintelligible, AAC may prove useful. Later, usually 1 year or more postonset, severe hypernasality, if present, may be treated through the fitting of a palatal lift prosthesis or through palatal surgery. Articulatory impairments are usually amenable to phonetic placement approaches or drill designed to increase gradually the length and complexity of phonetic units that a child can produce.

Developmental versus Remedial Logic

Depending on the age at which a child acquires aphasia, professionals may apply different models of recovery. Preschool children are likely to be learning fundamental syntactic and phonological skills at the time of their injury (Eisele & Aram, 1995). Consequently, a developmental model likely remains appropriate and may be used to select goals and teaching strategies for these children (Ylvisaker & Holland, 1984). With older children and adolescents, a model based on observed patterns of physiological recovery may be more useful. Table 10.5 displays a three-stage model of recovery and lists some of the symptoms and intervention strategies relevant to each stage.

Facilitating versus Compensatory Intervention

Many children with acquired aphasia are still in the process of learning language when their brain injury occurs. Although adolescents will have acquired many more language abilities, brain injury in the teenage years not only disrupts existing communication skills but can also affect further learning. Unlike their younger counterparts who sustain brain injury, these adolescents have much less of an advantage from neurological plasticity to help them. However, whether intervention is being planned for children or adolescents with acquired aphasia, the goals not only aim to restore what was lost but also to facilitate the new learning that was interrupted. Haley et al. (1990) describe this in terms of four objectives:

1. Restoration of function
2. Compensation for function
3. Adaptation of the environment to facilitate function
4. Normal acquisition of developmental skills

In the late stages of recovery the role served by the professional is to assist children and adolescents in compensating for skills that are lost or to help in adapting to the environment. Many techniques and strategies can be applied in this process, some of which are listed in Table 10.6.

TABLE 10.5   Stages of Recovery in Closed-Head Injury and Related Intervention Strategies

Stage	Symptoms	Intervention Strategies
Early	Responds to stimulation but can be easily overstimulated Disoriented to person, place, time, and own condition Inconsistent memory function, especially for recent events Inconsistent comprehension of speech Uses simple gestures to communicate Speech may be unintelligible, echolalic, perseverative, halting	Control amount and type of stimulation child receives: ■ Counsel family members ■ Determine and provide stimuli to which child is most appropriately responsive ■ Reassess frequently ■ Modify environment to suit needs of child; provide familiar pictures, objects, music, etc. ■ Verbally orient child to time and place
Middle	Alert and more oriented but still confused about schedules and own condition Limited attention span and concentration Information processing and language comprehension limited to small amounts and simple concepts and words Speaks but may require prompting Loses train of thought while talking and has difficulty with word retrieval	Begin practice of cognitive and communicative functions: ■ Structure child's day and provide ongoing orientation by means of schedule and log book ■ Schedule intervention in group and individual sessions ■ Work on attending behavior, memory function, and information processing by gradually increasing length and complexity of tasks ■ Ensure high success rate, vary activities, and use video to maintain child's motivation ■ Focus on improving comprehension of longer and more complex stimuli
Late	Well oriented as long as a routine is followed Difficulty in shifting from one task to another Capable of learning new skills and information, though slowly and with effort Difficulty with comprehension of nonliteral language (metaphors, jokes) Disorganization evident at all levels of language; has difficulty focusing on main points or staying on topic Few syntactic errors; mild word-finding problems	Begin to teach compensatory strategies and use of alternative communication devices: ■ Practice deductive reasoning and problem solving (e.g., "20 questions") ■ Vary activities and discussions to encourage cognitive flexibility (e.g., change rules of a game slightly) ■ Practice self-monitoring and require child to request clarification of information that is not understood ■ Compensate for poor memory with associative strategies and memo books ■ Practice analyzing information for major points

Source: Ylvisaker & Holland (1984).

Returning to School

Special education services designed primarily for children with intellectual disabilities, learning disabilities, or emotional disturbances may not be appropriate for children with acquired aphasia. On the other hand, full-time mainstreaming into a regular education class-

TABLE 10.6 Compensatory Teaching Strategies

Socialization and emotional support	Plan small group activities with unimpaired children to facilitate interaction skills.
	Schedule time for rest and emotional release. Encourage child to discuss problems as they come up.
Instruction	Give instructions both verbally and in writing. Repeat or paraphrase them as necessary. If understanding is critical, ask the student to repeat information or respond to a few questions about the instructions.
	Encourage student to self-monitor comprehension and to request repetition or rephrasing of instructions.
	Develop a verbal (e.g., calling student's name) or nonverbal system (e.g., posting a symbol or picture) for cueing the student to attend, respond, or change some aspect of behavior.
	Allow additional time for processing of instructions, responding to questions, and completing assignments.
	Provide child with a "buddy" to assist in following classroom directions, completing assignments, and traveling within the school.
Assistive devices	Allow and encourage the use of calculators, tape recorders, and computers.
	Have the student maintain a schedule and logbook in which are tracked all classes, appointments, assignments and due dates, and room locations. Include pictures of persons who are not readily identified.
	Provide maps for finding locations within the school.
Modification of materials	As far as possible, structure the physical environment to reduce distractions and allow freedom of movement.
	Use enlarged print in reading materials and supplement texts with pictures and other resources (vocabulary lists, outlines of key points) to facilitate comprehension.
	Cover parts of the page during reading and look at exposed areas systematically; use finger or index card to help in scanning.
	Modify assignments and tests according to the student's abilities by reducing the amount of reading or number of problems.

Sources: Blosser & DePompei (1994); New Zealand Guidelines Group (1998); and Ylvisaker et al. (1991).

room may be overwhelming for a child who has been in a hospital environment for several months (Blosser & DePompei, 1994; DePompei & Blosser, 1987; Savage & Wolcott, 1994; Ylvisaker, Hartwick, & Stevens, 1991). The rapid rate of recovery of many children with brain injuries means that their individualized educational plans (IEPs) must be reviewed and modified more frequently than those of other children (Savage, 1991; Ylvisaker et al., 1991).

To function effectively in school, children must be able to cope with demands for attention, concentration, and socialization. Cohen, Joyce, Rhoades, and Welks (1985) suggest that as a prerequisite to returning to school a child must be able to:

- Attend to a task for 10 to 15 minutes
- Tolerate 20 to 30 minutes of general classroom stimulation, such as movement, noises, and visual distractions

- Function within a group of two or more students
- Engage in meaningful communication through speech, gesture, or alternative/augmentative communication device
- Follow simple directions
- Show potential for learning

Successful return to school also requires the involvement and cooperation of professionals at both the hospital and school, as well as family members and individuals in the community (Taylor et al., 2002). Many areas will require planning and follow-up (New Zealand Guidelines Group, 1998; Ylvisaker et al., 1991):

1. The parents must be prepared for their role as advocates for their child's education. They must receive information about medical and social aspects of brain injury, entitlement to special education under federal laws, and cost sharing between schools and insurance companies.
2. Children with brain injuries must maintain peer relationships that are as close to normal as possible. Friends and classmates should be informed about the child's condition and how it affects and does not affect participation in various games and activities. Children who are willing can be involved in explaining their injuries to their peers.
3. Children should be prepared for the demands of school before they return. Environmental conditions, such as noisy classrooms and crowded hallways, can be simulated in the hospital, and children can be encouraged to visit their schools before they return full-time. Special instructional materials (e.g., large-print books, modified worksheets) and procedures should be tested and evaluated before they are used on a regular basis.
4. Teachers and other school staff should be educated about the child's condition, needs, and abilities. One individual should be appointed as case manager to coordinate services provided by the school.
5. The need for vocational rehabilitation should be considered from an early age. Efforts should be made to provide work experiences to children with brain injuries so that they develop normal expectations for and attitudes about employment.
6. Children who are discharged from the hospital during the summer months will require special planning to see them through the period until school begins.
7. Physical, health, or cognitive problems may prevent some children from attending school. In this case they are entitled to homebound services from the school system, which require special coordination efforts.

Plainly, the transition back to school is a challenge to friends, parents, school personnel, and, most of all, the child. Professionals should be ready to help organize and assist in this crucial process.

Summary

In this chapter, we have seen that

- Acquired aphasia is a condition in which a child begins to develop language and then loses all or part of that ability due to a brain injury.

- The major causes of acquired aphasia in children are closed-head injury, vascular lesions, and convulsive disorder (Landau-Kleffner syndrome).
- Besides causing aphasia, brain injuries can produce impairments of gross and fine motor skills, cognition, perception, and social behavior.
- Most children spontaneously recover a substantial portion of their premorbid communicative ability.
- During the acute period following injury, children with acquired aphasia may show a dramatic loss of language abilities. In the most severe cases they may be mute and completely unresponsive to speech stimuli.
- Most children recover much of their ability to comprehend and produce language during the first year following their injury. Thereafter, they are often plagued with residual communicative difficulties, often high-level language skills and/or pragmatic abilities, that can seriously affect academic and social performance.
- Assessment and intervention for children with acquired aphasia is a multidisciplinary endeavor. It must be planned with consideration of each child's intelligibility, behavior problems, preferred modality, and changing needs over the course of recovery.
- The aims of intervention are to assist in the restoration of some language functions and acquisition of skills for which development was interrupted and to help children compensate for other functions that remain impaired.
- The transition back to school is a complex undertaking that requires considerable cooperation, organization, and sensitivity to the host of physical, educational, and social problems a child will encounter.

Children with acquired aphasia pose special challenges to professionals working with language disorders. Over the course of recovery these children gradually exchange medical problems for social and educational ones. In most instances, professionals working in hospital settings hand over the intervention to school personnel. There is opportunity for confusion as these changes in service occur. The problem is best avoided by increasing everyone's awareness and understanding of these children's capabilities, disabilities, and needs.

11 Language and Other Special Populations of Children

STEVEN H. LONG

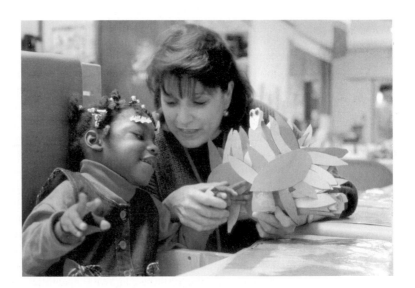

OBJECTIVES

After reading this chapter you should be able to discuss

- Definitions of giftedness and factors that affect estimates of its prevalence among children
- General characteristics of the spoken and written language of gifted children
- Issues in assessment and intervention with gifted children who also have disabilities or economic disadvantage
- Different factors involved in definitions of visual impairment
- Characteristics of the spoken language of blind children
- General principles of intervention with blind children and their parents
- The etiology and types of cerebral palsy and other neuromotor disorders
- General speech and language characteristics of children with cerebral palsy
- General aims of intervention for children with cerebral palsy
- Possible causes of delayed language development in children with cleft palate

This chapter takes a brief look at four populations of children whose language can be affected by their special conditions. Two of these populations are gifted children and children who are blind. It might be unexpected to see these sections included in a text about children with language disorders and, in fact, the language of these children is often overlooked. Yet, as will be discovered from reading the first half of this chapter, language ability plays an important role in their development. In the latter half of the chapter, we review language abilities of children with neuromotor impairments and those with cleft palate. While discussions of language and neuromotor impairments, in particular cerebral palsy, are more common in the literature, the language of children with cleft palate is not often a focus in descriptions and discussions of these children. Nevertheless, language is not exempt from being affected.

Language and Gifted Children

Some readers may be surprised to find a discussion of gifted children in a text about disorders of language. There are at least three reasons, however, why it is relevant to describe this population. First, gifted children, like children with language impairments, are exceptional. The psychometric procedures for identifying both groups of children are quite similar, and *gifted education* is commonly viewed either as a branch of *special education* or as a parallel division of education. Second, children with exceptional abilities are sometimes disruptive in the classroom because they are not sufficiently challenged by the style and pace of the curriculum (Cline & Schwartz, 1999; Webb, 1993). Hence, they may be referred for evaluation by a school psychologist, speech–language pathologist, or other professional. Third, and most important, the population of gifted children overlaps with three other groups: bilingual-bicultural children, children with physical or sensory impairments, and children with learning disabilities. One of the issues noted by experts in gifted education as most important to that field is how best to identify and serve gifted children who are economically disadvantaged or have some disabilities that limit the expression of their abilities (Cramer, 1991; Ford, 1996; Winebrenner, 2003). To some extent, therefore, professionals who serve children with language disorders have an important role to play in assessment and educational planning for children who are gifted.

An Overview of Giftedness

Definition. In popular thinking, there seems to be little argument that some individuals are more able than others. Our language has a number of words—*gifted, genius,* and *talented* among them—to distinguish those with exceptional abilities. Among scholars, however, there is considerable dispute over the concept of *giftedness* and whether it reflects anything more than just natural variation, the effects of practice, and the advantages of being raised in a privileged environment (Howe, Davidson, & Sloboda, 1998). One thing is clear: There is no single definition of *giftedness.* The difficulty in defining this term is much like the problem of defining *disordered* or *impaired.* Children may be viewed as disordered if they display characteristics that will hinder them from achieving socially valued goals such as getting along with peers, gaining an education, or finding a job. Similarly, children may be considered gifted if they show superior abilities in domains that society values: speech and language, writing, music, athletics, art, and others. As early as 1972, the U.S. Office of Education created the following definition of gifted and talented children that emphasized the idea of social value (Marland, 1972):

> Gifted and talented children are those identified by professionally qualified persons who by virtue of outstanding abilities are capable of high performance. These are children who require differentiated educational programs and services beyond those normally provided by the regular school program in order to realize their contribution to self and society.

This definition is deliberately broad and calls attention to the special educational needs of these children. Another definition of giftedness, based on opinions contributed by a panel of experts in the field, is shown in Table 11.1. This definition is more detailed and reflects the evolution of thinking among educators from the 1970s to the twenty-first century. Three major refinements have been made:

1. Giftedness is defined as a potential ability as well as a demonstrated ability. This subtle change is needed to justify efforts at early identification of gifted children whose skills are not yet well developed.
2. The definition contains a warning against biased judgments. This is consistent with the opposition to stereotyping and discrimination at all levels of education.
3. Separate characteristics are described for a gifted child and a gifted adult. The distinction is primarily one of potential versus performance. It is also suggested that a feature of giftedness in mature individuals is independent and creative work.

In principle, children may display giftedness in several different ways. They may score very highly on general tests of intelligence, suggesting that they are developmentally advanced in a number of areas. Or they may achieve high scores on tests of aptitude in only one or two domains, such as visuospatial abilities or mathematics. Another possibility is that they will not distinguish themselves on any formal test but will manifest their special abilities through their behavior in natural surroundings. Table 11.2 lists some of the behavioral

---

TABLE 11.1   A Consensus Definition of Giftedness by Experts in Gifted Education

1. Giftedness is the potential for exceptional development of specific abilities as well as the demonstration of performance at the upper end of a talent continuum; it is not limited by age, gender, race, socioeconomic status, or ethnicity.

2. A gifted child is one who is developmentally advanced in one or more areas; he or she has potential or demonstrated ability in general intellectual ability, specific academic aptitude, leadership, creative productive thinking, or the visual and performing arts; because of this potential or demonstrated ability, the child requires differentiated education services in order to function at the level appropriate to his or her potential.

3. A gifted adult is one who shows unusual skill, ability, or talent in one or more areas of intellect, leadership, or in the visual or performing arts; he or she makes independent and creative contributions to a field.

Sources: Cramer (1991); Ross (1993); and VanTassel-Baska (1998).

TABLE 11.2   Behavioral Characteristics of Gifted Children

Category	Behavior
Communication	Has unusually advanced vocabulary for age or grade level; uses terms in a meaningful way; has verbal behavior characterized by richness of expression, elaboration, and fluency
	Strong transmission and reception of signals or meanings through a system of symbols (codes, gestures, language, numbers)
	Demonstrates a flair for dramatic or oral presentations
Learning	Has quick mastery and recall of facts
	Quickly grasps new concepts and makes connections; senses deeper meanings
	Highly conscious, directed, controlled, goal-oriented thought
	Has rapid insight into cause–effect relationships; tries to discover the how and why of things; asks many thought-provoking questions (as distinct from information or factual questions)
	Logical approaches to figuring out solutions; effective (often inventive) strategies for recognizing and solving problems
	Determines alternatives to reach a desired goal
	Learns from experience and seldom repeats mistakes
	Transfers learning easily from one situation to another
	Exceptional ability to memorize, retain, and retrieve information; has large storehouse of information on school or nonschool topics
Motivation	Evidences strong desire to learn, satisfy a need, or attain a goal
	Becomes absorbed and involved in certain topics or problems; is persistent in seeking task completion; displays long attention span
	Strives toward perfection; is self-critical; is not easily satisfied with work
	Often is self-assertive (sometimes even aggressive); stubborn in beliefs
Creativity/ sensitivity	Displays a great deal of curiosity about many things; constantly asks questions about anything and everything; has strong insight; explores, experiments
	Displays much intellectual playfulness; fantasizes; imagines ("I wonder what would happen if . . ."), produces many ideas; is highly original
	Shows ability to form mental images of objects, qualities, situations or relationships which are not immediately apparent to the senses
	Is unusually aware of impulses and more open to the irrational (freer expression of feminine interest for boys, greater than usual independence for girls); shows emotional sensitivity
	May have intense (sometimes unusual) interests; activities and objects may have special worth or significance and are given special attention
Leadership	Carries responsibility well; can be counted on to fulfill promises and usually does it well
	Is self-confident with peers as well as adults; seems comfortable when asked to show work to the class
	Adapts readily to new situations; is flexible in thought and action and does not seem disturbed when the normal routine is changed
Humor	Conveys and picks up on humor well
	Shows ability to synthesize key ideas or problems in a humorous way; exceptional sense of timing in words and gestures

Sources: Adapted from Alexander & Muia (1982); Frasier et al. (1995); and Silverman, Chitwood, & Waters (1986).

characteristics of gifted children that can be observed informally. As with their performance on standardized tests, gifted children may display exceptional behaviors in all or just a few of the categories shown. Of particular relevance to this chapter is the number of references in the table to language and language-related skills.

Prevalence.   Neither of the definitions of giftedness just reviewed has any official or legal standing. They are merely attempts to delineate the concept in a way that is logical and consistent with observed characteristics. In many educational systems, however, giftedness is a category of placement. The responsibility for setting eligibility criteria is left to the states or, in some cases, to local school districts. Although not all gifted children perform well on tests, most states rely on standardized instruments for identification and placement in special educational programs (Ross, 1993).

Because of variation in definitions and eligibility criteria, prevalence estimates for giftedness can range from 2 percent to almost 90 percent (Fenstermacher, 1982; Gagne, 1998; Lilly, 1979). Very high estimates are nearly always based on definitions that focus on children's potential for achievement, not their actual achievement. Some educators, especially in the United States, are reluctant to recognize a category of gifted children because it smacks of elitism and therefore runs contrary to the inclusive, egalitarian principles (Mills & Durden, 1992; Runco, 1997). Individuals who share this view prefer to highlight the latent abilities all children have if provided stimulation and educational opportunity. This opinion is supported by psychological research indicating that most children's abilities can be accelerated beyond what is currently considered average by means of well-designed programs of instruction and encouragement (Howe, 1990). In the following discussion, we will be using *gifted* in its more narrow sense of children who appear to excel without special instruction.

Language Characteristics of Gifted Children

One of the most striking features of gifted children is their precocious language development. If provided with a typical home environment, many of these children talk early and learn to read before they start school (Freeman, 1986). Parents often note advanced language skills as one of the first indicators of giftedness in their children. As shown in Table 11.3, one survey found that the characteristic mentioned most frequently by parents was expressive language, and most surveys involved some aspect of language and/or language-related abilities.

Other than its faster rate, there is no evidence that the language learning of gifted children differs from that of typically developing children. Thus, it is likely that a developmental model can be used to predict their language skills. Gifted preschool children may produce and understand language at a level that would be expected of elementary school children, and gifted children between 5 and 10 years of age may show language skills that resemble those of middle and high school children.

It should be remembered, however, that advanced language ability is not a requirement of giftedness. A child may be gifted in musical, artistic, athletic, mathematical, or social skills and display ordinary verbal abilities. One of the main features of gifted children with disabilities is the discrepancy between their superior abilities in one domain and mediocre or even deficient skills in another (Waldron, Saphire, & Rosenblum, 1987). Therefore, we cannot speak of the "language of gifted children" as though they were a

TABLE 11.3 Skill Categories Mentioned Most Often by Parents of Gifted Preschool Children

Rank Item	Skill
1	Language: expressive–productive
2	Memory
3	Abstract thinking
4	Ahead of peers
5	Curiosity
6	Language: receptive–comprehensive
7	Motor
8	Nomination (comments by others)
9.5	Awareness of the environment
9.5	Special knowledge (e.g., dinosaurs, foreign language)
11	Early interest in books and reading
12	Word and symbol recognition

Source: Adapted from Louis & Lewis (1992).

homogeneous group. The following discussion refers only to those children who display precocious verbal skills as a component of their giftedness.

Oral Language.   Gifted children are often said to be precocious talkers. One frequently cited milestone is the age at which first words are spoken. For example, studies of gifted children have reported that the average age of first words is 9 months, and some children begin to talk as early as 6 months of age (Price, 1976; Rogers & Silverman, 1997). There are two problems, however, in interpreting the first-word phenomenon: (1) the source of information is usually the parents, who may be biased in their recall by their present belief that the child is gifted; and (2) there are no established criteria for what constitutes a first word, in contrast to a phonetically consistent form, a protoword, or any of the other vocalizations routinely produced by infants after about 7 months of age. What may be a more reliable indicator of advanced verbal development is the rate at which a child progresses from single words to word combinations or the rate at which vocabulary is acquired during the single-word period. Recall that typically developing children make the transition from single words to syntax over a period of about 6 to 12 months. Gifted children may exceed both of these expectations by moving rapidly beyond single words into syntax and/or by acquiring an exceptionally large vocabulary before they begin to combine words.

Once a child is producing syntax, the most conspicuous sign of verbal giftedness is the amount and sophistication of vocabulary. In all children, lexical development can be judged from a series of quantitative and qualitative changes that occur:

- The number of different words used increases.
- Word usage becomes more specific and adultlike.
- Vocabulary knowledge extends into an increasing number of semantic fields.
- There is greater knowledge of structural relationships among words, indicated by the production of synonyms, antonyms, definitions, and subordinate and superordinate terms.

Gifted children are likely to be advanced in all of these respects. Both their comprehension and production vocabularies will be larger than average. For example, early studies report that

- Fourth- to seventh-grade gifted students had an average vocabulary score of 130, two standard deviations above the test mean (Winne, Woodlands, & Wong, 1982).
- Gifted children are conspicuous by the fact that they produce fewer semantic mismatches (e.g., overextensions, underextensions, misnamings) (Guilford, Scheuerle, & Shonburn, 1981).
- Children who are gifted are less likely to rely on personal and indefinite pronouns to establish reference, being able instead to use the appropriate lexical item (Guilford et al., 1981).

Many factors influence the vocabulary that children learn, but a general developmental trend is for them to learn words across a wider range of semantic fields. For example, we expect that much of a child's early vocabulary will pertain to fields such as people (e.g., *mommy, brother, boy, policeman*), food (*banana, eat, cook*), and moving (*come, go, take*). Not until children are older do we find them using many words in fields such as business (*insurance, advertise, secretary*) or the world (*continent, soil, equator*). Gifted children, though, are often exceptions to this rule and will amaze adults by their command of such advanced vocabulary. A sophisticated vocabulary, though, is not always an indicator of giftedness. It is possible for a child's knowledge of words in particular categories to be accelerated through specialized instruction and practice (Howe, 1990). Parents may be impressed by an ability to name state capitals, colors, or insects, but such rote knowledge is commonly found in children who do not meet psychometric criteria for giftedness (Louis & Lewis, 1992).

As vocabulary is learned, children also begin to sort out the relationships among words. Thus, they become able not only to retrieve individual words (e.g., *big*) but also to retrieve words that are similar in meaning (*huge, giant*), that are opposite in meaning (*little, tiny*), or concepts that have some hierarchical relationship (size, dimension). This progression in vocabulary knowledge is often related to conceptual growth, particularly to the development of abstract thinking. Knowledge of antonyms, synonyms, and related vocabulary indicate that children have identified an abstract linkage among words. This paves the way for them to acquire higher-order vocabulary, such as *vehicle, furniture,* or *beverage.* Conceptual development is also reflected in the ability to define words. Very young children may define *clock* by pointing to the object. Later in development, they may describe its function ("It wakes you up") or attributes ("It's round and it's got hands"). Eventually, they are able to give both a class name and a specific attribute or property ("an instrument for telling time") (Nippold, 1998). Gifted children are frequently advanced in their knowledge of abstract vocabulary and of word relationships. This is shown in their spontaneous use of higher-order words, their ability to paraphrase, and their ability to define words, a task included in the verbal portion of many intelligence tests. In relation to precocious vocabulary development, advanced syntactic abilities may not be as dazzling but are further indications of oral language proficiency. Several measures have been used to examine the syntactic skills of gifted children. By asking children to explain the meaning of nonsense words embedded in sentences (e.g., "We saw a trog car"), researchers have found that gifted children are more sensitive to syntactic constraints on meaning (Williams & Tillman, 1968). Gifted children are better able to infer what the sense of a word must be based on its position within a sentence. They also perform superiorly on imitation tasks in which sentence stimuli are constructed to represent a wide range of sentence types (commands, questions, statements) and syntactic forms (passive sentences, complex sentences, expanded phrases, etc.) (Guilford et al., 1981). Studies of spontaneous speech have also shown evidence of precocious syntax. Four-year-old gifted children displayed a mean length of utterance (MLU) that is above the average for their age, while gifted children in the fifth grade used longer sentences and a higher proportion of complex sentences than their typically developing peers (Guilford et al., 1981; Jensen, 1973). Also impressive is the fact that 92 percent of the utterances spoken by gifted 4-year-olds were free of syntactic errors, compared to 74 percent of the utterances of their typically developing peers (Guilford et al., 1981; Lee, 1974). Gifted children appear to be accelerated in their mastery of what are potentially troublesome syntactic structures for typically developing children, such as determiners and irregular morphological markers.

Differences in language use are often mentioned as a characteristic of gifted children. As noted in Table 11.2, these children are distinguished by their persistent and insightful question asking and for their skill in producing narratives and other oral presentations. An early study involving formal analysis of language functions reported that gifted fifth-grade students were more likely to converse about general, scientific, or practical concerns, while their typically developing peers tended to talk about personal experiences, perceptions, and preferences (Jensen, 1973). There is little research directly comparing the pragmatic language skills of gifted and typically developing children. Following the general principle that gifted children show normal but accelerated development, we might anticipate that they would be superior in their skills of referential communication, conversational repair, and topic management.

Reading and Writing. Opinion is divided on the significance of early reading ability in giftedness. Some assert that early reading is characteristic of gifted children, but in a survey of parents of preschoolers believed to be gifted, only 16 percent mentioned an early interest in books and reading, and even when early reading was reported, it was not predictive of whether the child was actually gifted (Louis & Lewis, 1992). This is consistent with research suggesting that early reading is not strongly related to intellectual ability, does not always predict later levels of reading achievement, and is probably attributable in part to child-rearing practices (Jackson, 1988; Jackson & Kearney, 1995).

There is better agreement that, once they begin to read, many gifted children show an exceptional enthusiasm for books and quickly become extremely able readers. In a study of eighth-, tenth-, and twelfth-grade students, it was discovered that gifted students made more frequent use of effective strategies such as rereading, inferring, predicting, and relating to content area. Average readers, on the other hand, were more often concerned about word pronunciation and made more inaccurate summaries of what they were reading (Fehrenbach, 1991). The more effective strategies used by gifted children enable them to read with greater comprehension than their peers. This provides them with a tremendous advantage in all academic areas, especially as they advance in school and reading becomes a principal method for acquiring new information.

In comparison to their oral expression and reading skills, the writing ability of many gifted children is less impressive, although the content of what they write is frequently above average (Yates, Berninger, & Abbott, 1995). The form of their writing often resembles that of their typically developing peers. They may write in simple sentences and use a limited vocabulary (Mindell & Stracher, 1980). The discrepancy between writing and other language skills is usually explained in terms of motivation. Good writing requires a command of form—punctuation, spelling, organization—that is unnecessary for other language behaviors. Writing is also a motor skill that must be learned and integrated with the pace at which thinking occurs. Many gifted children appear to be put off by the work that is demanded for writing and by the way it slows self-expression (Freeman, 1979; McCluskey & Walker, 1986). Consequently, they may not practice their writing sufficiently to develop a level of skill equal to their other language abilities. Word processing is one possible alternative for these children.

Language in Disadvantaged or Disabled Gifted Children

One issue in gifted education is that of special populations of gifted children (Cramer, 1991). Three of the subgroups that have been identified are

1. Children from economically disadvantaged backgrounds, the majority of whom are members of racial/ethnic minorities
2. Children with intellectual, motor, or sensory disabilities
3. Children who are underachieving because of learning disabilities superimposed on a high level of intelligence

There has been little study of these subgroups, and they have proven difficult to identify and serve.

Disadvantaged children who are also gifted are frequently not recognized. Perhaps because they anticipate and actively look for signs of giftedness in their children, mainstream parents are far more likely to seek specialized evaluation and educational services for preschoolers (Louis & Lewis, 1992). The parents of disadvantaged children may not recognize giftedness, or they may lack the means or motivation to pursue special services. Cultural and linguistic factors also appear to play a role, as children from Asian American families tend to be overrepresented in giftedness programs relative to their population numbers and children from African American, Hispanic, and Native American families tend to be underrepresented (Cohen, 1990).

When they begin school, disadvantaged children should have an equal opportunity to be recognized as gifted. Research has shown, however, that teachers' judgments of individual students are swayed by gender, race, and social class background (Brophy & Good, 1974; Minner, 1990). Identification is also made difficult by differences in the verbal behavior or learning style of disadvantaged students, even those who are gifted, with gifted children from affluent families tending to use language in imaginative play and to comment on past or future events, but gifted disadvantaged children likely expressing needs, monitoring their own actions, and identifying present actions and objects (Frasier et al., 1995; Hale-Benson, 1986; Tough, 1977). Therefore, they may not adhere to the profile of a gifted child, which emphasizes verbal creativity and elaboration, as we have seen. Cultural differences, bilingualism, and test biases, as discussed in Chapter 9, may also inhibit Hispanic American, African American, and Asian American children from exhibiting their competencies fully.

Studies in the psychobiology of intelligence suggest that as a general principle, specific abilities can function independently of one another. Hence, it is possible for an individual to have a profile of abilities in which all are superior, or to have a few superior and the rest average, or even to have some superior, some average, and others inferior. An extreme and well-publicized example of discrepant ability levels is found in the idiot savant, an individual whose measured general intelligence is in the range of intellectual disability but who evidences a specific talent such as sculpture or music or feats of recall. In contrast to the individual's many deficiencies, the single high ability is astonishing. Another example of discrepancy is a child with a severe disabling condition, such as cerebral palsy or autism, who nonetheless possesses superior intellectual or other abilities. We are becoming increasingly aware of such individuals as we learn to assist their communication with augmentative/alternative communication (AAC) devices and techniques. Another central problem in identifying gifted children who are disabled has been to find a nonbiased means of assessment.

A different category of children with discrepant abilities are those described as underachievers. These children function at levels that are roughly age appropriate, but they are hindered by learning disabilities or adverse social or emotional conditions that prevent them from realizing their potential (Brody & Mills, 1997). Formally, these children are identified by the inconsistency between their scores on IQ or achievement tests and their actual classroom performance (National Joint Committee on Learning Disabilities, 1998). Informally, these children often call attention to themselves because of personality and behavioral disturbances. Researchers have found that gifted children who do not achieve often lack self-confidence, have lower self-concepts, may have difficulty forming social relationships, and exhibit aggression (Mendaglio, 1993; Olenchak, 1994; Schiff, Kaufman, & Kaufman, 1981). Those gifted underachievers who have learning disabilities are often verbally superior, in contrast to most children with learning disabilities who are linguistically deficient and perform better on nonverbal tasks. Perhaps as a result, gifted underachieving children are frequently not referred to be assessed for learning disabilities until they reach the third grade or beyond (Schiff et al., 1981).

Implications for Intervention

Professionals who serve children with language disorders have a different role to play with various subgroups of gifted children. With advantaged children who are verbally gifted, professionals in most educational settings defer to a teacher who has been charged with developing a gifted education program. That program will vary from one school to another but likely will consist of some combination of *acceleration* and *enrichment* approaches, which attempt to provide a curriculum that matches gifted children's abilities, and *grouping* approaches, which separate gifted children from other students during certain instructional periods so that they can work at a faster pace (VanTassel-Baska, 1992). Teaching methods tend to focus less on content, which gifted children find easy to master, and more on synthesis and creative processing of information (Shore & Delacourt, 1997).

With disadvantaged gifted students, professionals have more responsibility in evaluating their abilities and interpreting issues of language difference to other educators. Gifted children with linguistically-culturally diverse backgrounds require attention to matters of nonbiased assessment and nonstandard dialect, as discussed in Chapter 9. They also may need help in understanding and adjusting to their own giftedness. As we observed earlier, these children are much less likely to be identified by their families. Thus, many disadvantaged gifted children may never have been told that they are gifted and have received little reinforcement for their exceptional abilities. Because of their background as well as peer pressure, they may find it difficult to display their verbal abilities. This is a delicate issue that calls for sensitivity to a child's age, peer group, family, cultural, and ethnic group. For some children it may be prudent to let them develop their language skills quietly through reading and writing rather than force them into special programs that could create problems in psychosocial development.

Gifted children who have physical, sensory, or learning disabilities are frequently referred for intervention because of what they cannot do. Common sense dictates that professionals should try to take advantage of these children's giftedness in compensating for their deficiencies. For example, gifted children can often be taught *workaround* strategies, that is, alternative ways of accomplishing tasks they find difficult. Technology can assist these students in several ways. For children with physical or sensory disabilities, AAC devices may be the key to all teaching efforts. For those with learning disabilities, computers, calculators, and other specialized electronic devices offer assistance with vexing tasks such as spelling, calculating, and handwriting (Brown-Chidsey & Boscardin, 1999). The psychological profile of these students indicates that they are hindered by their own frustration and lack of confidence. They may benefit from cognitive training, discussed in Chapter 4, that reduces impulsive responding and promotes alternative methods of rehearsal and problem solving.

Language and Children with Visual Impairment

Judged by their progress through major language milestones, few children with visual impairment as their sole disability will meet the criteria for a language disorder. Because of their sensory deficit, however, these children acquire language differently from sighted children, which often leads to a request for professional evaluation and consultation. In addition, until complete developmental and sensory evaluations can be performed, there will be a concern that a child with visual impairment may also have hearing impairment, learning disabilities, or intellectual disabilities. In that event, the prognosis for normal development of language is considerably poorer. All children with intellectual disabilities will have difficulty with language; visual impairment adds to that problem and raises a serious obstacle to intervention efforts.

An Overview of Visual Impairment

A number of terms are used by professionals in medicine, education, and rehabilitation to describe loss of vision. *Blindness* has no fixed definition. It is possible to measure vision in different ways. The standard optometric test is a measure of visual acuity for objects at a distance. However, many individuals with visual impairment cannot see at a distance but do possess some near vision. Furthermore, vision does not operate independently of other sensory and cognitive systems. It is possible to have some functional vision if the nervous system is able to augment a very weak visual signal with information gained from other sensory channels and from previous experiences.

The American Foundation for the Blind recommends that the term *blind* be used to refer to individuals with no usable sight. Persons with usable vision, no matter how little, should be described as *visually impaired, partially sighted,* or *low vision.* Within the category of blindness, distinctions are made between individuals who do and do not have light perception and between those who can and cannot detect movement, as when a hand is waved in front of the face. Blindness may be congenital, with onset at birth or shortly after, or adventitious, occurring later in life. Children who become blind after 5 years of age retain visual memories and are able to visualize as an adjunct to thinking (Sardegna & Otis, 1991). Among children with visual impairment and no other deficits, language development is seriously affected only in children with congenital blindness who have no pattern recognition (Freeman & Blockberger, 1987). In the remainder of this section we will limit discussion to children who are congenitally blind. Children with lesser degrees of visual impairment can be expected to show greater parallels with the language development of sighted children. Children with visual impairment along with intellectual disabilities or physical disabilities will have wide-ranging language impairments.

Congenital blindness results from diseases or conditions that are either inherited or occur *in utero.* Damage may affect either non-neural (lens, cornea, iris) or neural (retina, optic nerve) portions of the visual system. Certain conditions, such as retinitis pigmentosa, are degenerative, so that vision will become worse as a child grows older. Recent improvements in obstetric and neonatal care now allow many extremely premature infants to survive. These infants, however, have a high incidence of impaired vision (Powls, Botting, Cooke, Stephenson, & Marlow, 1997). Data from a recent U.S. urban survey found that slightly less than 1 in 1,000 children between ages 3 and 10 had a vision impairment, mostly of prenatal origin (Mervis, Yeargin-Allsopp, Winter, & Boyle, 2000). In 1998 an estimated 93,600 visually impaired or blind students were enrolled in special education programs in the United States (Kirchner & Diament, 1999).

Language Characteristics of Blind Children

In general, what is observed in the language development of blind children is neither delayed nor deviant, but rather an alternative route to language acquisition that utilizes sensory and motor resources in a way different from sighted children (Perez-Pereira & Conti-Ramsden, 1999). Few developmental differences are observed between typically developing and blind children during the first 4 months of life. At that point, sighted children begin to attend to their hands, which in turn encourages manual exploration of the environment. In contrast, children who are blind rely on others to present objects for them to manipulate. They tend to mouth objects for a slightly longer time than sighted children, probably as a compensation for the loss of visual information about what they are holding (Sardegna & Otis, 1991). Blind children are generally delayed in walking and crawling and frequently do not spontaneously explore their environment (Troster, Hecker, & Brambring, 1993). If they are encouraged to become physically active, however, they will develop motor skills, though not quite at the level of sighted children (Bouchard & Tetreault, 2000). Without encouragement and opportunity, they may develop stereotypical movements such as rocking, head swaying, and poking or rubbing of the eyes (Sardegna & Otis, 1991).

To understand how language develops in blind children, it is crucial to consider the role that vision plays in typical language development. During the first year, sighted children develop preverbal communication routines that are mediated largely through sight. Recall that:

- Early exchanges between parents and infants are regulated through eye contact and head turning.
- Shared attention (joint attention) is achieved by the parent and infant each watching the other's eye movements.
- Systematic use of gesture is an important early form of intentional communication and overlaps with children's first use of meaningful words.

Blind children also develop routines with their parents, but they do so through a more laborious auditory–tactile process. For example, while it is possible to observe when a child is attending auditorily, the cues—cocking the head or becoming still—are subtle and easily missed (Baird, Mayfield, & Baker, 1997). Therefore, the mother tends to talk more and use more directives (Conti-Ramsden & Perez-Pereira, 1999), and may use touch and body contact to maintain a link with the child. Mother and child play games involving repetition and anticipation, comparable to peek-a-boo, but using touching, tickling, stroking, and other forms of contact instead of visual cues. The infant's vocalizations are actively encouraged to the point that idiosyncratic routines may develop. These vocal routines, though they also occur in sighted children, are especially important to the development of blind children because they serve as both an emotional link to the caretaker and a key sensory experience (Chen, 1996). Pointing and reaching for sources of sound are delayed in these children. Out of concerns for safety, parents may restrict the activities of their blind children, thereby limiting the children's opportunities for physical exploration of their environment (Rock, Head, Bradley, Whiteside, & Brisby, 1994). Not surprisingly, therefore, the onset of meaningful speech occurs slightly later than in sighted children.

Children who are blind become more developmentally heterogeneous as they grow older. Many factors have an impact on their language development, including the degree of visual loss, the presence of other impairments, and the response of caretakers to their impairment. Nevertheless, certain behaviors occur with sufficient frequency in these children to be considered generally characteristic.

Syntax.   The syntactic development of blind children differs little from that of sighted children. They are slightly delayed in beginning to use word combinations but, by age 3, their MLUs are comparable to those of their typically developing peers (Landau & Gleitman, 1985; Perez-Pereira & Conti-Ramsden, 1999). Utterance length may be less representative of syntactic competence than it is in typically developing children because of blind children's tendency to echo phrases they hear before they have productive control of the syntax of those phrases.

Semantics.   As vocabulary is learned, the contexts and functions of words tend to be restricted. Words first learned in the context of routine activities, such as eating or bathing, may not be used outside those contexts until a child is much older. Typically developing children commonly overextend the meanings of early words, for example, using *juice* to refer to all potable liquids. Most of these overextensions are based on visual similarities among objects. As might be expected, blind children rarely overextend the meanings of words they acquire (Andersen, Dunlea, & Kekelis, 1984).

A number of early developing concepts are closely linked to visual experiences. Thus, children who are blind may be slow to understand or use words such as *dirty, clean, open, shut, in, out, up,* and *down.* This delay appears to be due exclusively to the lack of sensory experience. Concepts and words that can be learned through other sense information, such as *sticky, sweet, hot, cold,* and *big,* are readily learned (Sardegna & Otis, 1991).

Blind children may display a type of egocentrism in the learning of words that are not substantial. Action words may be used only to refer to actions they are performing and not to actions involving other people or objects (Andersen et al., 1984). For example, the words *up* and *down* may be used only to request or describe the child's own movement and not as general locative terms (Urwin, 1984). Relational vocabulary, such as *more* or *no,* may find use only in expressing personal needs and not in commenting on changes of state in the environment (Andersen et al., 1984).

In typically developing children, vision facilitates awareness of themselves as separate from others and from their environment (Sardegna & Otis, 1991). Delays in a blind child's internal representation of self may be responsible for pronominal reversals and confusions they often display. For example, one child requested a drink by saying, "I want some juice. She wants some juice" (Kitzinger, 1984). Alternatively, pronoun confusion may be viewed as a problem with understanding deictic language, where meaning changes according to the speaker's perspective. Other deictic words, such as *here, there, this,* and *that,* also present difficulties to blind children (Andersen et al., 1984). Unlike children with autism, however, these problems with pronouns and interpersonal reference tend to be overcome by 7 years of age (Hobson, 1993).

Echolalia.   A characteristic of blind children's communication that draws frequent comment is their use of imitation. As in children with autism, this behavior is described as *echolalia* when it appears to occur in an automatic and unthinking way, that is, when the listener believes the speech was repeated without communicative intent. A high proportion of blind children's utterances may be echoic. In one study of a 3-year-old girl, the percentage of echoed utterances in spontaneous speech was 20.7 percent with her mother and 35.7 percent with an adult she knew slightly (Kitzinger, 1984).

Echoed utterances may appear more unusual than they really are. Lacking sight, blind children must find substitutes for many communicative behaviors that are typically accomplished with nonverbal visual signals. For example, repetition frequently serves the function of acknowledgment, which sighted children perform nonverbally by looking, nodding the head, changing facial expression, and so on. Sighted children are known to produce monologues that serve the purposes of verbal rehearsal, dramatic play, and direction of their own actions. Yet this speech is typically accompanied by movement, especially with the hands, that gives the words a context. Kitzinger (1984) gives an example and commentary about a blind girl's monologue in which she produces different voices but gives no other clues about the purpose of her language:

> Some of Betty's [the blind child's] echoed comments gave the impression that she had incorporated wholesale, without modification, aspects of others' speech:
> Betty is sitting on her potty and the following "conversation" takes place.
>
> **BETTY:** (with echoed intonation) Pull down your pants. You're too big for the potty.
>
> **BETTY:** (in her own voice) I'm too big for the potty.
>
> **MK** [the adult]:   Who says that?
>
> **BETTY:** (calling out) Ann! Ann!
>
> **MK:**   Does Ann say you are too big for the potty?
>
> **BETTY:** (with echoed intonation) Ann's toilet is never . . . (unintelligible) . . . on the potty.
>
> Betty seems to be relaying some former experience prompted by the context. It was said without any apparent intention of communicating something to me but had the quality of play of a sighted child, perhaps with a doll as a prop. Had she used such a prop a shared context would have been provided and the purpose of these utterances would have been clearer. (p. 142)

Pragmatics.   Blindness has some inevitable consequences for the way in which children use language. For example, although young blind children generally display a similar profile of communicative functions, they use language less often to name or request objects that are remote and cannot be touched. They produce fewer utterances describing the perceptions of others (that they cannot see) and more about ongoing or intended action (Perez-Pereira & Conti-Ramsden, 1999). Certain features of language may develop earlier or to a greater extent because they serve a compensatory role. Rising intonation may be used from an early age to keep a conversation going. Sighted children typically use eye contact for the same purpose. Blind children may show a greater knowledge and use of people's names, for this gives them an ability to initiate social interactions even when they cannot locate the conversational partner (Urwin, 1984).

Unusual nonverbal mannerisms may develop in blind children because they cannot observe certain behaviors during conversation. For obvious reasons, they have more difficulty in adjusting their vocal loudness to suit the distance of the listener. Therefore, they tend to speak at a constant, loud level (Freeman & Blockberger, 1987). Blind children tend to nod their heads less often but to smile more often. They may have eyebrow movements that appear inappropriate because they are not used to indicate interest or give emphasis to what is being spoken (Parke, Shallcross, & Anderson, 1980).

Phonology and Reading.   As discussed elsewhere in this text, reading disorders are viewed today from a developmental language perspective, emphasizing the relationship between reading and other language skills, especially in the domain of phonology. Sighted children must develop phonological awareness that allows them to decode the relationship between speech sounds and printed letters. Blind children must develop this same awareness, as braille is also based on the alphabetic principle. Research indicates that blind children who do not read at age level are delayed in their ability to understand and apply the sound structure of spoken language (Gillon & Young, 2002).

Implications for Intervention

Unlike many other groups of children with language disorders, there is some question whether language intervention is necessary for blind children. Most professionals agree, however, that intervention is needed to monitor and interpret the child's language acquisition because it can be expected to follow a different developmental path. Freeman and Blockberger (1987) suggest that intervention with blind children and their families should have three objectives:

1. Helping the child gain information through sources other than vision
2. Helping parents to interact with the child in ways that are stimulating and enjoyable
3. Modifying those behaviors of the child that bring negative attention and reduce communicative effectiveness

During the early years of life, the child will be more dependent on the parents for stimulation. Obviously, sound and touch must be used to fill in the gaps left by the child's lack of vision. With sighted infants it is possible to have interactions that are mostly nonverbal. While it should not be necessary to talk all the time, most parents of blind children do make conversational adjustments. They tend to initiate and repair conversations more actively, to talk more, produce more directive utterances, and make physical contact more often (Kekelis & Prinz, 1996; Moore & McConachie, 1994; Urwin, 1984).

The interests and concerns of a blind child's parents must be considered. Some parents may worry mainly about the child's physical independence and therefore emphasize early motor experiences. Other parents may focus on trying to normalize the child's learning by providing an enriched environment for manual exploration and auditory and tactile stimulation. Both sets of goals are important and can be used to facilitate the acquisition of language.

Superficially, some blind children may resemble children with autism because of their stereotyped movements, echolalia, and pronoun confusions. We have seen, however, that each of these behaviors is an understandable consequence of the lack of vision. In general, these will become less frequent as the children grow and become more independent. Professionals can be useful by providing an interpretation of the behaviors and by preventing negative reactions when they occur. For example, when blind children echo for no clear purpose, the natural reaction is to redirect the conversation. By doing this, however, we are not reinforcing the child's attempt to communicate through available means. It is important to try to discern the child's intent and then respond appropriately to it.

Blind children are a small population, and it is therefore difficult to develop good instincts for working with them and their families. Despite their training, many professionals may tend to overcompensate for the visual impairment rather than relying on a style of interaction that is generally effective with children. On the other hand, some necessary modifications are easily forgotten because visual ability is so easily assumed. Table 11.4 lists some suggestions that may facilitate interactions with blind children.

On the whole, progress in language acquisition cannot always be judged accurately by comparing blind children to the milestones observed in typically developing children.

TABLE 11.4   Suggestions for Interacting with Blind Children

Talk in a normal voice.

Provide verbal signals to substitute for nonverbal cues. For example, narrate what you are doing when you introduce or change materials.

Make sure that drawers, cabinet doors, and other obstacles are either fully open or shut.

Feel comfortable using "sighted" words such as *see, look,* or *pretty.* Blind children will interpret these appropriately in relationship to their abilities.

Tell the child when you are going to move to another part of the room.

Don't be surprised if the child reacts negatively to being suddenly held or picked up. This is not a rejection of affection but a response to being interrupted unexpectedly.

State your name when you approach the child, unless you are well known. Don't expect that the child will recognize your voice.

Don't use toy miniatures unless the child has previous experience with them.

Remember that most representational toys rely on visual analogy with the real objects.

Facilitate interaction between the child and one peer and then gradually increase the number of children in a play situation

Sources: Adapted from Rettig (1994); Sardegna & Otis (1991); and van Kleeck & Richardson (1988).

Some early communicative behaviors are delayed because they must be mediated through touch or hearing, which are less efficient sources of information. As a general guideline, professionals should always ask themselves whether a child's behavior is reasonable and even understandable in view of the sensory deficit.

Language and Children with Neuromotor Impairment

Unlike many of the other populations of children discussed in this text, children with neuromotor impairment do not present unique symptoms of language disorder. This does not mean that they are free of these difficulties. Their language problems, though, are not the direct result of the neuromotor disorders that interfere with posture and movement. Instead, these children are impaired communicators because of conditions that frequently coexist with neuromuscular disorders: intellectual disabilities, hearing impairment, visual impairment, and seizure disorders. They may also suffer from general delays because motoric disabilities interfere with their abilities to explore the environment and to speak, gesture, and engage in social interaction.

Children with Cerebral Palsy

The most common neuromotor disorder in children is cerebral palsy. This condition has no single cause and includes many different types and distributions of muscular impairment. The common elements in cerebral palsy are as follows.

- It is caused by an injury to the brain.
- It appears very early in life, either at birth or during the preschool years.

■ The damage to the brain does not become worse over time, though an individual's capability for functional movement may deteriorate.

Etiology and Types of Cerebral Palsy. The causes of cerebral palsy are classified by when they occur: during the pregnancy (prenatal), during birth (perinatal), or during the first few years of life (postnatal). Prenatal events, such as infection, physical injury, or substance abuse, may cause injury to the fetus or disrupt the normal development of the nervous system. During delivery, the major risks are lack of oxygen (anoxia), infection, and cerebral hemorrhage. Postnatal causes include cerebrovascular accidents, brain infection, and trauma. We see that there is overlap between the etiological categories of postnatal cerebral palsy and acquired childhood aphasia. The latter is discussed in Chapter 10.

About 8,000 babies and infants are diagnosed with cerebral palsy each year. In addition, some 1,200 to 1,500 preschool-age children are recognized each year to have the condition (United Cerebral Palsy, 2002). Recent studies indicate two opposite trends in the frequency of the disorder. The number of perinatal cases appears to be declining, probably as the result of improvements in obstetric care and fetal monitoring equipment used during delivery. On the other hand, improvements in neonatal medicine have increased the survival of low-birth-weight (premature) babies, who have an elevated risk of cerebral palsy (Pharoah, Cooke, Johnson, King, & Mutch, 1998; Skidmore, Rivers, & Hack, 1990).

Associated Problems. Rarely are the problems of children with cerebral palsy limited to their neuromotor difficulties. Table 11.5 summarizes information on some of the most commonly associated problems. In children with multiple disabilities, it is exceedingly difficult to judge the contribution of each impairment to the whole. For example, we might expect children with cerebral palsy to be slightly delayed in their cognitive development because of the limitations imposed on their physical exploration of the environment. If these children are also visually impaired, their ability to learn through observation will be compromised, leading to much greater restrictions on cognitive growth. And if these children are further affected by seizures, the pace of learning can slow markedly, or even regress, if the seizures are severe enough to produce brain damage.

Language Characteristics of Children with Cerebral Palsy. There is no pattern of communication deficits that is always identified with cerebral palsy. Every child with this condition has a profile of language skills that is derived from the severity of the neuromotor disorder, the number of associated problems, and the manner in which all of these impairments interact. Several other chapters in this text contain discussions of language characteristics that are potentially relevant to children with cerebral palsy. The characteristics of children with intellectual disabilities are described in Chapter 6; children with learning disabilities in Chapter 4; children with hearing impairment in Chapter 8; children with acquired aphasia in Chapter 10; and children with visual impairment in this chapter. If a child with cerebral palsy comes from a linguistically-culturally diverse background, then Chapter 9 is also pertinent.

A key to predicting the language deficits and potential of children with cerebral palsy is to assess their ability to compensate. Table 11.6 shows a simple outline of five resources for language learning and suggests how a child can compensate for the loss of each. For example, children with neuromotor disorders are denied normal opportunities for physical

TABLE 11.5   Associated Problems in Children with Cerebral Palsy

Intellectual disability	Many but not all are estimated to have intellectual disabilities. Testing is difficult or impossible with some children because of their inability to produce reliable verbal or other motor responses.
Orthopedic problems	Nearly all children have some orthopedic problem stemming from an imbalance in muscle forces. Physical therapy is prescribed to facilitate the development of motor reflexes and reduce the imbalances. Bracing is used to stabilize limbs, permitting greater mobility, and to counteract muscular pressure that leads to bone deformities. If these therapies are ineffective, surgery may be recommended to restore muscle balance or stabilize certain joints.
Feeding problems	Feeding problems result from abnormal development of oral reflexes and damage to the cranial nerves that supply the muscles of the face and mouth. Dental problems may also develop. Children will have difficulty with all phases of eating: sucking, chewing, and swallowing. Problems can be reduced through customized feeding programs that include precise positioning, relaxation and desensitization exercises, and special procedures for introducing food into the mouth (Gisel, Birnbaum, & Schwartz, 1998).
Hearing loss	Estimates of hearing loss vary, but prevalence can be sufficiently high, approximately 50%, to warrant vigilance. Both conductive and sensorineural losses are found, though severe sensorineural cases appear in less than 1% of children (Pharoah et al., 1998).
Seizures	Seizures occur commonly, especially in children of the spastic type. Anticonvulsant medications are often prescribed to control seizure activity. Some medications can adversely affect attention.
Visual impairment	Severe visual disability has been found in around 9% of children (Pharoah et al., 1998). Visual problems can result in an expressionless appearance and are associated with poor head control. Perception of color will be better than perception of shape. Spatial perception is frequently poor, causing difficulty in reaching for objects (Jan, Groenveld, Sykanda, & Hoyt, 1987).

TABLE 11.6   Compensation for Loss of Language Learning Resources

Resource	Compensation
Physical exploration	Hearing, sight, intelligence
Hearing	Sight, physical exploration, intelligence,
Sight	Hearing, physical exploration, intelligence
Intelligence	Social interaction
Social interaction	Intelligence

exploration of the environment. In typically developing children, this exploration increases their knowledge of the world and leads to preverbal communicative interactions. Children with cerebral palsy need to compensate through vicarious experience, which is most effective if they possess normal hearing, sight, and intelligence.

Children with both cerebral palsy and intellectual disabilities must work harder to compensate. As a rule, children with intellectual disabilities require additional language stimulation, which can be brought about through greater social interaction. However, social interaction will be made more difficult by the children's motor impairment. If adjustments are made—by providing extra time and structuring the interaction so that only simple motor responses are required—then a child with both of these conditions may still acquire considerable language.

Compensation becomes extremely difficult if, along with cerebral palsy and intellectual disability, a child also has a sensory impairment. Whether hearing or sight is impaired, two of the normal means of compensation—physical exploration and intelligence—are not fully available. Therefore, the child is reduced to a very small window of experience and can be expected to show severe problems in the acquisition of language.

Even when a child with cerebral palsy is capable of learning language, there remain serious problems in how that language can be encoded. Depending on the nature and extent of the child's neuromotor impairment, the ability to speak or use the hands to communicate (through gesture, writing, or signing) may be seriously compromised. The primary speech impairment in cerebral palsy is dysarthria, produced by neuromuscular damage affecting the systems for respiration, phonation, and articulation. The likelihood of dysarthria increases with the amount of upper-limb involvement. Thus, it is uncommon in children with hemiplegia (motor impairment on one side of the body) or paraplegia (motor impairment of the lower part of the body) and most frequent and severe for children with quadriplegia (motor impairment of all limbs). The major symptoms of dysarthria found in children with different types of cerebral palsy are shown in Table 11.7. There may also be articulatory symptoms, such as difficulty with speech initiation or inconsistent error patterns, that are better attributed to an apraxia of speech (a neurological disorder that affects the ability to plan speech movements). Regardless of the diagnosis, the effect on language acquisition will be to reduce the child's ability for self-expression. Communication may still be possible, but never at the speed or level of sophistication of the child's typically developing peers.

The role of speech practice in advancing the development of language is unclear. The rewards for language use are undoubtedly fewer for children with cerebral palsy, which may reduce motivation to learn. We do not know whether the ability to speak is also an important element in certain mechanisms of language learning, for example, imitation and verbal rehearsal. One study of adolescents with cerebral palsy found that they scored low on tests of receptive vocabulary and same–different phoneme discrimination. The investigators suggested that the children were less able to store phonological information because of their speech-production difficulties. This memory weakness may cause a specific impairment in the learning of vocabulary (Bishop, Byers Brown, & Robson, 1990). We need to keep in mind, however, that some children with cerebral palsy are able to develop high levels of language competence despite their limited speaking ability.

Implications for Intervention. Because children with cerebral palsy are likely to have multiple disabilities that require intervention, a number of professionals need to work together. The goals of language intervention can vary considerably, depending on the type, distribution, and severity of each child's neuromotor impairment and the number of associated problems. For instance, a child with mild hemiplegia and moderate hearing loss might require amplification and short-term articulation therapy. But a child with severe quadriplegia

TABLE 11.7 Symptoms of Developmental Dysarthria in Children with Cerebral Palsy

Subsystem	Nonspeech Problems	Speech Problems
Respiration	Reversed breathing (simultaneous muscle movements for inhalation and exhalation)	Short phrasing (small number of words spoken per breath)
	Rapid, shallow breathing	Frequent inspiration
	Involuntary movement of respiratory muscles	Decreased rate of speech
Phonation	Vocal folds do not come together fully	Breathy voice
	Involuntary spasms of vocal folds	
	Increased or decreased tension of vocal folds, depending on type of cerebral palsy	
Resonance	Inadequate velopharyngeal closure	Hypernasality
Articulation	Weakness in articulatory muscles	Mid vowels are most accurate, front and back vowels more difficult
	Reduced range of motion	Consonant manner errors predominate, especially with fricatives and affricates
	Variation in muscle tone	Final consonant sounds are more difficult
	Abnormal jaw and tongue reflexes	Individuals with athetosis present more severe problems than those with spasticity

and intellectual disabilities would most likely be a candidate for AAC. In all cases, language intervention has three purposes:

1. To compensate for impaired motor and sensory functions
2. To facilitate the development of motor speech skills and cognitive–linguistic abilities
3. To modify the environment so that the child is able to communicate more independently

Because cerebral palsy is usually detected at birth or soon afterward, early intervention is possible and desirable, especially for efforts at compensation and facilitation. Environmental adaptations that move a child in the direction of independence naturally become more important in later years.

A central component of all intervention for children with cerebral palsy is the development of a program for proper handling and positioning. Abnormal variations in muscle tone can result in undesirable movements and postures that inhibit skill development. By handling and positioning these children properly, muscle tone is more normalized and the body is better stabilized to allow standing and limb movement. Occupational and physical therapists will usually be in charge of developing the program, but everyone interacting with a child will be expected to assist in its implementation.

Compensation for sensory impairments must begin with auditory and visual assessment. Depending on the extent of any losses that are discovered, three avenues of intervention are available: (1) amplification of input by means such as hearing aids and glasses, (2) training to improve specific subskills such as visual tracking, scanning, use of peripheral vision, sound localization, and sound discrimination, and (3) use of alternative input sources, such as vibrotactile units that convert sound into vibrations felt on the skin (Marchant, 1992).

Motor speech skills can be facilitated in the context of feeding. Special exercises and feeding techniques have been developed to reduce the interference of oral reflexes during biting, chewing, and swallowing (Morris & Klein, 1987). These procedures are implemented during infancy, before a child would be expected to talk, in order to provide a better foundation of oral motor skills. Once the child's motor and sensory abilities have been attended to, language and cognitive development are promoted through a home program of stimulation and social interaction. The task of the professional is often to help interpret the child's communicative behaviors, which may be ambiguous at first glance, and to offer steadfast encouragement to the parents, who must continue to provide stimulation even when there may be little response in return.

A chief adaptation that can be made to help the communication of children with cerebral palsy is to introduce AAC. Further discussion of children with cerebral palsy and AAC is found in the next chapter. Considerations of AAC as an intervention generally are also discussed in that chapter.

Children with cerebral palsy require intervention in almost all aspects of their lives. Because the intervention is so pervasive, it imposes a particular burden on the family of the child. Professionals should be especially sensitive to parents' need to be the child's primary caretakers. Research suggests that parental distress as caretakers of children with cerebral palsy is related to their perception of unequal role distribution and lack of family support with day-to-day family tasks (Wiegner & Donders, 2000). Increasingly, professionals favor a family-centered approach to assessment and intervention (Crais & Wilson, 1996; Morris & Klein, 1987; Wilcox, 1989). Rather than the professional acting as an authority who dictates to the parents, the parents and professional work together on equal terms to identify and solve the child's problems. Parents are acknowledged as the best source of information about their child's daily abilities and problems. They are asked questions such as "What are your goals?" and "What would you like to see changed?" This approach has greater ecological validity in that it provides the professional with better access to information about the child's everyday routine. This should improve the outcome of language intervention, as well as letting the families participate more fully in decisions about the child.

Also not to be forgotten are the nonaffected siblings of a child with cerebral palsy. Given the demands made on the time and resources of the parents by the disabled child, siblings can easily develop feelings of resentment and jealousy. Increasing the nonaffected sibling's knowledge about cerebral palsy and its effects can help improve that child's behavior (Williams et al., 2002). In interactions between siblings, the nonaffected child tends to assume a directive role, regardless of age or birth order (Dallas, Stevenson, & McGurk, 1993). One solution may be to involve siblings as change agents. This approach has been used successfully to improve both the physical status and daily living skills of children with cerebral palsy (Craft, Lakin, Oppliger, Clancy, & Vanderlinden, 1990). Similar successes may be possible with communication goals.

Communication of Other Children
with Neuromotor Impairment

Although cerebral palsy is the most common form of neuromotor impairment, it is not the only one. Other neurological diseases and injuries can impair a child's ability to communicate. A brief summary of some of those conditions is presented here.

Muscular Dystrophy.   In contrast to cerebral palsy, muscular dystrophy is a progressive disorder that produces weakness and wasting of muscles (Cutler, 1992). The earliest signs of the condition are problems of balance and motor coordination. Over time, the arms, legs, and face are affected, so that eventually children are unable to walk or talk. There are more than twenty types of muscular dystrophy, most of which are genetically determined metabolic disorders that result in poor oxygenation and nutrition of muscle tissue. Duchenne muscular dystrophy, the most common type affecting children, has its onset in early childhood. Boys are affected almost exclusively, and most children are wheelchair bound by age 10. Children frequently die within 10 to 15 years after the first symptoms are observed, usually as the result of respiratory or acute infections (Muscular Dystrophy Campaign, 2002).

Most studies of children with Duchenne muscular dystrophy indicate that they generally have lowered intellectual functioning, but the findings are inconsistent (Cotton, Voudouris, & Greenwood, 2001). Verbal abilities appear consistently lower than performance abilities in young children, but there is more balance among some older children. This suggests that language deficits, especially in reading and spelling, persist in a portion of the children (Dorman, Hurley, & D'Avignon, 1988). Speech-production abilities are related to the progress of the disorder. As muscular degeneration occurs, it affects respiratory, phonatory, and articulatory systems, producing a gradually worsening dysarthria. Intervention is usually targeted at each child's specific language difficulties and at achieving the best possible compensation for the motor speech disorder. AAC may be used when intelligible speech becomes impossible.

Spina Bifida.   Spina bifida refers to a range of defects caused by a cleft in the spinal column. It is the most common central nervous system malformation. The spinal cord, the protective sheath around it, or the vertebrae of the spine can be affected. The defects usually occur in the lower portions of the spinal column. Milder forms of spina bifida do not affect the spinal cord itself and can, if necessary, be corrected by surgery. The most severe form of the disorder, spina bifida myelomeningocele, is caused by a large opening in the vertebral column through which the spinal cord and nerve roots protrude. Surgery, performed to repair the open defects, typically results in the loss of sensation and voluntary movement below the level of the vertebral anomaly. Most children with spina bifida myelomeningocele also have hydrocephalus and are therefore at risk for intellectual disabilities.

Speech and language disturbances in children with spina bifida result primarily from any associated intellectual disabilities (Byrne, Abbeduto, & Brooks, 1990; Tew, 1991). As in children with cerebral palsy, the motor impairment severely reduces the opportunities for physical exploration and may therefore also contribute to cognitive delays.

Spinal Cord Injury.   The most common cause of spinal cord injury is trauma from motor vehicle and sports accidents. Typically the injury results in fracture and dislocation of the cervical vertebra. The spinal cord is compressed, and the blood supply may be reduced by damage to the anterior spinal artery. Sudden quadriplegia can occur if the head is severely flexed or extended. Recovery can be improved by steroid treatment if it is administered shortly after the accident (Cutler, 1992). There are typically no direct effects on speech and language from a spinal cord injury. If a child sustains head trauma in the same accident, then acquired aphasia may result, as discussed in Chapter 10.

Language and Children with Cleft Palate

There is no question that children with cleft palate have unique problems in mastering phonetic skills. The patterns of articulation and resonance that are characteristic of these children are strongly related to the severity of the cleft and the adequacy of the result achieved by corrective surgery. This relationship is captured in the commonly used phrase, *cleft palate speech,* which indicates that the quality of speech is determined in most respects by the nature of the structural deficit. The question raised here is whether language impairments are also part of the communication problems these children experience.

An Overview of Cleft Palate

Cleft lip, cleft palate, and related disorders are congenital malformations of the midface and oral cavity. A variety of forms occur, ranging from a small notch of the lip to a total cleavage affecting the lip, bony palate, soft palate, and other facial structures. Genetic factors are the most important influence on the development of clefts, but certain drugs and environmental pollutants have also been implicated. In certain cases, clefting occurs as part of a larger syndrome, which can include intellectual disabilities and other disabilities as concomitant problems. In recent literature, a syndrome associated with clefting, velocardiofacial syndrome (VCF), has received considerable attention. Children with this genetic condition, which involves cardiac as well as cleft and facial abnormalities, often have language and learning disabilities that are not always related to intellectual disabilities that can be part of the syndrome (Carneol, Marks, & Weik, 1999; Scherer, D'Antonio, & Kalbfleisch, 1999).

Incidence figures vary, depending on the range of clefting that is included. The March of Dimes Birth Defects Foundation (2002) estimates that one child in every 1,000 is born with cleft lip, cleft palate, or both. The frequency of clefting is lowest for African Americans and grows progressively higher for white Americans, Asian Americans, and certain groups of Native Americans (Croen, Shaw, Wasserman, & Tolarova, 1998). Racial/ethnic differences may be caused by genetic variation across groups or by cultural practices, including diet and other habits, that affect environmental exposures during pregnancy (California Birth Defects Monitoring Program, 2002). The occurrence of combined cleft lip and palate is nearly twice as great for males, but females have a higher incidence of isolated cleft palate (Robert, Kallen, & Harris, 1996).

One of the major complications of palatal clefting for language ability is the elevated risk it brings for middle-ear disease and conductive hearing loss. This problem exists for most children both before and after surgical repair of the palatal opening. It is caused by a combination of impaired eustachian tube functioning and upper respiratory infection and inflammation (Paradise, Elster, & Lingshi, 1994). Vigilance in diagnosing and treating middle-ear disease in children with clefts appears to bring the frequency of conductive hearing loss in line with that of typically developing children (Broen, Doyle, Moller, & Prouty, 1991).

Language Characteristics of Children with Cleft Palate

From one perspective, the effect of cleft palate on language development can be conceived of as a set of interacting risk factors. Individually, the impact of these factors is probably quite limited. Collectively, however, they appear capable of disrupting the normal processes of language acquisition. The variables often identified as significant are listed and explained in Table 11.8.

Many studies on the language development of children with cleft palate over 50 years indicate that these children do display delays in language acquisition (Ceponiene et al., 2000; Richman & Eliason, 1993; Scherer & D'Antonio, 1997). In early childhood, both language comprehension and production are affected. After the preschool years the problems tend to become expressive. Vocabulary learning may be one of the more consistent areas of deficit. Compared to their typically developing peers, children with cleft palate who are just beginning to talk tend to use words that begin with different sounds. For some children this may reflect an avoidance of sounds they find difficult to produce (Broen, Devers, Doyle, Prouty, & Moller, 1998; Estrem & Broen, 1989). Of particular note is the finding that the early appearance of true stop consonants, either before or after early palatal surgery, is associated with better speech production and lexical development roughly nine months later (Chapman, Hardin-Jones, & Halter, 2003). Nevertheless, cumulative records of the vocabulary used during the second year of life have shown that children with clefts consistently lag behind in lexical acquisition (Broen et al., 1991). As children grow older, the gap in language abilities between those with clefts and those without gradually closes. The problems that remain often appear related to interpersonal factors, such as concerns about appearance and peer acceptance.

From another perspective, there are suspicions that not all language problems of children with clefts are due exclusively to early extrinsic factors associated with their medical, feeding, hearing, and experiential issues (Scherer & D'Antonio, 1997) and that such language problems do not resolve as the children mature. Besides early delays in vocabulary and morphosyntax (Broen et al., 1991; McWilliams, Morris, & Shelton, 1990), when children with clefts enter school, a greater proportion of the children than would be expected among typically developing children have been identified with learning disabilities, including reading problems (Broder, Richman, & Matheson, 1998; Richman & Eliason, 1993; Richman, Eliason, & Lindgren, 1988). Some suggest that about half of individuals with clefts have language and learning disabilities (Ceponiene et al., 2000). There is also evidence that language and learning disabilities are more prevalent among children with certain types of clefts, in particular children who have clefts of the palate only rather than clefts of both the lip and palate (Broder et al., 1998; Scherer & D'Antonio, 1997).

The reasons why some children with clefts might have language disorders not directly attributable to their craniofacial anomalies and the early efforts to cope with and treat their medical needs and related speech and hearing problems are not known. The reasons that caused the children's clefting in the first place are certainly suspect, including the possibility of subtle syndromes not yet identified. One line of research has begun to look at the brain morphology of individuals with clefts. Nopoulos and her co-workers (Nopoulos et

TABLE 11.8   Variables Potentially Disrupting Language Acquisition in Children with Cleft Palate

Variable	Explanatory Points
Intellectual disability	Risk of intellectual disability high only among children who have clefts as part of a syndrome that includes other anomalies, such as velocardiofacial syndrome (Gerdes et al., 1999).
Hearing loss	Risk of developing middle ear disease likely to lead to fluctuating conductive hearing loss.
	In one study, children followed from 9 to 24 months had depressed hearing on 16% of the days (Broen et al., 1991).
	Frequency of hearing loss probably higher for children who are not monitored so closely.
Surgery and recuperation	Surgery for cleft lip usually performed at about 10 weeks of age; repair of the palate commonly postponed until later but in most cases is completed before 12 months.
	Postsurgically, children somewhat limited in their activities in order to protect the wound and prevent infection.
	Effects of these experiences on language development not well known and seem likely to vary among children.
	Nevertheless, these appear to alter, at least temporarily, the normal patterns of parent–child interaction and motor exploration.
	During the first 2 years of life children with clefts show relative delays in cognitive and psychomotor development (Speltz et al., 2000).
	These developmental delays may slow progress in certain aspects of language acquisition.
Disruption in speech production	Palatal surgery performed most often during the period when children are babbling or beginning to use their first words.
	Studies of the prelinguistic vocalizations of babies with cleft palate show that they produce fewer oral sounds in general and fewer plosives in particular, and more nasal and glottal sounds (Devers & Broen, 1991; Grunwell & Russell, 1987; O'Gara & Logemann, 1988; Willadsen & Enemark, 2000).
	Following the surgery, which facilitates oral sound production, there is probably a reorganization of the motor schemes for producing speech (Broen et al., 1991). This may cause a delay in the acquisition and use of meaningful vocabulary.
Unintelligible speech	Nearly all children with cleft palate will have reduced speech intelligibility, especially until the cleft has been surgically corrected and they have had time to adjust to the changes in the speech mechanism.
	Poor intelligibility can hinder parents and other conversational partners from responding appropriately to children's speech attempts.
	The number of successful communicative interactions are diminished and language learning may be curbed.

al., 2000) found that the frontal lobes of men with orofacial clefts were larger and the temporal and occipital lobes were significantly smaller than those of the control subjects. Another line of research has investigated the ability of the brains of infants with clefts to detect changes in and retain auditory stimuli (Ceponiene et al., 1999, 2000). Results have indicated that neonates with clefts only, as opposed to other forms of clefting, may be born with differences in auditory cortex functioning that might be associated with language acquisition and later learning problems and that the early differences in auditory perceptual functioning may persist into later infancy.

To the extent that children with clefts are at risk for language problems not directly associated with their speech and other medical problems, professionals need to be careful not to attribute signs of early language delays to the wrong reasons. They also need to be prepared to provide early language as well as early speech intervention. If these children are in school and learning difficulties emerge, professionals need to be suspicious that these, too, may have a language basis and be an intrinsic part of the children's cleft palate condition.

Summary

In this chapter we have seen that

- Giftedness has no sanctioned definition. Experts generally describe it as either the potential or actual demonstration of exceptional abilities.
- Many but not all gifted children have exceptional verbal abilities. Those who do have exceptional abilities follow typical developmental paths but at an accelerated rate.
- Three special populations of gifted children are those from disadvantaged backgrounds, those with physical or sensory disabilities, and those with concomitant learning disabilities.
- Intervention with disabled gifted children is designed to help them compensate for their impairments. The superior intelligence of these children may facilitate the use of technology and cognitive teaching strategies.
- The major variables in visual impairment are degree of loss and age of onset. Children with no useful sight from birth are described as congenitally blind and show a different pattern of language development.
- The early language development of blind children is affected by the unavailability of vision to guide early mother–infant interactions.
- The major differences in blind children's language are semantic and pragmatic. Words are used more restrictively and may be acquired later if the underlying concept is visual. Language functions related to sight are also delayed. Unusual or inappropriate nonverbal behaviors may develop.
- Intervention with blind children should help to compensate for sensory loss, facilitate parent–child interaction, and reduce the frequency of inappropriate behaviors.
- Cerebral palsy is a set of nonprogressive neuromotor disorders caused by brain damage during fetal development or infancy.
- There is no standard profile of language disability in children with cerebral palsy. Problems result from the combined effect of neuromotor impairment, seizures, sensory loss, and intellectual disabilities.

- Language intervention in cases of nonprogressive neuromotor impairment aims to compensate for those motor and sensory functions that will remain impaired, to stimulate cognitive–linguistic abilities, and to modify the environment so that the child can function more independently within it.
- Neuromotor disorders other than cerebral palsy have different effects on speech and language abilities. Progressive disorders cause steady deterioration of function. Some disorders have little or no effect on communication
- Children with cleft palate who do not have other disabilities exhibit some delays in language acquisition. Some of these may be outgrown, but other children may continue to have language problems and experience learning disabilities when they enter school. Continuing language problems may be associated with cleft type. Congenital auditory perceptual problems have recently been suspected.
- Hearing loss, time spent in surgery and recuperation, structural changes in the speech mechanism, and unintelligible speech are conspicuous factors affecting the language development of children with clefts but may not account for all language problems these children can have.

In this chapter we have examined four groups of children who present very different language characteristics. Their needs for language intervention may range from comprehensive services to no services at all. Professionals must be prepared to encounter a variety of associated problems and ability levels. They should be careful not to assume that certain competencies are present. Neither should they restrict their expectations of what these children can accomplish.

12 Language and Augmentative and Alternative Communication (AAC)

SUSAN BALANDIN

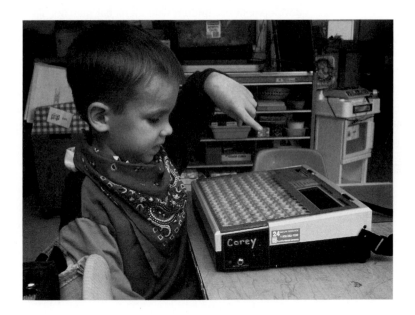

OBJECTIVES

After reading this chapter you should be able to discuss

- Augmentative and alternative communication (AAC) and complex communication needs and understand the importance of introducing AAC to some children with language impairment

- Types of AAC systems that may be appropriate for children with language impairment

- The role of AAC in the management of children's challenging behaviors

- Children for whom AAC might be appropriate

- Some of the issues related to AAC and language development

- Principles of AAC assessment and intervention for children with language impairment

Some children described in previous chapters could be likely candidates for augmentative and alternative communication (AAC) in order to provide them with opportunities to express their language and/or assist them with their language development. Because implementation of an AAC system is basically an intervention, we have chosen to locate this chapter at the beginning of the Language Intervention part of this text.

Despite the fact that AAC has been a well-established discipline since the mid-1980s, little continues to be known about the language development of children who use alternative communicative modes (von Tetzchner, 1999) or how the use of AAC may help children with language impairment develop their language (Blischak, Lombardino, & Dyson, 2003). This is due, in part, to a lack of research in this area and a dearth of case studies that describe how children using AAC develop language over time (von Tetzchner, 1999). Nevertheless, several studies indicate that the use of AAC does not hinder language development and may actually encourage individuals to develop and use more language (Iacono, Mirenda, & Beukelman, 1993; Iacono, Chan, & Waring, 1998; Iacono & Duncum, 1995; Romski & Sevcik, 1996; Romski, Sevcik, & Forrest, 2000; Sigafoos, Didden, & O'Reilly, 2003).

In this chapter we will explore who might be likely candidates for AAC, why, and what are some of the considerations in implementing AAC systems with these children. We will also discuss the role of AAC in challenging behavior of children and review some of the principles of AAC assessment. Throughout the chapter we consider factors in implementation of AAC with these children.

What Is AAC?

An Overview and Definitions

In order to consider AAC and its role with children with language impairments, it is important to define AAC and the populations most likely to use and benefit from AAC systems. The American Speech–Language–Hearing Association (ASHA, 1989) defined AAC as

> An area of clinical practice that attempts to compensate (either temporarily or permanently) for the impairment and disability patterns of individuals with severe expressive communication disorders (i.e., the severely speech-language and writing impaired). (p. 107)

This definition stresses that AAC is used with individuals with an expressive disorder. However, since 1989, when this definition was published, AAC has been recognized as being appropriate for use with individuals with a receptive language disorder, including children with autism (Mirenda & Schuler, 1988; von Tetzchner, 1999; von Tetzchner & Martinsen, 2000), who may use AAC systems to aid their comprehension and assist them to organize and make sense of their activities (Mirenda, 1997, 2001).

AAC is typically viewed as a system. One definition of an AAC system is that of ASHA (1991b) which states that AAC is

> an integrated group of components, including the symbols, aids, strategies and techniques used by individuals to enhance communication. The system serves to supplement any gestural, spoken, and/or written communication abilities. (p. 10)

As shown in Table 12.1, AAC systems may be unaided (e.g., signs) or aided (e.g., picture boards, alphabet boards, electronic communication aids) and are often referred to as being either high- or low-technology systems. High-technology communication systems, i.e., "high tech" (Sigafoos & Iacono, 1993) as they are commonly referred to, utilize micro-computers and specialized software. These have the capacity to provide printed and/or voice output. A device that has voice output is referred to as a voice output communication aid (VOCA) because it "speaks." The speech may be digitized (i.e., natural speech that has been recorded) or synthesized (i.e., synthetic speech produced from stored digital data). Low-technology communication systems, i.e., "low tech" (Sigafoos & Iacono, 1993), include communication boards, books, and object boards that may be made commercially or by a service provider or family member. These systems also include devices operated by electromechanical switches. Low-tech systems are used by beginning communicators, those who are unable to access high-tech systems because of severe physical disability, and as backup systems when an individual's high-tech system is under repair or unavailable. Many people who use AAC, as well as families and professionals, favor high-tech devices because they offer not only the power of voice output but can often be interfaced with other

TABLE 12.1   Summary of Features of Types of AAC Systems

	Features	
	Aided	*Unaided*
High technology	Utilizes microcomputers and specialized software	
	Synthesized or digitized speech, i.e., voice output communication aids (VOCAs)	
	May interface with a computer, environmental control system, or telephone	
	Accessed directly (e.g., using fingers or head pointer) or indirectly (e.g., scanning using a switch)	
	Requires a power source (battery)	
	Requires specialized repair	
	Expensive to purchase and maintain	
Low technology	No electronic parts but can include electromechanical switches	Manual signing
	Accessed directly (e.g., finger pointing, eye gaze) or indirectly using another person to ask which symbol is required	Examples:
	Examples:	■ Amerind
	■ Letter boards	■ American Sign Language
	■ Chat books	■ Signed English
	■ Object communication systems	■ Auslan
	■ Schedules	■ British Sign Language
	■ Symbol boards	
	Easy to maintain but setup and maintenance can be costly in time	

equipment (e.g., computers, environmental control systems). However, high-tech systems are not suitable for everyone, and low-tech systems must always be considered.

Symbol systems used on AAC systems vary in *transparency* (ease of deciphering what the symbol means), and it is important to match the symbol system to the user's level of cognitive ability and understanding (Mirenda & Locke, 1989). The easiest or most transparent symbols are real objects; the most difficult are written words. Many symbol systems are available commercially. These include pictures, line drawings, and symbol systems that are designed to provide fast and accurate access to language, for example, Minspeak (Baker, 1982) and Bliss symbols (Bliss, 1965). Practitioners in AAC must select the most appropriate system for the individual and be prepared to update the system if necessary. For example, early communicators may begin with an AAC system incorporating pictures and photos but may progress to a literacy-based system as their literacy skills develop.

One of the most common reasons for a child failing to use an AAC system is that the system is too difficult for the child to comprehend (Drager, Light, Speltz, Fallon, & Jeffries, 2003). Unfortunately, there has been a tendency for service providers to label children who are not using their systems as being unwilling to communicate rather than to recognize that the system may be unsuitable for the children. As we will discuss below, careful assessment of a child's abilities is of paramount importance when thinking about introducing AAC.

People who use AAC have only one thing in common: they are unable to use speech as a primary functional communication mode, although the reasons why this is so may vary. Beukelman and Mirenda (1998) noted that there is no typical person who uses AAC. It is important to remember that there are many people, including children with language impairments, who benefit from the introduction of AAC. ASHA (1991b) defined people who use AAC as

> ... those for whom gestural, speech, and/or written communication is temporarily or permanently inadequate to meet all of their communication needs. For those individuals, hearing impairment is not the primary cause of communication impairment. Although some individuals may be able to produce a limited amount of speech, it is inadequate to meet their varied communication needs. (p. 10)

It is not known how many children use AAC or how many might benefit from the introduction of an AAC system (Bax, Cockerill, & Carroll-Few, 2001). However, most children who do use AAC have congenital disabilities, including intellectual disabilities, cerebral palsy, autism, and/or severe developmental dyspraxia of speech (Mirenda & Mathy-Laikko, 1989). Some children may need AAC after acquiring a communication disorder (e.g., traumatic brain injury), and there has recently been interest in ensuring that individuals in hospitals, including children, have access to an AAC system if they are temporarily unable to speak because of extreme ill health or surgery (Costello, 2000).

In the early days of AAC, researchers advocated that AAC should only be introduced to a child after a number of criteria had been met (e.g., attained at least stage V of Piaget's cognitive skill, had some speech therapy) (Shane & Bashir, 1980). However, since the late 1980s it has been recognized that any child or individual who is unable to communicate using speech may benefit from the introduction of AAC, and that no prerequisite skills are necessary (Kangas & Lloyd, 1988). Indeed, every child has the right to the services and technology that can and are needed to enhance communication and assist in participating in both academic and community activities (National Joint Committee for the Communication Needs for Persons with Severe Disabilities, 2002).

The recognition that there are no prerequisite skills for the introduction of AAC was an important shift, because people with a severe physical disability have reported spending many years in intervention working on speech and language yet having no functional means of communication until they were introduced to AAC later in life (Merchen, 1984, 1990; Williams, 2000). For children with intellectual disability and autism, early introduction of AAC not only provides a functional means of communication but also reduces the likelihood of the use of disruptive and/or destructive behaviors as communicative acts (Beukelman & Mirenda, 1998; Mirenda, 1997; Peck, 1985; Sigafoos, Roberts, Kerr, Couzens, & Baglioni, 1994; Vicker, 1996).

Multimodal Communication

We have seen previously in this text that we all use a variety of modes to communicate. These include vocalizations, speech, facial expression, gestures, as well as written and electronic messages. It is important for service providers, family members, and people who use AAC to remember that no one mode of AAC will be optimal in all contexts. High-tech systems break down, low-tech systems may be lost or not contain needed vocabulary, children who sign may need to communicate with others who do not understand the signs. In addition, many who rely on AAC are also able to use their voices in some situations. Such situations include emergencies when a cry signals help is needed, interactions with familiar people (e.g., family members), or supplementing the use of AAC. Thus, those working with children with language disorders now emphasize the need for multimodal communication systems (Blischak & Lloyd, 1996; Iacono et al., 1993).

Not only does the use of multimodal communication help ensure that a person who uses AAC has a variety of systems that can be implemented as needed, it may foster further language development. Iacono and colleagues (Blischak & Lloyd, 1996; Iacono et al., 1993) suggested that the use of multimodal communication encouraged the two children with intellectual disabilities participating in their study to be more actively involved in communication and that multimodal communication was more effective in eliciting responses in one child. The multimodal system used in this research was a combination of signing and a VOCA. These researchers (Blischak & Lloyd, 1996; Iacono et al., 1993) did, however, caution that some AAC systems (e.g., sign) may place additional cognitive loads on children with intellectual disabilities. They suggested that while the use of signs may facilitate imitation, the use of a VOCA may actually facilitate spontaneous communication.

Who Provides AAC Intervention?

Several sources (Beukelman & Mirenda, 1998; Granlund, Björck Åkesson, Olsson, & Rydeman, 2001; Granlund, Björck-Åkesson, Brodin, & Olsson, 1995; Hunt, Soto, Maier, Müller, & Goetz, 2002; National Joint Committee for the Communication Needs for Persons with Severe Disabilities, 2002) agree that implementation of successful AAC services are provided by multidisciplinary teams that may include all or any of the following:

- Speech–language pathologist to provide communication assessment and intervention
- Occupational therapist to assist with seating and positioning

- Physical therapist to provide advice and therapy for motor problems
- Technical staff to assist with any high-tech systems and technology
- Regular and special educators to ensure that the child's educational and social needs are considered

Family members are, of course, part of every team. Other professionals (e.g., optometrist, audiologist) may also be involved if the child has additional sensory impairments that affect language development. Employing collaborative teams to provide AAC interventions, particularly in inclusive classroom settings, not only increases the potential for both academic achievement and social participation for children who use AAC (Hunt et al., 2002), but is consistent with federal education legislation and good practice.

Children Who Benefit from AAC

Children with Challenging Behavior

There are some children with limited language and speech production who demonstrate challenging behavior. *Challenging behavior* is a term used to refer to socially unacceptable behavior that includes self-injury, aggression toward self and others (e.g., biting, scratching), and disruption (e.g., prolonged screaming). Many of these children have intellectual disabilities or autism.

Since the mid-1980s there has been a recognition that challenging behavior is communicative (Carr & Durand, 1985; Donnellan, Mirenda, Mesaros, & Fassbender, 1984) and that such behavior should be treated as a communicative act. Researchers agree that it is important to assess the communicative functions of the behaviors (Carr & Durand, 1985; Carr et al., 1994; Mirenda, 1997; Sigafoos & Tucker, 2000) before teaching more acceptable communicative responses (Wacker, Berg, & Harding, 2002). The trick is to train new behaviors that fulfill the same functions as the challenging behaviors (i.e., the principle of functional equivalence) (Beukelman & Mirenda, 1998) and that are as easy to perform. In addition, communication partners must respond to the new behaviors consistently (i.e., principle of efficiency and response effectiveness) (Horner & Budd, 1985).

Challenging behavior can serve a variety of communicative functions:

- Escaping or avoiding an activity ("I don't like this place and want to leave now.")
- Having a break from situations ("I'm tired and want to take a rest before doing more.")
- Providing sensory stimulation to compensate for boredom or if a child is unable to occupy himself/herself in meaningful activities ("I'm bored and want something to do." "There's nothing else to do.")
- Gaining attention ("Hey, look")
- Obtaining a desired object ("I want that.")

Many studies have demonstrated that it is possible to teach an acceptable communicative act using AAC to obtain a desired goal (Brown, 1991; Carr & Durand, 1985; Durand, 1993; Horner & Budd, 1985; Mirenda, 1997; Peck, 1985; Sigafoos & Tucker, 2000).

It is also possible that some challenging behavior might serve another communicative function, that is, communication repair or communication clarification following communication failure. Brady and Halle (2002) recently suggested that when a child with poor communication skills makes a request that is not understood, he or she will keep trying until the request is understood and there is a response. This may result in behaviors becoming more extreme in attempts to gain the desired outcome. These authors give the example of a child ignored by a teacher while vocalizing softly and looking at the door. The child then touches the teacher and vocalizes but is still ignored. The child then screams loudly and the teacher immediately takes the child by the hand and asks what he or she wants. The child stops screaming and leads the teacher to the door. Thus, in this example screaming has been the successful repair strategy.

When AAC techniques, including manual sign, single message devices, and VOCAs, are used to reduce challenging behavior by providing effective and acceptable means of communication, this type of intervention is known as *functional communication training (FCT)*. FCT involves assessment of the function of the challenging behavior and systematic instruction of the new acceptable communicative behavior (Beukelman & Mirenda, 1998). New behaviors must be taught in natural contexts, and it is important that there be immediacy in the response of communication partners when the new behavior is first instigated. Behavior teams need to include an AAC specialist with experience in assessing the communicative function of challenging behaviors and with knowledge of a variety of communication systems. This helps ensure that the child with challenging behavior is furnished with a system suitable for his or her needs and level of skill. It is beyond the scope of this chapter and text to provide more detail on the variety of interventions available to deal with challenging behavior. There are, however, many excellent resources devoted to this topic (Brown, 1991; Carr & Durand, 1985; Durand, 1993; Emerson, McGill, & Mansell, 1994; Horner & Budd, 1985; Johnson & Reichle, 1993; Peck, 1985; Rauch, 1994; Sigafoos, Kerr, Roberts, & Couzens, 1994; Sigafoos & Tucker, 2000; Tucker, Sigafoos, & Bushell, 1998a, 1998b).

Children with Intellectual Disabilities

Many of the children who can benefit from using AAC have intellectual disabilities. Often, but not always, these children have fairly severe levels of intellectual impairment. However, use of AAC with some children with less severe intellectual disabilities may boost their acquisition of language (Launonen, 2003).

Children with Nonsymbolic Communication.   Some children do not easily develop the symbolic underpinnings of language and do not produce spoken language because of severe intellectual disabilities (Beukelman & Mirenda, 1998). Individuals who are unable to speak and who are unintentional communicators are commonly referred to as being "early communicators" (regardless of their chronological age) or as having nonsymbolic communication. They may communicate through a number of informal modes, including facial expression, body posture, changes in breathing rate, movements, and vocalizations (crying, laughing) (Siegel & Cress, 2002; Siegel-Causey & Guess, 1989). Children who begin with nonsymbolic communication may go on to develop the ability to learn a formal symbol system (e.g., sign, picture symbols, tangible symbols) (Rowland & Schweigert, 1989, 1990) or may remain at a nonsymbolic stage all their lives, depending on their level of cognitive ability and other factors including levels of seizure activity, state of alertness, and nutritional status.

One challenge is to try to attribute meaning to different communicative acts and to ensure that others involved with the individual respond to these acts appropriately (Beukelman & Mirenda, 1998). This helps children with intellectual disabilities to learn that they can influence the environment and fosters their development of meaningful communicative exchanges (Siegel & Cress, 2002). Those interacting with children who are early communicators need to support communication by attempting to interpret potential communicative acts (Keen, Woodyatt, & Sigafoos, 2002; Wetherby & Prizant, 1992). Personal communication dictionaries that describe idiosyncratic behaviors and their meanings are very helpful and assist in ensuring consistency in the responses of communication partners, including those who may not be familiar with the child. Such consistency is important in supporting the development of language and communication.

An additional challenge is to ensure that early communicators, whatever their chronological age, are provided with meaningful communicative experiences and that spoken language is supported by visual and tactile cues (Goossens & Crain, 1986; Goossens, Crain, & Elder, 1992; Musselwhite & St. Louis, 1988). As is the case with normally developing children, play and play activities foster communication, and it is important that parents and educators understand the potential of play to promote language and communicative acts in a functional setting (Launonen, 2003). The use of AAC systems in play situations has been shown to foster communication and support language development (Goossens & Crain, 1986; Goossens et al., 1992; Iacono et al., 1998; Iacono & Duncum, 1995). Thus, it is important that early communicators have access to a variety of AAC systems and that these systems are used by all those interacting in the situation to foster communication (Iacono et al., 1993, 1998; Iacono & Duncum, 1995; Romski & Sevcik, 1996; Romski et al., 2000).

Language Development and AAC.   The most comprehensive longitudinal research on the use of AAC to promote language and communication in children with intellectual disabilities has been conducted by Romski and Sevcik (Romski & Sevcik, 1996; Romski, Sevcik, & Adamson, 1997; Sevcik, Romski, & Adamson, 1999). These researchers have used the *System for Augmenting Language* (SAL) to successfully increase language production in elementary school children with intellectual disabilities, adolescents with intellectual disabilities in secondary school (Romski & Sevcik, 1996), and toddlers with intellectual impairments (Romski et al., 2000). The SAL has five integrated components:

1. A VOCA
2. A graphic symbol vocabulary individualized for each child and installed on the VOCA
3. Functional communication experiences throughout the day that allow the child to use the VOCA to communicate
4. An adult communication partner who uses the symbols on the VOCA during communicative interaction
5. A detailed feedback mechanism for parents and teachers

Both intrinsic factors (i.e., those that the child brings to acquiring language through AAC) and extrinsic factors (e.g., AAC system, teaching approach) are important to consider when creating a framework to understand language development using AAC (Romski et al.,

1997). Romski and colleagues (Romski et al., 1997) have suggested that children not only need to learn to understand the relationship between a spoken word and its referent but also between a visual symbol and the spoken word. Consequently, they have argued that children with limited comprehension must first learn the relationship between a visual symbol or manual sign and its referent before they can use AAC expressively. They have also noted that children who do not acquire speech may communicate using idiosyncratic gesture, vocalization, and physical manipulation of others in the environment. This has been discussed by other authors (Butterfield, Arthur, & Sigafoos, 1995; Siegel-Causey & Guess, 1989).

Despite limited research into AAC and language development, there is a great deal of research and information that indicates that children with intellectual disabilities, as well as children with autism, may benefit from the use of AAC (Bondy & Frost, 1994; Butterfield, Arthur, Linfoot, & Phillips, 1992; Butterfield et al., 1995; Carr & Felce, 2000; Carter, Hotchkis, & Cassar, 1996; Cutts & Sigafoos, 2001; Giorcelli, 1991; Goossens et al., 1992; Iacono et al., 1993; Iacono & Duncum, 1995; Musselwhite & St. Louis, 1988; Sigafoos et al., 2003; Stainton & Besser, 1998). Nevertheless, a number of barriers exist that may affect services to this group and thus delay children's introduction to functional communication systems (National Joint Committee for the Communication Needs for Persons with Severe Disabilities, 2002). Such barriers include a lack of professional staff knowledge (Balandin & Iacono, 1998) and lack of training for families and support staff (Light, Roberts, Dimarco, & Greiner, 1998).

Sign and Gesture.   Results of several studies have indicated that gesture is a precursor of spoken language in young children (Smith & von Tetzchner, 1986; Thal & Tobias, 1994), and children's natural gestures may be used to foster interactions between children with disabilities and their communication partners (Calculator, 2002). For example, in a recent study of three children with Down syndrome (Chan & Iacono, 2001), the children produced different gestures for a variety of communicative functions. Two children who produced a number of gestures for a variety of functions also demonstrated the emergence of single words by the end of the 5 months of the study. In contrast, a child who used only a few gestures did not develop any word use during the course of the study. Limited use of gestures coupled with a lack of clarity in children's communicative intent may predict poor spoken language and vocabulary development because adults have problems interpreting the children's gestures and other behaviors and therefore cannot provide language models appropriate to the children's communication attempts (Wetherby, Warren, & Reichle, 1998). Chan and Iacono (2001) reported that the children in their study demonstrated use of gesture common in children at a similar level of language development but did not develop speech concurrently, as do their peers without an intellectual disability. This study provided support for the argument that manual communication may be an advantage for children with Down syndrome, for whom speech may not be an accessible modality, particularly in light of work that has shown that there is a strong association between gestures and language development (Thal & Tobias, 1988, 1992, 1994; Thal et al., 1991).

The use of sign and gesture to support the language development of people with an intellectual disability is one of the earliest reported uses of AAC (Walker, 1976). However, some of the sign language systems used by the deaf community (e.g., American Sign Language) are not considered to be AAC systems but instead are languages in their own right. People with intellectual disability are unlikely to learn to be fluent users of a signed language but may benefit from the use of sign. Key-word signing (Beukelman & Mirenda, 1998; Grove & Walker, 1990; Windsor & Fristoe, 1989) is commonly used with children and adults who have language impairments and who may be helped by the visual representation of a word as an addition to the auditory stimulus. In key-word signing, only the most important content words in the utterance are signed. Frequently the signs are supplemented with natural gesture and may include idiosyncratic signs and gestures that are familiar to the individuals with a disability. Key-word signing is always accompanied by speech and is sometimes termed *simultaneous communication* (Beukelman & Mirenda, 1998). For example, the sentence, "It's time for us to go out now; go and get your coat," might be signed "time, out, you, get, coat," but the whole sentence would be spoken. Thus, the child is exposed to complete sentences in spoken language and at the same time has visual cues in the form of sign to support comprehension and learning.

As we know, sign systems vary across countries, and it is important that those who interact with the person with a disability use the signs consistently. It is also important that the person with a disability has the physical ability to make the signs (von Tetzchner & Martinsen, 2000). With deaf children, a common mistake is to assume that they will be able to understand sign language without regard to their cognitive and motor abilities. Similarly, a child with intellectual disability who is able to use key-word signing is not likely to be helped by an interpreter for the deaf in novel situations.

Children learning sign are likely to benefit from both implicit and explicit teaching (von Tetzchner & Martinsen, 2000). In *implicit teaching,* the child is exposed to a variety of signs that are meaningful within different contexts, but no effort is made to teach the signs directly. In *explicit teaching,* the relationship between the word and the sign is made explicit and the child is helped to learn the sign (Launonen, 2003). This teaching includes practicing and being prompted to use the sign and may also include hand-over-hand modeling. Children with impaired language have been taught to use signs not only to express themselves but also to aid their comprehension.

A number of studies have explored how best to select and teach signs to children who require a system other than speech to communicate (Fristoe & Lloyd, 1979, 1980; Iacono & Parsons, 1987; Reichle, Williams, & Ryan, 1981; Spragale & Micucci, 1990). The current focus on functional communication means that signs should be selected for the relevance they hold for an individual child within a given communicative context. Consequently, interventionists tend to teach signs that are most relevant and meaningful for a child and therefore are most easily learned. Although this focus on functional selection of signs means that there is no longer pressure to adhere to a developmental pattern of learning sign (Walker, 1976, 1985; Walker & Cooney, 1984), for young children, such sign vocabularies are likely to follow a developmental pattern; for older children and adults, these may not. In interventions aimed specifically to develop language skills in young children with intellectual disability, signs (as well as aided communication) have also been taught according to play scripts, which highlight relevant and meaningful vocabulary in specific contexts (Iacono & Duncum, 1995).

If signing is used as an aid to comprehension, it is important that all those interacting with the child use the signs consistently and that the child is rewarded for using sign. It can be argued that the onus is on those without a disability who interact with a child to learn signs and to use them in order to promote communication and language development. However, there appears to be some reluctance on the part of some to use sign, or its use may be dropped—for example, when new staff are employed in a group home or when a child changes class. This can occur despite the fact that signing might have been shown to be an effective communication tool with the particular child.

Children with Autism

The use of AAC may benefit people with autism who have no functional spoken language (approximately 50 percent) by supporting their receptive and expressive language needs (Light et al., 1998; Mirenda, 2001). Individuals with autism have described their experiences as young children struggling to develop language and to make sense of the variety of stimuli that they experienced (e.g., sounds, smell, touch, movement) (Grandin, 1995; Williams, 1996). This scenario contrasts with what is now known about AAC being used successfully not only to improve communication but also to support language development and reduce challenging behavior (Mirenda, 1997; Mirenda & Erickson, 2000; Mirenda & Schuler, 1988; Ogletree & Hahn, 2001; Sigafoos & Dempsey, 1992; Sigafoos, Kerr, et al., 1994; Sigafoos, Roberts, et al., 1994). Yet despite a strong focus on communication throughout the literature dealing with autism, there is still only a small empirically based research literature that reports the use and efficacy of AAC for people with autism (Mirenda, 2001; Ogletree & Hahn, 2001).

As we saw earlier in this book, echolalia, literalness of meaning, and idiosyncratic use of words are all common in children with autism who do develop speech. The use of AAC may be helpful in supporting the communication of children who exhibit these linguistic behaviors. Some children with autism appear to have superior visual memory and visual spatial skills that may result in unusual reading or spelling skills and the ability to perform tasks that are at odds with their overall level of functioning (e.g., the ability to find particular words in the telephone book). Such skills may mask a child's receptive language impairment, resulting in high levels of frustration for all concerned and limiting language and communication development. These children typically benefit from the use of AAC systems that support their comprehension and allow them to make sense of their world by using visual symbols (e.g., photographs, words, signs) to help them order their day (Mac-Duff, Krantz, & McClannahan, 1993), support their language comprehension (Wood, Lasker, Siegel-Causey, Beukelman, & Ball, 1998), and assist them to be independent within the contexts of both school and home.

Several AAC approaches have been used with children with autism. One of these is facilitated communication, which was introduced briefly in Chapter 7. *Facilitated communication* (FC) combines elements of physical support and positive expectations to allow individuals with autism to communicate by typing messages (Biklen, 1990; Crossley, 1994). FC is discussed in more detail later in this chapter, but it is important to mention it here because there are claims that the use of FC with children with autism has revealed that these individuals are literate and possess linguistic, cognitive, and social abilities hitherto unrecognized even by those who know them well. To date, however, there is little empirical evidence to support the use of FC, so caution is warranted when considering the use of FC (Beukelman & Mirenda, 1998; Calculator, 1999; Duchan, 1999).

Other forms of AAC used with children with autism include *aided language stimulation* (ALS) (Goossens et al., 1992) and SAL (Romski & Sevcik, 1996; Romski et al., 2000). In ALS the communication partner uses visual symbols coupled with the spoken word to support the message and assist comprehension. As described earlier, SAL (Romski & Sevcik, 1996; Romski et al., 2000) incorporates the use of a VOCA and has been shown to facilitate both receptive and expressive language, including learning how to make requests. Despite early success in using a VOCA to help individuals with autism develop spoken language, Schlosser and Blischak (2001) noted that the role of VOCAs in helping children with autism is not clear. They stress that this is an area that requires further research with a focus on the learning characteristics of people who are able to use this method of AAC and the benefits, not for the communication partner, but rather for the child.

The *Picture Exchange Communication System* (PECS) is another AAC system. There have been several anecdotal reports of the successful use of PECS with children with autism (Bondy & Frost, 1994; Frost & Bondy, 1994). The aim of PECS is to teach children with autism to use visual graphic symbols to make requests by exchanging the appropriate symbol for a preferred item (e.g., drink, cookie). Mirenda (2001) noted that the use of PECS may be helpful in facilitating speech development in young children with autism, but there is little research in this area to date.

Earlier in this chapter we saw that the AAC system referred to as *functional communication training* (FCT) has been used to reduce challenging behavior by replacing the behavior with functionally equivalent communication skills (e.g., signing, using a VOCA). With regard to its use with children with autism, successful use of FCT was reported as early as 1985 (Horner & Budd, 1985), when a young boy with autism was taught to use five manual signs to request items that he usually demanded by using problem behavior (e.g., yelling, grabbing). Since then a number of empirical studies have demonstrated that FCT is an effective way to reduce challenging behavior and at the same time teach children with autism to use functional communication (Mirenda, 1997, 2001). However, despite the emphasis on the need for communication partners to implement FCT strategies in order to promote successful and effective communication (Beukelman & Mirenda, 1998), there are few reports on the efficacy of training the communication partners of children with autism, which is surprising given the emphasis placed on training communication partners in the literature that focuses on AAC (Bruno & Dribbon, 1998; Buzolich & Lunger, 1995; Light, Datillo, English, Gutierrez, & Hartz, 1992).

This section highlights the need for ongoing research in the area of autism and AAC. Although a great deal of information is available on communication and children with autism, it is important that students and professionals be critical consumers of the literature and attempt to use literature that is empirically based rather than purely anecdotal.

Children with Physical Disabilities

Some children with physical disabilities have language impairments associated with intellectual disabilities. Others with physical disabilities have intact language abilities but may not have the physical abilities to express their language through speech. Children with cerebral palsy comprise the bulk of those with physical disabilities that affect speech as well as other physical skills. Like other children with physical disabilities, some of these children have concomitant intellectual disabilities, but many of them do not. Although many children with physical disabilities that affect their speech, with or without concomitant intellectual disabilities, are candidates for AAC, in this section we will focus our discussion more heavily on those children with physical disabilities who have little, if any, concomitant intellectual disability.

Despite some early research on the language of young children with physical disabilities who use AAC (Light, Collier, & Parnes, 1985a, 1985b, 1985c), the body of research in this area is limited (Paul, 1997a). Several researchers have conjectured about how knowledge of normal language development might be applied to this group of children using AAC to facilitate language (Gerber & Kraat, 1992; Iacono, 1992; Paul, 1997a), but there has been little research to test these theories.

Paul (1997a) surmised that research was limited because those who specialize in AAC have tended to focus on ensuring that children who need AAC have functional working systems rather than on empirical evaluation of the processes of serving the children. She suggested that some principles of normal language development are undoubtedly useful to consider when working with young children with physical disabilities who use AAC, but that there are challenges that are specific to these children. For example, if the levels of cerebral palsy of children are so severe that the children have little functional speech, they also have severe motor problems and are often unable to walk or indeed to move easily. Consequently, they must rely either on a wheelchair for mobility or on others to move them. They often require assistance with mealtime management and activities of daily living. As we noted in the previous chapter, this means that they are unable to explore their environment and learn by their own experience, two activities thought to be crucial to early language development (Light, 1997; von Tetzchner & Martinsen, 2000). Parents and caregivers of these children usually spend a great deal of time at medical centers, early intervention programs, and other appointments, and so have little time for the activities that are known to be critical in early language and reading development (e.g., play and activities that foster early literacy skills) (Beukelman & Mirenda, 1998; Koppenhaver, Coleman, Kalman, & Yoder, 1992; Koppenhaver, Pierce, Steelman, & Yoder, 1995; Light, 1997).

Any AAC system must be flexible enough for a child to transition from one level of linguistic complexity to another (Paul, 1997a), a difficult task when it is not known how these transitions take place for children with complex communication needs who are unable to produce speech. Paul (1997a) described the major transitions in child language and made suggestions about how children who use AAC might be assisted to make similar transitions. For example, she suggested that a communication device might be used to build on attempts at vocalization, thus proving a child with a means to transition from sounds to words. Indeed, the SAL (Romski & Sevcik, 1996; Romski et al., 2000) has been used successfully in this way. Nevertheless, to date few studies have reported on how children with physical disabilities using AAC make the transitions that are associated with normal language development.

Light (1997) posited that it is necessary to understand the physical, functional, language, social, and cultural contexts of language learning for the child who uses AAC in order to identify what facilitates and what impedes language learning. She suggested that children with physical disabilities who use AAC and who are acquiring language require facilitated access to their environments, particularly through play. She noted that children who use AAC are not able to play and communicate at the same time, which means that the very act of using an AAC system requires that the play activity must cease when the communicative act occurs (Light et al., 1985a, 1985b, 1985c). In addition, for children who use AAC, turn taking with natural-speaking partners is asymmetrical, with the speaking partners dominating conversations (Calculator & Dollaghan, 1982; Culp, 1987; Light et al., 1985a, 1985b, 1985c), taking more turns, and directing the child rather than following the child's lead (Light et al., 1985a, 1985b, 1985c). This reduces the child's opportunity to practice language and learn new linguistic skills.

Children who need AAC are exposed to spoken natural language in the home, but in most cases they do not produce any or only limited spoken language (Light, 1997). Consequently, they develop receptive skills in the spoken language of the home but must learn another code to express themselves. At the same time they are using as many oral expressive language skills in the home language as they are able. In other words, they may be in a similar situation to children who are learning language in a bilingual context.

Romski and Sevcik (1996; 2000) have utilized an electronic aid to reinforce receptive language (i.e., the natural-speaking partner uses the aid at the same time as speaking), and Goossens et al. (1992) have advocated the use of AAC to support language comprehension. To date, however, few studies have explored the impact of these approaches on the language of young children who require AAC and who are believed to have no cognitive disability. A major barrier to research in this area is that it may not be apparent that AAC is required until a child is about 2 years old or older, and assessment of children with complex communication needs and severe motor disability is extremely difficult.

Many symbol sets or AAC systems are not true language systems but rather words and phrases selected by caregivers or speech–language pathologists to support communication and meet the child's immediate communication needs (Light, 1997). These systems usually consist of nouns, and therefore the communication partner must use guessing, checks, and questions in order to assist the person who uses the system to complete a sentence (Balandin, 1994; Balandin & Iacono, 1993). Because these systems are developed by adults, they may use graphics that are adult rather than developmentally appropriate (e.g., help represented by a cross for the Red Cross) (Light, 1997). An additional problem is that adults, including speech–language pathologists, parents, and educators, may not be aware of all the vocabulary that young children use and require to support their play (Fried-Oken & More, 1992; Marvin, 1994; Marvin, Beukelman, & Bilyeu, 1994; Morrow, Mirenda, Beukelman, & Yorkston, 1993). Thus, for most children and indeed adults who use AAC, the system may not be adequate to meet all their communication needs. Despite studies that have indicated that AAC systems must be constantly updated and changed if they are to keep pace with the learner's needs (Balandin & Iacono, 1993; Beukelman, McGinnis, & Morrow, 1991), AAC systems are not always updated frequently enough to keep pace with the user's needs. This is particularly problematic because of the risk of actually promoting a plateau in a child's language development instead of facilitating advancement.

Researchers and practitioners agree that successful language intervention in AAC must include natural-speaking partners and there must be a focus on training the natural-speaking partners how best to facilitate language development and the use of AAC (Calculator, 1988, 1997; Granlund et al., 2001; Light et al., 1992, 1998). Instructing peers to interact appropriately with children using AAC has also been effective in increasing language and reducing challenging behavior (Hunt, Alwell, & Goetz, 1988, 1991). Finally, access to a suitable AAC system, which a child with a physical disability can use comfortably and without undue fatigue, is of paramount importance. Many children have AAC systems that they cannot easily reach, that they are unable to switch on by themselves, or that are not always available. Clearly these factors will impact negatively on language use and language development. If children with physical disabilities are to develop language using AAC, they must have a suitable system, training in the use of the system, communication partners who understand how to interact using the system, experiences that will foster language development, and vocabulary in the system that will enable them to express all the concepts and ideas that they generate.

Children with Acquired Language Disorders

Although there is a growing body of literature focusing on the use of AAC by adults with acquired language disorders, there is a dearth of information about AAC use with children with acquired aphasia, whom we discussed in Chapter 10. As we learned in that chapter, Landau-Kleffner syndrome (LKS) is commonly included in descriptions of acquired language disorder (Brown & Edwards, 1989) and is associated with seizures and severe communication impairment. Sieratzki et al. (2001) reported that a male diagnosed with this syndrome at 5 years of age learned British Sign Language at 13, and this remained his most efficient mode of communication. Similarly, a female diagnosed with LKS at 4½ years also used signed English as her preferred mode of communication. She was reported to have an intact language system but severe phonological impairment. The authors suggested that this resulted from deprivation of auditory input due to chronic auditory agnosia associated with the syndrome (Baynes, Kegl, Brentari, Kussmaul, & Poizner, 1998). Pearce and Darwish (1984) reported that a child with LKS learned Bliss symbols (Bliss, 1965) initially and, having learned 200 symbols, was introduced to sign language. By the age of 8 years he was able to produce utterances that were four or five signs long, whereas he could produce only ten to fifteen monosyllabic words in a structured setting.

Despite some literature on children with LKS using AAC, within the AAC research there are no data-based studies that focus on AAC use by children with LKS, although the use of AAC to facilitate language is well recognized (Paul, 1997a). Thus, the few cases in which successful use of AAC has been reported have been case studies or anecdotal reports (McNaughton, 1991).

Children Who Are Temporarily Unable to Speak

Although there is a small body of research that focuses on adults who are temporarily unable to speak (Dowden, Beukelman, & Lossing, 1986; Fried-Oken, Howard, & Roach Stewart, 1991), this is another area in which, to date, there has been limited research to explore how children who are temporarily unable to speak may benefit from the use of AAC (Costello, 2000). Often, these children are too sick to learn to use AAC, and neither the child nor the family has time to consider or prepare such a system. However, Costello (2000) described a program used at the Boston Children's Hospital with patients who were scheduled for surgery and who had time to prepare for being unable to speak after surgery and during some part of recovery. Patients were given the opportunity to learn to use a simple VOCA that could be programmed with messages and vocabulary chosen by the patients and family members. A strength of this program was that the patients' own voices were used to program the messages before their surgery, so that they could "speak" with their own voices on their VOCAs. Preliminary evaluation of this program indicates that not only do patients and families consider it beneficial, but staff in the hospital believe that having a communication system available immediately after surgery results in better postoperative care and a speedier recovery. The impact on the language development of children who are in hospital for long periods of time and who are unable to speak during this time (e.g., because they are intubated or have a tracheostomy) has yet to be explored, but preliminary research (Costello, 2000) suggests that all hospitals that have intensive care units or units that care for children who are temporarily unable to speak for any reason would benefit from implementation of the Boston Children's Hospital model.

Does AAC Prevent Speech Developing?

Many parents asked to consider using an AAC system with their child wonder if AAC will prevent or discourage the use of speech. As we have seen, there is no evidence that AAC inhibits the development of speech and language, and in fact there is some evidence that AAC can facilitate language development (Blischak et al., 2003). However, several other issues should be taken into account when considering introducing AAC. The first is that using AAC is slow; the second is that AAC, no matter which system is introduced, will never provide the ease of communication enjoyed by those who speak. As Light (1997) noted, AAC systems rarely contain all the vocabulary or concepts that a child needs to communicate all of his or her thoughts or ideas. The use of AAC systems also alters some of what are usual pragmatic expectations of spoken communication, such as the timing of conversational turns, eye contact, and other aspects of nonverbal communication, for example, use of vocal tone, gestures, and facial expression. Adults with physical disabilities who use AAC have commented on the difficulty they experience when not only their vocal tone but also their facial expressions may be hard to control because of spasms and consequently difficult to "read" (Merchen, 1990). On the other hand, the use of AAC does enable children to communicate, and there are many AAC users who succeed in mainstream education, complete postsecondary education, and lead fulfilling lives in the community. When considering AAC for children, parents and caretakers should be encouraged to focus on the child's opportunities for *communication* rather than *speech*.

A suitable AAC system should be introduced as soon as it is probable that speech is not a functional communication mode for the child (Bax et al., 2001). This includes children who are at risk for delayed language development (e.g., children with Down syndrome) and children who are at risk for problems with speech production (e.g., children with cerebral palsy). Because there are no reports of children preferring to use AAC to natural speech and there are several reports that indicate that AAC may be used to support the development of natural speech (Bondy & Frost, 1994; Iacono & Duncum, 1995; Romski et al., 2000) and receptive language skills (Mirenda, 1997, 2001; Mirenda & Schuler, 1988), it is unwise to wait to see if children develop speech and risk their having no functional communication system.

AAC Assessment

An AAC assessment involves more than assessing a child's current level of communication and suggesting a communication aid (Beukelman & Mirenda, 1998; Cockerill & Fuller, 2001). The goal of AAC assessment is not only to identify a system that will be functional for a child but also to select one that will allow the child to develop language skills and meet future communication needs (Beukelman & Mirenda, 1998). It is also important to remember that assessment is only a part of any AAC intervention. Providing a suitable communication system does not, in itself, ensure that a child will use it or will communicate more effectively. As noted above, training the child in the use of the system coupled with training of communication partners is important.

Like intervention with AAC, AAC assessment of children involves a team approach (Beukelman & Mirenda, 1998; Cockerill & Fuller, 2001; Costello, 2000; West & Bloomberg, 1997). Currently, the *Participation Model* of assessment (Beukelman & Mirenda, 1998) is used by many AAC teams. Table 12.2 describes the features of this model, which consists of three phases. As can been seen, this model stresses that assessment is an ongoing process, not an event that happens once for a child and a child's family. Beukelman and Mirenda (1998) state that "Assessment is not a one-time process. Assess to meet today's needs, then tomorrow's, and tomorrow's, and tomorrow's . . . " (p. 149). Because many individuals with complex communication needs can and do use some speech or vocalizations, it is also important to assess a child's potential to use natural speech as well as the child's language ability (Beukelman & Mirenda, 1998). However, assessing language is often problematic. For example, there are few standardized tests that are appropriate to use with children with severe physical disability who are unable to speak, may be unable to manipulate objects, and may have additional sensory problems. Morse (1988) suggested that norm-referenced standardized assessment tools may be used, but care must be taken to note any changes and adaptations made to the testing procedures, and of course, scores from standardized tests will not be valid

TABLE 12.2   **The Participation Model of AAC Assessment**

Phases	Features
Phase I: Initial assessment for today	*Aim:* To gain a picture of the child's current level of functioning in order to develop a communication system that will meet the child's immediate needs ■ Current communication needs assessed ■ Physical, cognitive, language, and sensory skills assessed
Phase II: Detailed assessment for tomorrow	*Aim:* To develop a system that will serve the child in a variety of contexts with varied communication partners ■ System needs to facilitate a variety of interactions (e.g., academic participation, social closeness) ■ Future interactions and participation considered
Phase III: Follow-up assessment	*Aim:* To ensure that the system continues to meet the child's needs as he or she matures and becomes involved in different activities across a variety of contexts and partners ■ Frequency of follow-up varies, depending on the needs of the individual ■ Young children developing language skills need more follow-up assessment; adolescents with developed language starting work need less frequent assessment

Source: Adapted from Beukelman & Mirenda (1998).

if adaptations were made. It is important to recognize that many individuals who use AAC have been wrongly diagnosed as having, for example, an intellectual disability when they do not, because the testing materials were unsuitable or the individuals were physically unable to perform the tasks. In contrast to using standardized, norm-referenced tests, professionals experienced with AAC are able to complete a full and accurate assessment using skilled observation and in-depth interviewing.

Observations and interviews with communication partners form a major part of every AAC assessment (Beukelman & Mirenda, 1998; Cockerill & Fuller, 2001; Morse, 1988). It is important to observe how different communication partners interact with the child. As already discussed, it is essential that communication partners know how to interact effectively with a child who uses AAC and that they do not limit the child by being overly directive or by denying the child a wide range of communication experiences (Light, 1997). It may also be helpful to view videotapes of the child interacting in a variety of contexts.

If a child is to use aided communication, the team will also need to assess the type of communication system and symbol system most suitable for the child (Mirenda & Locke, 1989). In the United States, communication devices are funded through Medicaid (National Joint Committee for the Communication Needs for Persons with Severe Disabilities, 2002), but in many countries the choice of device may be governed by the families' financial resources in terms of ability to purchase and maintain the devices. Some children who could use a high-tech device are unable to afford one and rely, instead, on low-tech devices (e.g., communication board, communication book).

AAC assessment is a complex and time-consuming process. It is likely to include a motor assessment as well as assessment of vision and hearing. Any child who uses AAC will require follow-up assessment to ensure that the system is still appropriate. This is particularly important not only because children's needs change but because technology, and AAC technology in particular, is a rapidly advancing field. Currently, new technology is enabling children with severe levels of disability ultimately to lead independent lives within the communities of their choice.

Facilitated Communication

Facilitated communication was developed by Crossley (1991) and has been used not only with children with autism, as noted previously, but with those with cerebral palsy and Down syndrome as well. The technique involves a child with a disability typing messages with the support of a facilitator. The facilitator supports, but is not supposed to guide, the typist's arm. Calculator (1999) noted that "FC is portrayed as a method of unlocking undisclosed social, intellectual, and communicative skills that previously laid dormant in individuals" (p. 408).

Facilitated communication is a controversial intervention, the main argument being one of authorship—that is, who is actually typing the message (Calculator, 1999). It is a method that has had some support, although on the whole not from speech–language pathologists. Professional organizations, researchers, and practitioners have urged that facilitated communication should be used with caution, as there is a lack of empirical studies and the validity and reliability of FC is as yet unproven (ASHA, 1995; Beukelman & Mirenda, 1998; Calculator, 1999). Calculator (1999) noted that there is currently not enough evidence to construct a theoretical basis for FC. He also suggested that there is insufficient information on the criteria for initiating, continuing, or terminating FC intervention and suggested that, if it is used, FC should be introduced concurrently with other independent AAC methods. At the same time, he stressed that the skills of both the facilitator and the person using FC should be monitored using experimentally controlled procedures. Despite this controversy, educators and clinicians report anecdotally that they have seen some clients apparently using facilitated communication successfully and expressing their own thoughts.

Beukelman and Mirenda (1998) warned that facilitated communication may not work for most people and suggested that care should be taken before instigating facilitated communication as an intervention technique. They suggested that facilitators must be properly trained and that multiple sources of evidence should be available to attempt to verify messages communicated using facilitated communication. Thus, those who are considering using facilitated communication techniques are advised to read all the arguments pertaining to the use of the technique and to apply stringent attempts to validate any messages that are produced.

Duchan (1999) summarized the dilemma that professionals encounter when asked to consider FC as an AAC technique. She noted that if FC is introduced, the professional risks using a technique that has no empirical or scientific basis. On the other hand, refusing to consider FC may deny someone access to the most efficient and effective communication system for that individual. Guidelines might assist professionals facing the dilemma of to use or not to use (Duchan, 1999). These guidelines would include informing families of the risks and possible benefits of FC and asking them to sign an informed consent that they are willing to take the risks of using a controversial approach. Duchan and her colleagues (Duchan, Calculator, Sonnenmeier, Diehl, & Cumley, 2001) suggested a framework for managing controversial practices that includes the following points:

- Identify the source of the controversy.
- Understand how the approach fits with more established practices.
- Use specifically designed informed consent procedures.
- Develop client-specific procedures for using the approach.
- Receive specialized training to implement the approach.
- Document and evaluate outcomes of the approach.
- Prepare for eventual challenges.

Duchan et al. (2001) cautioned that while professionals have a responsibility to ensure that the rights of clients and families to choose a controversial approach such as FC must be respected, they also have the responsibility to keep abreast of the research and new developments in order to provide their clients with the best possible service based on well-informed decisions.

Summary

In this chapter we have seen that

- There are several types of AAC.
- Children with a variety of permanent disabilities or temporary limitations are candidates for AAC.

- AAC can be effective for use with children with challenging behavior.
- It is important for all children to have functional communication systems, whatever their level of ability.
- All those working or interacting with children with a disability who use AAC have a responsibility to ensure that they are aware of the child's communication system, be it idiosyncratic gesture, body movements, sign, or an electronic communication system.
- AAC assessment is an ongoing process.
- Although relatively little is known about the impact of AAC on language development, a great deal is known about the effectiveness of AAC for those who are unable to communicate using speech.
- The family needs to be included in all parts of the intervention, from discussion of a child's communicative needs to the development and introduction of the AAC system and any teaching programs that are needed.
- There is no evidence that AAC use hinders speech and language development; there is some evidence that its use may facilitate speech and language development.
- The use of facilitated communication as a form of AAC is controversial, and the currently available empirical evidence does not indicate that it is an effective intervention.

It is also important that professionals, and in particular speech–language pathologists as "communication experts," have a good, up-to-date working knowledge of AAC and AAC assessment and intervention. All children have a right to communicate; AAC can provide the means for many to be heard.

13 Assessment

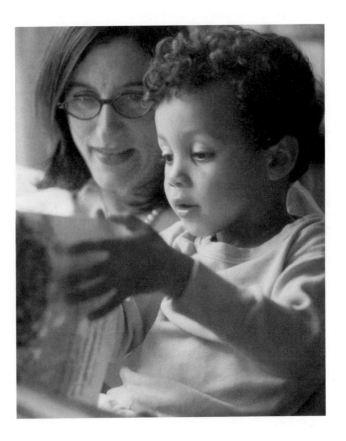

OBJECTIVES

After reading this chapter you should be able to discuss

- Objectives of the language assessment process and general issues related to achieving the objectives
- Differences between screening and assessment and issues relevant to sensitivity, specificity, positive predictive value, negative predictive value, false positive and false negatives arising from testing procedures

- Procedures and tools that can be used in the language assessment process and the ways in which these assist in achieving the process
- Dynamic assessment and criterion-referenced testing and their roles in the assessment process
- Strengths and weaknesses of norm-referenced standardized language testing
- Aspects of and issues related to language sampling and analysis
- Some of the approaches for assessing narrative and social discourse skills
- The role of intelligence testing as part of the assessment process for children with language disorders and identify several of the intelligence tests that psychologists might use

The assessment process is the first step in helping children with language disorders. Information obtained from the process is used to identify those children for whom language intervention is appropriate and to provide directions for that intervention. As Shipley and McAfee (1998) write:

> A valid assessment of an individual's communicative abilities and disabilities is the foundation on which all future clinical activities are based. . . . Clearly, all initial clinical decisions are based on information derived from the assessment process. (p. xiii)

In this chapter, a number of procedures and tools employed in the language assessment process are reviewed.

Approaches to and Objectives of the Language Assessment Process

Several authors (Darley, 1991; Miller, 1983, 1996) have suggested that there are two approaches to assessment, for which the purposes differ. One approach emphasizes the description, appraisal, and consequences of a child's language behaviors. With this approach, the aims are to identify problematic areas in the child's language performance and specify the patterns of language performance that the child possesses and those that are missing from the child's repertoire. The outcomes of such an approach are guidelines for developing appropriate intervention strategies. It is possible that in describing a child's language behaviors, other underlying or associated problems may be identified. That is, language behaviors may be indicators of primary or secondary etiological factors for which intervention, beyond just intervention for the language problem, is necessary.

The second approach emphasizes looking for a cause of a child's language problem. Implied in this approach is that knowing the etiology of the problem can lead to specific intervention plans. This approach is allied with the medical model, and the aim is to identify the etiology of a child's language disorder. Although the more descriptive or appraisal approach may lead to the identification of an underlying cause, the focus of the two approaches differs. With the causative approach, there is an emphasis on the "diagnosis" of the language disorder and its etiology. In reality, however, it may not always be possible to diagnose the etiology of a child's language disorder. In other instances, the etiology may indicate a larger condition of which a language disorder is only part, as in the case of microcephaly and concomitant brain damage that result in intellectual disability and an associated language problem. Such a diagnosis of the cause falls within the realm of medical practice. Knowing the etiology may or may not alter the intervention program significantly, or it may necessarily make intervention more effective, as many language characteristics overlap from one primary etiology to another.

There are, however, instances when diagnosing the cause of a problem, or at least identifying causal-related factors, can affect the intervention strategies and the professionals involved in implementing a coordinated intervention program. One obvious example is a language disorder stemming from a hearing loss. In another situation, recognizing a child's language behaviors as being characteristic of a specific "diagnostic category," such as those communication behaviors observed in children with autism, can lead to appropriate diagnostic team efforts and ultimately to effective medical, therapeutic, and/or educational intervention. Given what we are learning about genetics and potential implications for language performance, in other situations identifying the cause of a child's language disorder may lead to involving different teams of professionals and different directions for intervention. From this viewpoint, diagnosis and causation and the activities that go into searching for possible underlying causes are seen as important parts of the process, albeit not to the exclusion of describing a child's language behavior.

Within the framework of these two approaches, the assessment process aims to address several objectives. Because U.S. federal education legislation requires (and good practice in the absence of legal mandate indicates) that a child's assessment be carried out by a team of professionals, the different professionals will work together and bring together their information to achieve the same objectives. These include deciding whether a child has a language problem and/or whether a child qualifies for intervention, identifying what might be possible reasons or causes for a language problem if it exists or what factors might be contributing to and/or maintaining it, determining what language skills are and are not present in a child's language repertoire, profiling the child's strengths and weaknesses, and deciding what to recommend and directions for intervention if appropriate (Merrell & Plante, 1997; Nelson, 1998; Paul, 2001; Shipley & McAfee, 1998; Westby et al., 1996).

Determining If a Child Qualifies for Services

Not all children about whom several professionals might agree have language disorders qualify to receive intervention services. Whether a child is eligible to receive services from an agency or organization depends on the criteria set by that agency or organization. Consequently, this objective of assessment is, to some extent, separate from other objectives of the process, because it considers the service provider in addition to those of the child and his or her family. In contrast, the other objectives of the assessment process are child and family oriented. Issues such as standards for comparison, definitions of language impairment, normed cutoff scores, and what particular procedures and tests can be used to provide evidence for or against qualification for services come into play. Many of these issues have been discussed in other chapters.

The procedures needed to address this objective often involve the use of norm-referenced, standardized tests. In fact, use of norm-referenced tests is sometimes mandated by federal education legislation and/or service providers' guidelines. Although there have also been attempts to mandate use of *specific tests* to demonstrate that children do or do not qualify for services, this practice has run up against issues of professional ethics (the professional needing to be the one who determines what tests are most appropriate for individual children) and professional autonomy (the professional as the one who has the expertise and training to evaluate the quality of the tests and make appropriate selections). Consequently, the importance of these tools and their quality in the assessment process cannot be underestimated. In fact, of the objectives to be achieved in the assessment process, determining if a child qualifies for services is perhaps the one for which norm-referenced tests are most applicable and for which they are most used (Huang et al., 1997; Plante, 1996; Sabers, 1996). Professionals knowing the characteristics of available norm-referenced tests, knowing what evidence is available about the tests, and critiquing tests by applying psychometric principles are essential in being able to choose appropriate tests to use.

Deciding If a Child Has a Language Problem

Another objective of assessment is to determine if a language impairment exists (Merrell & Plante, 1997), because not all children who are seen for assessment have language impairments. Some children may have been referred by other professionals (e.g., physicians, psychologists, regular or special education teachers) or by their parents. Other children may have been identified as part of a screening program.

Screening. A screening typically involves a brief examination of several parameters of communication. Screening procedures are generally superficial and designed to serve large numbers of children in a short amount of time. Therefore, results of a screening cannot satisfy the objective of determining whether a child has a language problem. Rather, the purpose of a screening is to detect children whose language performances during this brief examination differ sufficiently from normal expectations to warrant concern and additional investigation. The results of a screening may raise concerns, but it can neither confirm nor reject those concerns. Having concerns raised, however, leads to referral for full assessment and diagnosis.

One reason for using screening programs is in an attempt to comply with federal education legislation that targets early identification of children with disabilities (Rescorla & Achenbach, 2002). A problem with screenings is the degree to which professionals can have confidence that a screening program is detecting the "right" children (Eisenberg et al., 2001; Fawcett & Nicolson, 2000; Gray, Plante, Vance, & Henrichsen, 1999; Klee, Pearce, & Carson, 2000; Klee et al., 1998). This issue involves the related concepts of:

- *Sensitivity* (percentage of tested children with language problems who are correctly identified)
- *Specificity* (percentage of tested children without language problems who are accurately identified)
- *Positive predictive value* (percentage of children identified as language disordered who subsequently turn out to be language disordered)
- *Negative predictive value* (percentage of children identified as not language disordered who subsequently turn out not to be language disordered)

In other words, children with normal language skills are not identified as candidates for full assessment, yet children with language problems are. When children with normal language skills are identified by a screening process as potentially language disordered, these results are termed *false positives,* and when children who do have language disorders are not identified, these results are termed *false negatives.*

No one screening procedure is infallible (Justice, Invernizzi, & Meier, 2002). An issue, therefore, becomes the direction in which we might be more professionally comfortable erring. A process that leads to too many false positives has the potential to swamp the service delivery system. As Tomblin and his colleagues (1991) point out, a screening process that results in a 60 percent false-positive error rate will generate, from a mass screening that identified 1,800 children as suspect and requiring full assessments, 1,350 children who turn out to have normal language skills and 900 who are found to have impaired language skills. A full assessment process takes a considerable amount of a professional's time. Therefore, completing full assessments on children who really did not need them consumes valuable professional resources. False negatives, on the other hand, risk missing children who need language intervention. If 1,000 children were screened but the screening process had a false-negative error rate of 10 percent, 100 children who had language impairments would be thought to have adequate language skills and likely not be provided with intervention. Given the now well-established relationship between language impairments and academic and social problems, this is a significant failure on the part of the system and has negative consequences for the children.

Another problem with screening processes is the degree to which more subtle language problems that can interfere with academic performance are detected. Most screening procedures consist of relatively gross and superficial measures of language performance. Otherwise, the screening procedures become too lengthy for professionals to see large numbers of children in a short amount of time. A recurring theme in this text has been the need to stress or challenge a child's language performance if these subtle problems are to be identified (Girolametto et al., 2001; Lahey, 1990; Nippold & Schwarz, 1996). When screening procedures fail to challenge children's language performances, professionals run the risk of increasing the false-negative rate. On the other hand, even normal children's language performances will deteriorate under conditions that stress their language systems too much. In such cases, professionals run the risk of increasing the false-positive rate. The answer is, of course, to determine the balance between too little and too much challenge to the child's system. Unfortunately, we do not know exactly what that balance should be or how to achieve it, although, as we have indicated previously in this text, narrative production may provide some of the answers to this dilemma for older preschool children and school-aged children and adolescents. It does not, however, provide all of the answers.

Evaluation.   Although a screening process might help as a first step in determining if a child has a language problem, a more complete evaluation that examines many different aspects of the child's abilities and considers the child's environment (e.g., home, school, preschool) is essential. Earlier we made the point that not all children referred for assessment have language impairments. We know that in some cases children may be seen for assessment because of false positives from screening processes. In other cases, a child may be referred by another professional as part of that individual's eliminative diagnostic process. That is, the referral source's operational plan may be that if a child does not have a language disorder, then the child does not have some other condition. Certain etiologies may then be eliminated from further consideration. Referrals may also come from people who are concerned about a child's communicative behavior but who are unaware of the language expectations for children at different ages. Some children seen for assessment may be "late bloomers," that is, children who are showing early but temporary delays in language development and who will outgrow their delays and do so without leaving residual problems.

In addressing the objective of determining whether a child has a language problem, it is necessary as part of the more comprehensive assessment process to find out whether a specific child is demonstrating language behaviors that deviate from those typically evidenced by children of that age and to ascertain whether any differences, if they exist, are significant ones that are likely not to be resolved if left alone. Westby and her colleagues (1996) propose that three questions need to be answered:

1. How does the child's level of performance compare with age or grade peers?
2. Where are the child's skills or developmental accomplishments within a predetermined hierarchy?
3. What perceptions of the child's status and progress are held by parents and professionals? (p. 145)

Procedures often involve exploring a child's performances on a variety of language tasks and in a variety of situations and comparing the performances to some standards or norms. Parental/caregiver reports of children's language performances are additionally important tools used to determine the presence or absence of a language disorder. These authors (Westby et al., 1996) also suggest that a different type of assessment procedure produces information for each of the three questions they proposed; norm-referenced procedures can address the first question, developmentally referenced procedures the second, and judgment-based procedures the third.

Identifying the Cause of the Problem

A third objective—to identify the cause of the problem—refers to our previous discussion of etiologies and the diagnostic approach, and we will not repeat it here. Information supplied by others, such as from interviews with a child's primary caregivers and/or teachers, a case-history questionnaire form, reports from other professionals, and/or information obtained from achieving other objectives of the assessment process, are usual methods of satisfying this objective, if it is possible to do at all. In some instances, attention to possible causes or causal-related factors can alert professionals to the need to make referrals to other professionals for additional examination.

In some instances, instead of being able to identify a cause or causal-related factors, it may be more realistic to identify maintaining factors. Although maintaining factors cannot be said to have caused or contributed to having caused a child's language problem, there are factors that can hinder a child's progress in language growth, even if intervention is commenced. Westby and coauthors (1996) indicate that the assessment question that, in part, addresses this objective is "What social and physical qualities of the child's developmental context (at home and school) affect performance?" (p. 145), and that ecologically based assessment procedures might be well used to answer the question. One example of a maintaining factor might be recurring ear infections. Another might relate to child–parent/ caregiver interactions, as discussed in Chapter 3. Even though the assessment process might not result in causal or causal-related factors being identified, highlighting maintaining factors that can be addressed in intervention may be an important outcome of the process.

Identifying Deficit Areas

Another objective is directed at determining the parameters of language that may be deficit for a child and the mode(s)—comprehension and/or production—in which the deficits occur. Some children may have difficulties producing age-appropriate sentences, although they may have no problems understanding syntactic constructions or comprehending and using the semantic and pragmatic systems. Other children may evidence problems in all aspects of language. Norm-referenced and criterion-referenced approaches to testing and observation in all parameters of language are the procedures typically employed to accomplish this objective. Knowledge of a child's specific deficit areas can help determine the broad focus or foci of an appropriate intervention plan for an individual child.

Describing the Regularities in the Child's Language

Although achieving the above objective may identify broad areas of language deficits, more specific, descriptive information about a child's language skills is necessary to develop an effective and comprehensive intervention plan (Fey, 1986; Lahey, 1988; Lund & Duchan, 1993; Paul, 2001). A further objective is aimed at describing patterns of language skills within each of the parameters of language. These are the regularities that comprise the child's language system, in terms of both the patterns present in the child's system and those absent from the system. Rarely can the results of norm-referenced tests lead to a description of a child's language patterns (Huang et al., 1997; Merrell & Plante, 1997), and even examining a child's performance on items within tests does not necessarily lead to correct decisions about the regularities in the child's language. There is evidence that item-analysis approaches using norm-referenced tests do not necessarily yield consistent results, with children passing some items and failing others that examine the same linguistic structure (Merrell & Plante, 1997). As Merrell and Plante (1997) point out from looking at the results of their investigation, "Inappropriately deriving therapy objectives from a child's item-level performance would lead to unnecessary social and economic costs" (p. 57).

Analyses of a child's language behaviors when communicative situations and stimuli are systematically varied typically result in information that is more useful in developing intervention strategies than that which comes from norm-referenced testing. To achieve this objective, criterion-referenced and nonstandardized procedures, such as observation of the child in context followed by in-depth analyses of the results, may be the most revealing procedures to employ (Westby et al., 1996). Paul (2001) suggests that these procedures also permit a baseline of a child's abilities to be determined, from which the child's future progress, with or without intervention, can be measured.

Another aspect of this objective is discovering a child's potential to improve performance, the extent to which a child can improve performance, and the circumstances under which improved performance can be obtained (Coggins, 1991; Gutiérrez-Clellen & Peña,

2001; Nelson, 1998; Olswang & Bain, 1996; Peña, 1996; Schneider & Watkins, 1996). Westby and her colleagues (1996) propose that the questions that need to be answered are:

> How responsive is the child to intervention? What repertoire of problem-solving processes does the child employ or not employ? By what means is change in the child's performance best effected? (p. 145)

The approach used to generate the information to answer these questions and achieve this objective is referred to as dynamic assessment.

The basis for dynamic assessment procedures is Vygotsky's (1978) concept of *zone of proximal development* (ZPD). The idea is that learning for a child occurs when the child attempts to function in this zone, which is the area of functioning between what the child is able to do without assistance from more capable individuals (e.g., parents, clinicians, teachers, higher-functioning peers) and what the child can do with considerable assistance from these individuals. According to Gutiérrez-Clellen and Peña (2001), in dynamic assessment, "the goal is to determine the 'size' of the [child's] zone of ZDP" (p. 212). The aim is to learn the *modifiability* of the child's language performance. There are several dynamic assessment approaches that have been described to ascertain the degree of modifiability (Gutiérrez-Clellen & Peña, 2001; Peña, 1996). Among these are:

1. *Test–teach–retest,* in which
   - A child's initial performance without prompts, as in a standardized testing situation, is determined
   - Essential components of the skill or task are taught, often in a brief teaching situation
   - The child's performance after teaching is tested again to determine change, if any, in performance

2. *Graduated prompting,* in which
   - A hierarchy of prompts in order of least amount of assistance to most amount of assistance is determined
   - Each prompt is provided one at a time, beginning with the least assistance, and the child's response to each is determined

3. *Limits testing,* in which
   - Usual procedures and instructions as to how to deliver stimuli during testing are modified in order to provide a child with a considerable amount of additional cues and reinforcement
   - Some of these modifications can include explaining the test tasks to the child and even providing some rationale as to how to approach them
   - The child's responses to the additional assistance are determined, in part to determine if the child understands the task itself

These approaches recognize that different contexts with differing amounts of cues and support can elicit better (or worse) language performance from a child and that the professional can systematically manipulate contextual support and/or cues for a child and observe what conditions, if any, result in more advanced (or lower-level) responses. As Olswang and Bain (1991) point out, support can be manipulated "by changing the consequences following a child's response, by changing the antecedent events preceding a child's response, or by modifying the task" (p. 260). It is possible that of these methods, changing the antecedent events is likely the most frequently used, the one that often results in changed performance, and the one that may provide the most information about what situations produce change (Olswang & Bain, 1991). Common ways in which antecedent events can be manipulated are shown in Table 13.1. The information gained from these procedures helps in knowing which children may benefit the most from intervention and change their behaviors most easily and what methods might best be used to facilitate change.

Deciding What to Recommend

The last objective is addressed by bringing together the information gained by the team of professionals involved in a child's assessment and involves more than just deciding whether a child needs intervention (Nelson, 1998; Olswang & Bain, 1991; Paul, 2001; Westby et al., 1996). The views, beliefs, and values of families and others involved in a child's education and care need to have significant influence in the decision about what to recommend (Karr, 1999; Westby et al., 1996). Again, not only does federal legislation require that the input of families be considered, it is good professional practice that can help increase the possibility that the child's family will be active participants in an intervention plan.

If intervention is warranted, part of deciding what to recommend involves deciding on the form of intervention (e.g., direct intervention delivered by a professional, indirect intervention delivered through another agent such as parents or teachers and guided and monitored by the professional, or a combination). It also involves deciding on the appropriate setting for intervention (e.g., in a separate room such as a resource room or clinic room, in a special class, in the classroom or preschool, in the home, a combination of settings) and, if in a separate resource/clinic room, whether the child should be seen individually, in a group, or a combination of both. When intervention is necessary, specific, sequential language goals that evolve directly from a child's deficit areas, the regularities in

TABLE 13.1   Examples of Manipulating Antecedent Events

Types of Manipulation	Explanations/Examples
Modality change	Present stimuli in a visual rather than auditory form.
Progressive addition of modalities	Present stimuli in one modality (e.g., auditory), add a second modality for bimodality stimuli (e.g., auditory plus visual), add a third modality for multimodality stimuli (e.g., auditory plus visual plus tactile).
Multiple presentations of stimuli before child response	Present stimuli one or more times (e.g., say the word or sentence several times) before asking the child to respond; can be combined with previous approach.
Provide models/hints for target response	Present an example of expected response for child to imitate; present first part (or last part) of the expected response; tell the child to think about producing the target before asking the child to produce it; tell the child a critical feature of the correct response.

Source: Adapted from Olswang & Bain (1991).

the child's language system, and the types of context/cues that result in improved performance and that take into account the possible causal and/or maintaining factor(s) must be identified. The goals form the framework of an intervention plan designed for an individual child. Recommendations need to specify a series of goals to be incorporated into a comprehensive plan if the intervention is to be successful. This should include timelines for achievement of goals as well as identifiable links to how the child's language affects his or her academic, social, emotional, and/or vocational functioning (Karr, 1999). Recommendations may also include referrals to other professionals who can assist the child or the child's caregivers. When intervention is not recommended, the plans for follow-up need to be determined. Children's progress without intervention is then monitored at regular intervals to ensure that the children are progressing adequately. The recommendations from the assessment process specify the follow-up times and the criteria against which progress will be evaluated. It is not enough simply to recommend or not recommend intervention.

Assessment is a continuing process. Those recommendations identified as a result of an initial diagnostic and assessment process cannot be considered "etched in stone." In situations where intervention has been recommended, it may be very inappropriate to adhere unbendingly to such recommendations once intervention commences. We learn more about a child as we work with that child over time than we can learn in the few hours spent during an initial assessment process. The child also changes. Because assessment is an ongoing process throughout intervention, we need to be prepared to change our minds or change our hypotheses as new information about a child comes to light. When intervention has not been initially recommended or when one form of intervention has been recommended, we also need to be prepared to change that initial recommendation if it is not working for the child.

Part of the ongoing nature of assessment is documenting the effectiveness of intervention. We need to monitor regularly how well the child is or is not meeting the intervention objectives (Hadley, 1999; Olswang & Bain, 1996; Paul, 2001). If the child is not making significant changes in language as a result of intervention, we need to do something different. Bain and Dollaghan (1991) write that a significant change

> . . . is a change in client performance that (a) can be shown to result from treatment rather than from maturation or other uncontrolled factors, (b) can be shown to be real, rather than random, and (c) can be shown to be important, rather than trivial. (pp. 264–265)

During intervention, a child's performance on intervention goals is probed at regular intervals in systematic ways on tasks that have not been directly targeted in intervention, that is, on exemplars of the desired behavior that have not been presented during intervention (Bain & Dollaghan, 1991; Fey, 1986). The child's performance on some behaviors that have not been intervention goals is also measured regularly. If performance improves on intervention objectives but not on behaviors that have not been targeted in intervention, the changes on the target objectives can be viewed as resulting from intervention and not from other factors. Determining whether a change is real or random is more difficult. It involves issues of using valid and reliable procedures to measure performance. However, the same norm-referenced standardized tests cannot be administered to a child repeatedly over short periods of time, because the child's performance on the test is likely to improve just from practice with the test, not because the ability or skill being measured has itself improved. The tests therefore no longer measure the behavior in question accurately, assuming they were an accurate measure initially. Professionals may need to use procedures they develop themselves, for which they cannot always ensure validity and reliability. Factors to consider in determining if a change is important include examining (Bain & Dollaghan, 1991)

- The magnitude of the change in relation to the amount of intervention time it took to facilitate the change and the child's unique characteristics
- The impact the change has on the child's life
- The opinions/ratings of unbiased adults who have had opportunities to observe the child's performance on the language behavior in question before and after intervention on the targeted objective

From the foregoing discussion, we can see that assessment is not truly distinct from intervention. Assessment and intervention are *dynamic, interactive processes* in all of our efforts to assist children with language disorders.

Tools and Procedures

A variety of tools and procedures are employed in the assessment process for children with suspected language disorders. In combination, the results obtained from these procedures and tools are used to accomplish the objectives of the process. One procedure or tool is insufficient for a thorough assessment. Instead, it is from analyzing and synthesizing the information obtained from a number of tools and procedures that the goals for an effective and comprehensive intervention program can be determined.

Gathering Information from Others

Gathering information about the child from others can help identify antecedent factors that might help resolve the questions about whether the child has a problem, the possible reasons for the problem, and/or what might be contributing to maintaining the problem. In many instances the information can assist in helping to determine what to recommend, what needs to be included in an intervention plan, and what might be the predicted outcome for the child over time. Parents (or other caregivers) are an obviously important source of information—for information about the child's birth history and early developmental milestones, about past and ongoing health problems, and about other assessments the child may have had. Given the increasing knowledge about familial and possible genetic factors associated with child language impairments and syndromes that affect language ability, information about the presence of communication or learning difficulties in other members of the child's immediate and extended family is important. Parents and caregivers are also an important source of information about cultural and linguistic influences that might be affecting the child's performance and what beliefs and values are factors to consider in planning for the child. These individuals are essential partners early in the assessment process. In fact, in the early identification of language impairments in children there is increasing use of parent report methods to provide information about their children's language (Dale, 1996; Girolametto, 1997; Klee, Pearce, & Carson, 2000; Rescorla & Achenbach, 2002). Information from parents can be obtained in a variety of ways, often used in combination. These include interviews, completion of child-related checklists (Klee et al., 2000; Rescorla & Achen-

415

bach, 2002), and/or completion of case-history questionnaires, of which there are many different forms (Paul, 2001; Shipley & McAfee, 1998).

Teachers are also essential partners who can provide invaluable information about how a child's language does or does not affect what the child can do academically and socially. Good practice, as well as mandated practice as a result of federal education laws, leads to their involvement in assessment. These professionals understand the curriculum demands, see the child try to deal with those demands given his or her language ability, and watch as the child interacts with peers and other adults. Experienced teachers also have encountered a large number of children over the years to whom they can compare how an individual child performs. These individuals can complete checklists in order to structure the information provided (Boyce & Larson, 1983; Damico, 1985; Semel, Wiig, & Secord, 1996a; Smith, McCauley, & Guitar, 2000), as well as being involved in discussions as members of an assessment team.

Information from all members of an assessment team is important in order to bring together assessment information. In some instances, professionals who are not members of a current team have evaluated and/or worked with a child, and their reports become valuable pieces of information in assessment. Examples of these might be psychologists' previous reports, those of medical professionals (e.g., neurologists, pediatricians), or audiologists' reports.

What to Assess

Before assessment information is obtained from interaction with or observation of a child, an initial plan about what behaviors, skills, and interactions to assess needs to be determined. It is important, however, that as an assessment progresses the plan is modified as needed. Most assessment procedures include evaluating a child's abilities with the syntactic, semantic, morphological, phonological, and pragmatic components of the language system, in terms of both the child's comprehension and production skills in these areas (Nelson, 1998; Paul, 2001; Shipley & McAfee, 1998). During the assessment, the situations in which the child demonstrates his or her skills with these different language parameters are systematically varied to provide a broad base of information regarding the child's areas of deficit and specific patterns of language competencies. Additionally, the effects of one component of language on the other language components, as the first component is assessed under several conditions, are examined. Trade-offs among the different aspects of language have been recognized both in children's normal language development and in children with language disorders (Masterson & Kamhi, 1992; Reed, 1992; Schwartz, Leonard, Folger, & Wilcox, 1980), and information about these patterns in a child's language profile can likely assist in planning intervention.

Observation of a child in a variety of settings is an essential feature of the assessment process. Because a child's language-learning environment can affect a child's language skills, an assessment of that environment is often included in the process. We indicated that information about a child's environment may provide clues as to the effectiveness or ineffectiveness of that environment for language learning. Observations of child–caregiver interactions and visits to the child's home may be included in the assessment process. Dialectal and sociological influences on a child's communicative behaviors need to be identified. Observations of a child in the classroom and during peer interactions can yield valuable information for making valid decisions about a child's communicative performance. Observation helps ensure that decisions about intervention and what intervention emphasizes are socially and ecologically valid for children.

Information about a child's abilities in areas other than language can help clarify the nature of the child's language problem and delineate a number of the recommendations to include in an intervention plan. For these reasons, a child's behavior and developmental gross and fine motor, perceptual, cognitive, adaptive, and general social skills may be assessed as part of the process. With teams of professionals involved in the assessment process, others may contribute considerable information about the child's abilities in these areas (Westby et al., 1996). Recall also from Chapter 3 that several of these areas of functioning may have predictive value in helping to know which toddlers with slow expressive language development are likely to catch up in their language development without intervention, and which are not.

Methods of Assessment

Several methods of obtaining information about the language behaviors of children in an assessment process are typically employed. Norm-referenced standardized tests, language sampling, and other criterion-referenced procedures are among the common methods. However, it is important that one method not be used to the exclusion of the other, and professionals need to be cognizant of the weaknesses of the procedures they are using as well as what the procedures can contribute to their decisions.

Norm-Referenced, Standardized Testing.   A standardized test is one in which there is a procedure for administration and analysis of responses is specified by the test developers in an attempt to achieve uniformity across individuals using the test in order to ensure reliability and validity. The idea is to reduce unwanted variations in procedures that could confound interpretation of results. For most standardized language tests, the stimuli for obtaining responses from a child are developed by the author(s) of the test and are included with the test itself. The procedures for using the stimuli, recording responses, and judging the adequacy of responses are specified in the administration instructions.

Most standardized tests are also norm-referenced. That is, they provide a means for comparing a particular child's score to some standard or norm that is based on a derived distribution of many individuals' performances assumed to represent a normal distribution of abilities. That is, a representative group of children without language disorders has typically been given the test, and their performances are those against which a specific child's score is then compared. To allow for comparison, the child's raw score (usually the number of correct responses or the number of errors) is generally converted to one or more other types of scores that reflect some sort of ranking or norm (e.g., age equivalencies, percentile ranks, or standard scores). The idea behind raw-score conversion is to give some indication of the child's performance compared to that of peers, so that an individual child's performance can be judged as falling within or outside the limits of this normal range. Previously in this text, however, we have discussed concerns regarding the use of age-equivalency scores as the standard to which we compare a child's performance (Bishop, 1997; Lahey, 1990).

There has been a proliferation of norm-referenced standardized language tests for use with young children. Numerous tests to measure children's comprehension of various aspects of the morphological, semantic, and syntactic systems are on the market. Tests designed to examine children's use of these systems are also available, as are tests to measure children's skills with the phonological system. There are fewer norm-referenced standardized tests in the area of pragmatics. Because the nature of pragmatics means that performance needs to change according to many different communicative variables interacting at one time, there are inherent difficulties in developing standardized procedures, and therefore tests, to tap this area than areas of syntax, morphology, and semantics.

There are several reasons for test proliferation. The assessment process for a child suspected of having a language disorder is a demanding, time-consuming task. Consequently, there is an ongoing search to find easier and quicker methods of achieving the objectives of the process. The use of tests is often viewed as a way of easing the assessment task. The emphasis on accountability, documentation, and qualifying children for services has also provided an impetus for test development, in the belief that numbers and norms suffice as evidence of fulfilling these responsibilities. Although good assessment requires the ability to make judgments, based on extensive knowledge, about a child's performance, those who lack the knowledge or the confidence in their knowledge and abilities to make these judgments may turn to tests as the answers to their dilemmas, thus creating a demand for norm-referenced standardized tests.

Although there are problems in an overdependence on the use of standardized, norm-referenced tests in the assessment process, these tools do serve several purposes. If selected carefully, employed correctly, and results interpreted properly, language tests can help determine whether a child has a language problem, assist in qualifying a child for services when appropriate, and, in some instances, provide preliminary information about language areas that might be deficit. However, tests must be selected that are appropriate to the individual child in terms of the characteristics of the norming population to which the child's performance is going to be compared. Careful consideration of the norming population is essential in selecting appropriate tests to use.

Tests must demonstrate validity and reliability if they are to be useful at all. These are not aspects of test selection that can be taken lightly. Several authors have provided guidelines that can be used in selecting standardized norm-referenced tests (Hutchinson, 1996; Sabers, 1996). However, even when tests might meet what are considered acceptable standards for acknowledged guidelines, they may not demonstrate acceptable diagnostic accuracy and therefore adequate validity. As an example from one study, only 38 percent of 21 child language tests met half of what are typically recognized psychometric criteria. Of the four tests that met the most of these criteria, only one adequately discriminated between children who did and those who did not have language impairments (Plante & Vance, 1994). As a further example, in an investigation of four vocabulary tests (Gray et al., 1999), the four tests did not equally identify children with specific language impairment from those with normal language, and the children's scores varied across the tests. Norm-referenced standardized tests must be chosen carefully, used carefully, and interpreted carefully. As Eisenberg and her colleagues (2001) remind us, "Ultimately, valid use of any assessment tool is up to the user" (p. 339).

And, *standardized tests are tools.* They do not direct or determine the assessment process. We select and use them because we want to accomplish an objective and we believe they will assist us with that objective. We do not use a particular test or any tests just because they are available. We use a hammer because we want to accomplish a carpentry objective and we believe the hammer is the tool we need to complete our objective. We are also aware that there are varying qualities of hammers. We use a measuring cup because we want to accomplish a cooking objective and we believe the cup is the tool we need. However, it could be that a saw of a particular quality would be a better tool for our carpentry objective or a food processor with particular features and of a particular quality would be better for our cooking objective. In the same way, a tool other than a norm-referenced standardized test or a different test could be better for accomplishing our specified objectives. Sometimes, we might have to use more than one tool to accomplish our objective (e.g., a hammer and a saw to complete the carpentry objective, or a measuring cup and a food processor to complete our cooking objective). This means, of course, that we must know clearly what our objectives are before selecting the tools to accomplish them. Some of the common errors and misconceptions about norm-referenced standardized test use are listed in Table 13.2. When it comes to using norm-referenced standardized tests, the quote, "Let the clinician beware" (Lieberman & Michael, 1986, p. 71) is apropos. However, even though there are serious concerns about many of the norm-referenced standardized tests and the ways in which they are used, Apel (1999b) concedes that their use is unlikely to disappear any time in the near future, in large part because of the need to have numbers to describe children's language performances in order to qualify them for services.

Norm-referenced standardized tests alone rarely yield enough information to describe a child's patterns or regularities of language behavior or to decide on the specifics of an intervention plan. For the most part, standardized tests do not contain a sufficient number of items examining a single feature in a wide variety of contexts to describe the content of performance or determine whether that feature should be a target for intervention (Miller, 1996). What norm-referenced standardized tests may indicate are those skills that appear to be suspect and that need to be examined in more detail. Because these tests rarely provide us with sufficient information to develop intervention objectives, a more detailed description of the child's language is needed. To accomplish the objectives of describing a child's language patterns and determining the specific intervention recommendations for the child, we use different tools, such as language sampling and/or other criterion-referenced procedures.

Language Sampling.   Our discussion focuses on general principles of language sampling and the use of the procedure with younger children. Although language sampling is a

---

TABLE 13.2   Common Errors and Misconceptions in Using Standardized Tests

1. Assuming that test scores demonstrate professional accountability.
2. Using tests to cover for insufficient knowledge or confidence.
3. Misinterpreting various types of test scores.
4. Using tests with children who are not represented in the norming sample.
5. Administering tests with inadequately demonstrated validity and reliability.
6. Using tests that do not measure the desired skills or abilities.
7. Employing tests without being clear about the objectives to be accomplished by using the tests.
8. Using tests to identify specific intervention objectives for children.

frequently employed tool, there is no universally agreed-on method for eliciting and analyzing a language sample. Although language sampling is a valued and purportedly ecologically valid tool, the lack of standardization in the procedures for collecting and analyzing samples creates problems with regard to replication of results across different children, for the same child at different times and in different situations, and across professionals (Eisenberg et al., 2001).

Eliciting the Sample.   One of the principles related to obtaining language samples is that the sample used for analysis must, as much as possible, be a realistic representation of what the child does and can do with language. Clinicians are often advised to use unstructured, free-play contexts and interactions to elicit samples of language from young children, keeping in mind that children with language disorders may be reticent to talk, especially to someone who is not familiar to them. However, different researchers have reported varying results with regard to the effect that the degree of examiner familiarity has on a child (Bornstein, Haynes, Painter, & Genevro, 2000; Kramer, James, & Saxman, 1979; Olswang & Carpenter, 1978). Some of the research has involved normally developing children and other studies have involved children with language disorders. What is uncertain is whether children with language impairments might be more susceptible to various degrees of familiarity of their conversational partners than children whose language is developing normally.

There are also differing opinions about what might be the better types of activities to use during play to elicit representative language samples from children. Some suggest that using items that can be manipulated by children may reduce their talking because they become engrossed in the activity (Kramer et al., 1979; Nelson, 1998; Olswang & Carpenter, 1978). Others (Miller, 1981; Owens, 1999) advise using such items and activities because a child might be more apt to communicate when the focus is on activities rather than on talking, when the activities are unstructured and of the child's own choosing, and when the adult's language relates to the child's utterances and the activities and contains few yes/no question forms and imperatives, such as "Tell me. . . ." The differing advice need not be too disconcerting. The choice of activities and even whether to present several toys or activities at a time to the child, or only one at a time, really depends on the child. Some children become overwhelmed, distracted, and therefore silent if too many activities or too many toys are available, whereas other children need several alternatives, especially if some are not interesting to them. If one strategy is not working, change to the other, remembering that it is always easier to add activities and toys than to take some away. Whatever activities are used, however, they need to be appropriate for a child's age and cognitive level. However, we can see how advice to be flexible in eliciting a sample could play havoc when consistency of sample elicitation across children or across examiners would be important, such as when wishing to compare a particular child's performance on some metric obtained from a sample to those obtained by other children of similar age.

Miller (1981) cautions that materials and activities must not serve "as a substitute for interaction with the child" (p. 11). For younger children, an appropriate scenario might be for the examiner and child to play and talk together in a relaxed, natural, child-directed free-play situation. The examiner can comment on what he or she is doing and what the child is doing, respond in a spontaneous way to the child's attempts at communication and to the child's activities, ask occasional open-ended questions about the child's activities and intentions, and even be silent periodically while engaging in play with the child. With older children, an appropriate scenario might be one in which there is greater emphasis on conversation and/or interview, which can take place around activities, but with much less emphasis on play.

Another caution about what materials and activities to use when eliciting a language sample comes from our knowledge about the effects of shared knowledge between listener and speaker on the level of language children use. When listeners do not share the same knowledge as a speaker, even child speakers, and when there is a limited number of contextual cues to use, speakers provide more information and tend to use more complex linguistic means to do so (Liles, 1985; Masterson & Kamhi, 1991).

Although the examiner's language should be natural for the situation, Lee (1974) suggests that the examiner attempt to elicit increasingly more complex language from the child by introducing more complex forms into his or her own language and creating situations in which a child's usual and logical responses would include these forms. This, of course, has the possible effect of introducing more structure into the sampling scenario. Some of the above discussion has suggested that low structure may encourage more reticent children to talk. However, there are other views that more structured contexts for eliciting language may be effective, particularly in eliciting certain types of language behaviors, and in some instances, may result in higher-level language use by a child while being more time efficient (Coggins, Olswang, & Guthrie, 1987; Evans & Craig, 1992; Wetherby & Rodriguez, 1992). Evans and Craig (1992) found that an interview technique as opposed to free play elicited more and longer utterances from school-age children. The level of semantic and syntactic complexity of language that was elicited was not compromised, with indications that the interview situation tended to elicit more of the more advanced structures.

An examiner also cannot always be sure that a sufficient number of occurrences of specific communicative behaviors will occur during a child-directed free play or even interview sample to allow for analysis. Consequently, it may be necessary to use contrived situations or impose certain linguistic forms and activities on the child to elicit these language behaviors. This can sometimes be accomplished by such techniques as an examiner setting up a repetitive play routine with accompanying models of a desired verbalization (repeatedly extracting toys one at a time from a bag and saying "I have a _____" and then handing the bag to the child with the expectation that the child would continue the pattern), puppet role playing of familiar scripts, or familiar guessing or requesting games ("Do you have a _____" in "Go Fish"). Contrived situations may also be helpful to assess a child's abilities to comprehend and use the range of intentions and the forms by which the intentions are conveyed (Roth & Spekman, 1984a). Sets of intentions and functions (Dore, 1975; Halliday, 1975) can be used as guidelines in examining how many different intentions and functions are present in a child's communicative patterns. Because intentions can be expressed by nonverbal and/or linguistic means, the manner by which a child codes the range of functions and intentions also needs to be determined. The degree of explicitness a child employs to express these, such as direct imperatives, permission directives, or hints, can also be examined. Contrived situations such as giving a child broken pencils or only one part of a toy to use or by putting desired objects in a closed, clear plastic container, may create opportunities to examine a child's range of communicative intentions and the degree of sophistication in expressing the intentions (Roth & Spekman, 1984b). Wetherby and Rodriguez (1992) have identified twelve situations they call "communicative temptations," which can be used to assess communicative intentions of young children. These are listed in Table 13.3 and may provide ideas for the types of strategies that can be employed with toddlers to elicit communicative intents. Of these situations, these authors suggest that the more effective communicative temptations may be the activities with the balloons, bubbles, jar, wind-up toy, books, and blocks in the box.

At some point during a sampling procedure it is necessary to challenge the child's language system (Girolametto et al., 2001; Hadley, 1998; Lahey, 1990). Although we may initially want to create a relaxed environment for a child with the idea of encouraging the child to "open up," such an environment may not place sufficient language demands on the child to tap the child's maximum potential or stress the language system to determine what, if any, linguistic breakdowns emerge (Hadley, 1998; Masterson & Kamhi, 1992). This means that the examiner will need to modify expectations and/or the language sample elicitation tasks for the child in order to encourage the child to use higher levels of language in

TABLE 13.3   "Communicative Temptations" to Elicit Communicative Intentions in Young Children

Communicative Temptation	Explanation
Desired food	Examiner eats a desired food item (e.g., cookie) as child watches but does not offer any to the child.
Wind-up toy	Examiner activates a wind-up toy, lets it wind down, and hands it to the child.
Blocks in a box	Child is given four blocks one at a time to drop in a box and is then immediately given a small animal figure to drop in the box.
Books	Examiner gives the child a book and encourages him or her to look at the book and turn pages; the examiner then repeats this with a second book.
Bubbles	Examiner opens a jar of bubbles, blows bubbles, closes the jar, and gives the closed jar to the child.
Social games	Examiner initiates a familiar and unfamiliar game (e.g., patty-cake, peek-a-boo) with the child and continues until the child expresses pleasure; examiner then discontinues the game and waits.
Balloon	Examiner blows up a balloon, deflates it slowly, either hands deflated balloon to the child or holds the deflated balloon to own mouth, and waits.
Disliked food/toy	Examiner offers the child a disliked food item or toy and waits.
Jar	In front of the child, examiner places a desired food item or toy in a clear jar/container that the child cannot open, closes the container, puts the container in front of the child, and waits.
Jello	The child's hands are placed in a cold, wet, sticky substance (e.g., Jello, paste, pudding).
Ball	Examiner rolls ball to the child and, after the child returns the ball three times, examiner rolls a different object to the child.
Bye-bye	Examiner waves and says "bye-bye" to objects as they are removed in the first four situations but does not do so when the items for remaining situations are removed.

Source: Adapted from Wetherby and Rodriguez (1992, p. 132).

more communicatively demanding contexts. This is particularly true for school-age children, some of whose language problems, particularly in the case of higher-level language difficulties, may be more subtle and not so readily apparent and detectable.

One way to increase language demands, as we know from previous chapters, is to ask the child to produce a narrative (Girolametto et al., 2001; Gummersall & Strong, 1999; Hadley, 1998). Use of a narrative task also has the advantage of allowing an examiner to analyze a child's use of the narrative genre, which we will discuss later in this chapter. Additionally, some language sample analysis procedures are based on narrative samples of children's language (Leadholm & Miller, 1992). The reference database for children between 3 and 13 years of age provided by Leadholm and Miller (1992) for narratives that are fictional retellings can be a valuable source to which to compare an individual's child's performance.

All narrative elicitation tasks, however, are not equal in the ways they challenge a child's language system (Coggins, Friet, & Morgan, 1998; Hughes et al., 1997; Strong, 1998). For example, a child's ability to retell a favorite fictional story is heavily influenced by the amount of exposure the child has had to the story as well as by the child's language ability and knowledge of the narrative genre. Asking a child to retell a story after the examiner's telling of the story is affected by how well the child can remember the story and can utilize the examiner's model. This task may not, however, tap as much knowledge about narrative structure, because a model was provided. If the person to whom the child is to retell the story is the same as the original storyteller, there is considerable shared knowledge between child and listener, so less complexity and detail may characterize the retelling in terms of both narrative complexity and linguistic complexity. Asking a child to make up a story and tell it is a very hard task that places considerable demands simultaneously on the child's language system, so if breakdowns occur the examiner may not know what part of the process was problematic. In contrast, asking a child to tell about a familiar routine or script or about something that happened to him or her (personal narrative) may be much easier but insufficiently challenging to the child's language system, depending on the child's age. While telling or retelling a story from a book reduces memory demands and addresses some of the story's familiarity issues, there can be considerable cues available to the child about narrative structure and sequence so that knowledge of narrative genre may not be well tapped. A rather unique approach to eliciting a narrative is video narration (Dollaghan, Campbell, & Tomlin, 1990). In video narration, a child talks about events in a video, either on-line as the video is shown or after the video is shown. Advantages of video narration (Dollaghan et al., 1990) include (1) content stability, which tends to standardize the content of language and reduces interference from extraneous and uncontrolled factors, (2) potentially high interest value, (3) all utterances produced by the child, rather than splitting speaking time between the child and the examiner, and (4) high processing demands that serve to stress the child's language system but include fewer demands on memory *per se.*

There is no one correct or universally accepted method for eliciting narratives from children. However, Hughes and her colleagues (1997) have provided some guidelines based on children's ages. For example, from preschool through about grade 6, personal narratives (descriptions of events experienced by the child) and scripts (descriptions of usual or typical routines such as getting ready for school in the morning) might be appropriate. At these ages, fictional narratives (stories) might also be elicited, but the amount of support provided to the child for this type of narrative in terms of pictures and whether the context of the narrative is or is not shared with the listener can be systematically varied depending on the child's age. These authors (Hughes et al., 1997) suggest that story generation (making up a novel story) not be elicited until a child is school age. Beyond grade 6, personal narratives might no longer be appropriate, but between grades 7 and 9 scripts might continue to be elicited. For fictional narratives, both story generation and story retelling with varying degrees of picture support with and without shared context might elicit narratives appropriate for the children's ages. Beyond grade 9, however, these authors (Hughes et al., 1997) recommend that narrative elicitation be limited to story generation and story retelling, but with no visual supports and in a context where the listener does not share the context of the story with the storyteller. It is important to remember that what an examiner is trying to ascertain is information about a child's language, and the child's age needs to serve as the guide for which method is selected.

Because an examiner is attempting to find out what a child can do with language while producing a narrative, principles of dynamic assessment might be applied. For example, Gummersall and Strong (1999) found that in a story retelling task, after an examiner had told the entire story to the children, asking the children to imitate each sentence in the narrative after the examiner increased the complexity of several syntax measures that the children used in their retellings when they were then asked to the retell the story again by themselves. The positive effect on syntactic complexity of the examiner's repetition of the story and the children's practice by repeating the sentences applied both to the story retellings of normally developing school-age children and school-age children with language disorders. Hughes (1998) used a different form of dynamic assessment. She employed a 1-minute wait period between children's, adolescents', and adults' exposure to a pictured story and their retellings of the story. When subjects utilized this wait period, not only was the overall length of the story retellings longer, but syntactically the utterances were longer than those of subjects who did not utilize the wait time but instead retold their stories immediately after viewing the pictures for the story.

Because of the nature of language in interactions, the examiner's language and the activities will place constraints on what language will be elicited from a child. As a result, some important aspects of language may not be elicited, especially with older children. This is always one of the real dangers in language sampling. However, busy professionals may not always feel they can devote the time needed to elicit multiple language samples from a child. Hadley (1998) developed a protocol in an attempt to ensure that several text-level discourse genres of school-age children could be sampled systematically in a time-efficient way. This approach was also designed to tax children's language abilities so that their abilities under different language performance conditions could be evaluated. The text-level discourse samples in this protocol were conversation, and not surprisingly, narrative, including different forms of narrative (personal narrative and fictional retelling) as well as expository discourse (explaining or giving instructions, such as how to play a game). In her description of the protocol, Hadley provides considerable details about its application, and further information can be found in her description (Hadley, 1998). As she (Hadley, 1998) writes,

> . . . if elicitation methods do not sufficiently tax older children's production systems, specific areas of weakness might not surface, and therefore, would not be "checked." Thus, the advantage of using these protocols, or other protocols based on these principles, lies in the comparison of strengths and weaknesses across different discourse types and under different situational task conditions, regardless of the analysis method used. (p. 139)

Whatever approaches an examiner ultimately selects, however, it is important to remember that one of the main principles of language sampling elicitation is that the materials, activities, and tasks are chosen on the basis of what we want to learn about child's language, rather than letting the materials, tasks, and activities tell us what we do learn.

Sample Length.   There is no one correct answer to the question of how long a sample should be for an adequate analysis, or whether length should be measured in time or by number of utterances. The length of the sample may depend on the child's language level, age, willingness to talk, and fatigue level, as well as the time that can be devoted to the task, the specific analysis techniques to be used, and the norm-referenced data to which a child's sample might be compared. Recommendations regarding the number of utterances that should be included in a sample range from 50 to 100 (Lahey, 1988; Lee, 1974; Miller, 1981; Owens, 1999; Retherford, 1993, 2000; Tyack & Venable, 1999). Fifty utterances is more or less agreed upon as the acceptable *minimum* (Miller, 1996). Generally, 30 minutes is suggested as about the amount of time to spend obtaining a language sample (Crystal, Fletcher, & Garman, 1989; Lahey, 1988; Miller, 1981). Miller (1981) writes that with "a transcript that includes everything the child and the adult said for 30 minutes we have the ability to perform several kinds of analyses, the choice of which will depend upon our specific goals for assessment" (p. 13). However, time is the lesser issue in considering sample size than number of utterances. Children with language disorders may not talk very much, so it may take longer to obtain the minimum number of utterances, and obtaining a sufficient number of utterances to have confidence in the sample from which assessment recommendations are going to be made is essential.

There are problems of validity and reliability of using sample sizes that do not consist of at least 50 utterances, and Gavin and Giles (1996) have reported that there is even a risk of low retest reliability with samples that do not consist of at least 100 utterances. Sample length is therefore important for accurate assessment. Unfortunately, in one report only 15 percent of the speech–language pathologists surveyed used samples of 100 or more utterances (Kemp & Klee, 1997), and in two other reports 25 percent (Hux, Morris-Friehe, & Sanger, 1993) and 43 percent (Loeb, Kinsler, & Bookbinder, 2000) of the speech–language pathologists surveyed indicated they used sample sizes consisting of fewer than 50 utterances. These are concerning practices.

Recording the Sample.   Rarely is it possible for an examiner who is busy interacting with a child to record in writing what the child says and does as the events are happening, yet a verbatim transcription that includes contextual information is essential for analysis. The usual method is to audiotape the interactions to preserve the events for later transcription and analysis. While audiorecording, it is essential that the examiner make handwritten notes on the contexts in which a child's utterances occur. These notes should contain information about the objects in the environment, the child's nonverbal behaviors, the events that happen before, during, and after the child's statements, and the time of each interaction. The information is used later to interpret the child's utterances in terms of communicative behaviors such as the functions, intentions, and semantic relations expressed. As smaller and easier-to-use videotaping equipment is becoming more accessible, its use can reduce the need to hand record contextual information and increase the accuracy with which pragmatically relevant information can be retained for later analyses. In fact, Nelson (1998) writes that "videotaping is *essential* [emphasis added] to capture the nonlinguistic context for very young or physically impaired children" (p. 303).

Transcription and Utterance Segmentation.   Once a language sample is recorded, one of the first tasks that needs to be completed is transcription of the recorded sample and the separation of the sample into units for analysis. The units used for analysis are typically referred to as *utterances,* and there are different definitions of what constitutes an utterance, many of which are specific to particular analysis approaches. Different language sample analysis approaches use different definitions to guide utterance segmentation. Given the varieties of language-sample analysis approaches, it is important to know what type of information is being sought from a procedure and what might be the reference data (norms) that will be used so these can be married with an appropriate approach. This also means that different ways of segmenting utterances may be used.

Four commonly used definitions of utterance that guide how language samples are separated into utterances for analysis are

- Tone unit (prosodic unit)
- Sentence, per Developmental Sentence Scoring (DSS)
- C-unit
- T-unit

The *tone unit* is the utterance segmentation approach commonly associated with the analysis technique known as the Language Assessment, Remediation and Screening Procedure (LARSP) (Crystal, 1982; Crystal et al., 1989), Miller's (1981) language sample analysis procedures, and to some extent Lee's (1974) Developmental Sentence Types (DST) analysis procedures for presentence utterances. This segmentation approach depends heavily on prosodic features of language (e.g., intonation patterns, pausing), as well as speakers' turns, to determine where utterances end and begin. Because there is no specified syntactic component to the definition, single words, phrases, and, except for the DST procedure, syntactic structures that contain a subject and finite verb (i.e., sentence or clause) can all be considered as individual utterances. The *DSS sentence procedure* (Lee, 1974) applies to segmentation of samples that consist primarily of utterances with subject–predicate structures (i.e., complete sentences) which corresponds with the DSS utterance definition and forms the basis of sample analysis according to DSS procedures. Hunt (1965) devised the *T-unit* as a way of segmenting samples of school-aged children's written work into units for analysis. One T-unit consists of an independent or main clause with all of its modifiers, including any dependent, or subordinate, clauses attached to it. This is similar to the DSS definition in that each utterance contains a subject and finite verb. In contrast, the *C-unit* was used by Loban (1976) to analyze spoken language. The definition of a C-unit is the same as that for the T-unit, except that in transcription of a sample, single words and phrases (i.e., not clauses, which have a subject and a finite verb) can be included in the sample to be analyzed if they are appropriate responses to an examiner's statements or questions. The T-unit and DSS definitions exclude these forms from analysis. For the T-unit, this was largely because it was devised for written language, which generally does not include such structures. T-unit and C-unit utterance definitions require that any utterance that contains a coordinating conjunction (e.g., *and, but*) used to conjoin two or more independent clauses be broken into separate utterance units for analysis. For example, "But the boy didn't like the pie and he ordered a different one the next time" would be two analysis units, "But the boy didn't like the pie" and "And he ordered a different one the next time." Therefore, no analysis unit can technically consist of a compound sentence. Although these different definitions of utterance and the resulting utterance segmentation procedures can be associated with particular analysis procedures, they are also often used to obtain common metrics of language ability, such as the average length of utterances, proportions of different types of clauses, or proportions of different words to number of words used.

The definition of utterance is not a trivial issue, because the different definitions have the potential to affect a number of the metrics of interest obtained from language samples (Reed, MacMillan, & McLeod, 2001). If the definition of utterance, and therefore the segmentation of utterances, is tied to a particular type of sample analysis and even possibly some reference databases (norms), then segmenting a sample in a different way from the utterance definition specified by the procedure potentially invalidates the results and interpretations that can be made about the sample. The definitions can also affect a number of the more generic metrics. Reed and her colleagues (2001) examined the effects of the four commonly used definitions of utterance noted above (tone unit, DSS sentence, C-unit, T-unit) in an attempt to illustrate some of the ways that frequently used metrics derived from language samples can vary based on the definitions of utterance. The difference in definition with regard to whether utterances could consist of two or more independent clauses was an issue that could be expected to affect language sample analysis results. This issue did, in fact, show up in the results of the study by Reed and colleagues (2001) with regard to metrics obtained for (1) length of utterances, (2) number of utterances derived from the same spoken samples of children that were considered to comprise samples for analysis, and (3) numbers of dependent and independent clauses per utterance. Because segmentation of utterances according to the definition of the DSS procedure (Lee, 1974) permitted some compound sentences to be included in a sample, this resulted in longer utterances and fewer numbers of utterances in samples and affected calculation of metrics based on number of utterances in the sample (e.g., average length of utterances, average number of dependent clauses used per utterance). That different definitions of utterance had a considerable impact on the number of utterances that ultimately comprised a sample is an important issue for validity, an issue we have noted above. Reliability of utterance segmentation across different examiners was another issue that emerged in the study. Reliability of utterance segmentation according to DSS, T-unit, and C-unit utterance definitions was high, but was sufficiently low for the tone unit definition to be concerning. As can be seen, decisions on how to segment utterances need to be made carefully.

Analysis.   Other decisions that need to be made once the sample is recorded are how the sample is going to be analyzed and what particular analysis approaches might be used. These decisions depend, in part, on the child's level of language and what types of samples have been elicited. We also need to have some metric of a child's language to guide us, and this frequently comes from the sample(s) obtained.

MLU.   An often-used metric to guide an examiner in selecting other language sample analysis approaches to use is mean length of utterance (MLU). MLU is based on Brown's (1973) early work that measured length in terms of morphemes and linked length of utterance to the emergence of specific grammatical morphological features (e.g., contractible copula, regular past tense). Brown's rules for calculating MLU are shown in Table 13.4. Miller (1981) subsequently developed stages of syntactic development to which the morphemes included in Brown's work could be assigned, that is, the Assigning Structural Stage (ASS) Procedure. Not only is MLU used as an indicator of how else an examiner might analyze a sample, it is used as a metric itself of a child's language ability.

Although MLU is a frequently used clinical metric (Loeb, Kinsler, & Bookbinder, 2000), Eisenburg and her colleagues (2001) have raised serious issues about the purposes for which MLU is used and the lack of standardization underpinning its use. These authors suggest that it may not be a valid and reliable measure and recommend that its use probably best be limited to the trait that it was originally intended to measure, that is, length of utterance (Sabers, 1996), as opposed to purposes for which it is sometimes used (e.g., as an indicator of syntactic complexity). Johnston (2001) found that, even as a measure of length, varying what kinds of utterances (e.g., discourse-dependent utterances such as elliptical responses, imitations) are included and what are excluded from analysis can change MLU measures by 3 to 49 percent and can change sample sizes by 20 percent. Johnston's (2001) work reflects one of the differences regarding what constitutes an utterance according C-unit and T-unit definitions that was also noted by Reed and her colleagues (2001) in their study. Others have found that MLU is particularly susceptible to variation depending on the

---

TABLE 13.4   Brown's Rules for Calculating MLU

A. Preferably use 100 utterances, although 50 may suffice for an estimate.

B. Determine total number of morphemes in language sample.

   1. Count as one morpheme:
   - Repetitions of words used for emphasis (*yes, yes, yes*)
   - Compound words (*birthday*)
   - Proper names (*Billy Boy* or *Sally Jones*)
   - Ritualized reduplications (*choo-choo*)
   - Diminutives (*doggie*)
   - Auxiliary verbs (*is* or *will*)
   - Irregular past-tense verbs (*ran* or *ate*)
   - Catenatives (*wanna* or *gonna*)

   2. Count as two morphemes all grammatical inflections, including:
   - Plural nouns (*dogs*)
   - Third-person singular present-tense verbs (*runs*)
   - Present progressive *-ing* (*running*)
   - Possessive nouns (*baby's*)
   - Regular past tense verbs (*jumped*)

   3. Do not count:
   - Stutterings or disfluencies, except for the one complete form (*I, I, I*)
   - Fillers (*um* or *oh*), except for *no, yeah, hi*

C. Divide the total number of morphemes by the number of utterances in the language sample.

Source: Adapted from Brown (1973).

context used to sample the language (Evans & Craig, 1992; Klee, Schaffer, May, Membrino, & Mougey, 1989), and as a measure of language development, it may be less reliable for children older than 3 to 3½ years of age (Klee, 1985; Klee & Fitzgerald, 1985; Scarborough, Wyckoff, & Davidson, 1986; Wells, 1985). Dollaghan and her colleagues (1999) have also found that children's MLUs vary as a function of their mothers' level of education. Johnston's (2001) work also raised other concerns about the validity of MLU as a metric of children's language. In reference to the use of MLU in identifying language impairment, Eisenberg and her coauthors (2001) write that "low MLU may be used as one piece of evidence supporting a diagnosis of language impairment in preschool children, but should never be used alone for this purpose" (p. 339). This advice is applicable to school-age children as well.

Analysis Approaches.   As indicated previously, a child's MLU might be used to guide an examiner in selecting other language-sample analysis approaches to use. For children at lower levels of language development, approaches that provide for analyses of the child's lexicon, semantic relations, grammatical morphemes, semantic intentions, and pragmatic functions reflected in the sample might be used. These might include, for example, Lahey's (1988) semantic relational analysis and/or Lee's (1974) DST presentence analysis procedure. To gather information about a child's lexical diversity from a language sample, two common approaches are a type–token ratio (TTR) (total number of different words divided by total number of words) and total number of different words (NDW) (Leonard, Miller, & Gerber, 1999; Watkins, Kelly, Harbers, & Hollis, 1995). More recently, use of a computer program (VOCD, a program of the CHILDES computerized language analysis system) (MacWhinney, 2000) provides for repeated random sampling of parts of a child's language sample to calculate multiple TTRs that are reported as D values. The idea is to find out the likelihood of a child using new vocabulary words in longer language samples. Because each sample yields multiple D values with this approach, a single, average D is reported. The D approach to estimating a child's lexical diversity has the purported advantages of being independent of sample size and addressing other problems related to usual TTR and NDW metrics. However, the findings of Owen and Leonard (2002) suggest that the measure is not completely free of the influence of the size of the language sample obtained.

For children at somewhat more advanced language levels, a child's lexicon again might be specified and analyses of semantic intentions, semantic relations, grammatical morphemes, and pragmatic functions would be included, with the addition of approaches that focus on analyses of morphosyntactic forms, including clause types and clausal connectors. Table 13.5 lists a number of different language-sample analysis approaches that are available. An emphasis on analysis of syntactic and morphological features of language is notable among these approaches, although several also include some procedures for analysis of semantic and pragmatic aspects of language, such as Retherford's (2000) *Guide to Analysis of Language Transcripts.*

From the above discussions, the prominence of analyzing language samples to determine what grammatical morphemes are present in children's language is evident. There are several reasons that most analyses include an analysis of grammatical morphemes. Earlier in this text we have seen that difficulties with use of grammatical markers, and in particular those related to tense marking, are characteristics of children, and possibly even young adolescents, with language impairments, and that these difficulties may even constitute a clinical marker

TABLE 13.5   Language Analysis Procedures

Author/Developer	Procedure
Crystal et al., 1989	Language Assessment, Remediation, and Screening Procedure—2 (LARSP—2)
Hannah, 1977	Applied Linguistic Analysis II
Leadholm & Miller, 1992	Language Sample Analysis: The Wisconsin Guide

Lee, 1974	Developmental Sentence Analysis:
	    Developmental Sentence Types (DST)
	    Developmental Sentence Scoring (DSS)

MacWhinney, 2000	The CHILDES System
Miller, 1981	Assessing Language Production in Children: Experimental Procedures
Mordecai & Palin, 1982	Lingquist 1 & 2
Pye, 1987	Pye Analysis of Language (PAL)
Retherford, 2000	Guide to Analysis of Language Transcripts (3rd ed.)
Scarborough, 1990	Index of Productive Syntax (IPSyn)
Tyack & Venable, 1999	Language Sampling, Analysis, and Training—3 (LSAT—3)

of specific language impairment. The work of Brown (1973), de Villiers and de Villiers (1973), and Miller (1981), which linked children's MLU development and the emergence of grammatical morphemes, has been used frequently in the identification of children with language disorders, and often a discrepancy between MLU and the presence or absence of particular grammatical morphemes is employed as an indicator of impairment (Leonard, 1998).

There are, however, some problems with grammatical morpheme analysis in the identification of language impairment that professionals need to take into account in their language sampling and analysis procedures. Among these are (1) the considerable variability from child to child in acquisition of grammatical morphemes, in particular the fourteen examined by Brown (1973), which has been identified more recently, and (2) the evidence that language samples may not contain sufficient instances of obligatory contexts for each of the morphemes to judge accurately whether children have acquired the individual grammatical markers (Balason & Dollaghan, 2002; Lahey, Liebergott, Chesnick, Menyuk, & Adams, 1992). In describing the findings of their study, Balason and Dollaghan (2002) write that the results "indicate that previous interpretations of relationships among age, language levels, and GM [grammatical morpheme] production based on group mean data are suspect, given the substantial variability in frequency of OCs [obligatory contexts] and percentage of GM production" (p. 967). Lahey (1994) has even questioned if we really know what the course and sequence is for children's acquisition of grammatical morphemes.

What this means is that in analyses of children's use of grammatical morpheme in their language samples, particularly in comparing morpheme acquisition to their MLUs, we need to be very careful that we have obtained sufficient evidence about a child's use of grammatical morphemes and that we are interpreting the evidence in relation to MLU thoughtfully. We may need to probe using contrived situations to elicit multiple opportunities for obligatory contexts of individual grammatical morphemes (Rice, Wexler, & Cleave, 1995; Rice, Wexler, & Hershberger, 1998), such as the 52-item task developed by Marchman and colleagues (1999) to assess past-tense marking and the 12-item task developed by Simkin and Conti-Ramsden (2001) to assess third-person singular verb marking. One standardized test, the Rice/Wexler Test of Early Grammatical Impairment (Rice & Wexler, 2001), which is based on the probes used in the authors' research, may include sufficient numbers of exemplars for each grammatical morpheme to make judgments about a child's use of each morpheme.

Whatever analysis procedures an examiner chooses to use, the regularities in the child's communicative behaviors must be abstracted in order to identify the specific target skills that need to be included in a language intervention plan. Different procedures provide different types of information, and it may be necessary to use several analyses.

Analysis of Mazes and Disruptions.   Recall from Chapter 5 that in Loban's (1976) longitudinal study of the language development of school-age children and adolescents, at all grade levels from first to twelfth grade, students who had poor language skills exhibited more maze behavior than those who had advanced language skills. In that chapter we suggested that maze behavior be considered in assessment of adolescents' language performance. The amount and type of maze behavior that occurs in language samples of younger children are also aspects of language performance that are frequently included in analyses and that can "supplement traditional language testing of children" with language impairment (Nettelbladt & Hansson, 1999, p. 495). As Hadley (1998) points out, "one indicator of linguistic vulnerability is excessive use of maze behavior (i.e., false starts, pauses, repetitions, and revisions)" (p. 134).

Dollaghan and Campbell (1992) developed a taxonomy of various disruptions or mazes that can occur in children's language samples and procedures to calculate them as a ratio of the number of disruptions to the number of unmazed words that occur in a sample. This ratio was used to control for samples of differing lengths. Four major types of disruptions are included in the taxonomy, with subtypes within each of the major types. Table 13.6 summarizes the types of disruptions identified by these authors (Dollaghan & Campbell, 1992). In a preliminary study investigating the utility of the taxonomy, Dollaghan and Campbell (1992) found that, in language samples elicited via a structured interview technique, the most frequently occurring types of disruptions for both normally achieving students and those with language impairment due to traumatic brain injury were pauses and repetitions, which together accounted for about 70 percent of all disruptions. Revisions and orphans (disruptions that lacked an obvious relationship to other elements in the utterance) each accounted for 15 percent of the remaining 30 percent of disruptions. However, only the frequency with which silent pauses of 2 seconds or more were used differentiated the two groups at a statistically significant level, with the students with language impairment using significantly more silent pauses than the normally achieving students. Although not significant, the data suggested a trend toward the students with language impairment using all types of pauses more frequently than the normally achieving students.

Hadley (1998) reminds us, however, that "different discourse types have been shown to tax children's language systems to different degrees" (p. 134), and we know that narratives can particularly stress children's language abilities. In explaining her protocol for sampling children's language in several text-level discourse contexts, the child in one case study that was presented clearly demonstrated a greater number of mazes during two narrative tasks (fictional retelling to a naïve listener and relating a known story to a naïve listener) than dur-

TABLE 13.6   Descriptions of Dollaghan and Campbell's Taxonomy for Classifying Disruptions/Mazes Occurring in School-Age Children's Utterances Produced During Language Samples Elicited Using Interview/Conversation

Major Type	Subtypes	Definitions/Examples
Pauses		
	Filled pauses	One-syllable, nonlexical vocalizations (e.g., *um*)
	Silent pauses	Silence for 2 seconds or longer
	Pause strings	Occurrence of more than one filled and/or silent pause in succession
Repetitions		
	Forward repetitions	Repeats an incomplete element and then completes it (e.g., "I I said we thought about it")
	Partial repetitions	Repeats an incomplete element but does not complete it (e.g., "I said we thought thought . . .")
	Exact repetitions	Repeat an already completed element (e.g., "I said we thought about it thought about it")
	Backward repetitions	Insertion of an element between an unaltered repetition (e.g., "I said I know I said we thought about it")
Revisions		
Each also coded for aspect(s) of language being revised (lexical, grammatical, phonological, or multiple aspects)	Correction of error	Correction of grammatical error (e.g., "I said we thinked thought about it")
	Addition of information	Addition of lexical information (e.g., "I said firmly said we thought about it")
	Deletion of information	Deletion of lexical information (e.g., "I firmly said I said we thought about it")
	Unknown	Reasons for revisions that affect several elements not apparent
Orphans		
(No apparent relationship to other elements)	Phonemes	"I said frrrr we thought about it"
	Words	"I said we girl thought about it"
	Strings (words or words and phonemes)	"I said frrrr girl we thought about it"

Source: Adapted from Dollaghan & Campbell (1992).

ing conversation (interview), relating a personal narrative, and expository discourse (explanation of games or sports). Given that Dollaghan and Campbell (1992) used samples obtained from interviews (conversations) rather than narratives, their sample-elicitation task may not have been sufficiently demanding to reveal greater differences in maze behavior between students with language impairments and those with normal language.

Another aspect of analyzing mazes from which examiners might obtain useful information involves the grammatical elements of utterances associated with the occurrences of mazes. If, as Hadley (1998) suggests, mazes reflect aspects of language performance that are vulnerable or wobbly, it is possible that the elements of language reflected in the mazes are those parameters of language with which a child may be struggling. For example, in Reed and Evernden's (2001) preliminary investigation comparing verb morphological performances of students with reading and language problems with their normally achieving peers, none of the mazes that occurred in the language samples of the normally achieving students involved verbs. This contrasted with the students with reading/language problems, for whom 13.5 percent of their mazes involved verbs, even though both students with reading/language problems and normally achieving students used about the same amount of maze behavior overall. Examiners might want to note what elements of language are involved in children's mazes, because it is possible these may be clues as to what could be specific weaknesses in a child's language system.

Narrative and Presuppositional Analyses.   Several different approaches are available for narrative analysis, some of which may be more helpful for analyzing narrative attempts of younger children, perhaps in the preschool years, whereas others might be more appropriate for use with older, school-age children. Different forms of analyses are also likely more appropriate for different types of narratives than others. Table 13.7 lists a number of approaches to narrative analysis and assessment and describes features of each. These analysis approaches provide different information about children's abilities with narrative production, so it is important for an examiner to select the analysis approach that fits what information is being sought.

Measures of cohesion for features that occur within narratives and that tie the elements together in meaningful ways can contribute to estimates of the quality and complexity of children's narratives. Some of the linguistic cohesive devices that occur in narratives are pronouns following initial nomination of the referent ("The boy ran. . . . *He* caught. . . ."), conjunctions and adverbial connectives ("*Unfortunately,* the boy. . . ."), and indefinite versus definite articles ("*A* child found. . . . *The* child returned. . . ."). Paul and her co-researchers (Paul et al., 1996) reported that one of the distinguishing features between the narratives of normally developing school-age children and their peers with language impairments was the use of linguistic devices that provided cohesive ties across the propositions presented in the narratives. Liles (1985) developed a system to score use of cohesive ties in children's narratives as a measure of narrative performance. This system uses a metric that is the proportion of complete (appropriate and accurate) cohesive ties to all cohesive devices attempted in a narrative sample. McFadden and Gillam (1996) found that the quality of children's narratives judged according to the author's holistic scoring procedure (Table 13.7) was associated with the text-level features (e.g., connectives) that appeared in the narratives, but not the sentence-level features (e.g., length of utterance). Such information suggests that an examiner might want to include analysis procedures that look at the quality and quantity of cohesive ties children use in their narratives.

Even though in this section we have been discussing methods of analyzing narrative samples as part of a larger language-sampling process, you might have noted in looking at Table 13.7 that several formal narrative assessment procedures and/or tests were included. Overall, there are only a few published formalized tests and assessments for narratives.

TABLE 13.7   Approaches for Analyzing and Assessing Narratives

Approach	Author(s)	Features
Narrative levels	Applebee, 1978	Six developmental levels in children's narratives 2 to 5 years old: heaps (no organization, bits of random information from whatever comes to a child's mind; approximately 2 years of age), sequences, primitive narratives, unfocused chains, focused chains, true narratives (plot with chain of events, themes or morals emerging; about 20% of 5-year-olds show evidence of true narratives)
		Additional levels identified in older children's narratives (6–17 years)
		Hutson-Nechkash's (1990) summary of Applebee's extensions: ■ Provide summaries and characterizing stories (about 7–11 years) ■ Provide analysis of narratives (approximately 13–15 years) ■ Provide generalizations about theme or moral of narrative (16+ years)
Story grammar	Stein & Glenn, 1979 Glenn & Stein, 1980	Focuses on development of the structural patterns and structural properties of narratives (i.e., types of sequences, types and number of episodes)
		Seven stages (in order from least to most complex): ■ Descriptive sequence (preschool): chain of setting statements with no temporal or causal links ■ Action sequence (preschool): setting statement with action statements functioning as attempts; action statements are chronologically but not causally chained ■ Reaction sequence (preschool): setting statement, an initiating event, and several action (attempt) statements in order of direct cause–effect relation, i.e., first action directly causes next action, but with no goal-direction ■ Abbreviated episode (about 6 years of age): setting statement and either an initiating statement followed by a consequence or an event statement followed by a consequence; goal-direction is either explicit or implicit ■ Complete episode (about 7–8 years of age): setting statement and two of three components (initiating event, internal response, attempt) followed by a consequence; goal-direction is present ■ Complex episode (about 11 years of age): multiple episodes or expansion of complete episodes; reaction statements and internal plans may be included ■ Interactive episode (11+ years): more than one character and separate episodes with each influencing the others

(continued)

TABLE 13.7   Continued

Approach	Author(s)	Features
Story grammar decision tree	Westby, 1998	A decision tree based on Stein and Glenn's story grammar
		At each stage, in developmental sequence, a decision is made as to whether a child's narrative represents the particular stage; if not, the stage assigned is the lower stage in the sequence; if yes, a decision is made about the next higher stage
		As an example, does the narrative evidence explicit planning or intentional behavior, characteristic of "abbreviated episode," per above; if not, child's stage is "reaction sequence"; if yes, the child's stage is either at the "abbreviated episode" stage or higher
Narrative stages	Lahey, 1988	Four sequential stages of narrative development
		Stages in order of development: ■ Additive chain (events that can occur in any order) ■ Temporal chain (event presented in temporal order) ■ Causal chain (cause–effect relationships presented in order) ■ Multiple causal chain (multiple causal relationships presented)
		Subcategories considered for narratives at or above causal chain stage ■ Initiating event ■ Setting ■ Reaction ■ Internal response (states or thoughts of characters) ■ Attempt ■ Resolution/consequence
Holistic analysis	McFadden & Gillam, 1996	Focuses evaluation of narrative on general impressions
		Not dependent on preset criteria or characteristics
		Narratives scored as "weak," "adequate," "good," or "strong"
		Elements at text level (e.g., connectives, constituents) as opposed to sentential level (length of utterance, predicate types) contribute to evaluation of quality
		Numerical values assigned, if needed, from 1 (weak) to 4 (strong)
Strong Narrative Assessment Procedure (SNAP)	Strong, 1998	Quality evaluation referenced to age of child
		Criterion-referenced, standardized procedure
		Uses story retelling tasks
		Initial model via audiotape of story and wordless picture book
		Retell to naïve listener without pictures
		Appropriate for elementary and middle school students
		Procedures for analyzing length and fluency of narrative production, cohesion, syntax, and story grammar

TABLE 13.7 Continued

Approach	Author(s)	Features
Story Construction Subtest, Detroit Tests of Learning Aptitude—4	Hammill, 1998	Standardized, norm-referenced subtest
		Three story creations each from a colored picture stimulus
		Stories scored for number and complexity of semantic themes
		Scores reflect story content rather than story form
		Percentile ranks, standard scores, age equivalents available
		Norms available for ages 6–17 years
Memory-for-Stories Subtest, Test of Memory and Learning	Reynolds & Bigler, 1994	Standardized, norm-referenced subtest
		Three story retells each after examiner reads a story
		Includes a delayed story retelling condition; the three stories retold after a wait of about 30 minutes
		Stories scored for characters and actions included the retells
		Scores reflect story content rather than story form
		Percentile ranks, standardized scores, and scaled scores available
		Norms available for ages 5 through 19 years

Consequently, professionals who need to give service providers scores and numbers to qualify children for intervention are often in a bind to locate standardized instruments, including those with norms, for narratives. Caution may, however, be appropriate in using some of the tests because of the concerns that (1) they may not identify well children who have problems with narratives *per se,* (2) scores can reflect more about story content than narrative form, and (3) high scores can be obtained for long stories with poor cohesion (Crais & Lorch, 1994; Gillam, Peña, & Miller, 1999).

In the same way that dynamic assessment procedures can be used with other aspects of language assessment, these procedures can be applied to narratives. For example, Gillam and colleagues (1999) have described a mediated learning experience, a form of the test–teach–retest method of dynamic assessment, to ascertain how much and what kinds of changes to elements of narrative production (e.g., increasing complexity of episodes, adding information about the characters) a child can make with only two intervention sessions. The amount of teaching effort that was required for the child to change is also evaluated. These authors (Gillam et al., 1999) suggest that children who make relatively rapid gains with short-term, mediated teaching are less likely to be language disordered.

One of the aspects of narratives that make them particularly demanding language tasks is that they require that the needs of the listener be considered and attended to so that the right amount of information unknown to the listener is provided but information that the listener knows is not made explicit. That is, children need to demonstrate *presupposition* abilities. However, presupposition is not limited to narrative tasks, but is an essential feature of interpersonal communication generally. Appropriate skills with presupposition can be assessed by systematically varying the conditions in which a child needs to communicate, that is, who the partners are and what they might know about what the child needs to communicate. The expectation is that the child will make modifications in terms of the content and form of the messages (Roth & Spekman, 1984a). One procedure that is frequently used is a modification of the barrier game mentioned in previous chapters, in which a child attempts to get a listener to choose an abstract object, construct a drawing, or arrange objects in a predetermined order only on the basis of the child's verbal instructions (Roth & Spekman, 1984b). This task does not, however, require the same level of presuppositional skills combined with effective use of cohesive devices as does narrative production.

Analyses of Organization of Social Discourse.   According to Roth and Spekman (1984a), one aspect of assessing a child's pragmatic abilities is to assess the child's "ability to function in, and contribute to, the ongoing stream of discourse or conversation" (p. 7). Specific behaviors to evaluate are the amount of a child's social speech (speech addressed to a listener) versus nonsocial speech (speech that does not obligate a listener to respond, such as monologues) and the child's abilities to maintain a topic of conversation, to initiate and terminate conversations, and to repair communication breakdowns. A child's turn-taking skills are also assessed. Dyadic communication portions of a language sample may provide the necessary information to assess many of these skills.

Several guides are available to assist in analyzing a child's discourse skills. In Chapter 3 we learned about one on-line method of assessment that can be used with young children in group situations to examine their social, interactive communication with peers (Rice, Sell, et al., 1990). Recall that Fey's (1986) interactionist approach (Chapter 3) emphasizes how children use language in social-conversational situations. Fey developed a coding system, based on those of Dore (1979) and Chapman (1981), to describe and classify each conversational act a child produces during an interactive interchange, with some acts reflecting assertiveness and others reflecting responsiveness. Examples from this coding system are: requests for information (RQIN), requests for attention (RQAT), statements (ASST), disagreements (ASDA), responses to requests for information (RSIN), responses to requests for clarification (RSCL), and responses to requests for attention (RSAT). The proportion with which these different acts occur during the interchange is used to classify a child into one of four profiles of social-conversational participation (e.g., active conversationalist, passive conversationalist, inactive communicator, verbal noncommunicator) (see Chapter 3). Retherford (2000) also presents systematic procedures for conversational analysis that examiners might find helpful.

The Breakdown Coding System (BCS) (Yont, 1998; Yont, Hewitt, & Miccio, 2000) was developed to provide a tool for analyzing preschoolers' communication breakdowns as these occurred in naturalistic interactions with their mothers. This system describes what is in a child's language that caused the listener (in this case mother) to signal a communication failure on the child's part. This system differs from others, therefore, in that it looks at the source of a child's communication breakdown, not the child's ways of attempting or not attempting to repair communication breakdown. What the child did that caused a breakdown is determined by what the listener communicates to the child about the nature of the breakdown. That is, the classification of the problem is based on what the listener did not understand. The BSC is presented in Figure 13.1. As can be seen, there are five ways in

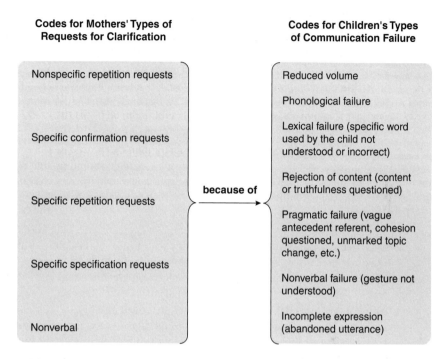

Codes for Mothers' Types of Requests for Clarification

- Nonspecific repetition requests
- Specific confirmation requests
- Specific repetition requests
- Specific specification requests
- Nonverbal

because of

Codes for Children's Types of Communication Failure

- Reduced volume
- Phonological failure
- Lexical failure (specific word used by the child not understood or incorrect)
- Rejection of content (content or truthfulness questioned)
- Pragmatic failure (vague antecedent referent, cohesion questioned, unmarked topic change, etc.)
- Nonverbal failure (gesture not understood)
- Incomplete expression (abandoned utterance)

FIGURE 13.1

Coding Communication Breakdowns in Preschool Children's Conversations with Their Mothers—The Breakdown Coding System (BCS)

Source: Adapted from Yont, Hewitt, and Miccio (2000).

which mothers can request clarifications of what their children tried unsuccessfully to communicate and seven types of child communication failures that the mothers could identify with their clarification requests. In a preliminary study using this coding system, differences between children with specific language impairment and normally developing children were apparent in the types and frequency of breakdowns the children had (Yont & Hewitt, 1999). Yont and her colleagues (2000) suggest that the system can assist in identifying individual children's profiles of communication breakdown and potentially point the way to developing intervention objectives.

When samples of "naturalist" dyadic communication have failed to elicit discourse elements of interest, role playing and contrived communicative situations may be needed to create opportunities to assess a child's skills. For example, an examiner may purposefully give vague instructions to a child or use a nonverbal cue indicating a lack of understanding, such as a puzzled expression, to evaluate a child's reactions (Roth & Spekman, 1984b).

Computer-Assisted Analysis.   Increasingly, the computer is being used as a tool in assessment and in intervention. Several computer programs have been developed to assist in analyzing language samples. Among these are: *Systematic Analysis of Language Transcripts (SALT)* (Miller & Chapman, 2000), *Lingquest 1 & 2* (Mordecai & Palin, 1982), the *CHILDES* system (MacWhinney, 1996, 2000), *Pye Analysis of Language (PAL)* (Pye, 1987), and *Computerized Profiling (CP)* (Long, Fey, & Channell, 2000). These programs generally provide for analyses of a variety of morphosyntactic aspects of language, and several also provide for analyses of some semantic and pragmatic characteristics.

In using computerized programs, the utterances for analysis are entered into the computer according to the format specified by the program. The advantage of computerized analyses is that these can be performed more quickly and generally more accurately than by hand (Long, 1999a). Long and Channell (2001) write that, "all of these programs have the ability to produce detailed analyses far faster than they could be done by hand" (p. 180), which means that the argument for not using language sampling, that is, that it took more time for analyses than busy professionals could devote to the process, is no longer valid.

The primary difference between different computerized analysis programs deals with what the examiner needs to do and what the computer does (Long, 1999b). Some of the programs assist mostly by retrieving, counting, and categorizing data after a human examiner has entered a transcript into the computer with necessary codings for the utterances. The examiner uses his or her metalinguistic knowledge, such as segmenting utterances, identifying mazes, and coding occurrences of morphological markers in assigning the requisite codes. This means that some degree of analysis of each utterance is required by the examiner as it is entered. Unless these structures are coded initially, the computer cannot perform further analyses accurately. Accuracy in entering the initial data is essential. Other programs can assist the examiner by interacting symbiotically with the human transcriber so that the program analyzes many aspects of the transcript, such as word boundaries, word types, syntactic categories. More recently, computer programs have used algorithms to increase the level of automatic analyses they are able to do, so that the human effort can be decreased further (Channell, 1998; Channell & Johnson, 1999). This approach means that the computer programs simulate and execute some of a human's "metalinguistic knowledge." Long and Channell (2001) examined the accuracy of results for automatically generated metrics for four analyses—MLU, LARSP, DSS, and IPSyn. Results were promising, suggesting that generally the generated analyses were equally as accurate as a human completing the analyses. These authors (Long & Channell, 2001) concluded that

> . . . at least for certain procedures, software can produce analysis results that rival those achieved by hand. This should not be seen as cause for alarm. Rather, it should impel us to reconsider the purpose of clinical language analysis. Now, and increasingly in the future, the burden of generating an analysis will become lighter. This will, thankfully, permit us to focus our attention on *how* that information should be used in our evaluation and treatment decisions. (p. 187)

Future developments, including those in voice recognition, should add to the benefits offered by computerized language sampling analyses.

Criterion-Referenced Testing.   Criterion-referenced testing is designed to probe whether a child's performance with regard to a particular language skill, such as ability to mark regular past-tense verbs with different allomorphs appropriately, attains a specified level of performance—the criterion. In some instances, the child is compared to his or her own performance at different times, for example, before targeting an intervention objective and then at some time later after a period of intervention; in other instances, as McCauley (1996) writes, a child's performance might be "interpreted in terms of established performance levels" (p. 122), such as when a child's MLU is compared to Brown's stages (1973). In fact, language sampling is perhaps the most common criterion-referenced procedure used in child language assessment, but is likely not often recognized, or at least not labeled as, a criterion-referenced procedure (McCauley, 1996).

Criterion-referenced testing in child language assessment is not really new. Quite some time ago, at least in terms of the history of the study of child language disorders, Leonard, Prutting, Perozzi, and Berkley (1978) wrote about the value of this type of testing and proposed three reasons for employing criterion-referenced, clinician-constructed tasks as a supplement to standardized norm-referenced testing:

1. *Few standardized norm-referenced tests assess a sufficient number of items for a specific linguistic feature to determine whether that feature is truly present or absent in the child's language patterns.* For example, the Patterned Elicitation Syntax Test with Morphological Analysis (Young & Perachio, 1993) contains only two items that examine regular plural morphemes and one item that examines irregular past tense.

Therefore, criterion-reference testing might be used as a form of extension testing. In using a criterion-referenced approach to assessing a child's skills with morphological markers, for example, with regular noun plural morphemes, more regular noun plural items could be selected so that root word endings are varied and more opportunities to respond to items examining all three regular allomorphs are provided for the child. Items might include *drums, dogs, cakes, lips, horses,* and *dishes.* Tasks could be designed in an attempt to be as consistent as possible with the format of the test, which prompted extension criterion testing.

2. *A range of standardized norm-referenced tests is not available to examine some aspects of language, so choice of what to use is limited.* For example, assessment of pragmatic skills and narrative abilities are areas relatively untapped by tests. Several of the approaches previously discussed in this chapter would be examples of using criterion-referenced tests to fill a gap in range of available tests, such as, narrative assessment.

3. *The tasks or stimuli used to assess a feature may create problems for the child rather than the child actually having a problem with the feature itself.* This is what Sabers (1996) referred to as the techniques used to measure a trait affecting the degree to which the intended trait is actually measured. For example, previously in this chapter we discussed how different approaches to assessing children's narrative skills might place different forms of constraints on what skills with narrative the child might be able to demonstrate. The same issue applies to standardized, norm-referenced tests.

In order to discern the reasons for a child's problem, a task or stimulus different from the ones used on a norm-referenced, standardized test to assess the feature can be devised. This is actually a form of dynamic assessment we discussed earlier in this chapter. For example, the pictures provided with a test may be unclear or confusing. It is also possible that changing the pictorial stimuli may elicit correct responses. In one study (Barrow, Holbert, & Rastatter, 2000) of the effects of colored versus black-and-white stimuli on the picture-naming speed and accuracy of normally developing children 4 to 8 years of age, the addition of color increased naming speed for vocabulary words that were within an emerging period for the children (i.e., words most likely to be in the process of being learned).

When the vocabulary words were well within the repertoires of the children or beyond their developmental level, colored pictures held no advantage over black-and-white pictures. For more advanced vocabulary words, the addition of color helped the children name the pictures depicting the words more accurately. As another example, a child may not be able to deal with sentence-completion tasks, such as "Here is a dog. Here are two _____," which are types of tasks used in several standardized tests. However, the same child may be able to use the same morphological forms in other types of tasks.

As we can see, many of these suggestions sound like elements of dynamic assessment.

Nonword repetition ability has gained prominence as a potential clinical marker of specific language impairment (SLI) in children (Conti-Ramsden, 2003; Dollaghan & Campbell, 1998; Edwards & Lahey, 1998; Ellis Weismer et al., 2000; Gathercole, 1995; Gathercole, Willis, Baddeley, & Emslie, 1994; Gray, 2003a; Marton & Schwartz, 2003). It is important, therefore, that assessment includes tasks designed to evaluate children's abilities to repeat nonsense words of increasing complexity. Standardized criterion-referenced tasks, such as those of Dollaghan and Campbell (1998) and Gathercole and colleagues (1994), are frequently used. Because these tasks have typically been used with school-age children, Gray (2003a) has explored the "usefulness of nonword repetition as a diagnostic measure of SLI in younger children" (p. 134), and in particular, preschool children. Her results suggest that her tasks hold promise for use with preschoolers. As this aspect of assessment has become more important, increasing numbers of formal measurement tools, such as the Comprehensive Test of Phonological Processing (CTOPP) (Wagner, Torgesen, & Rashotte, 1999), which include nonword repetition tasks, are also being developed.

Intelligence Testing

Results of intelligence quotient (IQ) tests administered by qualified psychologists are often part of a comprehensive assessment process for a child with a suspected language disorder, and in previous chapters we have discussed relationships among children's cognitive abilities, mental age, and language. The use of IQ tests has been inextricably tied to identification of children with language disorders and frequently to qualifying children with language impairments for intervention services. As we have seen, in most cases the concept of match/mismatch between intellectual ability/cognitive ability and language ability is core to these identification and qualifying procedures. However, the practice of using IQ tests in these ways has increasingly been seen as untenable (Francis, Fletcher, Shaywitz, Shaywitz, & Rourke, 1996; Stanovich & Siegel, 1994), in part because of the recognition that factors that affect performance on IQ tests probably also affect language abilities. Nevertheless, as Francis and his colleagues (1996) acknowledge, the use of IQ tests for identifying discrepancy between intellectual and language levels "is firmly entrenched in public policy and clinical practice" (p. 132). It is likely that changes in the policy and practice will be slow to come and hindered by the lack of agreed-on alternatives.

What is surprising is that the extent to which IQ testing has become so established in assessment, identification of children with language disorders, and practices to qualify children for services given its dubious past record for accomplishing these purposes. For example, in the past, children with normal or above cognitive abilities but with language differences or disorders—such as hearing-impaired children and linguistically-culturally diverse children with cerebral palsy—have been misdiagnosed as intellectually disabled and placed in classrooms for cognitively low-functioning children. A major reason for these misdiagnoses stems from the nature of some of the intelligence tests that were used. Historically, the Stanford-Binet Intelligence Scale (Terman & Merrill, 1973) originally yielded a single IQ score and was recognized as heavily based on language and language-related abilities. When given to a child with a language problem or difference, the resulting IQ score reflected more directly the child's language skills rather than the child's cognitive level. More recent editions have attempted to address concerns about gender and ethnic biases, but there is still a relatively heavy language component. In contrast, the Wechsler Intelligence Scale for Children—III (WISC—III) (Wechsler, 1991) and the Wechsler Preschool and Primary Scale of Intelligence—III (WPPSI—III) (Wechsler, 2002) yield separate IQ scores for performance and verbal portions, as well as a full-scale combined IQ score, which at least try to address some of the issues surrounding IQ testing with children with language impairments. As with the Stanford-Binet, the verbal scale tends to reflect a child's language abilities or disabilities. The performance scale may be a more accurate indication of a language-disordered child's intellectual level, although cautions are even appropriate in interpreting the performance IQ as valid (Francis et al., 1996). One reason for caution, but not the only reason, is that instructions are given orally, and a child with language comprehension problems can be at a severe disadvantage in completing the performance tasks accurately because the instructions may not be understood. For example, in one study involving the previous version of the WISC, WISC—R performance IQ scores of hearing-impaired children increased about 20 points when the examiner's oral instructions were supplemented with manual communication (Sullivan, 1978). Similarly, Braden (1994) has reported that, on performance IQ tests where hearing-impaired children are shown what to do, their scores do not differ from those of children without hearing losses, but when the instructions on performance IQ tests need to be presented orally to the children, they score significantly poorer than their hearing peers, even though their scores can still be within normal limits.

An extremely unfortunate situation for language-different and language-disordered children was the description and subsequent use of an early edition of the Peabody Picture Vocabulary Test (PPVT) (Dunn, 1965) as a measure of intellectual functioning. Rather than assessing intellectual level, the PPVT and its newer edition, the Peabody Picture Vocabulary Test—III (PPVT—III) (Dunn & Dunn, 1997), actually assess receptive single-word vocabulary. Fortunately, the authors of the PPVT-III no longer refer to the test as a measure of intelligence, although some texts on psychological assessment continue to list it as an intelligence test. The Kaufman Assessment Battery for Children (K-ABC) (Kaufman & Kaufman, 1983) is increasingly becoming a popular intelligence test, especially its nonverbal scale. It assesses children's abilities, in children as young as 2½ years, to problem solve using simultaneous or sequential mental processes. Achievement tests for areas such as reading and arithmetic are also included. There are several alternative intelligence tests that minimize the language loading seen in some of the tests. Two such tests are the third edition of the Columbia Mental Maturity Scale (Burgemeister, Blum, & Lorge, 1971) and the Universal Nonverbal Intelligence Test (UNIT) (Bracken & McCallum, 1998). Other tests of nonverbal intelligence include the Test of Nonverbal Intelligence (TONI—3) (Brown, Sherbenou, & Johnsen, 1997) and the Comprehensive Test of Nonverbal Intelligence (CTONI) (Hammill, Pearson, & Wiederholt, 1996). The Raven's Progressive Matrices (Raven, 1998), a set of tests based mostly on visual perception, are also sometimes used with communicatively impaired or language-different children. Where children with language impairments are concerned, Conti-Ramsden and her colleagues (2001) suggest that the use of the Raven's matrices as tests of children's intellectual functioning may have some particular advantages over other nonverbal or performance intelligence tests that can include timed tasks and those requiring memory skills. Because the tasks in the Raven's matrices rely primarily on visual perception and reasoning/logic tasks and are not timed, children with language impairment, who are frequently believed to have problems with working memory and/or slowed general processing abilities, may be better able to demonstrate their intellectual abilities when these matrices are used rather than other nonverbal intelligence tests (Conti-Ramsden et al., 2001).

Although standardized tools for assessment of intelligence are supposed to be given in very specific ways with little room for deviation from stated protocols, their uses with language-disordered or language-different children may require special precautions in giving the tests or modifications of instructions, materials, or administration procedures if relatively accurate estimates of intelligence are to be obtained. For example, for a child with cerebral palsy with severe oral and motor involvements, testing materials may need to be cut apart and placed so the child can respond only by having to look at the stimuli to respond. Or, the examiner may need to change the procedures to allow for multiple-choice responses instead of oral or motor target responses. A number of intelligence tests have timed subtests that are inappropriate for children with motor handicaps, and many of the tests that minimize language loading emphasize the visual modality, which then render them unsuitable for children with visual impairments. In some cases, children with sensory impairments may be given only one scale of the WISC—III or the WPPSI—III, for example, the verbal scale to children with visual impairments, the performance scale to children with hearing impairments. For a hearing-impaired child who is visually oriented, appropriate visual cues may help the child perform optimally, but distracting visual information may adversely affect the child's performance. In administering test items that use a picture–response format, an examiner should avoid looking at any specific picture after giving a test stimulus or placing his or her hand in such a way as to direct inadvertently the hearing-impaired child's responses. These are only a few examples of the modifications and precautions necessary when testing these special children. Of course, most intelligence tests are standardized, so changing administration procedures to accommodate these children potentially invalidates the results. On the other hand, to administer tests to children whose communicative and other abilities spuriously affect results about their intellectual functioning is equally invalid. Given the intertwining of language with intelligence tests, children with language impairments are exceptionally special.

Summary

In this chapter we have seen that

- Language assessment needs to accomplish a number of objectives, and several procedures and tools are employed to achieve these objectives.
- Screenings are brief examinations of children's communicative performances, the results of which can raise concerns about children's language but cannot determine if

children have language problems; issues of test sensitivity, specificity, positive predictive value, negative predictive value, false positive and false negative results are important issues in assessment and test use.

- The regularities in a child's language need to be identified to develop intervention objectives; language sampling, criterion-referenced testing, and clinician-constructed tasks are valid procedures to use in achieving this.
- Assessment is an ongoing process; evaluation of intervention efficacy is part of this ongoing process.
- Norm-referenced, standardized tests are tools and do not suffice as sole methods to be used in achieving the objectives of assessment; professionals must be careful not to misuse nor misinterpret standardized tests.
- Factors to consider in language sampling include methods used to elicit the sample, the settings and communicative partners involved in eliciting the sample, the length of the sample, the ways to record the sample, and transcription and analysis procedures to be used.
- Assessing interactive discourse, pragmatic, and narrative skills is essential as part of the assessment process and generally requires using nonstandardized approaches.
- Intelligence testing is generally a part of a child's total assessment; obtaining valid results when children have language problems is a challenging task for psychologists and requires careful test selection and may involve modification of usual procedures.

The language assessment process for a child with a suspected language problem involves gathering information about the child from a variety of sources and procedures. All of these lead to accomplishing the objectives of the assessment process. One of these objectives is determining the directions that intervention for a child with a language problem should take.

14 Considerations for Language Intervention

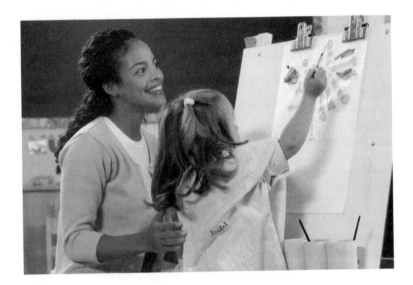

OBJECTIVES

After reading this chapter, you should be able to discuss

- Considerations in planning and implementing language intervention and how these affect intervention decisions
- Various approaches to intervention and the ways in which the approaches overlap and affect other decisions about language intervention
- Methods of highlighting intervention targets in order to increase their saliency
- Facilitation and elicitation techniques that can be employed in language intervention

In previous chapters, we discussed a number of intervention considerations. Many of these intervention strategies are appropriate for other children and situations and should be viewed as having applications beyond the specific instances cited. However, no two language-disordered children are exactly alike in the language abilities and disabilities they manifest. Therefore, each child's language intervention plan is developed individually and is initially based on the results of the assessment process and later on the ongoing assessment that is part of any intervention program. There is no one recipe for language intervention. Instead, multiple factors and approaches must be considered in planning.

Fey and Proctor-Williams (2000) list four aims of intervention for grammatical targets:

1. Attend to a new or unmastered language form or operation in the input;
2. Recognize the semantic, pragmatic, and/or grammatical functions of the new form;
3. Relate the new form or operation to their existing grammatical systems and modify their grammars accordingly; and/or
4. Access and produce the new structure more quickly and reliably after it is generated by their underlying grammars. (p. 178)

It seems that these aims could as easily apply to intervention for pragmatic or semantic targets. The following sections provide guidelines for how these aims of intervention might be achieved for children with language impairments, regardless of the specific targets for a child at a particular point in time.

Considerations in Intervention

Normal versus Not So Normal Processes

Many approaches in language intervention are based on language behaviors and developmental patterns observed in normal children. This implies that what is good and works for children who are acquiring language normally is good and will work for children with language disorders. The problem is, of course, that children with language problems are not learning language normally, and it is possible that what works for normal language-learning children may not work for language-disordered children and vice versa (Connell, 1987; Connell & Stone, 1992; Kiernan & Snow, 1999).

Several approaches to intervention place an emphasis on naturalistic child-directed environments that resemble normal language-learning interactions of mothers and their children (Girolametto et al., 1996; Yoder, Kaiser, & Alpert, 1991). These approaches are based, in large part, on the knowledge that normal children learn language by actively exploring their environments and communicatively interacting with others. However, it is possible that not all language-impaired children will benefit optimally from such a strategy, because some children with language problems begin intervention as passive or unresponsive (Fey, 1986) and/or whatever is the reason for their language problems affects their ability to make efficient use of the ambient language-learning environment (Proctor-Williams, Fey, & Loeb, 2001). These children may not be able to take good advantage of such a "naturalist" environmental strategy. It is likely that at least some language-disordered children need "not so normal" intervention approaches in order to benefit most from intervention. What this means is that we may need to modify the "normal process" of intervention somewhat in order to effect language change as efficaciously as possible. Doing more of what is normal by applying the "normal process" model fully to language intervention for language-disordered children may not be entirely appropriate (Olswang & Bain, 1991).

Developmental and Nondevelopmental Intervention

A consideration of intervention somewhat related to the previous discussion is that of using normal child language-development information to guide planning and implementation of intervention. Language intervention plans are often heavily grounded in normal language development. We have encountered this notion elsewhere in this text. Normal language-developmental patterns can guide the sequences of objectives planned for language-disordered children. A rationale behind a developmental approach is that a particular language skill has antecedents that provide the bases for the acquisition of the higher-level skill. New language skills are built on previously acquired skills, and earlier acquired abilities influence the learning of later-developing skills. Information from normal language development assists us, therefore, in deciding what skills need to be learned before other skills can be acquired.

In many cases, a developmental approach to language intervention is warranted. Besides providing a rationale for selecting initial goals of intervention, it serves as a way of guiding ongoing intervention for children. Examples of using a developmental approach in choosing intervention goals for syntax or morphology include (1) focusing on relative clauses to modify objects of sentences before relative clauses to modify subjects of sentences for which an embedding process is required, (2) emphasizing the present progressive verb inflection (-*ing*) before past-tense verbs or third-person present-tense regular verb inflections (*runs*), or (3) introducing the allomorph /z/ to pluralize nouns before the allomorphs /s/ and /əz/. Because normal language-learning children generally use semantic relations that express nomination, recurrence, and nonexistence before those indicating attributes of objects, we might use this information to guide intervention goals in the semantic area; thus we might emphasize the former types of semantic relations in intervention before entity + attributive ("car big") and attributive + entity ("big car") relations. For intervention focusing on pragmatic aspects of language, utterances that encode only one function per utterance might be stressed before asking children to encode two or more functions per utterance. Intervention for conversational turn-taking skills might begin with the language precursors of reciprocal interactions at the nonverbal level, if the child lacks these skills, before introducing verbal turn-taking activities. In helping children learn to maintain a topic in conversation, intervention might first include objectives aimed at having the children use one, possibly two, contingent responses and later include objectives for several contingent responses. Furthermore, contingent responses involving repetitions of part of an adult's previous utterance (focus/imitation devices) might be encouraged before contingent responses involving the addition of new information (substitution/expansion devices).

Normal developmental data need to be viewed, however, as providing guidelines rather than prescriptions for language intervention. Furthermore, although a developmental approach is probably the more frequently used strategy for planning intervention, there may be occasions when deviations from usual developmental sequences are appropriate. As we saw in Chapter 7, intervention with children with autism may not always follow developmental sequences. Individual characteristics of other children with language disorders, such as a child's cognitive level, level of comprehension for a particular language skill, or response to intervention, may indicate the use of nondevelopmental strategies. In other instances, a child or the child's parents/caregivers or teachers may have immediate communication needs that support the choice of a nondevelopmental approach.

Rules and Regularities

Because some children with language disorders seem to have particular difficulties figuring out the principles, rules, and regularities of language (e.g., semantic maps of super- and subordinate classifications of words, use of verb allomorphs, preposing and transposing patterns for question form, appropriate and inappropriate conversational topics with teachers), one principle of language intervention is that intervention should help children to discover these (Fey, Long, & Finestack, 2003). One objective of intervention, therefore, is to create and/or capitalize on situations and experiences so that the child can discover the regularities. Presenting multiple repetitions of systematically controlled, but varied, exemplars of intervention targets may help facilitate the desired discoveries. Even if the source of a child's problem is not in figuring out the rule and regularities but instead in limitations or difficulties in processing information, the use of multiple and systematically controlled exemplars can be an effective intervention strategy. In this case, the repetitious patterning associated with this intervention approach can reduce the processing demands for these children and therefore reduce the complexity of the task demands for them.

To illustrate, if a goal was to help a child discover the meaning of *more* to express recurrence, one activity might involve a musical Jack-in-the-box controlled by an adult. After an initial presentation of the toy's action, hopefully to the child's delight, the adult allows the child to play with it momentarily, then closes the lid, gives it back to the child for a moment, and finally asks the child, *More? More?* After a slight pause, the adult repeats the sequence. After the whole process is repeated several times, the adult can begin to pause for longer periods of time between saying *more* and opening the box, with the aim that the child will request *more.* Should that happen, the adult immediately opens the box. Although the child may begin to use *more* in this situation, we cannot be sure exactly what the child has discovered about the meaning. It may be that the child has linked the little doll, the action of popping up, or the action of winding the handle with the word. Consequently, other events that highlight the regularities of *more* need to be introduced into intervention. The Jack-in-the-box activity might be followed by a treat, such as juice, during which the child is given sip-sized amounts of juice in a glass. After the child drinks the juice, the adult asks *More?* and more is poured. The intention is that the child will start to use the expression appropriately after the adult begins to pause between asking if the child wants more and supplying it. Additional events clearly illustrating the desired discoveries are also necessary. A pragmatic emphasis is inherent in such an intervention approach. In this example, the inclusion of communicative intents in the form of Halliday's (1975) regulatory function or Dore's (1975) requesting action intention is obvious. The child discovers that the behaviors of others can be regulated and desires can be met through the appropriate use of language.

To discover the rules and regularities, a child will probably need to be helped to use both inductive and deductive processes. *Induction* involves discovering a general rule from observing multiple individual cases; *deduction* is applying a general or known rule to a new or unknown situation. However, different types of intervention objectives (e.g., semantic objectives, morphological or syntactic objectives, pragmatic objectives) may require different approaches in helping children discover the rules and regularities. Connell (1989), for instance, reported that an intervention approach that employed induction facilitated semantic objectives, but an intervention approach that employed deduction facilitated a morphosyntactic target.

Although this principle of assisting children to discover the regularities applies to language intervention for preschoolers, school-aged children, and adolescents alike, it is especially applicable for younger children who have not acquired metalinguistic skills in order to talk about and analyze language. For older children and adolescents with some metalinguistic abilities, explanations of the regularities to be discovered may help them focus on the rules. Incorporating some use of writing or written practice may even assist older children in identifying the regularities and reinforce the interaction between oral and written language (Fey et al., 2003). However, these explanations and analyses complement, not substitute for, actual practice in contextually appropriate situations.

Controlling and/or Reducing Language Complexity

If we are going to focus on rules and regularities, it makes some sense to try to control complexity in such a way that a child can figure out what the rules and regularities are. In the previous discussion, the procedures used to help children discover the rules and regularities of language were also described as potentially helping to reduce the complexity of the task of learning language for them. Given the current thrust in the literature indicating that many children with language impairments may have limited or impaired processing capacities (Ellis Weismer, 1996; Ellis Weismer & Evans, 2002; Gillam, Cowan, & Marler, 1998; Leonard, 1998; Merzenich et al., 1996; Miller, Kail, Leonard, & Tomblin, 2001; Montgomery, 2002b), it seems that important considerations in intervention should be controlling and reducing the complexity of the language demands of a language target we are asking children to acquire, and controlling and reducing the complexity of the stimulation we provide to children to learn the relevant language targets.

With regard to controlling the complexity of the language demands for the child, when intervention focuses on one aspect of language, it is important to control the complexity of the other aspects that are simultaneously included. We do not expect a language-disordered child to use a new word in a multiword utterance containing a new syntactic form to express a new function all at the same time. Even children who are acquiring language normally do not do this. They tend to use simpler, earlier-acquired syntactic structures to encode new ideas or content and to express earlier-acquired content in new syntactic forms (Bloom, Lightbown, & Hood, 1974; Slobin, 1973) and newly acquired intentions and functions in old, well-established linguistic forms to express well-known content. There is substantial evidence that aspects of language interact with each other and that there are trade-offs in what children can do with the demands of language of various language tasks at any point in time (Ellis Weismer & Evans, 2002; Gershkoff-Stowe & Smith, 1997; Lahey & Bloom, 1994; Leonard, 1998; Leonard, Schwartz, Morris, & Chapman, 1981; Masterson, 1997; Namazi & Johnston, 1996; Schwartz & Leonard, 1982; Schwartz, Leonard, Folger, & Wilcox, 1980), depending on the degree of difficulty of the combination of tasks, the robustness of the children's knowledge of the tasks, and/or the facility of their mental operations are at handling the tasks.

In using this information for intervention, we would make an attempt to reduce the complexities seen in usual language-learning situations so that the children's tasks in identifying the rule and regularities for the intervention target and in being able to use the target are simplified. For example, a new morphological or syntactic structure would initially be presented in a situation where the child could use well-established words in highly stabilized, perhaps even routinized, contexts. For semantics, intervention would first involve new words or new semantic relations used in familiar morphosyntactic forms and contexts. For improvement of pragmatic skills, the child would initially be encouraged to apply the new pragmatic skills in situations when the child could use old linguistic forms in familiar interactions. Even controlling the phonological content of words being taught in intervention focusing on semantics may influence how easily the words are acquired. As a child starts to demonstrate acquisition of the new target language behavior, less established aspects of the other language components can be gradually and systematically introduced.

There is evidence indicating that it is also important to control the complexity of the language input or stimuli we provide to the child as we are attempting to assist the child to acquire a particular feature of language. Some of this evidence comes from studies of mothers talking to their normally developing children. Not only do mothers reduce their rates of speech and vary prosodic features of the language, they also reduce the overall complexity of their language by using short, simple utterances. From an intervention perspective, for example, in a program to help toddlers between about 2 and 2½ years of age with slow expressive language development but most with age-appropriate receptive language vocabulary to acquire new lexical targets (words), Girolametto and colleagues (1996) taught the children's mothers to reduce their rate of speech to their children, the length of utterances they used, and their lexical diversity, as well as to increase the frequency with which they modeled lexical targets. The children whose mothers reduced the complexity of their language input made gains not only with the intervention targets but in a variety of other language areas. Similar gains were not evidenced in children whose mothers had not made these changes in their interactions with their children. Such approaches to reducing input complexity may also be effective in highlighting the systematic patterns from which a child is to learn the guiding rules and regularities if the child is having difficulties figuring these out. Instead of adults using long, complex utterances that can hide the elements to be discerned or overload a child's processing facilities, pairing short, simple utterances with appropriate content and context appears to be a logical approach. In addition to controlling the length and morphosyntactic complexity of language models, an adult needs to use words in the utterances that are well within a child's semantic repertoire. If the child does not understand the meaning of an adult's model, it is doubtful the child will discern much of anything from the utterance.

The point is: Complexity matters, and controlling it matters even more (Ellis Weismer & Schraeder, 1993).

Comprehension or Production

Most children with language disorders have problems both using and comprehending language. Therefore, a common issue is whether to focus first on comprehension and then move to production or to start with areas of production that need to be addressed. We need to recall that comprehension does not always precede production (Miller & Paul, 1995). Another important consideration is that the process of working on production, if carried out in meaningful contexts and with as much pragmatically appropriately grounding, is likely to bring along comprehension and knowledge of the language target (Lahey, 1988; Leonard, 1998; Paul, 2001). As Leonard (1998) suggests, "in gaining practice in the production of the target forms, the children are also learning the appropriate contexts in which they are used" (p. 194). It is hard to see how helping children to discern rules and regularities, as discussed above, could be carried out without helping a child to understand. However, having children produce specific forms by rote, without understanding the utterances' meanings or purposes, certainly does not lay the groundwork for generalization to everyday use.

Although it might be defensible to decide to focus on production with the aim of concurrently developing comprehension, there is some evidence suggesting that comprehension work alone is not sufficient to result in production for children with language disorders, even though such an approach might work for normally developing children. Here we can see the relevance of our discussion at the beginning of this chapter about "normal versus not so normal processes." Two studies can be used to illustrate this point. In one of these studies, Dollaghan (1987) investigated normal and language-impaired children's abilities to fast map the meanings of words. She found that both the normal and language-impaired children were equally able to infer word meaning from limited, structured exposures. However, the language-impaired children could not produce the words following limited exposure, whereas the majority of the normal language-learning children could. Connell and Stone's (1992) study focused on morphological acquisition. In their study, normal and language-impaired children were taught several morphemes. The normal and language-disordered children both learned to comprehend the meaning of the morphemes. Unlike the normal children, however, the language-impaired children were able to use the morphemes only if they had previously been asked to produce utterances containing the morphemes. These studies suggest that children with language impairments may need to be given opportunities to produce intervention targets in order for them to be realized in their expressive language. For these children, it seems that training involving comprehension resulted in comprehension of the targets; training involving comprehension alone did not result in production; production practice resulted in using the targets.

We are not sure why this may be so for children with language disorders. It may be that the task of production adds more practice, experience, and/or time with intervention targets generally. It might be a quantity factor. That is, the quantity of work with the targets is greater because the children must do something more than they might if work were limited to comprehension. It could also be a quality factor in that the process of production activates learning or reduces resource demands for the children.

Having suggested that production might actually aid acquisition compared to comprehension work alone, it is also possible the act of production itself might require too many resources for a child. That is, the act of production may be sufficiently taxing for the current abilities of a child so that it is beyond what the child is able to do. This might apply particularly in the early stages of learning a new language skill, and results from dynamic assessment processes might provide us with this information. If this is the case, considerations related to reducing complexity might take precedence and we would chose to focus initially on comprehension and move to production later in intervention.

Comprehension difficulties, however, are major problems for some children and adolescents and, in fact, these may be more debilitating than their expressive language delays.

If school-age children cannot comprehend easily and quickly what their teachers say, they cannot learn, and if they cannot comprehend what their teachers or peers say, they are likely to respond inappropriately and sometimes say or do some very strange things as a result. Even for preschoolers, comprehension problems are seen to affect interpersonal relationships with peers. Gertner, Rice, and Hadley (1994) found that for preschoolers with specific language impairment, their level of receptive vocabulary knowledge predicted their being named or not named as a friend by their preschool peers, and those with lower comprehension vocabulary were less likely to be nominated as friends. From this perspective, intervention must include attention to comprehension abilities.

Focus of Intervention and Picking Intervention Targets

Decisions about whether the language targets or objectives of initial intervention focus on a child's pragmatic, semantic, and/or morphosyntactic skills depend on an individual child's needs as identified through the assessment process. Very young, prelinguistic children may first need to develop intentional and nonverbal communicative interactions and cognitive skills associated with language learning, such as participation in joint action and joint attention routines or symbolic play with accompanying symbolic gestures, or gestural requests for objects. For other children, developing social interactive discourse skills may be most immediate. Discovering morphological or syntactic rules and regularities may be the appropriate focus of intervention for other language-disordered children, whereas developing semantic skills may be most important for still others. Children often need intervention in more than one area and/or need to strengthen their associations among the areas (Fey et al., 2003). Intervention for the specific language patterns presented by a child is individualized for each child.

Results from dynamic assessment procedures can help in decisions about what to target and often in what order (Bain & Olswang, 1995; Olswang & Bain, 1996; Schneider & Watkins, 1996). If the concepts associated with Vygotsky's (1978) zone of proximal development are used, then those skills that fall within this zone for the child, determined as a result of dynamic assessment, will be probable candidates as intervention targets. Skills that might fall in this zone include ones for which the child was stimulable during dynamic assessment, had receptive knowledge of but did not produce, or used only some of the time. However, if a child is using targets correctly in more than half of the opportunities to do so, then those skills might not be as high of a priority for intervention as others that the child uses sometimes but not the majority of the time (Fey, 1986). The logic is that the child is likely to acquire skills in the former category with less intervention, whereas those in the latter category might be within the zone of proximal development and amenable to improvement with adequate intervention. For intervention for grammatical forms, we might be able to select from either those that children use some of the time or do not use at all since, according to the findings of Nelson and colleagues (Nelson, Camarata, Welsh, Butkovsky, & Camarata, 1996), either responds to intervention about equally as well. A caveat, however, might be that a child's receptive knowledge of targets, even if they are not used, could affect the suitability of those as the focus of intervention.

Although it may be appropriate to focus intervention on one aspect of language, this does not preclude attention to the other aspects of language. Intervention plans need to attend to all aspects of language simultaneously, even though one aspect may receive greater emphasis. It also makes little sense in intervention to have a child produce syntactic sequences, for example, that contain words whose meanings are unknown to the child, or to use sentences in which the semantic relations among the words are typically nonsensical (e.g., "The tree is walking."). It is also likely that language targets taught using nonsense forms will not generalize very well (Connell & Stone, 1992; Swisher & Snow, 1994; Swisher, Restrepo, Plante, & Lowell, 1995). Intervention with a syntactic focus also needs to help a child realize the ways in which linguistic forms can be used for communication. Even when intervention has a pragmatic focus, form and content must match the aspects of use being emphasized. Similarly, intervention with a semantic focus must include relationships among meanings of words as expressed in morphological and syntactic forms and use of the word meanings in appropriate contexts. When all aspects of language are kept in mind in planning and executing intervention, a primary focus on one aspect may well facilitate a child's learning of other, secondary aspects concurrently. This is likely to be true, however, only if intervention is not limited solely to "drill work." Instead, intervention needs to encourage a child's use of a specific target in human interactions (Fey et al., 2003).

Although intervention may begin with a greater focus on one aspect of language than others, the focus and targets of intervention may shift several times during a child's continuing intervention program. Ongoing intervention for a child is a fluid process, the focus of which changes to meet the child's changing needs. This means that it is essential to probe regularly and to reassess systematically along the way. And, as the focus of intervention changes for a child, the strategies must also change.

Usefulness of Intervention Content

Language-disordered children must learn to communicate, not just learn the forms and content of language. Almost all individuals working with children with language impairments agree that intervention needs to have as much of a pragmatic focus that demonstrates the usefulness of particular language targets as possible. Among the many helpful principles of intervention that Paul (2001) lists are several that reinforce the importance of making the content of intervention useful. Among these are

- Make the language informative (p. 77).
- Increase the motivation to communication within the task (p. 77).
- Obligate pragmatically appropriate responses (p. 81).

Regardless of what specific language skills are targets of intervention, we want children to learn that with appropriate language they can better control their environments and what happens to them, influence other people, establish and maintain relationships with others, and gain information.

In planning content and forms to stress in intervention, the ways in which children can employ them in their daily environments are always considered (Fey et al., 2003). Teaching children about how to communicate may, in fact, be the primary focus of intervention in some instances. Recall that some language-impaired youngsters seem to be uninterested in communication and communicative interactions. Helping these children to discover that language is useful for a variety of functions and intentions and then teaching them how to employ language to accomplish these purposes can be important intervention objectives in and of themselves.

When it is appropriate to emphasize syntax and morphology in intervention, the usefulness of the forms for the child is an equally important consideration in selecting what grammatical features to teach. This includes the unique and definitive meanings the forms can encode for a child, the efficiency with which certain forms can accomplish communication (e.g., one utterance encoding two ideas, as in a sentence with a relative clause, "I like the boy who plays nicely" rather than two utterances to express the ideas, "I like the boy. He plays nicely."), and the variety of ways the forms can provide for encoding functions and intentions (e.g., direct versus indirect requests).

Reinforcement and Generalization

Reinforcement is a powerful factor in language intervention, and several different types of reinforcement can promote language learning. Some of these are natural consequences of a communicative act. In our earlier example with *more,* using the word *more* can have natural and very reinforcing consequences for children. In intervention we can both capitalize on the natural reinforcing consequences of communicative acts and create opportunities for reinforcing consequences to occur. The more these can be employed in intervention, the more likely it is that children will find what they are doing useful and be inclined to do more of it. Some refer to naturally occurring reinforcers or consequences of communicative events as *intrinsic reinforcement* because these are inherent to the interaction. Another kind of reinforcement occurs outside usual communicative interactions in situations where a child might be given a star, tally mark, stamp, or verbal praise ("Good word," "Nice sentence," "Nice asking"). These are *extrinsic reinforcers,* which can be used as effectively in language intervention as they are in other aspects of children's lives, for example, parents' praise, school, and grades. There are also occasions in language intervention with some children when only extrinsic reinforcers are effective. On a long-term basis, language intervention should probably not depend solely on extrinsic reinforcers. Because they are artificial, it is unlikely that they will retain their reinforcing properties, in contrast to naturally occurring intrinsic reinforcers.

If extrinsic forms of reinforcement are employed in language intervention, there needs to be a consistent move toward eventually replacing them with more natural intrinsic ones. This can be accomplished either by gradually fading the extrinsic reinforcements and introducing the naturalistic reinforcements or by pairing the extrinsic and intrinsic reinforcers so that the naturalistic forms take on the characteristics of the extrinsic reinforcers. Achieving generalization of targets can also be more difficult with extrinsic than intrinsic reinforcers because naturalistic reinforcers tend to facilitate generalization, which is one reason for the general preference for emphasizing intrinsic reinforcer with their natural consequences of communication.

Generalization of language skills learned in intervention to effective use in everyday situations is the major objective in developing language intervention plans. Unfortunately, a lack of generalization is too often a problem. All too often children are observed to use language skills focused on in intervention only in those situations, and not to use the same skills in other contexts. Not surprisingly, the types of reinforcements employed, as just discussed, may be one reason that generalization fails to occur. Another problem that can limit generalization is lack of deep learning of targeted language skills; overlearning is needed for children with language disorders, and without it they may not generalize. Lack of continuity in building language skills systematically across years of intervention and intervention plans that lack social validity are other barriers to generalization. Generalization needs to be considered at all stages of intervention and from the beginning of intervention.

It is possible that children will spontaneously generalize use of specific language skills to other skills that closely resemble the skill emphasized in intervention and to contexts that differ only slightly from the situation used in intervention to teach a language skill. For example, a child who receives intervention targeting the copula *is* may generalize its use to the auxiliary *is* in similar types of sentences, even though the latter skill was not an intervention target. For this to occur, the nontargeted skills may need to share many of the same topographical features, such as phonological and grammatical similarities, as the targeted skill in order for generalization to occur.

Although some limited spontaneous response class generalization and generalization to slightly different contexts may be observed for some language skills, attention needs to be given to several specific aspects of intervention to promote generalization. That is, intervention needs to use:

1. Different stimuli to elicit the targeted language behavior.
2. A variety of contexts in which the targeted language behavior is to be used.
3. Different people with whom the targeted behavior is to be used. These people may include other children, parents, classroom teachers, and other adults.

In effectively employing parents and other adults in an intervention plan, it is likely that these people will need specific training in how best to facilitate generalization. As we have seen previously in this text, parents/caregivers are essential partners in intervention.

Child Characteristics

Most certainly, the individual characteristics of each child influence not only what the focus of intervention may be, but many of the other decisions that are made about intervention (Cleave & Fey, 1997; Cole, 1995; Paul, 2001). For a child with attention difficulties, we may decide that a nondistracting intervention environment may be appropriate. For a child with communicative interactive difficulties without attention problems, we may decide that a group setting, classroom, or preschool setting may be appropriate. The combinations are numerous, but among the child characteristics often considered, beyond the children's profiles for specific language skills, are age, nonverbal intelligence level, and amount of verbal behavior generally, in addition to types of language needs or the focus of intervention (Cole & Dale, 1986; Connell, 1987; Friedman & Friedman, 1980; Yoder, Kaiser, & Alpert, 1991). Clearly, these are not discrete child characteristics but can instead be expected to interact. For example, older children can be expected to have greater language functioning, and therefore intervention might need to focus on morphosyntactic structures. Similarly, more cognitively advanced children can be expected to have greater language functioning. Unfortunately, we have only limited empirically derived information to provide guidelines for matching specific child characteristics with intervention approaches and/or strategies, and for the present, we do not know exactly how level of functioning, type of intervention objective, and intervention approach may interact (Leonard, 1998). We do know, however, that we need to consider such interactions in making decisions about intervention for individual children.

Another child characteristic to be considered in intervention relates to the child's interests, which affect the activities to be employed. Activities need to reflect the child's interests and cognitive level. When a child is presented with alternative toys and situations, it may be possible for the adult to follow the child's lead in what is interesting and stimulating for the child at the moment and create logical opportunities for use of a targeted language skill in that context (Cole, 1995). In what has become a classic example of taking advantage of children's interests, Holland (1975) wrote:

> I observed a therapy session in which a gifted clinician was teaching "more." She had prepared for the session by amassing quantities of similar small items to use in conjunction with her own utterance "more _____" and had plans eventually to demand the word from the child. However, the child, hyperactive and of limited verbal skills, became fascinated by a box of Kleenex in the room. The clinician began pulling tissues from the box, accompanying each pull with her utterance "more Kleenex." Eventually, when clinician and child had scattered tissues around the room the clinician introduced the utterance "more throw," accompanied by the two of them creating a snowfall of tissues. In this manner the child learned "more." (pp. 517–518)

Unfortunately, some language-disordered children demonstrate so little interest in their environments that an approach focusing on child-centered activities is useless, at least in early stages of intervention. For these children, the adult may need to create the interesting situations artificially through structured reinforcement schedules, parallel and intersecting play activities, and/or careful control of stimuli presentations. In other instances, specific targeted language behaviors, such as some morphosyntactic structures, may necessitate more adult-centered activities. The point is that both child-centered and adult-centered activities can be appropriate, depending on the individual child's status and the language behavior to be emphasized. Successful language intervention depends, in part, on the ability to determine which approach is appropriate under particular circumstances and a willingness to employ each as the situations demand.

Metalinguistics

We have seen that toddlers and preschoolers possess only rudimentary metalinguistic skills and that the beginning of relatively sophisticated metalinguistic skills emerges in the early school years. Therefore, for young children it is inappropriate to base intervention strategies solely on metalinguistic skills. That is, we do not teach a word's meaning, a discourse rule, or a morphosyntactic structure only by explaining the meaning or the rule to a toddler or preschooler. Rather, we teach by example. This does not mean, however, that we must avoid referring to a regularity. In fact, such reference may actually help a young child focus on the regularity and promote development of metalinguistic skills, as well as provide direct instruction about a language feature. Such reference is not unusual in parent–preschooler interactions, although it may not correspond to parent–toddler interactions. Parents of normal preschoolers often comment to their children that certain words have specific meanings, some things can be said to some people and not others, and some ways of saying a sentence are right and others are wrong (Demetras, Post, & Snow, 1986; Yont, 1998; Yont et al., 2000). What the developmental information about toddlers' and preschoolers' metalinguistic skills does imply is that intervention strategies that depend only on metalinguistic skills are not appropriate. In contrast, intervention for school-aged children and adolescents may not only include metalinguistics as an intervention strategy but may actually focus on improving metalinguistic abilities as intervention objectives themselves.

Highlighting Intervention Targets

For whatever reasons, language-disordered children have not learned and do not learn language incidentally in the same ways as normal children. When a specific language feature is chosen as a target for intervention, it may be necessary to highlight the regularities of the feature in order for a language-disordered child to discover the general rule from exposure to particular instances and/or keep the feature in the child's immediate environment long enough for the child to process and/or retain it. Lahey (1988) has referred to this approach as enhancing the salience of the language patterns, a principle of intervention also emphasized by Fey and his colleagues (2003). There are several techniques that can be employed to increase the salience of language features. Earlier we indicated that some use of techniques involving metalinguistic skills might help to emphasize the critical features for a child. Other techniques discussed here are multiple exposures to the language feature targeted, suprasegmental and rate variations, and input modality variations.

Multiple Exposures

Paul (2001) cleverly used the adage, "If I've said it once, I've said it a hundred times" (p. 80), to make the point about the need for children with language disorders to be exposed to multiple exemplars of whatever the language target is. More is better; redundancy is essential. In reviewing the research on the efficacy of treatment for children with specific language impairment, Leonard (1998) concluded that "the most successful approaches were those that encouraged production and provided *multiple* [emphasis added] yet natural cues for the desired response" (p. 203).

Research related to one intervention technique that we will discuss later in this chapter (i.e., recasting in which an adult's response after a child's utterance is referentially contingent with the child's but adds or modifies one or more language elements to what the child said) illustrates the point about frequency of exposure. The combination of findings from several studies and the literature that have looked at the use of this particular technique (Baker & Nelson, 1984; Camarata & Nelson, 1992; Camarata, Nelson, & Camarata, 1994; Farrar, 1990; Fey & Proctor-Williams, 2000; Fey et al., 1993; Fey et al., 1997; Fey et al., 1999; Nelson, Carskaddon, & Bonvillian, 1973; Nelson, Camarata, Welsh, Butkovsky, & Camarata, 1996; Proctor-Williams et al., 2001) led Proctor-Williams and colleagues (2001) to write that "for children with SLI . . . increased exposure to recasts may indeed be necessary for language development to proceed at rates that approach those of their typically developing peers" and that "unless rates of target-specific recasts approach .8 per minute, the rate used in the experiment of Camarata et al. (1994), it may be unreasonable to expect success" (p. 166) in intervention. This is basically one recast per minute during adult–child interactions. With training aimed at parents of preschool children with language impairment, researchers have shown that they can increase the frequency of parental recasts to rates up around two per minute (Fey et al., 1993, 1997, 1999). This compares to other research that has suggested that estimates of the average number of parents' recasts in their interactions with their young, typically developing children range from 0.06 to about 1 per minute (Conti-Ramsden, 1990; Conti-Ramsden et al., 1995; Farrar, 1990; Fey et al., 1999). In summarizing, Fey and Proctor-Williams (2000) write that, if intervention for young children with language impairments is to have a significant impact, then

> . . . it appears not to be enough just to recast the children's utterances at rates found in their environment. Instead, successful intervention efforts involving recasts have increased the rates by approximately 2–4 times those observed in naturalistic contexts. (p. 180)

This line of reasoning is consistent with the finding of Gray (2003b) in her research on word learning of preschoolers with specific language impairment. These children needed twice the number of exposures than children with normal language to learn the meaning of new words and double the number of opportunities to use new words before using them independently.

Clearly, for language-disordered children, controlling their exposure to exemplars of the desired language targets and increasing the frequency of the children's exposures to these are ways to enhance salience. The technique of multiple exposures can be used for any aspect of language targeted for intervention in order to assist a child to discover the appropriate rules or retain and process the information from the exemplars. To illustrate, in targeting the early developing regulatory function, a game similar to "Simon Says" can be employed. The adult can first direct the activities of the child via utterances such as "You hop," "You jump," or "Hop, jump." After multiple examples, the child becomes the director and orders the adult, who obeys readily. A subsequent activity can employ dolls, one for the child and one for the adult. During play, the adult repeatedly tells the doll to perform acts, such as "Go to bed," and follows each command with the consequent action, such as putting the doll in a cradle. After multiple sequences, the adult can cue the child by asking "What do you want your doll to do? Tell him" or "Tell my doll what to do."

Gentle sabotage can be an effective intervention technique. When things do not go just according to plan, the most efficient and effective way of correcting the situation is with language. A caution is warranted, however. Although gentle sabotage may work, sabotage that creates frustration in the child will not work and is unfair to the child. Gently sabotaging a child's play with cars and trucks by moving another vehicle to block the movement of the child's can help the child realize that his or her verbalizations can regulate the adult's behavior. The adult can say "Move" or "Don't" and then move the vehicle. Desirable toys can be placed in sight but out of reach of the child. The adult can even talk about the seen but unreachable toys. If the child points to one of them, a gestural regulatory behavior, the adult can reach for a toy, pause, cue the child with "Get toy?" and pause again to wait momentarily for the child's order. In a 30-minute period with activities such as these, it may be possible to generate 60 to 100 examples of the regulatory function paired with linguistically appropriate structures and corresponding content, or a rate of 2 to 3 exposures per minute.

The examples given at the beginning of this chapter to illustrate discovery of the meaning of *more* can also be used to demonstrate the technique of multiple exposures in semantically focused intervention. In a morphological or syntactic focus to intervention, such as one targeting the copula *is* to form interrogatives, multiple exposures to the target can be accomplished during guessing games ("Is it a dog?" "Is it red?"). For example, the adult and child can take turns hiding objects in a box. After each object is hidden, the adult can engage in a sequence, such as asking "Is it blue?" looking in the box, saying "No," asking "Is it red?" looking again, saying "No," asking "Is it green?" looking again, saying "Yes," and finally removing the green object. (This activity assumes, of course, that the child knows colors!)

Another way to increase children's exposures to language targets is to increase the number of intervention opportunities or sessions they receive. However, very little is known about what is the optimal number of sessions children with language impairments need to receive in order to facilitate the greatest amount of progress in the least amount of time. One study does, however, provide us with some preliminary guidance. Jacoby and his colleagues (2002) found that the more intervention sessions young children received, the greater their progress was. Of particular interest was the finding that, for about 75% of the children, 20 hours of intervention was needed for them to improve at least one functional communication level and no children improved more than two levels with fewer than 20 hours. These findings suggest a relationship between amount of intervention and amount of progress; we suspect that the greater the amount of intervention, the more exposure children have to language targets.

The point is: More matters.

Suprasegmental and Rate Variations

Lahey (1988) and others (Hargrove, 1997; McGregor, 1997a) have suggested that suprasegmental or prosodic features, such as stress, and modifying rate of input to a child can influence children's language learning. Varying these may increase the salience of a selected language target. Some of these suggestions have been based on observations of mothers' talk to their normally developing children, in which they have been found to speak more slowly and increase the number of words that receive primary stress in their utterances (Berko-Gleason & Weintraub, 1978; Broen, 1972).

Some of the suggestions about the possible effectiveness of rate and suprasegmental variations have been demonstrated in recent research. For example, the findings from the work of Ellis Weismer and her colleagues (Ellis Weismer, 1997; Ellis Weismer & Hesketh, 1993, 1996, 1998; Ellis Weismer & Schraeder, 1993) have suggested that several different prosodic modifications in an adult's language during intervention, such as increased vocal stress on language targets and slower speech rate in presenting language targets, have positive effects in facilitating the language learning of children with language impairments for lexical and possibly grammatical targets. Ellis Weismer and Schraeder (1993) also found that increased wait time between requests to a child and the child's response facilitated children's narrative production. This finding with regard to wait time improving narrative performance is consistent with that of Hughes (1998), which we presented in the previous chapter on assessment as an example of a dynamic assessment approach for evaluating narrative production. Wait time was also suggested as an intervention strategy for adolescents in Chapter 5. Although Evans and her colleagues (1997) did not find that a response latency (pause) before formulating their response in their turn during conversation predicted the length of the response used by school-age children with specific language impairment, the children's use of a verbal filler (e.g., *um, uh*) before their responses, which was another way of "buying" response formulation time, did predict their use of longer responses. Recall also that earlier in this chapter we reported that Girolametto and colleagues (1996) found that when mothers reduced their rate of speech to their toddlers with language delay, along with making other changes in their language-stimulation techniques, the toddlers made more progress than toddlers whose mothers did not make this and other changes in their language input. An important aspect of the work of Ellis Weismer and her coauthors (Ellis Weismer, 1997; Ellis Weismer & Hesketh, 1993, 1996, 1998; Ellis Weismer & Schraeder, 1993) is that the suprasegmental and rate variations investigated tended to be more effective in improving children's language performances when the language tasks were more challenging or difficult for them, that is, when the tasks were more taxing on the children's language abilities and resources and/or increased the language processing demands for the children. Often, this was in tasks where the children were asked to use the targets rather than simply indicating their comprehension of them. Again, we see level of complexity implicated as an aspect to consider in language intervention.

We could use the target of interrogative reversal and answer sequences to illustrate how stress might be used in intervention to increase salience of the target. For example, an adult could stress the *is* in the syntactic sequence ("*Is* it blue? Yes it *is*"; "*Is* it red? Yes it *is*"; "*Is* it green? Yes it *is*") both to highlight its presence and contrast its location. A finding from one study (Swanson & Leonard, 1994) about the duration of what is a frequent target of intervention for young children, the uncontracted copula *is,* could also be helpful in manipulating duration, and therefore stress and saliency, to assist children's language learning. In this study, when the verb was in the final position of sentences, its length in mothers' speech to young children was 250 milliseconds (ms), compared to the much shorter duration of 60 ms for the verb when the mothers used it in sentence initial positions, as in "*Is* it blue?" or in the middle of sentences, as in "The baby *is* big." Some morphological markers, such as possessive, plural, and third-person singular present-tense verb inflections that we know have both low semantic and perceptual salience, lend themselves to being prolonged as well as stressed.

It may also be important to control stress in another way to increase effectiveness of intervention. We know that many of the language features that are especially challenging for children often occur in relatively unstressed contexts, such as the *is* in "*Jim*my is *eat*ing," in which italics indicate the two stressed syllables that make up the five-syllable utterance. Yet, for children learning English, there seems to be a bias for better production when weak syllables come after stressed ones (Gerken, 1994; Gerken & McGregor, 1998; McGregor, 1997a). Because, as McGregor (1997a) suggests, "manipulation of prosodic-phonological contexts should aid grammatical morpheme acquisition" (p. 63), initially we might ask children to produce a particular language target in unstressed contexts where it follows a stressed syllable, such as the *is* in "*Jim* is *eat*ing" rather than "*Jim*my is *eat*ing" (Bedore & Leonard, 1995; Gerken & McGregor, 1998). However, children need to maintain their use of the targets in other contexts. This means that there may be a logical way to build in extension and generalization by manipulating the stress patterns of required utterances so that the children are gradually asked to use the targets in the less facilitating and supportive stress patterns, such as when the targets follow an unstressed syllable, as in "*Kat*ie is *run*ning" and "The *ba*by is *cry*ing."

Input Modality Variations

In Chapter 5 we suggested that, for adolescents with language disorders, use of intransient and stable visual or graphic stimuli in intervention could reduce the information-processing demands of language-learning tasks by keeping information needed to complete the tasks in the immediate environment while processing could take place. We have also seen elsewhere in this text (e.g., Chapter 1 describing aspects of normal communication process, Chapter 12 on AAC) that communication is, in fact, multimodal. These ideas can be applied to language intervention for younger children. Some children can benefit from intervention that employs input modalities in addition to the auditory modality. For example, adults' use of gestures paired with specific linguistic forms has been shown to increase language-impaired school-children's comprehension of novel words (Ellis Weismer & Hesketh, 1993).

The words *here, there,* and *give* provide excellent examples of how meaning can be enhanced by the combined use of the words and supporting gestures. Gestures can highlight a number of pragmatic intents and functions, such as reaching for desired objects as "I want the _____" or "Want _____" is said. Gestures can also reinforce turn-taking skills. In intervention designed to pair "all gone," "no, no _____," or "gone" with the object relations of disappearance and nonexistence, an adult can raise his or her hands in the classic "I don't know"/"Where is it?" gesture, adopt a puzzled facial expression, and move his or her head in a searching manner as the appropriate linguistic forms are modeled. Recall that children will often follow an adult's eye gaze. Negative headshakes can also highlight negative markers in targets such as "The dog is *not* big."

Graphically displayed symbols have also been used occasionally to enhance the salience of a specific target. The symbols are typically presented in conjunction with auditory input and then gradually faded as a child begins to demonstrate awareness of the target. The Fokes Sentence Builder (Fokes, 1976, 1977) is an example of such a method. However, such an approach is probably most appropriately used with older language-disordered children and for morphosyntactic intervention goals, ensuring that sentences that are created are semantically plausible.

Procedures and Techniques to Facilitate Learning of Language Targets

In reading about the following procedures and techniques, it is important to keep in mind that the previous discussion of ways to highlight language targets can be used with these facilitating techniques. On a continuum, illustrated in Figure 14.1, these techniques can range from those that are quite indirect and "natural" (i.e., used by parents naturally with their normally developing children), unintrusive (not interfering with or interrupting the flow of a normal adult–child interaction), and quite child centered, to those that are more didactic and directive, intrusive on the flow of adult–child interactions, and adult centered. Some of the techniques have evolved from observations of mothers' verbal behaviors that seem to promote language learning in their normally developing children; others come from behavioral orientations and related learning theories.

These techniques can be divided into those that are used before a child's response, in order to set up or stimulate the occurrence of the response, and those that occur after a child's utterance, in order to modify or encourage the child toward the desired target for the next time the child has an opportunity to use it. The following sections divide the techniques into those that are *a priori* and those that are *post hoc* to a child's utterance.

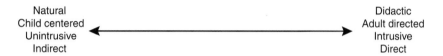

FIGURE 14.1 Continuum Representing Degrees of Naturalness and Directiveness of Procedures and Techniques to Facilitate Children's Learning of Language Targets

There is no preferential or hierarchical order in the presentation of the techniques. More often than not, intervention utilizes combinations of the techniques, and in some instances, various labels have been used in the literature to refer to what are essentially the same or similar techniques. Examples of each technique are given below. However, because the examples are designed to illustrate a specific technique, they may appear more stilted and exaggerated here than their uses would be in true language intervention situations.

Before the Child's Utterance

Self-Talk and Parallel Talk.   In using self-talk, an adult talks aloud about objects in the immediate environment and about actions that are occurring at the moment. It is important that the topics for the talk be in context at the moment, to parallel the situations in which children typically first begin to talk. The language the adult uses needs to correspond closely to the child's language level in terms of both grammatical and semantic complexity. In other words, the adult's vocabulary and linguistic structures should neither greatly exceed the child's language capacity nor be at a level too simplistic for the child.

Self-talk can emphasize very specific aspects of language that a child needs to acquire, or it can be used as a more general language-stimulation approach. The idea is for the child to hear the target language behaviors frequently. However, the purpose of self-talk is not to have the child repeat the targets. Therefore, the child is not overtly directed to talk. The following three examples illustrate how self-talk might be utilized during interactions with a child. In the first two examples, a specific language target is emphasized. The targets are repeated many times although in slightly different ways. The last example represents a more general self-talk activity. The language level in the last example is aimed at using two- and occasional three-word combinations.

Example 1
TARGET: *am + verb + ing*

SITUATION: Adult and child are looking at a book.
Oh, I am looking at the book. . . . I am opening the book . . . am opening the book. . . .
I am looking at the picture. . . . I am pointing to the dog. . . . I am turning the page. . . .
Oh, there is a new picture. . . . I am pointing to the ball. . . . I am looking at the cat. . . .
I am pointing to the cat. . . . I am closing the book now. . . . Now, I am putting the
book away . . . am putting the book away. . . . I am putting the book away.

Example 2

TARGET: The color "red"

SITUATION: Adult and child are playing with toys of various colors, many of which are red.

I see the red car. . . . I have the red car . . . the red car. . . . My car is red . . . red. . . . Oh, here is a red ball. . . . The red ball. . . . My ball is red. . . . Like the apple. . . . The apple is red, too. . . . I want the red apple. . . . Oh, here is a red block. . . . I'll put my red block with my red apple . . . and my red car. . . . These are all red. . . . Red toys. . . . The toys are red.

Example 3

TARGET: Two- and three-word combinations

SITUATION: Adult and child are cleaning up a room.

Clean the room. . . . Put toys away. . . . Put the toys away. . . . The ball's away. . . . Find the book. . . . Where's the book? . . . Where's the book? . . . Oh . . . the book's over there. . . . There's the book. . . . Put the book away. . . . Now, where's the glue? . . . Put the glue away. . . . There, the glue's away. . . . All gone. . . . What now? . . . I see the paper. . . . I'll get the paper. . . . The paper's put away. . . . Where's the block? . . . Oh . . . I see blocks. . . . Blocks on the table. . . . On the table. . . . There's the block. . . . Blocks on the table. . . . Get the blocks. . . . Put the blocks away.

In contrast to self-talk, in which adults describe what they are doing, parallel talk emphasizes what the child is doing or what is about to happen to the child or in the child's environment. Again, the purpose is not to have the child repeat the utterances used by the adults but to put the language, at the appropriate complexity level, in the child's auditory environment as the child is acting on the environment. Like self-talk, parallel talk activities can be used to emphasize specific language skills or to encourage language learning more generally. The following two examples illustrate parallel talk.

Example 1

TARGET: Use of elliptical responses to maintain conversation

SITUATION: Adult and child are playing with dolls, a dollhouse, and its furnishings.

Who has the chair? . . . Oh, she does. . . . Here it is. . . . Where is the table? . . . Oh yes, over there. . . . You get it. . . . Who wants it? . . . You do? . . . Me, too. . . . We'll both get it. . . . Where was it? . . . Oh, over there. (In this example, we also see the adult using deictic terms—*here* and *there*—and presuppositions in the form of the pronoun *it*.)

Example 2

TARGET: Three- and four-word phrases

SITUATION: Child is putting an animal puzzle together.

What do you have? . . . You have a horse. . . . Putting the horse there. . . . Putting the horse there. . . . Good, the horse goes there. . . . What goes there? . . . Oh, you have a dog. . . . A little dog. . . . Oh, oh, the dog fell down. . . . Picking up the dog. . . .

Putting the dog in. . . . The dog is in. . . . Looking for the duck. . . . Where's the duck? . . . Can't find the duck. . . . Oh, there's the duck. . . . Putting the duck in. . . . All done now. . . . The puzzle is done. . . . All done now. . . . The puzzle is done.

Self-talk and parallel talk can be used together during adult–child intersecting and cooperative interactions. The next example incorporates both language facilitation techniques.

Example

TARGET: Performative intents encoded with "going to"

SITUATION: Adult and child are playing with various toys.
Oh, I'm going to get the toy. . . . You're going to get the car. . . . Going to get the car. . . . You're going to get the car. . . . You're going to go. . . . I'm going to color. . . . You're going to color. . . . You're coloring. . . . I'm going to cut. . . . You're going to cut. . . . You are going to fall. . . . Oops, you fell. . . . You are going to get up.

Imitation, Modeling, and Priming.   A number of terms have been used to refer to imitation and modeling. As a result, some confusion as to their meanings has arisen. For our purposes, *imitation* and *mimicry* can be used synonymously. These terms refer to responses that are basically similar, if not identical, to a previously presented stimulus and that occur temporally in close proximity to the stimulus. The use of mimicry or imitation implies a "one-to-one process of literal matching" (Courtright & Courtright, 1976, p. 655). An interchange, such as the following one, involves imitation on a child's part:

ADULT: Look at what the girl is doing now. Tell me, "The girl is running."

CHILD: Girl is running.

Imitation may prove to be a valuable facilitating technique (Camarata & Nelson, 1992; Courtright & Courtright, 1976; Fey & Proctor-Williams, 2000; Hegde, 1980; Hegde, Noll, & Pecora, 1979), particularly in the early stages of language intervention for a specific targeted language behavior. Dependence on imitation, however, is reduced as a child becomes more able to use the targets (Fey & Proctor-Williams, 2000; Leonard, 1981). From this perspective, imitation can be seen as a facilitating technique that may be helpful to start a child's acquisition of a language target but not a technique that is continued once the path to acquisition in under way. Some have also objected to imitation because it violates normal language-learning interactions. Although this may be true, the counterargument is that children with language impairments have not been successful in learning language via normal child–adult interaction. It is also possible to create situations where imitation can be used in reasonably pragmatically appropriate interchanges and interactions.

In contrast to imitation, *modeling* is a technique in which an adult (or sometimes other children) provides several examples of slightly different utterances, each of which contains the same critical language feature to be acquired by a child. This is one of the several techniques commonly included in an approach to intervention that is often referred to as *focused stimulation.* The expected response to these models may not match the models exactly, but the aim is that it will contain the common critical element(s) in the models. The following interchange represents a modeling approach:

> ADULT: This dog is big. That cat is big. The elephant is big. That lion is big. Oh look, a pig.
>
> CHILD: Pig is big.

Many exemplars are provided for a child before a situation is created to which a child might respond. There is no hard-and-fast rule about how many exemplars should be provided before moving on, but some suggest ten to twenty (Fey & Proctor-Williams, 2000). In some uses of modeling, there is no direct request or command (or a mand) for the child to respond, although it is certainly hoped that the child will. In other uses of modeling, an evoked response may be part of the technique. That is, the child is directed to respond, as in the example below, which is a modification of the example above.

> ADULT: This dog is big. That cat is big. The elephant is big. That lion is big. Tell me about this pig.
>
> CHILD: Pig is big.

We can see from the child's response in both of these examples that common elements of the adult's utterances have been included to produce a similar but not exact response. Often, at least one other person (adult or child) may be included in intervention when a modeling approach is used. The third person models the target behaviors in response to the adult's stimuli. Positive reinforcements may be provided for the third person's appropriate responses, as the child observes both the responses and the reinforcements. Such an approach is consistent with social learning theory (Bandura, 1971, 1977). If we examine the examples for self-talk and parallel talk, we can see how much modeling of target language behaviors occurs. The following examples illustrate how modeling can be used. In light of our previous discussion about increasing the saliency of the target, the models of the target language behavior may receive a little extra stress as the examples are modeled and/or be presented at a slightly slower rate.

Example 1

TARGET: *a* + noun

SITUATION: Adult and child are looking at picture cards.

> ADULT: Oh look, *a* dog! This is *a* dog. Look, *a* dog. This is *a* cat. This is *a* cat. This is *a* cat. *A* ball. Here is *a* ball. Oh, *a* top! *A* top. This is *a* top. This is *a* cup. Oh, *a* new picture. What is this?
>
> CHILD: A coat.

Example 2

TARGET: Meaning and use of *in*

SITUATION: Adult and child are playing with a number of small toys and a paper bag, a box, and an old purse.

ADULT: Here's a block. Let's put the block *in* the purse. Look *in* the purse. Put the block *in* the purse. Where's the block?—Oh, look *in* the purse (Both adult and child look.) *In* the purse. Look, here's a ball. We'll put the ball *in* the bag. Look *in* the bag. The ball's *in* the bag. Where's the ball?—Look *in* the bag. *In* the bag. Now, let's put the car *in* the box. Good, you put it *in* the box. *In* the box. Here's a spoon. Here it goes. *In* the box. Where's the spoon?—See, *in* the box. Oh, here's a horse. I'll put the horse *in* the box. Where's the horse?

CHILD: In box.

Basing their work on that of Bock and her co-workers (Bock & Loebell, 1990; Bock, Loebell, & Morey, 1992), Leonard and his colleagues (Leonard et al., 2000, 2002) have begun to examine the role of structural *priming* in increasing the likelihood that the sentences of children with language impairment will include particular language features if their previous utterance contained the same features. The scenarios to elicit responses from the children in this research required the children first to imitate a sentence containing a specific target (e.g., uncontractible auxiliary *is* in present progressive sentences such as "The mouse is eating the cheese") in response to a picture and then to provide a spontaneous (nonimitated) response to a new picture that also required the same structure, although a plural subject could be depicted (e.g., uncontractible auxiliary *are* in present progressive sentences such as "The dogs are chasing the ball"). Results have confirmed the tendency of children to be more accurate in using the target forms under the priming condition as opposed to situations where they first produced a sentence with a different target structure, such as a past-tense verb. This trend with regard to different target structures held even when the first priming sentence contained a phonologically identical but grammatically different verb (such as *is* as a copula in "The dog is fat") for a target nonimitated sentence with the uncontractible auxiliary *is* as in present progressive sentences ("The mouse is eating the cheese"), suggesting the superiority of the syntactic form over the phonological form in priming.

Although these investigations were not designed as intervention studies, to the extent that these findings are replicated over time in further research, there may be implications for facilitating language learning in children with language impairments. That is, manipulating situations in which children are first required to imitate a targeted structure and then to provide an immediately subsequent nonimitated, novel response with the same essential grammatical constituents might be an effective intervention approach. Suprasegmental variations could be used in presenting the target to be imitated in order to increase its saliency. Research is needed, however, to confirm or reject the effectiveness of priming as an intervention technique. The example below illustrates how a dialogue between an adult and child might incorporate priming.

Example
TARGET: *are* + verb + *ing*

SITUATION: Adult and child are looking at pictures.

ADULT: Look at this picture. Tell me what is happening. Tell me, The boys *are chasing* the ball.

CHILD: Boys are chasing the ball.

> ADULT: Now tell me about the horse.
>
> CHILD: Horse is jumping the fence.
>
> ADULT: Tell what is happening here. Tell me. The mouse *is eating* the cheese.
>
> CHILD: Mouse is eating cheese.
>
> ADULT: Tell about the cats.
>
> CHILD: Cats are catching the bug.

After the Child's Utterance

Reauditorization.   Reauditorization is a language-stimulation technique in which an adult repeats what a child has said. In contrast to the previous language-facilitating techniques, which are employed before a child responds, reauditorization occurs in response to the child's statements. The concept behind this approach is to keep the auditory models of target language behaviors in a child's auditory environment. This language-facilitating technique is rarely used by itself. Instead, it is typically combined with other techniques, such as modeling. Following is an example of reauditorization combined with modeling using an evoked-response technique. In this example, positive verbal reinforcement is also incorporated with the language-stimulation techniques.

> ### Example
> *TARGET:*   *are* + verb + *ing*
>
> *SITUATION:*   Adult and child are on a playground.
>
> ADULT: You *are swinging.* We *are swinging.* I like it. Oh, now you *are running.* You *are running.* We *are running.* We *are jumping* now. You *are jumping.* We *are jumping.* Now, you *are hopping.* Me, too. What are we doing?
>
> CHILD: We are hopping.
>
> ADULT: We *are hopping* (reauditorization). Good. We *are hopping* up and down. You *are hopping.* We *are hopping* (reauditorization).

Recasting.   In the above example, recasts occurred in the adult's two utterances following the positive verbal reinforcement, *Good,* and before the second reauditorization. As we indicated earlier, recasting is a facilitating technique in which an adult's response after a child's utterance maintains the topic, content, and reference of the child's utterance (i.e., is referentially contingent) but in some way adds or modifies one or more language elements to what the child said. This technique has also been known in the literature as *expansion* or sometimes *expatiation.* (The differences between techniques are not always obvious.) The adult models for the child a slightly more complex or linguistically appropriate way of saying what the child has said and/or extends what the child has said to a slightly different context with slightly different content by adding information. What the adult chooses to include in the recast is typically the target of intervention for the child. The overall complexity of the recast, however, cannot be so difficult that the aspects of language that are the targets of intervention get lost in the adult's response. Recasting is often used with other language-stimulation techniques, such as imitation, modeling, and reauditorization. The following three examples show various combinations of recasting, modeling, reauditorization, as well as positive verbal reinforcement.

Example 1

TARGET: Attributive *big* + noun

SITUATION: Adult and child are putting toys away.

ADULT: We need to clean up. We need to put our toys away. Clean up now. Put the *big ball* away. No, not the little ball—the *big ball*. The *big ball*. I'll take the little ball. Good, you put the *big ball* away. Now, you have the *big truck*. I'll take the little truck. You put the *big truck* away. Good. Now, what do you have?

CHILD: Big car.

ADULT: *Big car* (reauditorization). That's right. You have the *big car* (recast). The *big car* (recast). I want the *big car* (recast). *Big car* (reauditorization). The *big car* (recast). Now, I'll take the *big boat* (model). Here's the *big boat* (model). You take the *big boat* (model). Put the *big boat* away (model). Good. What do you have now?

Example 2

TARGET: Regular past-tense verbs

SITUATION: Child and adult are looking at a storybook of "Jack and the Beanstalk."

CHILD: He climb up.

ADULT: He *climbed* up (recast). Jack *climbed* up the tree (recast). He *looked* around (model). He *looked* for a house (model). Jack *called* for help (model). He *called* and he *called* (model). He *yelled* and he *yelled* (model). He *wanted* to go home (model). He *climbed* down the beanstalk (model). What did he do? (mand)

CHILD: He climbed down.

ADULT: He *climbed* down (reauditorization). Yes, he *climbed* down the beanstalk (recast).

Example 3

TARGET: *will* + verb

SITUATION: Adult and child are decorating a bulletin board for Valentine's Day.

ADULT: I *will put* a heart here (model). I *will put* it here (model). I *will pin* it here (model). Where will you put your heart? (Notice the adult's question contains a varied form of the target and is also phrased so that the child's response could include the target.)

CHILD: I put it here.

ADULT: You *will put* it here? (recast) You *will pin* it here? (recast) That *will be* a good place. I *will glue* my arrow there, too (model). I *will glue* it on (model). Where will you glue yours?

CHILD: Will glue there.

ADULT: *Will glue* there (reauditorization). Good, that's right. You *will glue* it. (recast). You *will glue* your arrow there (recast). I *will get* the glue and I *will get* the other arrow (model and recast). And, I *will get* another arrow (model). Now, we *will glue* our arrows (model). What will we do?

CHILD: We *will glue* arrows.

ADULT: We *will glue* arrows (reauditorization). Good. You *will glue* your arrow and I *will glue* mine (recast).

Response Dialogues

When a child's specific language response is inadequate in terms of a target response, engaging the child in systematic types of interchanges may help elicit a response that more closely approximates the target. Lee and colleagues (1975) have proposed seven different interchange techniques: complete model, reduced model, expansion request, repetition request, repetition of error, self-correction request, and rephrased question. These interchanges, or response dialogues, were originally developed as part of the Interactive Language Development Teaching (ILDT) (Lee et al., 1975) strategy. This language-teaching strategy is built around stories, usually with accompanying pictures, with different stories facilitating various aspects of language. These response dialogues are not completely unrelated to some of what we saw in Leonard's (Leonard et al., 2000, 2002) work on priming effects, in that the stories set up the grammatical structure for the child and then systematically respond to the child's attempt in such a way to try to prime the child to use a correct structure in the next attempt. Fey and Proctor-Williams (2000) cite ILDT as one example of the way some of the less "natural" facilitating techniques such as imitation and modeling might be made more pragmatically appropriate for children.

In this approach, which is often used with a small group of children, the professional presents a small portion of a story and, using specific targeted language features, questions the children about the story. Additional portions of the story are then presented and dialogue routines completed. Each question is designed to elicit a specific structure. In reviewing the ILDT, Leonard (1998) wrote that the stories not only focused on "particular grammatical forms but also served as a means of teaching new lexical items, narrative cohesion, and other grammatical forms" (p. 206).

Some children need more assistance than others to modify initially inadequate responses in the direction of more complete responses. Therefore, these different interchange techniques are designed to provide varying amounts of help. Some give children considerable assistance in modifying initial responses; others offer very little help. These interchange techniques are described below. They are presented in decreasing order of assistance given to children in approximating target responses.

Complete Model.   In light of our previous discussion of modeling as a facilitating technique, this use of the term *model* is a misnomer. As used to describe this interchange technique, it requests an imitative or mimicked response from the child. After an inadequate response from the child, an adult provides an example of the exact target utterance that the child is expected to duplicate. Following is an example of this interchange technique.

Example
TARGET: Past-tense verbs formed by adding the allomorph /t/ *(kicked)*

ADULT: Yesterday, we read a story about a rabbit. What did the rabbit do in the story?
CHILD: He hop into a basket.
ADULT: *He hopped into a basket.*
CHILD: He hopped into a basket.
ADULT: Good. What else did the rabbit do?
CHILD: The rabbit kick the fence.
ADULT: *The rabbit kicked the fence.*
CHILD: The rabbit kicked the fence.
ADULT: Good. What else did the rabbit do?

Reduced Model. In a reduced model, the elements of a target utterance that have been omitted are included in an adult's response. The partial model cues a child as to the exact element(s) that need special focus in a reformulation. As Lee and her colleagues (1975) explain, a partial model is "not imitation but rather reformulation of an utterance" (p. 18). The following example illustrates an interchange using reduced, or partial, models.

Example
TARGET: Noun + *is* + verb + *ing*
ADULT: What is the boy doing?
CHILD: Boy jumping.
ADULT: *Is*
CHILD: Boy jumping.
ADULT: *Is jumping.*
CHILD: Boy is jumping.
ADULT: Good. Boy is jumping (reauditorization).

Partial models can include only the missing parts of the target or the missing elements plus closely associated grammatical units, as in the adult's second partial model in the example above. The last adult utterance provides a reauditorization of the child's correct response. Such an utterance could additionally include a recast.

Expansion Request. In an expansion request, the adult informs the child that the response is not adequate and more information is needed. However, the adult does not provide the missing information. The child must decide, without the adult's identifying the missing element(s), what has been omitted, and then supply a complete structure on reformulation. There are several ways of requesting an expansion. These include "Tell me the whole thing," "Tell me more," "I didn't hear all of it," or "There's more." The following example illustrates expansion requests.

Example
TARGET: *Do* + subject + verb ("Do you want some food?")
ADULT: We are going to pretend we're in a restaurant. You are the waiter. You have to ask us what we want to eat.

CHILD: You want hamburger?

ADULT: *Tell me the whole thing.*

CHILD: Do you want hamburger?

ADULT: Good. Yes, I do want hamburger.

CHILD: Want milk?

ADULT: *Say the whole thing.*

CHILD: You want milk?

ADULT: *More.*

CHILD: Do you want milk?

ADULT: Good. Yes, I do want milk. I do want milk to drink (recast). I do want milk to drink with my hamburger (recast). What else do you have?

Repetition Request.   According to Lee and colleagues (1975), a repetition request does not let a child know whether the response was adequate. As such, this interchange can be used to stabilize a correct response by having the child say it again or to reformulate adequately an incorrect response. In this latter use, a child has to reauditorize internally the first utterance, compare it to an internal standard auditory model, and restructure the utterance. We see examples of repetition requests in the following.

Example
TARGET: Use of polite requests

CHILD: Close the door.

ADULT: *What did you say? Say that again.*

CHILD: Close the door.

ADULT: *What did you say?*

CHILD: Can you close the door?

ADULT: Good. Yes, I will close the door now.

Repetition of Error.   In some ways, this appears to be a form of providing a stimulus for a child to imitate. However, the adult is actually supplying an incorrect model. This is often accompanied by a questioning intonation or an unpleasant facial grimace. The child's task is to recognize the nonverbal cues that the response was inadequate, identify the error, and reformulate the response. However, if this interchange is used too early in intervention with a child, the child will mistakenly interpret the adult's utterance as a correct model to be imitated (Lee et al., 1975). Consequently, accurate interpretation of this approach is a more complex task than those listed earlier. Following is an example of this interchange technique.

Example
TARGET: Use of *red* to describe objects appropriately

ADULT: I have an apple. What color is the apple?

CHILD: The apple green.

ADULT:	*The apple is green?*
CHILD:	Apple green.
ADULT:	*Green?*
CHILD:	Apple red.
ADULT:	You're right. The apple is red (recast).

Self-Correction Request.   As the name of this technique implies, the adult asks a child to self-evaluate an utterance. In some instances, this approach may be employed even though a child's response was correct. The purpose is to reinforce and stabilize use of the target. In other instances, the technique can be used when the child's response is inaccurate. Despite the situation in which it is utilized, the purpose is to have the child self-monitor language productions in much the same way as adult speakers monitor their own productions. Use of self-correction interchanges is illustrated in the following example.

Example

TARGET: Irregular third-person present-tense singular verbs

CHILD:	He haves some toys.
ADULT:	*Is that right?*
CHILD:	He has some toys.
ADULT:	*Is that okay?*
CHILD:	Yes.
ADULT:	What else does he have?
CHILD:	He has some shoes.
ADULT:	*Is that right?*
CHILD:	Yes.

Rephrased Question.   This interchange may be especially effective when a number of other interchanges have occurred in order to elicit an adequate target response from a child (Lee et al., 1975). Rephrasing the original question may help the child stabilize use of the target language behavior. The following example shows this technique used in combination with the techniques of repetition request and repetition of an error.

Example

TARGET: *is* + verb + in*g*

ADULT:	What is the boy doing?
CHILD:	Boy crying.
ADULT:	Boy crying? (repetition of error)
CHILD:	Boy is crying.
ADULT:	Good. Tell me again (repetition request)
CHILD:	Boy is crying.
ADULT:	*Is the boy laughing?*
CHILD:	No, boy is crying.

In many instances, several of these techniques are used in combination in any one set of successive utterances between child and adult, as the last example illustrates. As we indicated earlier, other language-facilitating techniques, such as modeling, reauditorization, and recasts, can also be incorporated. The following example demonstrates several interchange techniques and language-facilitation approaches. An important feature in this example is that every time the child gave an inadequate response, the adult's subsequent interchange technique was one that provided more help or is lower in the hierarchy. It is important that a child not become frustrated as a result of giving several inaccurate responses in a row. The adult must be aware of this possibility and modify the situation so that the child will succeed.

Example

TARGET: Interrogative reversal of copula *is*

SITUATION: Adult and child are guessing the contents of a large box filled with various toys.

ADULT: What is in the box? (self-talk) Let's guess. Is it a ball? (model) I don't know (self-talk). Is it a ball? (model) Yes, it is a ball (self-talk). What else is in the box?

CHILD: It a car?

ADULT: What did you say? (repetition request)

CHILD: It a car?

ADULT: Is it (reduced model)

CHILD: Is it a car?

ADULT: Is it a car? (reauditorization) Good. Let's look to see if you guessed right. Yes, it is a car (recast). It is a big, red car (recast). Is it a big, red car? (recast). Yes, it is a big, red car (self-talk). It is my turn to guess (self-talk). Let's see (self-talk). Is it a . . . (model). Is it a horse? (model). No, it is not a horse (selk-talk). Your turn.

CHILD: It a pig?

ADULT: It a pig (repetition of error—accompanying facial grimace).

CHILD: Is it a pig?

ADULT: Is it a pig? (reauditorization). Good. Let's see if it is a pig. Is it a pig? (reauditorization). Yes, it is a pig (recast). It is a little pig (recast). Is it a little pig? (recast) Yes, it is a little pig (self-talk). My turn (self-talk). Is it a . . . (model). Is it a duck? (model) No, it is not a duck (self-talk). Your turn.

CHILD: It a truck?

ADULT: Did you say that right? (self-correction request)

CHILD: It a truck?

ADULT: Tell me the whole thing (expansion request)

CHILD: Is it a truck?

ADULT: Did you say that right now? (self-correction request)

CHILD: Yes.

ADULT: What is in the box? (rephrased question).

CHILD: Is it a truck?

ADULT: Is it a truck? (reauditorization). Good question. Let's look.

So Which Ones Should We Use?

To date, we have no clear evidence as to the superiority of one technique over others for different language targets at children's different stages of communicative development. Different techniques have been subjected to empirical scrutiny, for example, the work of Connell and Stone (1992), Courtright and Courtright (1976), Ellis Weismer and Murray-Branch (1989), and Skarakis-Doyle and Woodall (1988) for modeling or the work of Camarata and Nelson (Camarata & Nelson, 1992; Camarata et al., 1994; Nelson, Camarata, Welsh, Butkovsky et al., 1996) for recasting of children's utterances. In some studies one technique has compared with another, for example, recasting compared to imitation (Camarata & Nelson, 1992; Camarata et al., 1994; Nelson et al., 1996) or modeling compared to imitation (Connell & Stone, 1992; Courtright & Courtright, 1976; Friedman & Friedman, 1980). There have also been studies that have tried to match children's characteristics with particular techniques, such as level of nonverbal intelligence and imitation versus techniques involving recasting and modeling (Cole & Dale, 1986; Friedman & Friedman, 1980; Yoder et al., 1991). However, as Leonard (1998) summarizes for us, we are not yet at the point where we can match children and their characteristics with language targets with particular facilitating techniques and procedures. What we do know, however, is that intervention works and we should probably try to elicit responses, that is, get the children to talk and to use their targets, rather than settle for letting the children only listen to their targets. For the most part, however, the decisions about which of the techniques may be effective are left to the adult facilitating language learning for a specific child. Certainly, some approaches seem more appropriate for some children at specific points in an intervention sequence than others. There needs to be sufficient flexibility so that when one technique or combination of techniques is not working, other techniques can be selected. And, several techniques are typically used with a child at a time.

Approaches to Intervention

In this section we discuss various approaches to intervention. Although we divide this section into four subsections, it will become apparent that the topics are not completely discrete. Rather, aspects of each discussion interact with aspects of the others.

Direct and Indirect Intervention

Previously in this text, reference has been made to direct and indirect approaches to intervention. The basic difference between the two approaches is who acts as the primary agent of language change for a child (Olswang & Bain, 1991). In *direct intervention,* the professional assumes the role as the primary change agent. The professional plans the objectives of intervention, the strategies to be employed in accomplishing the objectives, and implements the strategies by direct interaction with the child. Others, such as parents/caregivers and teachers, are typically involved in the planning and may even assist the professional in implementation, but the professional retains the role as the major change agent. In *indirect intervention,* the professional also plans the objectives of intervention, again typically with the involvement of parents/caregivers and/or teachers, and decides on specific strategies for implementation. However, individuals other than the language professional, such as parents/caregivers and/or teachers, carry out the plans. The professional works with these individuals to show them how to carry out the plans and monitors the implementation and the child's progress. The professional generally does not work directly with the child. In Chapter 3 we discussed the necessity to train parents/caregivers for indirect intervention with toddlers and preschoolers. The same is true when teachers or day-care providers are the primary agents of change. In some cases, a combination of direct and indirect intervention may be warranted, or intervention may change from one approach to another as the objectives of intervention and the child's language behavior change.

There are few empirical data to help us in deciding which approach is most effective under what conditions. Olswang and Bain (1991) point out that identifying the purpose of intervention at a specific point in time may assist in deciding which approach may be more effective. They suggest that direct intervention may be more appropriate when the aim is to establish a new language behavior, and that indirect intervention may be more appropriate when the aim is to stabilize, generalize, or extend a language behavior that the child already demonstrates or that has been established as a result of direct intervention.

Group and Individual Intervention

In Chapter 5 we suggested that, for adolescents with language impairment, group intervention may be more effective than individual, or one-to-one, intervention. This belief is somewhat counter to a more traditional view that a one-to-one setting is the more effective format for language intervention. With a one-to-one format, extraneous environmental distractions can be controlled to allow a child to focus attention on the desired stimuli. Language learning, it is believed, will be promoted quickly.

The rationale behind a one-to-one structure for language intervention may, in part, be valid. Reducing distractions can increase the salience of the provided stimuli, and more opportunities for exemplars and responses might be possible. However, language is an interactive, interpersonal behavior. As such, many of the reasons cited for employing group intervention for language-disordered adolescents apply to intervention for younger children (Bunce, 1995; Rice & Wilcox, 1995; Swenson, 2000). Young children learn language by interacting with their environments and the people in them. A one-to-one intervention format often limits the number of events and contexts in which language teaching can occur and restricts the number of people with whom the language can be used. In contrast, small-group intervention formats for young language-disordered children can provide situations for language learning that are not present in individual intervention settings. In light of our previous discussions of reinforcement and generalization, we can see how a group format might furnish opportunities for naturalistic reinforcers to occur and promote generalization. Each child in a small group is exposed to a variety of stimuli, experiences, contexts, and people that are not available in one-to-one situations. A number of adults, including parents, often participate with the children in group situations, thereby providing the children opportunities to use language with different adults as well as with other children. Such a format can also be used to help train parents and teachers in strategies to be employed in indirect intervention.

The decision as to whether a child will benefit more from a group setting or an individual format depends on the specific child. Some children, particularly those who are hyperactive, distractible, or inattentive or those who show little interest in interacting with people, may initially require one-to-one intervention. For other children, a small-group setting may be the most appropriate. Furthermore, the type of setting from which a specific child will benefit more may change as the child's behaviors and language skills change. Children who initially required individual intervention can progress so that a group setting is warranted. Children initially seen in a group setting may progress to needing intervention for very specific skills best accomplished in an individual format. Again, there is no fixed rule as to which format must be used throughout a child's entire intervention program. Instead, flexibility in providing a child with the appropriate setting at a particular point in intervention is the key.

The decision regarding the structure of a child's intervention does not always have to involve a choice between a group or individual format. In many instances, a combination of the two can be effective (Cleave & Fey, 1997). Targeted language skills can be presented in an undistracting, one-to-one situation and then extended to a variety of contexts with a variety of people present in a group setting.

Three Language Teaching Methods

Beyond considering the degree of "naturalism" of facilitating techniques that can be used in language intervention, as illustrated in Figure 14.1, the larger structure of intervention can vary along a continuum of "naturalness." Some can be quite didactic, while others are quite unstructured and focus exclusively on child-centered approaches. Each, however, has strengths and weaknesses, so many professionals have tried to adopt methods somewhere between the extremes. Fey (1986) terms these "hybrid" methods. These attempt to bring to intervention environments and/or activities that are as natural as possible but still provide sufficient opportunities for the adults to control and manipulate the teaching situations in order to ensure adequate exemplars, opportunities for response, practice, and generalization.

Olswang and Bain (1991) have described three commonly adopted language-teaching methods: milieu teaching, joint action routines, and inductive teaching. As the authors explain, these methods share some similar features and incorporate procedures found in other methods as well. However, they vary in terms of the degree of structure involved. The various facilitating techniques discussed in the previous section will be used within the formats of these three language-teaching methods. However, it is logical to assume that some techniques will be more compatible with one or two of the teaching approaches than another.

Milieu Teaching.   Of the three methods, milieu teaching employs the least amount of structure. Natural consequences of communication as reinforcements, activities determined by the child's interests and attention, conversational contexts for teaching, and intervention in the child's usual environment (home, preschool, classroom) are characteristics of the milieu teaching approach. Opportunities for targeted language behaviors are dispersed throughout a session. Three procedures are used in milieu teaching (Olswang & Bain, 1991), although these procedures can also be employed in other teaching approaches. The procedures are incidental teaching, mand-model teaching, and delay.

Incidental Teaching.   In incidental teaching, the child determines the activity or topic and the adult works the language teaching into it. The activity or topic lasts only as long as the child is interested in and reinforced by it. During the activity, the adult may use a variety of the facilitating techniques discussed previously to elicit specific language behaviors. Incidental teaching was also discussed briefly in Chapter 6.

Mand-Model.   This procedure was also introduced in Chapter 6. Unlike incidental teaching, it is a more adult-directed procedure. The adult chooses a time to direct the child's attention to an object or activity, asks for (mands) a response from the child or provides a prompt for a response. If the child gives an appropriate response verbally, the adult reinforces the child's response and then gives the child the desired object or allows the activity to proceed. If the child's response is incomplete or incorrect, models of the target response or other elicitation techniques are used.

Delay.   When a child wants an object out of reach or desires certain events to occur, the adult looks questioningly at the child but waits, usually for about 15 seconds, before responding to the child. Obviously, the adult is waiting for an appropriate response from the child before complying. If the child does not respond, the adult may provide a model of the target response or use other elicitation techniques and wait again. Generally, the sequence is repeated only twice before complying with the child's desires. Too many repetitions without a successful outcome may do nothing more than increase a child's frustration. However, if too many unsuccessful outcomes are occurring, immediate reevaluation of the teaching approaches and strategies being employed is warranted.

   Delay is an important intervention procedure even when it is used with other language teaching methods. Language-disordered children may not be able to respond as quickly as normal language-learning children. They may very well need more time to understand what is expected, to process the stimuli, and/or to retrieve and generate a response.

   One of the major difficulties with the milieu teaching method is the dispersed nature of the opportunities for learning.

Joint Action Routines.   This teaching method is sometimes known as *script therapy.* The idea behind joint action routines is to create interactive, systematic repetitions of events in which each partner has predictable language and behavioral patterns to complete. The routines can reflect usual events in a child's environment, or they can be created (Constable, 1986; DeKroon, Kyte, & Johnson, 2002; Kim & Lombardino, 1991; McCormick, 1997; Robertson & Ellis Weismer, 1997). These routines are socially based and incorporate the need to communicate. They focus on specific themes or topics, such as craft activities in which the adult and child interact and the child has to ask for needed materials, or they may be centered around pretend play routines. Joint action routines are purported to reduce demands on a child so that the child can focus on the language tasks required (Ellis Weismer, 2000). As the child becomes familiar with specific routines, the expectations for language use gradually change to more advanced skills. A problem with the joint action routine method of language teaching is the manner in which the routines are or are not modified to increase the level of language expected from a child and the strategies employed to elicit the higher-level language behaviors. Generalizing the routines to novel situations can sometimes also be problematic.

Inductive Teaching. Inductive teaching is the most structured and adult-centered method discussed here. The adult manipulates meaningful communicative interactions so that the child begins to identify patterns (or regularities). The three elements of inductive teaching are (Olswang & Bain, 1991)

1. The communicative interactions are arranged to allow the child to discover that a pattern exists.
2. The child discovers that the meaningful context or communicative interaction is associated with the pattern and, in fact, explains the pattern. The child learns that the patterns involved affect meaning.

The child hypothesizes "the rule that captures the nature of the correspondence between the observed pairs of stimuli. The assumption of this procedure is that the induction process is an innate one so that by this step, if the preceding ones have been arranged correctly, hypothesizing the rule will occur automatically" (Olswang & Bain, 1991, pp. 81–82).

In practice, it is not unusual to see professionals using elements of all three methods. Each has its merits and its drawbacks. The merits need to be matched to the child and the intervention objectives. The different methods or elements of the methods may suit different children and different language objectives. What we do not know yet is how to match these variables unfailingly. We do know that we need to try.

Service Delivery Models

Previously in this text, we have introduced ideas related to different models of delivering language intervention services to children. In addition to findings from research, forms of service delivery are influenced by setting in which intervention is to occur, policies and orientations of different service providers, and legislative mandates.

Increasingly, however, it is clear that the trend has been to provide language intervention in children's classrooms or their other usual environments. Settings consistent with this trend are sometimes referred to as *inclusive, integrated,* or *mainstreamed.* These services are sometimes delivered by an adult other than the professional, in which case they can be considered indirect interventions, per our previous discussion. These also probably fall into the category of consultation services because of the consultative role that the language professional plays. In some situations, children may be provided language intervention by the language professional in the children's classrooms during activities taking place at various times of the day, such as free reading time, art, and group discussions. These services are considered direct intervention and not necessarily consultative. In still other cases, the language professional delivers the services in the classrooms, generally in collaboration with the regular educator or other professionals, aides, or parents/caregivers in the environment, that is, collaborative service delivery. Forms of delivery in these instances may include team teaching or turn teaching with the teachers. Strengths that have been attributed to collaborative, and even consultative, service delivery models are the ecological validity of the language intervention and the promotion of generalization. However, there is considerable variation in how different service delivery models are implemented, prompting Ferguson (1992) to comment that "Program designs are as individual as those who participate in their development; there is no single correct program" (p. 361).

In the midst of the trend toward increasing use of collaborative and/or consultative service delivery models, use of what has come to be known as the "traditional pull-out" model of service delivery, even in school settings, has not been abandoned, even in settings where collaborative/consultation models have also been implemented. Pull-out means that a child leaves the activities of the typical educational routine to receive services from a specialist. At the extreme, the pull-out might be complete, in which case the child receives all of his or her education in a self-contained classroom or more recently even in self-contained schools, given an increase in the number of such special schools, from which the child might again be pulled out for other special services, such as language intervention (Conti-Ramsden & Botting, 1999; Conti-Ramsden et al., 2001; Hirst & Brittion, 1998). More usually, however, pull-out means that the child participates in the usual educational routine for most of the time, leaves it temporarily for special services, and then returns. In Chapter 5, we discussed why this model was not appropriate at the secondary school level for adolescents with language disorders. Factors related to this model were also raised in discussion of service delivery for children with language-learning disabilities in Chapter 4. Two of the biggest criticisms of the model relevant to language intervention have been the limited contextual support for language learning and the difficulties in generalizing language skills into naturalistic environment.

Others have interpreted pull-out to mean that a child is seen individually by the professional. However, pull-out does not equate to individual intervention and does not preclude group intervention, which can take place within a pull-out model. Therefore, the issues related to pull-out are not essentially issues related to individual versus group intervention approaches. It is likely that some language-disordered children at certain times during their language intervention benefit from language teaching that takes place in a less distracting environment in which the targeted rules and regularities can be made more salient and language-teaching techniques can be used more consistently.

Most professionals now agree that, as a sole model of intervention, a pull-out model is insufficient. It can, however, be used successfully in combination with both consultative and collaborative models. Service delivery does not have to be "all or nothing" with regard to models. Rather, it needs to be viewed as requiring several service delivery models, with each contributing differently to different children with differing language needs at different times.

Putting It Together

We have reviewed many of the factors that go into planning and implementing language intervention. Each of these represents a decision point in the planning process, but each decision is not independent. We have seen that the factors frequently interact with each other. The decisions, therefore, interact. Figure 14.2 illustrates some of these factors and the interactions, as well as the complexity involved in the intervention decision-making process. There is no claim that the model includes all of the factors affecting intervention decisions. Furthermore, as we learn more about intervention and children with language disorders, more factors will probably be added. It is also possible that some factors will combine with others. Ultimately, the factors and the decisions will combine to produce an individual child's intervention plan. Planning and implementing language intervention for individual children is a complex decision-making process.

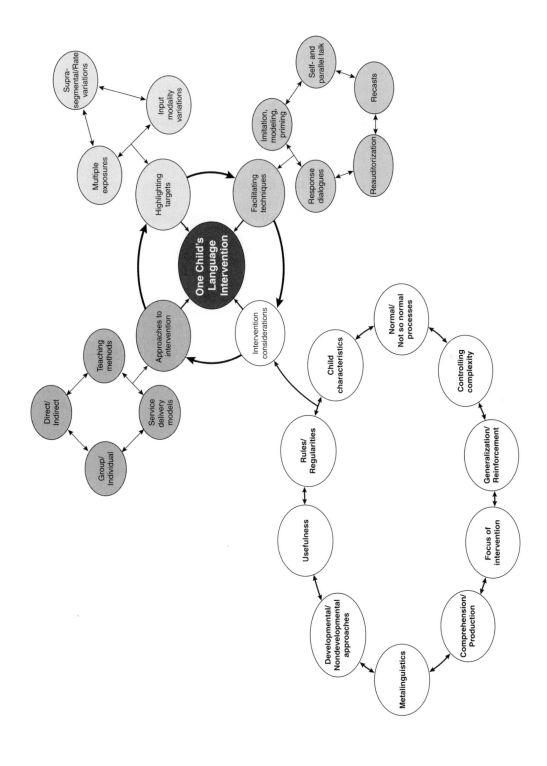

FIGURE 14.2   A Model of Language Intervention

Summary

In this chapter we have seen that

- Normal language processes generally guide much of what we do in language intervention, but there are some suggestions that children with language disorders may need intervention that modifies normal processes in order to realize language features productively.
- Language intervention aims to help children discover rules and regularities and/or provide opportunities for the children to process relevant information about what it is they need to learn.
- Language intervention needs to stress the usefulness of language.
- Developmental approaches are more frequently used to guide the sequencing of intervention objectives, although nondevelopmental approaches may sometimes be appropriate.
- Comprehension of a language target is sometimes emphasized before production; in other instances, comprehension and production are emphasized concomitantly. It may be that language-disordered children need to have practice in producing targeted language behaviors in order to learn to use them most efficiently.
- The focus of intervention depends on an individual child's needs and likely changes throughout the child's total intervention program.
- It is important to control all aspects of language complexity when planning for and requiring a response from a child.
- Reinforcement and generalization are important considerations in planning intervention; generalization may be promoted more successfully when naturalistic reinforcers and varied contexts are incorporated into the implementation of intervention.
- The characteristics of each child affect the intervention approaches and strategies chosen, but we still do not know how to match most efficaciously child characteristics and intervention approaches and/or strategies.
- Language intervention for young children does not depend heavily on metalinguistic approaches but does not avoid incorporating metalinguistics. In contrast, for older children, improving their metalinguistic abilities may be a focus of intervention and metalinguistic approaches are sometimes employed as teaching strategies.
- Intervention can be direct or indirect and can be provided via several language-teaching strategies and service delivery models.
- Exposure to language targets needs to be more frequent and made more salient for children with language impairment.
- Many direct and indirect facilitating and elicitation techniques can be employed.
- Planning and implementing language intervention is a complex decision-making process in which multiple factors interact.

Each language-disordered child has unique needs that require flexibility in planning intervention. Unless intervention is viewed as an individually designed, dynamic, fluid process, language-disordered children will be fortunate if their needs are met at least some of the time.

REFERENCES

Abbeduto, L. (1991). Development of verbal communication in persons with moderate to mild mental retardation. *International Review of Research in Mental Retardation, 17,* 91–115.

Abbeduto, L., Benson, G., Short, K., & Dolish, J. (1995). Effects of sampling context on the expressive language of children and adolescents with mental retardation. *Mental Retardation, 33*(5), 279–288.

Abbeduto, L., Davies, B., Solesby, S., & Furman, L. (1991). Identifying the referents of spoken messages: The use of context and clarification requests by children with mental retardation and by nonretarded children. *American Journal on Mental Retardation, 95,* 551–562.

Abbeduto, L., Furman, L., & Davies, B. (1989). Relation between the receptive language and mental age of persons with mental retardation. *American Journal on Mental Retardation, 93,* 535–543.

Abbeduto, L., & Hesketh, L. J. (1997). Pragmatic development in individuals with mental retardation: Learning to use language in social interactions. *Mental Retardation and Developmental Disabilities Research Reviews, 3,* 323–333.

Abbeduto, L., Pavetto, M., Kesin, E., Weissman, M. D., Karadottir, S., O'Brien, A., et al. (2001). The linguistic and cognitive profile of Down syndrome: Evidence from a comparison with fragile X syndrome. *Down Syndrome: Research and Practice, 7,* 9–15.

Abbeduto, L., & Rosenberg, S. (1980). The communicative competence of mildly retarded adults. *Applied Psycholinguistics, 1,* 405–426.

Abbeduto, L., & Short, K. (1994). Relation between language comprehension and cognitive functioning in persons with mental retardation. *Journal of Developmental & Physical Disabilities, 6*(4), 347–369.

Abbeduto, L., Short-Meyerson, K., Benson, G., & Dolish, J. (1997). Signaling of noncomprehension by children and adolescents with mental retardation: Effects of problem type and speaker identity. *Journal of Speech, Language, and Hearing Research, 40,* 20–32.

Abbeduto, L., Short-Meyerson, K., Benson, G., Dolish, J., & Weissman, M. (1998). Understanding referential expressions in context: Use of common ground by children and adolescents with mental retardation. *Journal of Speech, Language, and Hearing Research, 41*(6), 1348–1362.

Abbeduto, L., Weissman, M. D., & Short-Meyerson, K. (1999). Parental scaffolding of the discourse of children and adolescents with intellectual disability: The case of referential expressions. *Journal of Intellectual Disability Research, 43*(6), 540–557.

Abel, E. (1998). *Fetal Alcohol Abuse Syndrome.* New York: Plenum Press.

Abrahamsen, E. P., & Sprouse, P. T. (1995). Fable comprehension by children with learning disabilities. *Journal of Learning Disabilities, 28,* 302–308.

Achenbach, T. (1970). Standardization of a research instrument for identifying associative responding children. *Developmental Psychology, 2,* 283–291.

Achenbach, T. (1991a). *Manual for the Child Behavior Checklist/4–18.* Burlington: University of Vermont Press.

Achenbach, T. (1991b). *Manual for the Teacher Report Form.* Burlington: University of Vermont Press.

Achenbach, T. (1992). *Manual for the Child Behavior Checklist/2–3 and 1992 Profile.* Burlington: University of Vermont, Department of Psychiatry.

Adams, M. J. (1990). *Beginning to read: Thinking and learning about print.* Cambridge, MA: MIT Press.

Alexander, P. A., & Muia, J. A. (1982). *Gifted education: A comprehensive roadmap.* Rockville, MD: Aspen.

Almli, C. R., & Finger, S. (1992). Brain injury and recovery of function: Theories and mechanisms of functional reorganization. *Journal of Head Trauma Rehabilitation, 7,* 70–77.

American Association on Mental Retardation. (2002). *Definition of mental retardation.* Retrieved February 7, 2004, from www.aamr.org/Policies/faq_mental_retardation.shtml.

American Educational Research Association, American Psychological Association, & National Council on Measurement and Education. (1999). *Standards for educational and psychological testing.* Washington, DC: American Psychological Association.

American Psychiatric Association. (1980). *Diagnostic and statistical manual of mental disorders* (3rd ed.). Washington, DC: American Psychiatric Association.

American Psychiatric Association. (1994). *Diagnostic and statistical manual of mental disorders (DSM-IV)* (4th ed.). Washington, DC: American Psychiatric Association.

American Psychiatric Association. (2000). *Diagnostic and statistical manual of mental disorders* (4th edition, Text Revision ed.). Washington, DC: American Psychiatric Association.

Andersen, E. S., Dunlea, A., & Kekelis, L. S. (1984). Blind children's language: Resolving some differences. *Journal of Child Language, 11,* 645–664.

Anderson, R. (1996). Assessing the grammar of Spanish-speaking children: A comparison of two procedures. *Language, Speech, and Hearing Services in Schools, 27,* 333–345.

Anderson, V., Morse, S. A., Klug, G., Catroppa, C., Haritou, F., Rosenfeld, J., et al. (1997). Predicting recovery from head injury in young children: A prospective analysis. *Journal of the International Neuropsychological Society, 3*(6), 568–580.

Andolina, C. (1980). Syntactic maturity and vocabulary richness of learning disabled children at four age levels. *Journal of Learning Disabilities, 13,* 27–32.

Apel, K. (1999a). An introduction to assessment and intervention with older students with language-learning impairments: Bridges from research to clinical practice. *Language, Speech, and Hearing Services in Schools, 30,* 228–230.

Apel, K. (1999b). Checks and balances: Keeping the science in our profession. *Language, Speech, and Hearing Services in Schools, 30,* 98–107.

Applebee, A. (1978). *The child's concept of story.* Chicago: University of Chicago Press.

Aram, D. (1988). Language sequelae of unilateral brain lesions in children. In F. Plum (Ed.), *Language, communication, and the brain* (pp. 171–198). New York: Raven Press.

Aram, D. (1991). Comments on specific language impairment as a clinical category. *Language, Speech, and Hearing Services in Schools, 22,* 84–87.

Aram, D. (1998). Acquired aphasia in children. In M. T. Sarno (Ed.), *Acquired aphasia* (3rd ed., pp. 451–480). San Diego, CA: Academic Press.

Aram, D., & Eisele, J. (1994). Limits to a left hemisphere explanation for specific language impairment. *Journal of Speech and Hearing Research, 37,* 824–830.

Aram, D., Ekelman, B., & Nation, J. (1984). Preschoolers with language disorders: 10 years later. *Journal of Speech and Hearing Research, 27,* 232–244.

Aram, D., Ekelman, B. L., & Whitaker, H. (1986). Spoken syntax in children with acquired left and right hemisphere lesions. *Brain and Language, 27,* 75–100.

Aram, D., Ekelman, B. L., & Whitaker, H. (1987). Lexical retrieval in left and right lesioned children. *Brain and Language, 31,* 75–100.

Aram, D., Hack, M., Hawkins, S., Weissman, B., & Borawski-Clark, E. (1991). Very-low-birthweight children and speech and language development. *Journal of Speech and Hearing Research, 34,* 1169–1179.

Aram, D., & Nation, J. E. (1982). *Child language disorders.* St. Louis, MO: Mosby.

Archwamety, T., & Katsiyannis, A. (2000). Academic remediation, parole violation, and recidivism rates among delinquent youths. *RASE: Remedial and Special Education, 21*(3), 161–170.

Armour-Thomas, E., & Allen, B. (1990). Componential analysis of analogical-reasoning performance of high and low achievers. *Psychology in the Schools, 27,* 269–275.

Arnold, K. S., & Reed, L. (1976). The Grammatic Closure Subtest of the ITPA: A comparative study of black and white children. *Journal of Speech and Hearing Disorders, 41,* 477–485.

Arnold, L. E. (1996). Sex differences in ADHD: Conference summary. *Journal of Abnormal Child Psychology, 24,* 555–569.

ASHA. (1973). *Task force report on speech pathology and audiology service needs in prison.* Washington, DC: American Speech-Language-Hearing Association.

ASHA. (1976). ASHA Taskforce on Central Auditory Processing Consensus Development: Central auditory processing: current status of research and implications for clinical practice. *American Journal of Audiology, 5*(2), 41–54.

ASHA. (1989). Competencies for speech-language pathologists providing services in augmentative communication. *Asha, 31*(3), 107–110.

ASHA. (1991a). A model for collaborative service delivery for students with language-learning disorders in the public schools. *Asha, 33*(Suppl. 5), 44–50.

ASHA. (1991b). Report: Augmentative and alternative communication. *Asha, 33*(Suppl. 5), 9–12.

ASHA. (1995). Position statement on facilitated communication. *Asha, 37*(Suppl. 5), 9–12.

ASHA. (1996). Inclusive practices for children and youths with communication disorders: Position statement and technical report. *Asha, 38*(Suppl. 16), 35–44.

ASHA. (1997). *Preferred practice patterns for the profession of speech-language pathology.* Rockville, MD: American Speech-Language-Hearing Association.

ASHA. (1998). Provision of English-as-a-second-language instruction by speech-language pathologists in school settings; Position statement and technical report. *Asha, 40*(Suppl. 18).

ASHA. (2002a). *Annual member counts for the period January 1 through June 30, 2002.* Rockville, MD: American Speech-Language-Hearing Association.

ASHA. (2002b). *Demographic profile of the ASHA constituents for the period January 1 through June 30, 2002: Table 5.* Rockville, MD: American Speech-Language-Hearing Association.

ASHA. (2002c). *Omnibus survey caseload report: SLP.* Rockville, MD: American Speech-Language-Hearing Association.

ASHA Committee on the Status of Racial Minorities. (1983). Social dialects position paper. *Asha, 25,* 23–24.

ASHA Committee on the Status of Racial Minorities. (1985). Clinical management of communicatively handicapped minority language populations. *Asha, 27,* 29–32.

Asher, S., & Gazelle, H. (1999). Loneliness, peer relations, and language disorder in childhood. *Topics in Language Disorders, 19*(2), 16–33.

Axtell, R. E. (1991). *Gestures: The do's and taboos of body language around the world.* Baltimore, MD: Wiley.

Baddeley, A. (1986). Working memory and comprehension. In D. Broadbent, J. McGaugh, M. Kosslyn, N. Mackintosh, E. Tulving, & L. Weiskrantz (Eds.), *Working memory.* Oxford, UK: Oxford University Press.

Bae, Y., Choy, S., Geddes, C., Sable, J., & Snyder, T. (2000). *Trends in the educational equity of girls and women.* Washington, DC: U.S. Department of Education, National Center for Education Statistics.

Baer, D. M., & Guess, D. (1973). Teaching productive noun suffixes to severely retarded children. *American Journal of Mental Deficiency, 77,* 498–505.

Bagnato, S. J., Mayes, S. D., Nichter, C., Domoto, V., Hamann, L., Keener, S., et al. (1988). An interdisciplinary neurodevelopmental assessment model for brain-injured infants and preschool children. *Journal of Head Trauma Rehabilitation, 3,* 75–86.

Bain, B., & Dollaghan, C. (1991). The notion of clinically significant change. *Language, Speech, and Hearing Services in Schools, 22,* 264–270.

Bain, B., & Olswang, L. (1995). Examining readiness for learning two-word utterances by children with specific expressive language impairment: Dynamic assessment. *American Journal of Speech-Language Pathology, 4,* 81–91.

Baird, S. M., Mayfield, P., & Baker, P. (1997). Mothers' interpretations of the behavior of their infants with visual and other impairments during interactions. *Journal of Visual Impairment and Blindness, 91*(5), 467–483.

Baker, B. (1982). Minspeak: A semantic compaction system that makes self expression easier for communicatively disabled individuals. *Byte, 7,* 186–202.

Baker, L., & Cantwell, D. (1982). Psychiatric disorder in children with different types of communication disorders. *Journal of Communication Disorders, 15,* 113–126.

Baker, L., & Cantwell, D. (1983). Developmental and behavioral characteristics of speech and language disordered children. In S. Chess & T. Thomas (Eds.), *Annual progress in children development* (pp. 205–216). New York: Brunner-Mazel.

Baker, N., & Nelson, K. (1984). Recasting and related conversational techniques for triggering syntactic advances by young children. *First Language, 5,* 3–22.

Balandin, S. (1994, October). Symbol board vocabularies. Paper presented at the Sixth Biennial Conference of the International Society for Augmentative and Alternative Communication, Maastricht, The Netherlands.

Balandin, S., & Iacono, T. (1993). Symbol vocabularies: A study of vocabulary found on communication boards used by adults with cerebral palsy. In The Crippled Children's Association of SA Inc. (Ed.), *Australian Conference on Technology for People with Disabilities* (pp. 85–87). Adelaide, Australia: The Crippled Children's Association of SA Inc.

Balandin, S., & Iacono, T. (1998). AAC and Australian speech pathologists: A report on a national survey. *Augmentative and Alternative Communication, 14,* 239–249.

Balason, D., & Dollaghan, C. (2002). Grammatical morpheme production in 4-year-old children. *Journal of Speech, Language, and Hearing Research, 45,* 961–969.

Ball, M., & Lowry, O. (2001). *Methods in clinical phonetics.* London, UK: Whurr.

Baltaxe, C., & Guthrie, D. (1987). The use of primary sentence stress by normal, aphasic, and autistic children. *Journal of Autism and Developmental Disorders, 17,* 255–271.

Baltaxe, C., & Simmons, J. Q. (1985). Prosodic development in normal and autistic children. In E. Schopler & G. Mesibov (Eds.), *Communication problems in autism.* New York: Plenum Press.

Baltaxe, C., & Simmons, J. Q. (1988). Communication deficits in preschool children with psychiatric disorders. *Seminars in Speech and Language, 8,* 81–90.

Bandura, A. (1971). *Psychological modeling.* Chicago: Aldine-Atherton.

Bandura, A. (1977). *Social learning theory.* Englewood Cliffs, NJ: Prentice-Hall.

Bangs, T. (1975). *Vocabulary comprehension scale.* Hingham, MA: Teaching Resources.

Baranek, G. T. (1999). Autism during infancy: A retrospective video analysis of sensory-motor and social behaviors at 9–12 months of age. *Journal of Autism and Developmental Disorders, 29,* 213–224.

Barnes, M. A., & Dennis, M. (2001). Knowledge-based inferencing after childhood head injury. *Brain and Language 76, 3,* 253–265.

Baron-Cohen, S. (1988). Social and pragmatic deficits in autism: cognitive or affective? *Journal of Autism and Developmental Disorders, 18,* 379–402.

Baron-Cohen, S. (1991). Do people with autism understand what causes emotion? *Child Development, 62,* 385–395.

Barr, M. L., & Kerinan, J. A. (1988). *The human nervous system: An anatomical viewpoint.* (5th ed.). Philadelphia: Lippincott.

Barrett, M., Huisingh, R., Zachman, L., Blagden, C., & Orman, J. (1992). *The listening test.* East Moline, IL: LinguiSystems.

Barrow, I., Holbert, D., & Rastatter, M. (2000). Effect of color on developmental picture-vocabulary naming of 4-, 6-, and 8-year-old children. *American Journal of Speech-Language Pathology, 9,* 310–318.

Bashir, A. S. (1989). Language intervention and the curriculum. *Seminars in Speech and Language, 10,* 181–191.

Bashir, A. S., & Scavuzzo, A. (1992). Children with language disorders: Natural history and academic success. *Journal of Learning Disabilities, 25,* 53–65.

Bates, E. (1976). *The emergence of symbols: Cognition and communication in infancy.* New York: Academic Press.

Bates, E., Benigni, L., Bretherton, I., Camaioni, L., & Volterra, V. (1977). From gesture to the first word: On cognitive and social prerequisites. In M. Lewis & L. Rosenblum (Eds.), *Interaction, conversation, and the development of language.* New York: Wiley.

Bates, E., Benigni, L., Bretherton, I., Camaioni, L., & Volterra, V. (1979). *The emergence of symbols: Cognition and communication in infancy.* New York: Academic Press.

Bates, E., & Roe, K. (2001). Language development in children with unilateral brain injury. In C. A. Nelson & M. Luciana (Eds.), *Handbook of developmental cognitive neuroscience* (pp. 281–307). Cambridge, MA: MIT Press.

Bauman, M. L., & Kemper, T. L. (Eds.). (1994). *The neurobiology of autism.* Baltimore, MD: Johns Hopkins University Press.

Bauman-Waengler, J. (2000). *Articulatory and phonological impairments: A clinical focus.* Boston: Allyn & Bacon.

Bax, M., Cockerill, H., & Carroll-Few, L. (2001). Who needs augmentative and alternative communication and when? In L. Carroll-Few & H. Cockerill (Eds.), *Communication without speech: Practical communication for children* (pp. 65–72). Cambridge, UK: Mac Keith Press.

Bayley, N. (1993). *Bayley Scales of Infant Development Mental Development—Revised* (2nd ed.). San Antonio, TX: The Psychological Corporation.

Baynes, K., Kegl, J. A., Brentari, D., Kussmaul, C., & Poizner, H. (1998). Chronic auditory agnosia following Landau-Kleffner Syndrome: A 23 year outcome study. *Brain and Language, 63,* 381–425.

Bear, G. G., & Proctor, W. A. (1991). Self-perceptions of non-handicapped children and children with learning disabilities in integrated classes. *Journal of Special Education, 24,* 409–426.

Beaumanoir, A. (1992). The Landau-Kleffner syndrome. In J. Roger, C. Dravet, M. Bureau, F. E. Dreifuss, & P. Wolf (Eds.), *Epileptic syndromes in infancy, childhood and adolescence* (2nd ed., pp. 231–244). London, UK: John Libbey Eurotext.

Beautrais, A. (2000). Risk factors for suicide and attempted suicide among young people. *Australian & New Zealand Journal of Psychiatry, 34,* 420–436.

Becker-Bryant, J. (2001). Language in social contexts: Communicative competence in the preschool years. In J. Berko-Gleason (Ed.), *The development of language* (5th ed., pp. 213–253). Boston: Allyn & Bacon.

Bedore, L., & Leonard, L. (1995). Prosodic and syntactic bootstrapping and their applications: A tutorial. *American Journal of Speech-Language Pathology, 4,* 66–72.

Bedrosian, J., & Prutting, C. A. (1978). Communicative performance of mentally retarded adults in four conversational settings. *Journal of Speech and Hearing Research, 21,* 79–95.

Beisler, J. M., Tsai, L. Y., & Vonk, D. (1987). Comparisons between autistic and nonautistic children on the Test for Auditory Comprehension of Language. *Journal of Autism and Developmental Disorders, 17,* 95–102.

Beitchman, J., Adlaf, E., Douglas, L., Atkinson, L., Young, A., Johnson, C., et al. (2001). Comorbidity of psychiatric and substance use disorders in late adolescence: A cluster analysis approach. *American Journal of Drug and Alcohol Abuse, 27,* 421–440.

Beitchman, J., Brownlie, E., Inglis, A., Wild, J., Ferguson, B., Schachter, D., et al. (1996). Seven-year follow up of speech/language impaired and control children: Psychiatric outcome. *Journal of Child Psychology and Psychiatry, 37,* 961–970.

Beitchman, J., Wilson, B., Brownlie, E., Walters, H., & Lancee, W. (1996). Long-term consistency in speech/language profiles: I. Developmental and academic outcomes. *Journal of the American Academy of Child and Adolescent Psychiatry, 35,* 804–814.

Beitchman, J., Wilson, B., Brownlie, E., Walters, H., Inglis, A., & Lancee, W. (1996). Long-term consistency in speech/language profiles: II. Behavioral, emotional, and social outcomes. *Journal of the American Academy of Child and Adolescent Psychiatry, 35,* 815–825.

Beitchman, J., Wilson, B., Douglas, L., Young, A., & Adlaf, E. (2001). Substance use disorders in young adults with and without LD: Predictive and concurrent relationships. *Journal of Learning Disabilities, 34,* 317–332.

Beitchman, J., Wilson, B., Johnson, C., Atkinson, L., Young, A., Adlaf, E., et al. (2001). Fourteen-year follow up of speech/language-impaired and control children: Psychiatric outcome. *Journal of the American Academy of Child and Adolescent Psychiatry, 40,* 75–82.

Belenchia, T., & Crowe, T. (1983). Prevalence of speech and hearing disorders in a state penitentiary population. *Journal of Communication Disorders, 16,* 293–300.

Bender, W., Rosenkrans, C., & Crane, M. (1999). Stress, depression, and suicide among students with learning disabilities: Assessing the risk. *Learning Disability Quarterly, 22*(2), 143–156.

Benedict, H. (1979). Early lexical development: Comprehension and production. *Journal of Child Language, 6,* 183–200.

Bennett, F. S., Ruuska, S. H., & Sherman, R. (1980). Middle ear effusion in learning disabled children. *Pediatrics, 66,* 254–260.

Bennett-Gates, D., & Zigler, E. (1998). Resolving the developmental-difference debate: An evaluation of the triarchic and systems theory models. In J. A. Burack, R. M. Hodapp, & E. F. Zigler (Eds.), *Handbook of mental retardation and development* (pp. 115–131). New York: Cambridge University Press.

Berger, J., & Cunningham, C. C. (1983). Development of early vocal behaviors and interactions in Down's syndrome and nonhandicapped infant-mother pairs. *Developmental Psychology, 19,* 322–331.

Berko, J. (1958). The child's learning of English morphology. *Word, 14,* 150–177.

Berko-Gleason, J. (Ed.). (2001). *The development of language* (5th ed.). Boston: Allyn & Bacon.

Berko-Gleason, J., & Weintraub, S. (1978). Input language and the acquisition of communicative competence. In K. Nelson (Ed.), *Children's language* (Vol. 1). New York: Gardner Press.

Berlin, C. (2000). *Managing patients with auditory neuropathy/auditory dys-synchrony.* Retrieved July 17, 2003, from www.medschool.lsumc.edu/otor/dys.html

Berlin, C., Bordelon, J., St. John, P., Wilensky, D., Hurley, A., Kluka, E., & Hood, L. (1998). Reversing click polarity may uncover auditory neuropathy in infants. *Ear and Hearing, 19,* 37–47.

Bernstein, D., & Levey, S. (2002). Language development: A review. In D. K. Bernstein & E. Tiergerman-Faber (Eds.), *Language and communication disorders in children* (5th ed., pp. 27–94). Boston: Allyn & Bacon.

Bernstein, D., & Tiegerman-Farber, E. (1997). *Language and communication disorders in children* (4th ed.). Boston: Allyn & Bacon.

Berry, P. (1972). Comprehension of possessive and present continuous sentences by non-retarded, mildly retarded, and severely retarded children. *American Journal of Mental Deficiency, 76,* 540–544.

Bess, F. H., Klee, T., & Culbertson, J. L. (1986). Identification, assessment and management of children with unilateral sensorineural hearing loss. *Ear and Hearing, 7,* 43–51.

Bess, F. H., & Tharpe, A. M. (1988). Performance and management of children with unilateral sensorineural hearing loss. *Scandinavian Audiology.* Suppl., *30,* 75–79.

Bettelheim, B. (1967). *The empty fortress: Infantile autism and the birth of the self.* New York: Free Press.

Beukelman, D., McGinnis, J., & Morrow, D. (1991). Vocabulary selection in augmentative and alternative communication. *Augmentative and Alternative Communication, 7*(3), 171–185.

Beukelman, D., & Mirenda, P. (1998). *Augmentative and alternative communication: management of severe communication disorders in children and adults* (2nd ed.). Baltimore, MD: Paul H. Brookes.

Beveridge, M. (1976). Patterns of interaction in the mentally handicapped. In P. Berry (Ed.), *Language and communication in the mentally handicapped.* Baltimore, MD: University Park Press.

Bidder, R., Bryant, G., & Gray, O. (1975). Benefits to Down's syndrome children through training their mothers. *Archives of Disease in Childhood, 50,* 383–386.

Bigelow, B. (2000). Delinquency. *Current Opinion in Psychiatry, 13,* 64–70.

Biklen, D. (1990). Communication unbound: Autism and praxis. *Harvard Educational Review, 60,* 291–314.

Bishop, D. V. M. (1985). Age of onset and outcome in "acquired aphasia with convulsive disorders." *Developmental Medicine and Child Neurology, 27,* 705–712.

Bishop, D. V. M. (1989). Autism, Asperger's syndrome and semantic-pragmatic disorder: Where are the boundaries? *British Journal of Disorders of Communication, 24,* 107–121.

Bishop, D. V. M. (1994). Grammatical errors in specific language impairment: Competence or performance limitations? *Applied Psycholinguistics, 15,* 507–550.

Bishop, D. V. M. (1997). *Uncommon understanding: Development and disorders of language comprehension in children.* East Sussex, UK: Psychology Press.

Bishop, D. V. M., Byers Brown, B., & Robson, J. (1990). The relationship between phoneme discrimination, speech production, and language comprehension in cerebral-palsied individuals. *Journal of Speech and Hearing Research, 33,* 210–219.

Bishop, D., & Edmundson, A. (1987). Language-impaired 4-year-olds: Distinguishing transient from persistent impairment. *Journal of Speech and Hearing Disorders, 52,* 156–173.

Bishop, D. V. M., North, T., & Donlon, C. (1995). Genetic basis of specific language impairment: Evidence from a twin study. *Developmental Medicine and Child Neurology, 37,* 56–71.

Bishop, D. V. M., Price, T., Dale, P., & Plomin, R. (2003). Outcomes of early language delay: II. Etiology of transient and persistent language difficulties. *Journal of Speech, Language, and Hearing Research, 46,* 561–575.

Blachman, B. (1984). Relationship of rapid naming ability and language analysis skills in kindergarten and first-grade reading achievement. *Journal of Educational Psychology, 76,* 610–622.

Black, B., & Hazen, N. (1990). Social status and patterns of communication in acquainted and unacquainted preschool children. *Developmental Psychology, 26,* 379–387.

Black, B., & Logan, A. (1995). Links between communication patterns in mother-child, father-child, and child-peer interactions and children's social status. *Child Development, 66,* 255–271.

Blackman, J. A. (2000). Attention-deficit/hyperactivity disorder in preschoolers. *Pediatric Clinics of North America, 46,* 1011–1025.

Blagden, C., & McConnell, N. (1984). *Interpersonal language skills assessment.* Moline, IL: LinguiSystems.

Blake, A. (1992). Speech-language pathologists in schools. *Asha, 34,* 82.

Blamey, P., Sarant, J. Z., Paatsch, L. E., Barry, J. G., Bow, C. P., Wales, R. J., et al. (2001). Relationships among speech perception, production, language, hearing loss, and age in children with impaired hearing. *Journal of Speech, Language, and Hearing Research, 44*(2), 264–285.

Blank, M. (1990). Sentence master [computer program]. Winooski, VT: Laureate Learning.

Blank, M., Rose, S., & Berlin, L. (1978). *Preschool Language Assessment Instrument (PLAI).* San Antonio, TX: Psychological Corporation.

Bleile, K., McGowan, J., & Bernthal, J. (1997). Professional judgements about the relationship between speech and intelligence in African American preschoolers. *Journal of Communication Disorders, 30*(5), 367–383.

Bleile, K., & Schwarz, I. (1984). Three perspectives on the speech of children with Down's syndrome. *Journal of Communication Disorders, 17,* 87–94.

Bleile, K., & Wallach, H. (1992). A sociolinguistic investigation of the speech of African-American preschoolers. *American Journal of Speech-Language Pathology, 1,* 44–52.

Blischak, D., & Lloyd, L. (1996). Multimodal augmentative and alternative communication: Case study. *Augmentative and Alternative Communication, 12*(1), 37–46.

Blischak, D., Lombardino, L. J., & Dyson, A. T. (2003). Use of speech-generating devices: In support of natural speech. *Augmentative and Alternative Communication, 19,* 29–35.

Bliss, C. K. (1965). *Semantography.* Sydney, Australia: Semantography (Blissymbolics).

Bliss, L., Allen, D., & Walker, G. (1978). Sentence structures of trainable and educable mentally retarded subjects. *Journal of Speech and Hearing Research, 21,* 722–731.

Bloom, L. (1970). *Language development: Form and function in emerging grammars.* Cambridge, MA: MIT Press.

Bloom, L. (1973). *One word at a time: The use of single-word utterances before syntax.* The Hague: Mouton.

Bloom, L. (1988). What is language? In M. Lahey (Ed.), *Language disorders and language development.* Columbus, OH: Merrill/Macmillan.

Bloom, L., & Lahey, M. (1978). *Language development and language disorders.* New York: Macmillan.

Bloom, L., Lahey, M., Hood, L., Lifter, K., & Fiess, K. (1980). Complex sentences: Acquisition of syntactic connectives and the semantic relations they encode. *Journal of Child Language, 7,* 235–262.

Bloom, L., Lightbown, P., & Hood, L. (1974). Structure and variation in child language. *Monographs for the Society for Research on Child Development, 40*(2), 1–97.

Bloom, L., Rocissano, L., & Hood, L. (1976). Adult-child discourse: Developmental interaction between information processing and linguistic knowledge. *Cognitive Psychology, 8,* 521–552.

Blosser, J., & DePompei, R. (1994). *Pediatric traumatic brain injury.* San Diego, CA: Singular.

Bochner, S., Price, P., & Jones, J. (1997). *Child language development: Learning to talk.* London, UK: Whurr.

Bock, J., & Loebell, H. (1990). Framing sentences. *Cognition, 35,* 1–39.

Bock, J., Loebell, H., & Morey, R. (1992). From conceptual roles to structural relations: Bridging the syntactic cleft. *Psychological Review, 99,* 150–171.

Bolton, P., Pickles, A., Murphy, M., & Rutter, M. (1998). Autism, affective and other psychiatric disorders: Patterns of familial aggregation. *Psychological Medicine, 28,* 385–395.

Bondy, A., & Frost, L. (1994). The Picture Exchange Communciation System. *Topics in Language Disorders, 19,* 373–390.

Boone, D. R. (1985). Disorders of language in adults. In P. Skinner & R. Shelton (Eds.), *Speech, language, and hearing: Normal processes and disorders* (2nd ed.). New York: Wiley.

Boone, D. R., & McFarlane, S. C. (2000). *The voice and voice therapy* (6th ed.). Boston: Allyn & Bacon.

Boothroyd, A. (1982). *Hearing impairments in young children.* Englewood Cliffs, NJ: Prentice-Hall.

Boothroyd, A. (1993). Profound Deafness. In R. Tyler (Ed.), *Cochlear Implants.* San Diego, CA: Singular.

Bornstein, M., Haynes, O., Painter, K., & Genevro, J. (2000). Child language with mother and with stranger at home and in the laboratory: A methodological study. *Journal of Child Language, 27,* 407–420.

Bouchard, D., & Tetreault, S. (2000). The motor development of sighted children and children with moderate low vision aged 8–13. *Journal of Visual Impairment and Blindness, 94*(9), 564–573.

Boudreau, D., & Chapman, R. S. (2000). The relationship between event representation and linguistic skill in narratives of children and adolescents with Down syndrome. *Journal of Speech and Hearing Research, 43*(5), 1146–1159.

Boudreau, D., & Hedberg, N. (1999). A comparison of early literacy skills in children with specific language impairment and their typically developing peers. *American Journal of Speech-Language Pathology, 8,* 249–260.

Bountress, N., & Richards, J. (1979). Speech, language, and hearing disorders in an adult penal institution. *Journal of Speech and Hearing Disorders, 44,* 293–300.

Bower, A., & Hayes, A. (1994). Short term memory deficits and Down syndrome: A comparative study. *Down Syndrome: Research and Practice, 2*(2), 47–50.

Bowers, L., Huisingh, R., Barrett, M., Orman, J., & LoGiudice, C. (1991). *Test of Problem Solving—Adolescent.* East Moline, IL: LinguiSystems.

Bowers, L., Huisingh, R., Orman, J., & LoGiudice, C. (1998). *The Expressive Language Test.* East Moline, IL: LinguiSystems.

Boyce, N., & Larson, V. (1983). *Adolescents' communication: Development and disorders.* Eau Claire, WI: Thinking Publications.

Bracken, B., & McCallum, R. S. (1998). *Universal Nonverbal Intelligence Test (UNIT).* Itasca, IL: Riverside Publishing.

Braden, J. P. (1994). *Deafness, deprivation and IQ.* London, UK: Plenum Press.

Brady, N. C., & Halle, J. W. (2002). Breakdowns and repairs in conversations between beginning AAC users and their partners. In J. Reichle, D. Beukelman, & J. Light (Eds.), *Exemplary practices for beginning AAC users and their partners* (pp. 323–352). Baltimore, MD: Paul H. Brookes.

Branigan, G. (1979). Some reasons why successive single word utterances are not. *Journal of Child Language, 6,* 411–421.

Bray, C. (1995). Developing study, organization, and management strategies for adolescents with language disabilities. *Seminars in Speech and Language, 16*(1), 65–83.

Brice, A. (2001). *The Hispanic child: Speech, language, culture, and education.* Boston: Allyn & Bacon.

Brice, A., & Anderson, R. (1999). Code mixing in a young bilingual child. *Communication Disorders Quarterly, 21*(1), 17–22.

Brinton, B., & Fujiki, M. (1982). A comparison of request-response sequences in the discourse of normal and language-disordered children. *Journal of Speech and Hearing Disorders, 47,* 57–62.

Brinton, B., & Fujiki, M. (1984). Development of topic manipulation skills in discourse. *Journal of Speech and Hearing Research, 27,* 350–357.

Brinton, B., Fujiki, M., & McKee, L. (1998). Negotiation skills of children with specific language impairment. *Journal of Speech, Language, and Hearing Research, 41,* 927–940.

Bristol, M. M., Cohen, D. J., Costello, E. J., Denckla, M., Eckberg, T. J., Kallen, R., et al. (1996). State of the science in autism: Report to the National Institutes of Health. *Journal of Autism and Developmental Disorders, 26,* 121–154.

Broder, H., Richman, L., & Matheson, P. (1998). Learning disability, school achievement, and grade retention among children with cleft: A two-center study. *Cleft Palate-Craniofacial Journal, 35,* 127–131.

Brody, L. E., & Mills, C. J. (1997). Gifted children with learning disabilities: A review of the issues. *Journal of Learning Disabilities, 30*(3), 282–286.

Broen, P. (1972). The verbal environment of the language learning child. *Monographs of the American Speech and Hearing Association, 17.*

Broen, P., Devers, M., Doyle, S., Prouty, J., & Moller, K. (1998). Acquisition of linguistic and cognitive skills by children with cleft palate. *Journal of Speech, Language, and Hearing Research, 41,* 676–700.

Broen, P., Doyle, S., Moller, K., & Prouty, J. (1991, November). Early language development in children with cleft palate. Paper presented at the Annual Convention of the American Speech-Language-Hearing Association, Atlanta, GA.

Brookshire, B. L., Chapman, S. B., Song, J., & Levin, H. S. (2000). Cognitive and linguistic correlates of children's discourse after closed head injury: A three-year follow-up. *Journal of the International Neuropsychological Society, 6*(7), 741–751.

Brophy, J., & Good, T. (1974). *Teacher–student relationships.* New York: Holt, Rinehart & Winston.

Brown, B. B., & Edwards, M. (1989). *Developmental Disorders of Language.* London, UK: Whurr.

Brown, F. (1991). Creative daily scheduling: A nonintrusive approach to challenging behaviors in community residences. *Journal of the Association for Persons with Severe Handicaps, 16*(2), 75–84.

Brown, L., Sherbenou, R., & Johnsen, S. (1997). *Test of Nonverbal Intelligence—3.* Austin, TX: Pro-Ed.

Brown, R. (1973). *A first language: The early stages.* Cambridge, MA: Harvard University Press.

Brown-Chidsey, R., & Boscardin, M. L. (1999). *Computers as accessibility tools for students with and without learning disabilities.* Amherst: University of Massachusetts.

Brownell, R. (2000a). *Expressive One-Word Picture Vocabulary Test—2000.* Novato, CA: Academic Therapy Publications.

Brownell, R. (2000b). *Receptive One-Word Picture Vocabulary Test—2000.* Novato, CA: Academic Therapy Publications.

Bruno, J., & Dribbon, M. (1998). Outcomes in AAC: Evaluating the effectiveness of a parent training program. *Augmentative and Alternative Communication, 14*(2), 59–70.

Bryan, T., Donahue, M., & Pearl, R. (1981). Learning disabled children's peer interactions during a small-group problem-solving task. *Learning Disability Quarterly, 4,* 13–22.

Bryant, J. (2001). Language in social contexts: Communicative competence in the preschool years. In J. Berko-Gleason (Ed.), *The development of language* (5th ed., pp. 213–253). Boston: Allyn & Bacon.

Bryson, S. E. (1997). Epidemiology of autism: Overview and issues outstanding. In D. J. Cohen & F. R. Volkmar (Eds.), *Handbook of autism and pervasive developmental disorders* (2nd ed., pp. 41–46). New York: Wiley.

Buckley, S. (1993). Language development in children with Down's syndrome: Reasons for optimism. *Down Syndrome: Research and Practice, 1,* 3–9.

Buckley, S. (1995). Improving the expressive language skills of teenagers with Down's syndrome. *Down Syndrome: Research and Practice 3,* 110–115.

Buckley, S., & Bird, G. (1993). Teaching children with Down's syndrome to read. *Down Syndrome: Research and Practice, 1,* 34–39.

Buffington, D. M., Krantz, P. J., Poulson, C. L., & McClannahan, L. E. (1998). Procedures for teaching appropriate gestural communication skills to children with autism. *Journal of Autism and Developmental Disorders, 28,* 535–545.

Buium, N., Rynders, J., & Turnure, J. (1974). Early maternal linguistic environment of normal and Down's syndrome language-learning children. *American Journal of Mental Deficiency, 79,* 52–58.

Bunce, B. (1995). *Building a language-focused curriculum for the preschool classroom: A planning guide* (Vol. II). Baltimore, MD: Paul H. Brookes.

Bunch, G. W., & Melnyk, T. (1989). A review of the evidence for a learning-disabled, hearing-impaired sub-group. *American Annals of the Deaf, 134,* 297–300.

Burack, J. A. (1990). Differentiating mental retardation: The two-group approach and beyond. In R. M. Hodapp, J. A. Burack, & E. Zigler (Eds.), *Issues in the developmental approach to mental retardation* (pp. 27–48). New York: Cambridge University Press.

Burd, L., Gascon, G., Swenson, R., & Hankey, R. (1990). Crossed aphasia in early childhood. *Developmental Medicine and Child Neurology, 32,* 539–546.

Burgemeister, B., Blum, L., & Lorge, I. (1971). *Columbia Mental Maturity Scale* (3rd ed.). San Antonio, TX: Psychological Corporation.

Buschbacher, P. W., & Fox, L. (2003). Understanding and intervening with the challenging behavior of young children with autism spectrum disorder. *Language, Speech, and Hearing Services in Schools, 34,* 217–227.

Butt, J., & Benjamin, C. (2000). *A new reference grammar of modern Spanish* (3rd ed.). London, UK: Edward Arnold.

Butterfield, N., Arthur, M., Linfoot, K., & Phillips, S. (1992). *Creating Communicative Contexts: An instruction manual for teachers of students with severe intellectual disability.* Sydney, Australia: NSW Department of School Education.

Butterfield, N., Arthur, M., & Sigafoos, J. (1995). *Partners in everyday communicative exchanges.* Sydney, Australia: Maclennan & Petty.

Buttrill, J., Niizawa, J., Biemer, C., Takahashi, C., & Hearn, S. (1989). Serving the language learning disabled adolescent: A strategies-based model. *Language, Speech, and Hearing Services in Schools, 20,* 185–203.

Buzolich, M. J., & Lunger, J. (1995). Empowering system users in peer training. *Augmentative and Alternative Communication, 11*(1), 37–45.

Bybee, J., & Zigler, E. (1999). Outerdirectedness in individuals with and without mental retardation: A review. In E. Zigler & D. Bennett-Gates (Eds.), *Personality development in individuals with mental retardation* (pp. 165–205). Cambridge, UK: Cambridge University Press.

Byrne, A., Buckley, S., MacDonald, J., & Bird, G. (1995). Investigating the literacy, language and memory skills of children with Down's syndrome. *Down Syndrome: Research and Practice, 3,* 53–58.

Byrne, K., Abbeduto, L., & Brooks, P. (1990). The language of children with spina bifida and hydrocephalus: Meeting task demands and mastering syntax. *Journal of Speech and Hearing Disorders, 55,* 118–123.

Byrne, S., Constance, A., & Moore, G. (1992). Making transitions from school to work. *Educational Leadership, 49*(6), 23–26.

Bzoch, K., & League, R. (1991). *Receptive-Expressive Emergent Language Test* (2nd ed.). Austin, TX: Pro-Ed.

Cacace, A. T., & McFarland, D. J. (1998). Central auditory processing disorder in school-aged children: A critical review. *Journal of Speech, Language, and Hearing Research, 41*(2), 355–373.

Calculator, S. N. (1988). Promoting the acquisition and generalization of conversational skills by individuals with severe disabilities. *Augmentative and Alternative Communication, 4*(2), 94–103.

Calculator, S. N. (1997). Fostering early language acquisition and AAC use: Exploring reciprocal influences between children and their environments. *Augmentative and Alternative Communication, 13*(3), 149–157.

Calculator, S. N. (1999). Look who's pointing now: Cautions related to the clinical use of facilitated communication. *Language, Speech, and Hearing Services in Schools, 30*(4), 408–414.

Calculator, S. N., & Dollaghan, C. (1982). The use of communication boards in a residential setting: An evaluation. *Journal of Speech and Hearing Disorders, 47,* 281–287.

Calderon, R., & Greenberg, M. (1997). The effectiveness of early intervention for deaf children and children with hearing loss. In M. Guralnik (Ed.), *The effectiveness of early intervention* (pp. 455–482). Baltimore, MD: Paul H. Brookes.

Calhoon, M., & Fuchs, L. (2003). The effects of peer-assisted learning strategies and curriculum-based measurement on the mathematics performance of secondary students with disabilities. *Remedial and Special Education, 24,* 235–245.

California Birth Defects Monitoring Program. (2002). *Oral clefts: Racial/ethnic variation.* Retrieved December 2, 2002, from www.cbdmp.org/bd_clefts_racial.htm

Camarata, S., Hughes, C., & Ruhl, K. (1988). Mild/moderate behaviorally disordered students: A population at-risk for language problems. *Language, Speech, and Hearing Services in Schools, 19,* 191–200.

Camarata, S., & Nelson, K. (1992). Treatment efficiency as a function of target selection in the remediation of child language disorders. *Clinical Linguistics and Phonetics, 6,* 167–178.

Camarata, S., Nelson, K., & Camarata, M. (1994). Comparison of conversational recasting and imitative procedures in children with specific language impairment. *Journal of Speech and Hearing Research, 37,* 1414–1423.

Camarata, S., & Schwartz, R. (1985). Production of object words and action words: Evidence for a relationship between phonology and semantics. *Journal of Speech and Hearing Research, 28,* 323–330.

Campbell, T., & Dollaghan, C. (1990). Expressive language recovery in severely brain-injured children and adolescents. *Journal of Speech and Hearing Disorders, 55,* 567–581.

Campbell, T., Dollaghan, C., Needleman, H., & Janosky, J. (1997). Reducing bias in language assessment: Processing-dependent measures. *Journal of Speech, Language, and Hearing Research, 40,* 519–525.

Cantwell, D., & Baker, L. (1991). *Psychiatric and developmental disorders in children with communication disorder.* Washington, DC: American Psychiatric Press.

Caplan, P. J., & Kinsbourne, M. (1974). Sex differences in response to school failure. *Journal of Learning Disabilities, 7,* 232–235.

Capute, A., Palmer, F., Shapiro, B., Wachtel, R., Schmidt, S., & Ross, A. (1986). Clinical linguistic and auditory milestone scale: Prediction of cognition in infancy. *Developmental Medicine and Child Neurology, 28,* 762–771.

Cardoso-Martins, C., & Mervis, C. B. (1985). Maternal speech to prelinguistic children with Down syndrome. *American Journal of Mental Deficiency, 89,* 451–458.

Cardoso-Martins, C., Mervis, C. B., & Mervis, C. A. (1985). Early vocabulary acquisition by children with Down syndrome. *American Journal of Mental Deficiency, 90,* 177–184.

Carlisle, J., & Chang, V. (1996). Evaluation of academic capabilities in science by students with and without learning disabilities and their teachers. *Journal of Special Education, 30*(1), 18–34.

Carlson, N. R. (1987). *Psychology: The science of behaviour* (2nd ed.). Boston: Allyn & Bacon.

Carneol, S., Marks, S., & Weik, L. (1999). The speech-language pathologist: Key role in the diagnosis of velocardiofacial syndrome. *American Journal of Speech-Language Pathology, 8,* 23–32.

Carr, D., & Felce, D. (2000). Application of stimulus equivalence to language intervention for individuals with severe linguistic disabilities. *Journal of Intellectual and Developmental Disability, 25,* 181–205.

Carr, E. G., & Durand, V. M. (1985). Reducing behavior problems through functional communication training. *Journal of Applied Behavior Analysis, 18,* 111–126.

Carr, E. G., & Kemp, D. C. (1989). Functional equivalence of autistic leading and communicative pointing: Analysis and treatment. *Journal of Autism and Developmental Disorders, 19,* 561–578.

Carr, E. G., Kologinsky, E., & Leff-Simon, S. (1987). Acquisition of sign language by autistic children III: Generalized descriptive phrases. *Journal of Autism and Developmental Disorders, 17,* 217–229.

Carr, E. G., Levin, L., McConnachie, G., Carlson, J. I., Kemp, D. C., & Smith, C. E. (1994). *Communication-based intervention for problem behavior.* Baltimore, MD: Paul H. Brookes.

Carr, J. (1995). *Down's syndrome: Children growing up.* New York: Cambridge University Press.

Carrow, E. (1973). *Test for Auditory Comprehension of Language.* Austin, TX: Learning Concepts.

Carrow-Woolfolk, E. (1996). *Oral and Written Language Scales.* Circle Pines, MN: American Guidance.

Carrow-Woolfolk, E. (1998). *Comprehensive Assessment of Spoken Language.* Circle Pines, MN: American Guidance.

Carrow-Woolfolk, E., & Lynch, J. (1982). *An integrative approach to language disorders in children.* New York: Grune & Stratton.

Carter, M., Hotchkis, G., & Cassar, M. (1996). Spontaneity of augmentative and alternative communication in persons with intellectual disabilities: A critical review. *Augmentative and Alternative Communication, 12,* 97–109.

Casby, M. (1997). Symbolic play of children with language impairment. *Journal of Speech, Language, and Hearing Research, 40,* 468–479.

Castrogiovanni, A. (2002). Special populations: Prison populations—2002 edition. Rockville, MD: American Speech-Language-Hearing Association.

Catroppa, C., & Anderson, V. (1999). Recovery of educational skills following pediatric head-injury. *Pediatric Rehabilitation, 3*(4), 167–175.

Catroppa, C., & Anderson, V. (2003). Children's attentional skills 2 years posttraumatic brain injury. *Developmental Neuropsychology, 23,* 359–373.

Catts, H. (1986). Speech production/phonological deficits in reading-disordered children. *Journal of Learning Disabilities, 19,* 504–508.

Catts, H. (1989). Speech production deficits in developmental dyslexia. *Journal of Speech and Hearing Disorders, 54,* 422–428.

Catts, H. (1991). Phonological processing deficits and reading disabilities. In A. Kamhi & H. Catts (Eds.), *Reading disabilities: A developmental language perspective.* Boston: Allyn & Bacon.

Catts, H. (1997). The early identification of language-based reading disabilities. *Language, Speech, and Hearing Services in Schools, 28,* 86–89.

Catts, H., Fey, M., Tomblin, J. B., & Zhang, X. (2002). A longitudinal investigation of reading outcomes in children with language impairments. *Journal of Speech, Language, and Hearing Research, 45,* 1142–1157.

Catts, H., Fey, M., Zhang, X., & Tomblin, J. B. (2001). Estimating the risk of future reading difficulties in kindergarten children: A research-based model and its clinical implications. *Language, Speech, and Hearing Services in Schools, 32,* 38–50.

Catts, H., & Kamhi, A. (Eds.). (1999). *Language and reading disabilities.* Boston: Allyn & Bacon.

Ceponiene, R., Hukki, J., Cheour, M., Haapanen, M., Koskinen, M., Alho, K., & Naatanen, R. (2000). Dysfunction of the auditory cortex persists in infants with certain cleft types. *Developmental Medicine and Child Neurology, 42,* 258–265.

Ceponiene, R., Hukki, J., Cheour, M., Haapanen, M., Ranta, R., & Naatanen, R. (1999). Cortical auditory dysfunction in children with oral clefts: Relation with cleft types. *Clinical Neurophysiology, 110,* 1921–1926.

Chan, J., & Iacono, T. (2001). Gesture and word production in children with Down syndrome. *Augmentative & Alternative Communication, 17,* 73–87.

Channell, R. (1998). GramCats (Version 1.0) [MS-DOS computer software]. Provo, UT: Department of Audiology and Speech-Language Pathology, Brigham Young University.

Channell, R., & Johnson, B. (1999). Automated grammatical tagging of child language samples. *Journal of Speech, Language, and Hearing Research, 42,* 727–734.

Chao, R. (1996). Chinese and European American mothers' beliefs about the role of parenting in children's school success. *Journal of Cross-Cultural Psychology, 27,* 403–423.

Chapman, K., Hardin-Jones, M., & Halter, K. (2003). The relationship between early speech and later speech and language performance for children with cleft lip and palate. *Clinical Linguistics and Phonetics, 17,* 173–197.

Chapman, R. (1981). Exploring children's communicative intents. In J. Miller (Ed.), *Assessing language production in children: Experimental procedures* (pp. 111–138). Boston: Allyn & Bacon.

Chapman, R., & Hesketh, L. J. (2001). Language, cognition, and short-term memory in individuals with Down syndrome. *Down Syndrome: Research and Practice, 7,* 1–7.

Chapman, R., Kay-Raining Bird, E., & Schwartz, S. E. (1990). Fast mapping of words in event contexts by children with Down syndrome. *Journal of Speech and Hearing Disorders, 55,* 761–770.

Chapman, R., Schwartz, S. E., & Kay-Raining Bird, E. (1991). Language skills of children and adolescents with Down syndrome: I. Comprehension. *Journal of Speech and Hearing Research, 34,* 1106–1120.

Chapman, R., Seung, H. K., Schwartz, S. E., & Kay-Raining Bird, E. (1998). Language skills of children and adolescents with Down syndrome: II. Production deficits. *Journal of Speech, Language, and Hearing Research, 41*(4), 861–873.

Chapman, S. B., Levin, H. S., Wanek, A., Weyrauch, J., & Kufera, J. (1998). Discourse after closed head injury in young children. *Brain and Language, 61*(3), 420–449.

Chen, D. (1996). Parent-infant communication: Early intervention for very young children with visual impairment or hearing loss. *Infants and Young Children, 9,* 1–13.

Cheng, L. L. (1987a). *Assessment and remediation of Asian language populations.* Rockville, MD: Aspen.

Cheng, L. L. (1987b). Cross-cultural and linguistic considerations in working with Asian populations. *Asha, 29,* 33–38.

Cheng, L. L. (1998). *Enhancing the communication skills of newly-arrived Asian American students.* Retrieved December 2, 2002, from http://ericcass.uncg.edu/virtuallib/diversity/1026.html

Chomsky, N. (1957). *Syntactic structures.* The Hague: Mouton.

Chomsky, N. (1965). *Aspects of the theory of syntax.* Cambridge, MA: MIT Press.

Chomsky, N. (1981). *Lectures on government and binding.* Dordrecht, The Netherlands: Foris.

Choudhury, N., & Benasich, A. (2003). A family aggregation study: The influence of family history and other risk factors on language development. *Journal of Speech, Language, and Hearing Research, 46,* 261–272.

Cipani, E. (1989). Providing language consultation in the natural context: A model for delivery of services. *Mental Retardation, 27,* 317–324.

Cirrin, F. M. (1991). Issues in determining eligibility for service: Who does what to whom? In A. Kamhi & H. Catts (Eds.), *Reading disabilities: A developmental language perspective* (pp. 345–368). Boston: Allyn & Bacon.

Clahsen, H. (1989). The grammatical characterization of developmental dysphasia. *Linguistics, 27,* 897–920.

Clarkson, R., Eimas, P., & Marean, G. (1989). Speech perception in children with histories of recurrent otitis media. *Journal of the Acoustical Society of America, 85,* 926–933.

Cleave, P., & Fey, M. (1997). Two approaches to the facilitation of grammar in children with language impairments: Rationale and description. *American Journal of Speech-Language Pathology, 6,* 22–32.

Clements, S. D. (1966). *Minimal brain dysfunction in children: Terminology and identification.* Washington, DC: U.S. Department of Health, Education, and Welfare.

Cline, S., & Schwartz, D. (1999). *Diverse populations of gifted children.* Columbus, OH: Prentice-Hall.

Cockerill, H., & Fuller, P. (2001). Assessing children for augmentative and alternative communication. In L. Carroll-Few & H. Cockerill (Eds.), *Communication without speech: Practical communication for children* (pp. 73–87). Cambridge, UK: Mac Keith Press.

Coggins, T. (1979). Relational meaning encoded in the two-word utterances of Stage I Down's syndrome children. *Journal of Speech and Hearing Research, 22,* 166–178.

Coggins, T. (1991). Bringing context back into assessment. *Topics in Language Disorders, 11,* 43–54.

Coggins, T., Carpenter, R., & Owings, N. O. (1983). Examining early intentional communication in Down's syndrome and nonretarded children. *British Journal of Disorders of Communication, 18,* 98–106.

Coggins, T., & Frederickson, R. (1988). Brief report: The communicative role of a highly frequent repeated utterance in the conversations of an autistic boy. *Journal of Autism and Developmental Disorders, 18,* 687–694.

Coggins, T., Friet, T., & Morgan, T. (1998). Analysing narrative productions in older school-age children and adolescents with fetal alcohol syndrome: An experimental tool for clinical applications. *Clinical Linguistics and Phonetics, 12,* 221–236.

Coggins, T., & Morrison, J. A. (1981). Spontaneous imitations of Down's syndrome children: A lexical analysis. *Journal of Speech and Hearing Research, 24,* 303–308.

Coggins, T., Olswang, L., & Guthrie, J. (1987). Assessing communicative intents in young children: Low structured observation or elicitation tasks? *Journal of Speech and Hearing Disorders, 52,* 44–49.

Coggins, T., & Stoel-Gammon, C. (1982). Clarification strategies used by four Down's syndrome children for maintaining normal conversational interaction. *Education and Training of the Mentally Retarded, 17,* 65–67.

Cohen, L. M. (1990). *Meeting the needs of gifted and talented minority language students.* Retrieved July 2002, from www.ed.gov/databases/ERIC_Digests/ed321485.html.

Cohen, N., Davine, M., Horodezky, N., Lipsett, L., & Isaacson, L. (1993). Unsuspected language impairments in psychiatrically disturbed children: Prevalence and language behavioral characteristics. *Journal of the American Academy of Child and Adolescent Psychiatry, 32,* 595–603.

Cohen, S. B., Joyce, C. M., Rhoades, K. W., & Welks, D. M. (1985). Educational programming for head injured students. In M. Ylvisaker (Ed.), *Head injury rehabilitation: Children and adolescents.* Austin, TX: Pro-Ed.

Cole, E., & Paterson, M. (1984). Assessment and treatment of phonologic disorders in the hearing impaired. In J. Castello (Ed.), *Speech disorders in children.* San Diego, CA: College Hill Press.

Cole, K. (1995). Curriculum models and language facilitation in the preschool years. In M. Fey, J. Windsor, & S. Warren (Eds.), *Language intervention: Preschool through the elementary years* (Vol. 5, pp. 39–60). Baltimore, MD: Paul H. Brookes.

Cole, K., & Dale, P. (1986). Direct language instruction and interactive language instruction with language delayed preschool children: A comparison study. *Journal of Speech and Hearing Research, 29,* 206–217.

Cole, K., Mills, P., & Kelley, D. (1994). Agreement of assessment profiles used in cognitive referencing. *Language, Speech, and Hearing Services in Schools, 25,* 25–31.

Cole, K., Schwartz, I., Notari, A., Dale, P., & Mills, P. (1995). Examination of the stability of two methods of defining specific language impairment. *Applied Psycholinguistics, 16,* 103–123.

Comkowycz, S. M., Ehren, B. J., & Hayes, N. H. (1987). Meeting classroom needs of language disordered students in middle and junior high schools: A program model. *Journal of Childhood Communication Disorders, 11,* 199–208.

Connell, P. (1986). Teaching subjecthood to language-disordered children. *Journal of Speech and Hearing Research, 29,* 481–493.

Connell, P. (1987). An effect of modeling and imitation teaching procedures on children with and without specific language impairment. *Journal of Speech and Hearing Research, 30,* 105–113.

Connell, P. (1989). Facilitating generalization through induction teaching. In L. McReynolds & J. Spradlin (Eds.), *Generalization strategies in the treatment of communication disorders.* Philadelphia: B. C. Decker.

Connell, P., & Stone, C. (1992). Morpheme learning of children with specific language impairment under controlled instructional conditions. *Journal of Speech and Hearing Research, 35,* 844–852.

Connor, D. F. (2002). Preschool attention deficit hyperactivity disorder: A review of prevalence, diagnosis, neurobiology, and stimulant treatment. *Journal of Developmental and Behavioral Pediatrics, 23,* S1–S9.

Constable, C. (1986). The application of scripts in the organization of language intervention contexts. In K. Nelson (Ed.), *Event knowledge: Structure and functions in development* (pp. 205–230). Hillsdale, NJ: Lawrence Erlbaum.

Conti-Ramsden, G. (1990). Maternal recasts and other contingent replies to language-impaired children. *Journal of Speech and Hearing Disorders, 55,* 262–274.

Conti-Ramsden, G. (2003). Processing and linguistic markers in young children with specific language impairment (SLI). *Journal of Speech, Language, and Hearing Research, 46,* 1029–1037.

Conti-Ramsden, G., & Botting, N. (1999a). Characterisitics of children attending language units in England: A national study of 7-year-olds. *International Journal of Language and Communication Disorders, 34,* 359–366.

Conti-Ramsden, G., & Botting, N. (1999b). Classification of children with specific language impairment: Longitudinal considerations. *Journal of Speech, Language, and Hearing Research, 42,* 1195–1204.

Conti-Ramsden, G., Botting, N., Simkin, Z., & Knox, E. (2001). Follow-up of children attending infant language units: Outcomes at 11 years of age. *International Journal of Language and Communication Disorders, 36,* 207–219.

Conti-Ramsden, G., Crutchley, A., & Botting, N. (1997). The extent to which psychometric tests differentiate subgroups of children with SLI. *Journal of Speech, Language, and Hearing Research, 40,* 765–777.

Conti-Ramsden, G., & Dykins, J. (1991). Mother-child interactions with language-impaired children and their siblings. *British Journal of Disorders of Communication, 26,* 337–354.

Conti-Ramsden, G., Hutcheson, G., & Grove, J. (1995). Contingency and breakdown: Children with SLI and their conversations with mothers and fathers. *Journal of Speech and Hearing Research, 38,* 1290–1302.

Conti-Ramsden, G., & Jones, M. (1997). Verb use in specific language impairment. *Journal of Speech, Language, and Hearing Research, 40,* 1298–1313.

Conti-Ramsden, G., & Perez-Pereira, M. (1999). Conversational interactions between mothers and their infants who are congenitally blind, have low vision, or are sighted. *Journal of Visual Impairment and Blindness, 93,* 691–703.

Cooper, J. A., & Flowers, C. R. (1987). Children with a history of acquired aphasia: Residual language and academic impairments. *Journal of Speech and Hearing Disorders, 52,* 251–262.

Copeland, A. P., & Weissbrod, C. S. (1983). Cognitive strategies used by learning disabled children: Does hyperactivity always make things worse? *Journal of Learning Disabilities, 16,* 473–477.

Coplan, J. (1993). *Early Language Milestone Scale—2.* Austin, TX: Pro-Ed.

Cornett, R. (1985). Diagnostic factors bearing on the use of cued speech with hearing impaired children. *Ear and Hearing, 6*(1), 33–35.

Costello, J. M. (2000). AAC intervention in the intensive care unit: The Children's Hospital Boston model. *Augmentative and Alternative Communication, 16,* 137–153.

Cotton, S., Voudouris, N. J., & Greenwood, K. M. (2001). Intelligence and Duchenne muscular dystrophy: Full-scale, verbal, and performance intelligence quotients. *Developmental Medicine and Child Neurology, 43*(7), 497–501.

Council of Economic Advisers. (1998). *Changing America: Indicators of social and economic well-being by race and Hispanic origin.* Retrieved December 2, 2002, from www.access.gpo.gov/eop/ca/index.html

Courtright, J., & Courtright, I. (1976). Imitative modeling as an instructional base for instructing language-disordered children. *Journal of Speech and Hearing Research, 19,* 655–663.

Craft, M. J., Lakin, J. A., Oppliger, R. A., Clancy, G. M., & Vanderlinden, D. W. (1990). Siblings as change agents for promoting the functional status of children with cerebral palsy. *Developmental Medicine and Child Neurology, 32,* 1049–1057.

Crago, M. (1990). Development of communicative competence in Inuit children: Implications for speech-language pathology. *Journal of Childhood Communication Disorders, 13,* 73–83.

Crago, M., & Gopnik, M. (1994). From families to phenotypes: Theoretical and clinical implications of research into the genetic basis of specific language impairment. In R. Watkins & M. Rice (Eds.), *Specific language impairment in children* (pp. 35–51). Baltimore, MD: Paul H. Brookes.

Craig, H. (1993). Social skills of children with specific language impairment. *Language, Speech, and Hearing Services in Schools, 24,* 206–215.

Craig, H., & Evans, J. (1989). Turn exchange characteristics of SLI children's simultaneous and nonsimultaneous speech. *Journal of Speech and Hearing Disorders, 54,* 334–347.

Craig, H., & Gallagher, T. (1986). Interactive play: The frequency of related verbal responses. *Journal of Speech and Hearing Research, 29,* 206–215.

Craig, H., Thompson, C., Washington, J., & Potter, S. (2003). Phonological features of child African American English. *Journal of Speech, Language, and Hearing Research, 46,* 623–635.

Craig, H., & Washington, J. (1993). Access behaviors of children with specific language impairment. *Journal of Speech and Hearing Research, 36,* 322–337.

Craig, H., & Washington, J. (2000). An assessment battery for identifying language impairments in African American children. *Journal of Speech, Language, and Hearing Research, 43,* 366–379.

Craig, H., & Washington, J. (2002). Oral language expectations for African American preschoolers and kindergartners. *American Journal of Speech-Language Pathology, 11,* 59–70.

Crais, E. (1992). Fast mapping: A new look at word learning. In R. Chapman (Ed.), *Processes in language acquisition and disorders.* St. Louis, MO: Mosby Year Book.

Crais, E., & Chapman, R. (1987). Story recall and inferencing skills in language/learning-disabled children. *Journal of Speech and Hearing Disorders, 52,* 50–55.

Crais, E., & Lorch, N. (1994). Oral narrative in school-age children. *Topics in Language Disorders, 14*(3), 13–28.

Crais, E., & Wilson, L. B. (1996). The role of parents in child assessment: Self-evaluation by practicing professionals.

Infant-Toddler Intervention: the Transdisciplinary Journal, 6(2), 125–143.

Cramer, R. H. (1991). The education of gifted children in the United States: A Delphi study. *Gifted Child Quarterly, 35,* 84–91.

Crawford, J. (2003). *Language legislation in the U.S.A.* Retrieved January 1, 2003, from http://ourworld. compuserve.com/homepages/JWCRAWFORD/langleg. htm

Creaghead, N. A. (1990). Mutual empowerment through collaboration: A new script for an old problem. *Best Practices in School Speech-Language Pathology, 1,* 109–116.

Creaghead, N. A. (1992). Classroom interactional analysis/ script analysis. *Best Practices in School Speech-Language Pathology, 2,* 65–72.

Croen, L. A., Shaw, G. M., Wasserman, C. R., & Tolarova, M. M. (1998). Racial and ethnic variations in the prevalence of orofacial clefts in California, 1983–1992. *American Journal of Medical Genetics, 79*(1), 42–47.

Crossley, R. (1994). *Facilitated communication training.* New York: Teachers College Press.

Crowe, T., Byrne, M., & Henry, A. (1999). Prison services: The Parchman project. *Asha, 41*(6), 50–54.

Crystal, D. (1982). *Profiling linguistic disability.* London, UK: Edward Arnold.

Crystal, D. (1984). *Linguistic encounters with language handicap.* New York: Basil Blackwell.

Crystal, D. (1997). *The Cambridge encyclopedia of language* (2nd ed.). New York: Cambridge University Press.

Crystal, D., & Davy, D. (1975). *Advanced conversational English.* London, UK: Longman.

Crystal, D., Fletcher, P., & Garman, M. (1989). *The grammatical analysis of language disability: A procedure for assessment and remediation* (2nd ed.). London, UK: Cole & Whurr.

Crystal, D., & Varley, R. (1998). *Introduction to language pathology* (4th ed.). London, UK: Whurr.

Culp, D. M. (1987). Outcome measurement: The impact of communication augmentation. *Seminars in Speech and Language, 8*(2), 169–185.

Curcio, F., & Paccia, J. (1987). Conversations with autistic children: Contingent relationships between features of adult input and children's response adequacy. *Journal of Autism and Developmental Disorders, 17,* 81–93.

Cutler, R. W. P. (1992). Neurology. In E. Rubentein & D. D. Federman (Eds.), *Scientific American medicine.* New York: Scientific American.

Cutts, S., & Sigafoos, J. (2001). Social competence and peer interactions of students with intellectual disability in inclusive high school. *Journal of Intellectual and Developmental Disability, 26,* 127–141.

Dagenais, D. J., & Beadle, K. R. (1984). Written language: When and where to begin. *Topics in Language Disorders, 4,* 59–85.

Dahl, E. K., Cohen, D. J., & Provence, S. (1986). Clinical and multivariate approaches to the nosology of pervasive developmental disorders. *Journal of the American Academy of Child Psychiatry, 25,* 170–180.

Dahle, A. J., & Baldwin, R. L. (1992). Audiologic and otolaryngologic concerns. In S. M. Pueschel & J. K. Pueschel (Eds.), *Biomedical concerns in persons with Down syndrome* (pp. 1–12). Baltimore, MD: Paul H. Brookes.

Dale, P. (1996). Parent report assessment of language and communication. In K. Cole, P. Dale, & D. Thal (Eds.), *Assessment of communication and language* (pp. 161–182). Baltimore, MD: Paul H. Brookes.

Dale, P., Bates, E., Reznick, S., & Morisset, C. (1989). The validity of a parent report instrument of child language at twenty months. *Journal of Child Language, 16,* 239–250.

Dale, P., Price, T., Bishop, D. V. M., & Plomin, R. (2003). Outcomes of early language delay: I. Predicting persistent and transient language difficulties at 3 and 4 years. *Journal of Speech, Language, and Hearing Research, 46,* 544–560.

Dale, P., Simonoff, E., Bishop, D. V. M., Eley, T., Oliver, B., Price, T., et al. (1998). Genetic influences on language delay in two-year-old children. *Nature Neuroscience, 1,* 324–328.

Dale, P., & Thal, D. (1989, November). Assessment of language in infants and toddlers using parent report. Paper presented at the Annual Convention of the American Speech-Language-Hearing Association, St. Louis, MO.

Dallas, E., Stevenson, J., & McGurk, H. (1993). Cerebral-palsied children's interactions with siblings: I. Influence of severity of disability, age and birth order. *Journal of Child Psychology & Psychiatry & Allied Disciplines, 34*(5), 621–647.

Damico, J. (1985). Clinical discourse analysis: A functional language assessment technique. In C. Simon (Ed.), *Communication skills and classroom success: Assessment of language-learning-disabled students.* San Diego, CA: College-Hill Press.

Damico, J. (1988). The lack of efficacy in language therapy: A case study. *Language, Speech, and Hearing Services in Schools, 19,* 51–66.

Damico, J. (1993). Language assessment in adolescents: Addressing critical issues. *Language, Speech, and Hearing Services in Schools, 24,* 29–35.

Dapretto, M., Woods, R. P., & Bookheimer, S. Y. (2000). Enhanced cortical plasticity early in development: Insights from an fMRI study of language processing in children and adults. Paper presented at the Annual Meeting of Neuroscience Society, Los Angeles.

Darley, F. (1991). A philosophy of appraisal and diagnosis. In F. Darley & D. Spriestersbach (Eds.), *Diagnostic methods in speech pathology* (2nd ed., pp. 1–23). Prospect Heights, IL: Waverton Press.

Davis, A., Sanger, D., & Morris-Friehe, M. (1991). Language skills of delinquent and nondelinquent adolescent males. *Journal of Communication Disorders, 24,* 251–266.

Davis, B. L., Jakielski, K. J., & Marquardt, T. P. (1998). Developmental apraxia of speech: Determiners of differential diagnosis. *Clinical Linguistics and Phonetics, 12,* 25–46.

Davis, H., Stroud, A., & Green, L. (1988). Maternal language environment of children with mental retardation. *American Journal on Mental Retardation, 93,* 144–153.

Davis, J. M. (Ed.). (1990). *Our forgotten children: Hard-of-hearing pupils in the schools* (2nd ed.). Washington, DC: Self-Help for the Hard of Hearing.

Davis, J. M., Elfenbein, J. L., Schum, R., & Bentler, R. A. (1986). Effects of mild and moderate hearing impairments on language, educational and psychosocial behaviour of children. *Journal of Speech and Hearing Disorders, 51,* 53–62.

Davis, J. M., & Hardick, E. (1981). *Rehabilitative audiology for children and adults.* New York: Wiley.

Dawson, P. W., Blamey, P., Dettman, S. J., Barker, E., & Clark, G. M. (1995). A clinical report on receptive vocabulary skills in cochlear implant users. *Ear and Hearing, 16,* 287–294.

de Bode, S., & Curtiss, S. (2001). Exploring neuronal plasticity: Language development in pediatric hemispherectomies. Paper presented at the 23rd Annual Conference of the Cognitive Science Society, Edinburgh, Scotland.

de Feu, M. (1997). Mental health in children with hearing problems. *Health Visitor, 70*(7), 257.

De Houwer, A. (1995). Bilingual language acquisition. In P. Fletcher & B. MacWhinney (Eds.), *Handbook of child language* (pp. 219–250). London, UK: Blackwell.

De Houwer, A. (1999). *Two or more languages in early childhood: Some general points and practical recommendations.* Retrieved December 2, 2002, from www.cal.org/ericcll/digest/earlychild.html

De Renzi, A., & Vignolo, L. A. (1962). Token Test: A sensitive test to detect receptive disturbances in aphasics. *Brain, 85,* 665–678.

de Villiers, J., & de Villiers, P. (1973). A cross-sectional study of the acquisition of grammatical morphemes in child speech. *Journal of Psycholinguistic Research, 2,* 267–278.

Deal, V., & Rodriquez, V. (1987). *Resource guide to multicultural tests and materials in communicative disorders.* Rockville, MD: American Speech-Language-Hearing Association.

Deal-Williams, V. (2002). *Celebrating our differences.* Retrieved December 2, 2002, from http://professional.asha.org/news/020402a.cfm

DeKroon, D., Kyte, C., & Johnson, C. (2002). Partner influences on the social pretend play of children with language impairments. *Language, Speech, and Hearing Services in Schools, 33,* 253–267.

Delgado, C., Mundy, P., Crowson, M., Markus, J., Yale, M., & Schwartz, H. (2002). Responding to joint attention and language development: A comparison of target locations. *Journal of Speech, Language, and Hearing Research, 45,* 715–719.

Demetras, M., Post, K., & Snow, C. (1986). Feedback to first language learners: The role of repetitions and clarification questions. *Journal of Child Language, 13,* 275–292.

Denning, C. B., Chamberlain, J. A., & Polloway, E. A. (2000). An evaluation of state guidelines for mental retardation: Focus of definition and classification practices. *Education and Training in Mental Retardation, 35*(2), 226–232.

Dennis, M. (1980). Strokes in childhood I: Communicative intent, expression, and comprehension after left hemisphere arteriopathy in a right-handed nine-year-old. In R. W. Rieber (Ed.), *Language development and aphasia in children.* New York: Academic Press.

Dennis, M. (1992). Word finding in children and adolescents with a history of brain injury. *Topics in Language Disorders, 13,* 66–82.

Dennis, M., & Barnes, M. A. (2001). Comparison of literal, inferential, and intentional text comprehension in children with mild or severe closed head injury. *Journal of Head Trauma Rehabilitation, 16*(5), 456–468.

Dennis, M., Barnes, M. A., Wilkinson, M., & Humphreys, R. P. (1998). How children with head injury represent real and deceptive emotion in short narratives. *Brain and Language, 61*(3), 450–483.

Dennis, M., Purvis, K., Barnes, M. A., Wilkinson, M., & Winner, E. (2001). Understanding of literal truth, ironic criticism, and deceptive praise following childhood head injury. *Brain and Language, 78*(1), 1–16.

Denton, K., & Zarbatany, L. (1996). Age differences in support processes in conversations between friends. *Child Development, 67,* 1360–1373.

DePompei, R., & Blosser, J. (1987). Strategies for helping head-injured children successfully return to school. *Language, Speech, and Hearing Services in Schools, 18,* 292–300.

Dermody, P., Katsch, R., & Mackie, K. (1983). Auditory processing limitations in low verbal children. *Ear and Hearing, 4,* 272–277.

Dermody, P., Mackie, K., & Katsch, R. (1983). Dichotic listening in good and poor readers. *Journal of Speech and Hearing Research, 26,* 341–348.

Deshler, D., & Schumaker, J. (1988). An instructional model for teaching students how to learn. In J. Graden, J. Zins, & M. Curtis (Eds.), *Alternative educational delivery systems: Enhancing instructional options for all students* (pp. 391–411). Washington, DC: National Association of Secondary Principals.

Despain, A., & Simon, C. (1987). Alternative to failure: A junior high school language development-based curriculum. *Journal of Childhood Communication Disorders, 11,* 139–179.

Dever, R. (1972). A comparison of the results of a revised version of Berko's Test of Morphology with the free speech of mentally retarded children. *Journal of Speech and Hearing Research, 15,* 169–178.

Devers, M., & Broen, P. (1991, November). Prelinguistic vocalizations of infants with and without cleft palate. Paper presented at the Annual Convention of the American Speech-Language-Hearing Association, Atlanta, GA.

Dewart, H. (1979). Language comprehension processes of mentally retarded children. *American Journal of Mental Deficiency, 84,* 177–183.

DiMeo, J., Merritt, D., & Culatta, B. (1998). Collaborative partnerships and decision making. In D. Merritt & B. Culatta (Eds.), *Language intervention in the classroom* (pp. 37–98). San Diego, CA: Singular.

Docking, K., Jordan, F., & Murdoch, B. (1999). Interpretation and comprehension of linguistic humour by adolescents with head injury: A case-by-case analysis. *Brain Injury, 13*(12), 953–972.

Docking, K., Murdoch, B., & Jordan, F. (2000). Interpretation and comprehension of linguistic humour by adolescents with head injury: A group analysis. *Brain Injury, 14*(1), 89–108.

Dodd, B. (1975). Recognition and reproduction of words by Down's syndrome and non-Down's syndrome retarded children. *American Journal of Mental Deficiency, 80,* 306–311.

Dodd, B. (1976). A comparison of the phonological systems of mental age matched normal, severely subnormal, and Down's syndrome children. *British Journal of Disorders of Communication, 11,* 27–42.

Dodd, B., McCormack, P., & Woodyatt, G. (1994). Evaluation of an intervention program: Relation between children's phonology and parents' communicative behavior. *American Journal of Mental Retardation, 98*(5), 632–645.

Dollaghan, C. (1985). Child meets word: "Fast mapping" in preschool children. *Journal of Speech and Hearing Research, 28,* 449–454.

Dollaghan, C. (1987). Fast mapping in normal and language-impaired children. *Journal of Speech and Hearing Disorders, 52,* 218–222.

Dollaghan, C., & Campbell, T. (1992). A procedures for classifying disruptions in spontaneous language samples. *Topics in Language Disorders, 12*(2), 56–68.

Dollaghan, C., & Campbell, T. (1998). Nonword repetition and child language impairment. *Journal of Speech, Language, and Hearing Research, 41,* 1136–1146.

Dollaghan, C., Campbell, T., Paradise, J., Feldman, H., Janosky, J., Pitcairn, D., et al. (1999). Maternal education and measures of early speech and language. *Journal of Speech, Language, and Hearing Research, 42,* 1432–1443.

Dollaghan, C., Campbell, T., & Tomlin, R. (1990). Video narration as a language sampling context. *Journal of Speech and Hearing Disorders, 55,* 582–590.

Donahue, M. (1986). Linguistic and communicative development in learning-disabled children. In C. Ceci (Ed.), *Handbook of cognitive, social, and neuropsychological aspects of learning disabilities* (Vol. 1). Mahwah, NJ: Lawrence Erlbaum.

Donahue, M., Pearl, R., & Bryan, T. (1980). Learning disabled children's conversational competence: Responses to inadequate messages. *Applied Psycholinguistics, 1,* 387–403.

Donahue, M., Pearl, R., & Bryan, T. (1982). Learning disabled children's syntactic proficiency on a communicative task. *Journal of Speech and Hearing Disorders, 47,* 397–403.

Donahue, M., Szymanski, C., & Flores, C. (1999). When "Emily Dickinson" met "Steven Speilberg": Assessing social information processing in literacy contexts. *Language, Speech, and Hearing Services in Schools, 30,* 274–284.

Donnellan, A. M., Mirenda, P., Mesaros, R. A., & Fassbender, L. L. (1984). Analysing the communicative functions of aberrant behavior. *Journal of the Association for Persons with Severe Handicaps, 9*(3), 201–212.

Dore, J. (1975). Holophrase, speech acts, and language universals. *Journal of Child Language, 2,* 21–40.

Dore, J. (1979). Conversational acts and the acquisition of language. In E. Ochs & B. Schieffelin (Eds.), *Developmental pragmatics.* New York: Academic Press.

Doren, B., Bullis, M., & Benz, M. (1996). Predicting arrest status of adolescents with disabilities in transition. *Journal of Special Education, 29,* 363–380.

Dorman, C., Hurley, A. D., & D'Avignon, J. (1988). Language and learning disorders of older boys with Duchenne muscular dystrophy. *Developmental Medicine and Child Neurology, 30,* 316–327.

Douglas, V. I. (1988). Cognitive deficits in children with attention deficit disorder with hyperactivity. In L. M. Bloomingdale & J. A. Sergeant (Eds.), *Attention deficit disorder: Criteria, cognition, intervention* (pp. 65–82). London, UK: Pergamon Press.

Dowden, P., Beukelman, D., & Lossing, C. (1986). Serving nonspeaking patients in acute care settings: Intervention outcomes. *Augmentative and Alternative Communication, 2,* 38–44.

Dowell, R., & Cowan, R. (1997). Evaluation of benefit: Infants and children. In G. Clark, R. Cowan, & R. Dowell (Eds.), *Cochlear implantation for infants and children: Advances* (pp. 205–222). San Diego, CA: Singular.

Drager, K., Light, J., Speltz, J. C., Fallon, K., & Jeffries, L. (2003). The performance of typically developing

2½-year-olds on dynamic display AAC technologies with different system layouts and language organizations. *Journal of Speech, Language, and Hearing Research, 46,* 298–312.

Duchan, J. F. (1983). Autistic children are noninteractive: Or so we say. *Seminars in Speech and Language, 4,* 53–61.

Duchan, J. F. (1999). Views of facilitated communication: What's the point? *Language, Speech, and Hearing Services in Schools, 30,* 401–408.

Duchan, J. F., Calculator, S. N., Sonnenmeier, R., Diehl, S., & Cumley, G. D. (2001). A framework for managing controversial practices. *Language, Speech, and Hearing Services in Schools, 32,* 133–141.

Duhaime, A. C., Christian, C. W., Rorke, L. B., & Zimmerman, R. A. (1998). Nonaccidental head injury in infants—the "shaken-baby syndrome." *New England Journal of Medicine, 338*(25), 1822–1829.

Dukes, P. (1981). Developing social prerequisites to oral communication. *Topics in Learning and Learning Disabilities, 1,* 47–58.

Dulaney, C. L., & Ellis, N. R. (1997). Rigidity in the behavior of mentally retarded persons. In W. E. MacLean, Jr. (Ed.), *Ellis' handbook of mental deficiency, psychological theory and research* (3rd ed., pp. 175–195). Mahwah, NJ: Lawrence Erlbaum.

Dunn, L. (1965). *Peabody Picture Vocabulary Test.* Circle Pines, MN: American Guidance Service.

Dunn, L. M., & Dunn, L. M. (1981). *Peabody Picture Vocabulary Test—revised.* Circle Pines, MN: American Guidance Service.

Dunn, L., & Dunn, L. (1997). *Peabody Picture Vocabulary Test—III.* Circle Pines, MN: American Guidance Service.

Durand, J. (1990). *Generative and non-linear phonology.* London, UK: Longman.

Durand, M. (1993). Functional communication training using assistive devices: Effects on challenging behavior and affect. *Augmentative and Alternative Communication, 9*(3), 168–176.

Durand, V. M., & Crimmins, D. B. (1987). Assessment and treatment of psychotic speech in an autistic child. *Journal of Autism and Developmental Disorders, 17,* 17–28.

Durham, S. R., Clancy, R. R., Leuthardt, E., Sun, P., Kamerling, S., Dominguez, T., et al. (2000). CHOP infant coma scale ("Infant Face Scale"): A novel coma scale for children less than two years of age. *Journal of Neurotrauma, 17,* 729–737.

Dyer, K., Williams, L., & Luce, S. C. (1991). Training teachers to use naturalistic communication strategies in classrooms for students with autism and other severe handicaps. *Language, Speech, and Hearing Services in Schools, 22,* 313–321.

Edwards, J., & Lahey, M. (1998). Nonword repetitions of children with specific language impairment: Explo-

ration of some explanations for their inaccuracies. *Applied Psycholinguistics, 19,* 279–309.

Edwards, S., Fletcher, P., Garman, M., Hughes, A., Letts, C., & Sinka, I. (1999). *Reynell Developmental Language Scales—III.* Windsor, UK: NFER-Nelson.

Eheart, B. (1982). Mother-child interactions with nonretarded and mentally retarded preschoolers. *American Journal of Mental Deficiency, 87,* 20–25.

Ehren, B. J. (1994). New directions for meeting the academic needs of adolescents with language-learning disabilities. In B. Wallach & K. Butler (Eds.), *Language-learning disabilities in school-age children and adolescents: Some principles and applications* (pp. 393–417). Boston: Allyn & Bacon.

Ehren, B. J. (2002). Speech-language pathologists contributing significantly to the academic success of high school students: A vision for professional growth. *Topics in Language Disorders, 22*(2), 60–80.

Ehren, B. J., & Lenz, B. K. (1989). Adolescents with language disorders: Special considerations in providing academically relevant language intervention. *Seminars in Speech and Language, 10,* 192–203.

Eilers, R. E., Cobo-Lewis, A. B., Vergara, K. C., & Oller, D. K. (1997). Longitudinal speech perception performance of young children with cochlear implants and tactile aids plus hearing aids. *Scandinavian Audiology. Supplementum, 26*(Suppl. 47), 50–54.

Eisele, J., & Aram, D. (1995). Lexical and grammatical development in children with early hemisphere damage: A cross-sectional view from birth to adolescence. In P. Fletcher & B. MacWhinney (Eds.), *The Handbook of Child Language* (pp. 664–689). Oxford, UK: Basil Blackwell.

Eisenberg, S., Fersko, T., & Lundgren, C. (2001). The use of MLU for identifying language impairment in preschool children: A review. *American Journal of Speech-Language Pathology, 10,* 323–342.

Eisenson, J. (1972). *Aphasia in Children.* New York: Harper & Row.

Elfenbein, J. L., Hardin-Jones, M., & Davis, J. M. (1994). Oral communication skills of children who are hard of hearing. *Journal of Speech and Hearing Research, 37*(1), 216–225.

Elliott, R. O., Hall, K., & Soper, H. V. (1991). Analog language teaching versus natural language teaching: Generalization and retention of language learning for adults with autism and mental retardation. *Journal of Autism and Developmental Disorders, 21,* 433–447.

Ellis, E. (1993). Integrative strategy instruction: A potential model for teaching content area subjects to adolescents with learning disabilities. *Journal of Learning Disabilities, 26,* 358–383, 398.

Ellis, E. (1994). Integrating writing strategy instruction with content-area instruction: Part I: Orienting students to organizational devices. *Intervention in School and Clinic, 29*(3), 169–179.

Ellis Weismer, S. (1991). Hypothesis-testing abilities of language-impaired children. *Journal of Speech and Hearing Research, 34,* 1329–1338.

Ellis Weismer, S. (1996). Capacity limitations in working memory: The impact on lexical and morphological learning by children with language impairment. *Topics in Language Disorders, 17*(1), 33–44.

Ellis Weismer, S. (1997). The role of stress in language processing and intervention. *Topics in Language Disorders, 18,* 41–52.

Ellis Weismer, S. (2000). Intervention for children with developmental language delay. In D. V. M. Bishop & L. Leonard (Eds.), *Speech and language impairment in children: Causes, characteristics, intervention and outcome* (pp. 157–176). East Sussex, UK: Psychology Press.

Ellis Weismer, S., & Evans, J. (2002). The role of processing limitations in early identification of specific language impairment. *Topics in Language Disorders, 22*(3), 15–29.

Ellis Weismer, S., Evans, J., & Hesketh, L. (1999). An examination of verbal working memory capacity in children with specific language impairment. *Journal of Speech, Language, and Hearing Research, 42,* 1249–1260.

Ellis Weismer, S., & Hesketh, L. (1993). The influence of prosodic and gestural cues on novel word acquisition by children with specific language impairment. *Journal of Speech and Hearing Research, 36,* 1013–1025.

Ellis Weismer, S., & Hesketh, L. (1996). Lexical learning by children with specific language impairment: Effects of linguistic input presented at varying speaking rates. *Journal of Speech and Hearing Research, 39,* 177–190.

Ellis Weismer, S., & Hesketh, L. (1998). The impact of emphatic stress on novel word learning by children with specific language impairment. *Journal of Speech, Language, and Hearing Research, 41,* 1444–1458.

Ellis Weismer, S., & Murray-Branch, J. (1989). Modeling versus modeling plus evoked production training: A comparison of two language intervention methods. *Journal of Speech and Hearing Disorders, 54,* 269–281.

Ellis Weismer, S., Murray-Branch, J., & Miller, J. (1994). A prospective longitudinal study of language development in late talkers. *Journal of Speech and Hearing Research, 37,* 852–867.

Ellis Weismer, S., & Schraeder, T. (1993). Discourse characteristics and verbal reasoning: Wait time effects on the performance of children with language learning disabilities. *Exceptionality Education Canada, 3,* 71–92.

Ellis Weismer, S., Tomblin, J. B., Zhang, X., Buckwalter, P., Chynoweth, J., & Jones, M. (2000). Nonword repetition performance in school-age children with and without language impairment. *Journal of Speech, Language, and Hearing Research, 43,* 865–878.

Emerson, E., McGill, P., & Mansell, J. (Eds.). (1994). *Severe learning disabilities and challenging behaviours.* London, UK: Chapman & Hall.

Entwisle, D., & Astone, N. (1994). Some practical guidelines for measuring youth's race/ethnicity and socioeconomic status. *Child Development, 65,* 1521–1540.

Eskes, G. A., Bryson, S. E., & McCormick, T. A. (1990). Comprehension of concrete and abstract words in autistic children. *Journal of Autism and Developmental Disorders, 20,* 61–73.

Espin, C. A., Scierka, B. J., Skare, S., & Halverson, N. (1999). Curriculum-based measures in writing for secondary students. *Reading and Writing Quarterly, 15,* 5–27.

Espinosa, L. (1995). *Hispanic parent involvement in early childhood programs.* Retrieved July 2002, from http://ericeece.org/pubs/digest/1995/espino95.html.

Estabrooks, W. (Ed.). (1994). *Auditory verbal therapy for parents and professionals.* Washington, DC: A. G. Bell Association for the Deaf.

Estrem, T., & Broen, P. (1989). Early speech production of children with cleft palate. *Journal of Speech and Hearing Research, 32,* 12–23.

Evans, J., & Craig, H. (1992). Language sample collection and analysis: Interview compared to freeplay assessment contexts. *Journal of Speech and Hearing Research, 35,* 343–353.

Evans, J., Viele, K., & Kass, R. (1997). Response latency and verbal complexity: Stochastic models of individual differences in children with specific language impairments. *Journal of Speech, Language, and Hearing Research, 40,* 754–764.

Ewing-Cobbs, L., Fletcher, J. M., Landry, S. H., & Levin, H. S. (1985). Language disorders after pediatric head injury. In J. K. Darby (Ed.), *Speech and language evaluation in neurology: Childhood disorders.* Orlando, FL: Grune & Stratton.

Ewing-Cobbs, L., Levin, H. S., & Fletcher, J. M. (1998). Neuropsychological sequelae after pediatric traumatic brain injury: Advances since 1985. In M. Ylvisaker (Ed.), *Traumatic brain injury rehabilitation: Children and adolescents* (2nd ed., pp. 11–26). Boston: Butterworth-Heinemann.

Ezell, H. K., & Goldstein, H. (1991a). Comparison of idiom comprehension of normal children and children with mental retardation. *Journal of Speech and Hearing Research, 34,* 812–819.

Ezell, H. K., & Goldstein, H. (1991b). Observational learning of comprehension monitoring skills in children who exhibit mental retardation. *Journal of Speech and Hearing Research, 34,* 141–154.

Fabbrini, G. (1989). Speech perception in children with histories of recurrent otitis media. *Journal of the Acoustical Society of America, 85*(2), 926–933.

Fagundes, D., Haynes, W., Haak, N., & Moran, M. (1998). Task variability effects on the language test performance of Southern lower socioeconomic class African American and Caucasian five-year-olds. *Language, Speech, and Hearing Services in Schools, 29,* 148–157.

Fairbanks, G. (1960). *Voice and articulation drill book.* New York: Harper & Row.

Farber, J., & Klein, E. (1999). Classroom-based assessment of a collaborative intervention program with kindergarten and first grade children. *Language, Speech, and Hearing Services in Schools, 30,* 83–91.

Farrar, M. (1990). Discourse and the acquisition of grammatical morphemes. *Journal of Child Language, 17,* 607–624.

Fawcett, A., & Nicolson, R. (1991). Vocabulary training for children with dyslexia. *Journal of Learning Disabilities, 24,* 379–383.

Fawcett, A., & Nicolson, R. (2000). Systematic screening and intervention for reading difficulty. In N. Badian (Ed.), *Prediction and prevention of reading failure* (pp. 57–85). Timonium, MD: York Press.

Fayne, H. (1981). A comparison of learning disabled adolescents with normal learners on an anaphoric pronominal reference task. *Journal of Learning Disabilities, 14,* 597–599.

Fazio, B. (1994). The counting abilities of children with specific language impairment: A comparison of oral and gestural tasks. *Journal of Speech and Hearing Research, 37,* 358–368.

Fazio, B. (1996). Mathematical abilities of children with specific language impairment: A 2-year follow-up. *Journal of Speech and Hearing Research, 39,* 839–849.

Feagans, L. (1980). Children's understanding of some temporal terms denoting order, duration, and simultaneity. *Journal of Psycholinguistic Research, 9,* 41–57.

Fehrenbach, C. R. (1991). Gifted/average readers: Do they use the same reading strategies. *Gifted Child Quarterly, 35,* 125–127.

Felberg, R. A., Burgin, W. S., & Grotta, J. C. (2000). Neuroprotection and the ischemic cascade. *CNS Spectrums, 5*(3), 52–58.

Felsenfeld, S., & Plomin, R. (1997). Epidemiological and offspring analyses of developmental speech disorders using data from the Colorado Adoption Project. *Journal of Speech and Hearing Research, 40,* 778–791.

Feng, J. (1994). *Asian-American children: What teachers should know.* Retrieved July 2002, from www.ed.gov/databases/ERIC_Digests/ed369577.html.

Fenson, L., Dale, P., Reznick, J., Bates, E., Thal, D., & Pethick, S. (1994). *The MacArthur Communicative Development Inventories: Short Form Versions.* Unpublished manuscript.

Fenson, L., Dale, P., Reznick, J., Hartung, J., & Burgess, S. (1990). Norms for the MacAurthur Communicative Development Inventories. Paper presented at the International Conference on Infant Studies, Montreal, Canada.

Fenson, L., Dale, P., Reznick, J., Thal, D., Bates, E., Hartung, J., et al. (1993). *Guide and technical manual for the MacArthur Communicative Development Inventories.* San Diego, CA: Singular.

Fenstermacher, G. D. (1982). To be or not to be gifted: That is the question. *Elementary School Journal, 82,* 299–303.

Ferguson, M. (1992). Implementing collaborative consultation: An introduction. *Language, Speech, and Hearing Services in Schools, 23,* 361–362.

Ferretti, R. P., & Cavalier, A. R. (1991). Constraints on the problem solving of persons with mental retardation. *International Review of Research in Mental Retardation, 17,* 153–192.

Fey, M. (1986). *Language intervention with young children.* Boston: Allyn & Bacon.

Fey, M., Catts, H., & Larrivee, L. (1995). Preparing preschoolers for the academic and social challenges of school. In M. Fey, J. Windsor, & S. Warren (Eds.), *Language intervention: Preschool through the elementary years* (pp. 3–37). Baltimore, MD: Paul H. Brookes.

Fey, M., Cleave, P., & Long, S. (1997). Two models of grammar facilitation in children with language impairments: Phase 2. *Journal of Speech, Language, and Hearing Research, 40,* 5–19.

Fey, M., Cleave, P., Long, S., & Hughes, D. (1993). Two approaches to the facilitation of grammar in language-impaired children: An experimental evaluation. *Journal of Speech and Hearing Research, 36,* 141–157.

Fey, M., Krulik, T., Loeb, D., & Proctor-Williams, K. (1999). Sentence recast use by parents of children with typical language and specific language impairment. *American Journal of Speech-Language Pathology, 8,* 273–286.

Fey, M., Leonard, L., & Wilcox, K. (1981). Speech style modifications of language-impaired children. *Journal of Speech and Hearing Disorders, 46,* 91–96.

Fey, M., Long, S., & Finestack, L. (2003). Ten principles of grammar facilitation for children with specific language impairments. *American Journal of Speech-Language Pathology, 12,* 3–15.

Fey, M., & Proctor-Williams, K. (2000). Recasting, elicited imitation and modelling in grammar intervention for children with specific language impairments. In D. V. M. Bishop & L. Leonard (Eds.), *Speech and language impairment in children: Causes, characteristics, intervention and outcome* (pp. 177–194). East Sussex, UK: Psychology Press.

Figueroa, R., & Hernandez, S. (2000). *Testing Hispanic students in the U.S.: Technical and policy issues.* Washington, DC: President's Advisory Commission on Educational Excellence for Hispanic Americans.

Finch-Williams, A. (1984). The developmental relationship between cognition and communication: Implications for assessment. *Topics in Language Disorders, 5,* 1–13.

Fischel, J., Whitehurst, G., Caulfield, M., & DeBaryshe, B. (1989). Language growth in children with expressive language delay. *Pediatrics, 28,* 218–227.

Fitzgerald, E. (1949). *Straight language for the deaf: A system of instruction for deaf children.* Washington, DC: Volta Bureau.

Flax, J., Realpe-Bonilla, T., Hirsch, L., Brzustowicz, L., Bartlett, C., & Tallal, P. (2003). Specific language impairment in families: Evidence for co-occurrence with reading impairments. *Journal of Speech, Language, and Hearing Research, 46,* 530–543.

Fleischman, H., & Hopstock, P. (1993). *Descriptive study of services to limited English proficient students. Volume 1: Summary of findings and conclusions.* Development Associates, Inc. Retrieved July 2002, from www.ncbe.gwu.edu/miscpubs/siac/descript/part2.htm.

Flowers, A., Costello, M., & Small, V. (1970). *Manual for the Flowers-Costello Test of Central Auditory Abilities.* Dearborn, MI: Perceptual Learning Systems.

Fokes, J. (1976). *Fokes Sentence Builder.* Hingham, MA: Teaching Resources.

Fokes, J. (1977). *Fokes Sentence Builder Expansion.* Hingham, MA: Teaching Resouces.

Foley, R. (2001). Academic characteristics of incarcerated youth and correctional educational programs: A literature review. *Journal of Emotional and Behavioral Disorders, 9,* 248–259.

Folstein, S. E., & Rutter, M. L. (1988). Autism: Familial aggregation and genetic implications. *Journal of Autism and Developmental Disorders, 18,* 3–30.

Ford, D. Y. (1996). *Reversing underachievement among gifted black students: Promising practices and programs.* New York: Teachers College Press.

Fowler, A. E. (1988). Determinants of language growth in children with Down syndrome. In L. Nadel (Ed.), *The psychobiology of Down syndrome* (pp. 217–245). Cambridge, MA: MIT Press.

Fowler, A. E. (1990). Language abilities in children with Down syndrome: Evidence for a specific syntactic delay. In D. Cicchetti & M. Beeghly (Eds.), *Children with Down syndrome: A developmental perspective* (pp. 302–328). New York: Cambridge University Press.

Fowler, A. E., Gelman, R., & Gleitman, L. R. (1994). The course of language learning in children with Down syndrome. In H. Tager-Flusberg (Ed.), *Constraints on language acquisition: Studies of atypical children.* Hillsdale, NJ: Lawrence Erlbaum.

Fowles, B., & Glanz, M. (1977). Competence and talent in verbal riddle comprehension. *Journal of Child Language, 4,* 433–452.

Francis, D., Fletcher, J. M., Shaywitz, B., Shaywitz, S., & Rourke, B. (1996). Defining learning and language disabilities: Conceptual and psychometric issues with the use of IQ tests. *Language, Speech, and Hearing Services in Schools, 27,* 132–143.

Frankel, F., Simmons, J. Q., & Richey, V. E. (1987). Reward value of prosodic features of language for autistic, mentally retarded, and normal children. *Journal of Autism and Developmental Disorders, 17,* 103–113.

Frankenberger, W., & Harper, J. (1988). States' definitions and procedures for identifying children with mental retardation: Comparison of 1981–1982 and 1985–1986 guidelines. *Mental Retardation, 26,* 133–136.

Frankenburg, W., Dodds, J., Archer, P., Bresnick, B., Maschka, P., Edelman, N., & Shapiro, H. (1990). *Denver II: Screening manual.* Denver, CO: Denver Developmental Materials.

Frasier, M. M., Hunsaker, S. L., Lee, J., Mitchell, S., Cramond, B., Krisel, S., et al. (1995). *Core attributes of giftedness: A foundation for recognizing the gifted potential of economically disadvantaged students.* Storrs, CT: The National Research Center on the Gifted and Talented, University of Connecticut.

Freedman, P., & Carpenter, R. (1976). Semantic relations used by normal and language-impaired children at stage I. *Journal of Speech and Hearing Research, 19,* 784–795.

Freeman, B., & Parkins, C. (1979). The prevalence of middle ear disease among learning impaired children. *Clinical Pediatrics, 18,* 205–212.

Freeman, J. (1979). *Gifted children: Their identification and development in a social context.* Baltimore, MD: University Park Press.

Freeman, J. (1986). Up-date on gifted children. *Developmental Medicine and Child Neurology, 28,* 77–80.

Freeman, R., & Blockberger, S. (1987). Language development and sensory disorder: Visual and hearing impairments. In W. Yule & M. Rutter (Eds.), *Language development and disorders.* Philadelphia: Lippincott.

Fria, T. J., Cantekin, E. I., & Eichler, J. A. (1985). Hearing acuity of children with otitis media with effusion. *Otolaryngology—Head and Neck Surgery, 111,* 10–16.

Friedman, P., & Friedman, K. (1980). Accounting for individual differences when comparing the effectiveness of remedial language teaching methods. *Applied Psycholinguistics, 1,* 151–170.

Fried-Oken, M., Howard, J. M., & Roach Stewart, S. (1991). Feedback on AAC intervention from adults who are temporarily unable to speak. *Augmentative and Alternative Communication, 7,* 43–50.

Fried-Oken, M., & More, L. (1992). An initial vocabulary for nonspeaking preschool children based on developmental and environmental language sources. *Augmentative and Alternative Communication, 8,* 41–56.

Friel-Patti, S., & Finitzo, T. (1990). Language learning in a prospective study of otitis media with effusion in the first 2 years of life. *Journal of Speech and Hearing Research, 33,* 188–194.

Fristoe, M., & Lloyd, L. (1979). Signs used in manual communication training with persons having severe communication impairment. *AAESPH Review, 4*(4), 364–373.

Fristoe, M., & Lloyd, L. (1980). Planning an initial expressive sign lexicon for persons with severe communication impairment. *Journal of Speech and Hearing Disorders, 45,* 170–180.

Frith, U. (1989). A new look at language and communication in autism. *British Journal of Disorders of Communication, 24,* 123–150.

Fromkin, V., Rodman, R., Collins, P., & Blair, D. (1996). *An introduction to language* (3rd ed.). Marrickville, Australia: Harcourt Brace.

Frost, L., & Bondy, A. (1994). *PECS: The picture exchange communication system training manual.* Cherry Hill, NJ: Pyramid Educational Consultants.

Fujiki, M., Brinton, B., & Clarke, D. (2002). Emotion regulation in children with specific language impairment. *Language, Speech, and Hearing Services in Schools, 33,* 102–111.

Fujiki, M., Brinton, B., Hart, C. H., & Fitzgerald, A. (1999). Peer acceptance and friendship in children with specific language impairment. *Topics in Language Disorders, 19*(2), 34–48.

Fujiki, M., Brinton, B., Morgan, M., & Hart, C. (1999). Withdrawn and sociable behavior of children with langauge impairment. *Language, Speech, and Hearing Services in Schools, 30,* 183–195.

Fujiki, M., Brinton, B., Robinson, L., & Watson, V. (1997). The ability of children with specific language impairment to participate in a group decision task. *Journal of Childhood Communication Development, 18,* 1–10.

Fujiki, M., Brinton, B., & Todd, C. (1996). Social skills of children with specific langauge impairment. *Language, Speech, and Hearing Services in Schools, 27,* 195–201.

Fulk, B. M. (1994). Mnemonic keyword strategy training for students with learning disabilities. *Learning Disabilities Research and Practice, 9,* 179–185.

Fulkerson, S. C., & Freeman, W. H. (1980). Perceptual-motor deficiency in autistic children. *Perceptual and Motor Skills, 50,* 331–336.

Fung, F., & Roseberry-McKibbin, C. (1999). Service delivery considerations in working with clients from Cantonese-speaking backgrounds. *American Journal of Speech-Language Pathology, 8,* 309–318.

Gaddes, W. H., & Crockett, D. J. (1975). The Spreen-Benton aphasia tests, normative data as a measure of normal language development. *Brain and Language, 2,* 257–280.

Gagne, F. (1998). The prevalence of gifted, talented, and multitalented individuals: Estimates from peer and teacher nominations. In R. C. Friedman & K. B. Rogers (Eds.), *Talent in context: Historical and social perspectives on giftedness* (pp. 101–126). Washington, DC: American Psychological Association.

Gallagher, T. (1977). Revision behaviors in the speech of normal children developing language. *Journal of Speech and Hearing Research, 20,* 303–318.

Gallagher, T. (1999). Interrelationships among children's language, behavior, and emotional problems. *Topics in Language Disorders, 19*(2), 1–15.

Gallagher, T., & Darnton, B. (1978). Conversational aspects of the speech of language-disordered children: Revision behaviors. *Journal of Speech and Hearing Research, 21,* 118–135.

Gardner, H. (1974). Metaphors and modalities: How children project polar adjectives into diverse domains. *Child Development, 45,* 84–91.

Gardner, H., Kircher, M., Winner, E., & Perkins, D. (1975). Children's metaphoric productions and preferences. *Journal of Child Language, 2,* 125–141.

Gardner, M. (1979). *Expressive One-Word Picture Vocabulary Test.* Novato, CA: Academic Therapy.

Gardner, M. (1983). *Expressive One-Word Picture Vocabulary Test Upper Extension.* Novato, CA: Academic Therapy.

Gardner, M. (1993). *Test of Auditory Reasoning and Processing Skills.* Novato, CA: Academic Therapy.

Garnett, K. (1986). Telling tales: Narratives and learning-disabled children. *Topics in Language Disorders, 6,* 44–56.

Gathercole, S. (1995). Nonword repetition: More than just a phonological output task. *Cognitive Neuropsychology, 12,* 857–861.

Gathercole, S., & Baddeley, A. (1990). The role of phonological memory in vocabulary acquisition: A study of young children learning new names. *British Journal of Psychology, 81,* 439–454.

Gathercole, S., Hitch, G., Service, E., & Martin, A. (1997). Phonological short-term memory and new word learning in children. *Developmental Psychology, 33,* 966–979.

Gathercole, S., Willis, C., Baddeley, A., & Emslie, H. (1994). The Children's Test of Nonword Repetition: A test of phonological working memory. *Memory, 2,* 103–127.

Gaub, M., & Carlson, C. L. (1997). Gender differences in ADHD: A meta-analysis and critical review. *Journal of the American Academy of Child and Adolescent Psychiatry, 36,* 1036–1045.

Gavin, W., & Giles, L. (1996). Temporal reliability of language sample measures. *Journal of Speech and Hearing Research, 39,* 1258–1262.

Geers, A. (2002). Factors affecting the development of speech, language, and literacy in children with early cochlear implantation. *Language, Speech, and Hearing Services in Schools, 33*(3), 172–183.

Geers, A. (2003). Predictors of reading skill development in children with early cochlear implantation. *Ear and Hearing, 24*(1 Suppl.), 59S–68S.

Geers, A., & Brenner, C. (2003). Background and educational characteristics of prelingually deaf children implanted by five years of age. *Ear and Hearing, 24*(1 Suppl.), 2S–14S.

Geers, A., Brenner, C., & Davidson, L. (2003). Factors associated with development of speech perception skills in children implanted by age five. *Ear and Hearing, 24* (1 Suppl.), 24S–35S.

Geers, A., & Moog, J. (1994a). Spoken language results: Vocabulary, syntax, and communication. *Volta Review, 96*(5), 131–148.

Geers, A., & Moog, J. (1994b). The effectiveness of cochlear implants and tactile aids for deaf children. A report of the CID sensory aids study. *Volta Review, 96*(5), 1–232.

Geers, A., Nicholas, J., & Sedey, A. (2003). Language skills of children with early cochlear implantation. *Ear and Hearing, 24*(1 Suppl.), 46S–58S.

Geers, A., Spehar, B., & Sedey, A. (2002). Use of speech by children from total communication programs who wear cochlear implants. *American Journal of Speech Language Pathology, 11*(1), 50–58.

Gerber, S. E. (1990). Chromosomes and chromosomal disorders. *Asha, 32*(9), 39–41, 47.

Gerber, S., & Kraat, A. (1992). Use of a developmental model of language acquisition: Applications to children using AAC systems. *Augmentative and Alternative Communication, 8*(1), 19–32.

Gerdes, M., Solot, C., Wang, P. P., Moss, E., LaRossa, D., Randall, P., et al. (1999). Cognitive and behavior profile of preschool children with chromosome 22q11.2 deletion. *American Journal of Medical Genetics, 85*(2), 127–133.

Gerken, L. (1994). Young children's representations of prosodic phonology: Evidence from English-speakers' weak syllable productions. *Journal of Memory and Language, 33*, 19–38.

Gerken, L., & McGregor, K. (1998). An overview of prosody and its role in normal and disordered child language. *American Journal of Speech-Language Pathology, 7*, 38–48.

German, D. (1979). Word-finding skills in children with learning disabilities. *Journal of Learning Disabilities, 12*, 176–181.

German, D. (1982). Word-finding substitutions in children with learning disabilities. *Language, Speech, and Hearing Services in Schools, 13*, 223–230.

German, D. (1990). *Test of Adolescent/Adult Word Finding.* Austin, TX: Pro-Ed.

German, D. (1991). *Test of Word Finding in Discourse.* Austin, TX: Pro-Ed.

German, D. (1992). Word-finding intervention for children and adolescents. *Topics in Language Disorders, 13*, 33–50.

German, D. (2000). *Test of Word Finding—2.* Austin, TX: Pro-Ed.

German, D. (2001). *It's on the tip of my tongue, word finding strategies for remembering names and words you often forget.* Chicago: Word Finding Materials.

German, D., & Simon, E. (1991). Analysis of children's word-finding skills in discourse. *Journal of Speech and Hearing Research, 34*, 309–316.

Gershkoff-Stowe, L., & Smith, L. (1997). A curvilinear trend in naming errors as a function of early vocabulary growth. *Cognitive Psychology, 34*, 37–71.

Gertner, B., Rice, M., & Hadley, P. (1994). Influence of communicative competence on peer preferences in a preschool classroom. *Journal of Speech and Hearing Research, 37*, 913–923.

Gesell, A., & Thompson, H. (1934). *Infant behaviour: Its genesis and growth.* New York: McGraw-Hill.

Gibbs, D. P., & Cooper, E. B. (1989). Prevalence of communication disorders in students with learning disabilities. *Journal of Learning Disabilities, 22*, 60–63.

Gillam, R., & Carlile, R. M. (1997). Oral reading and story retelling of students with specific language impairment. *Language, Speech, and Hearing Services in Schools, 28*, 30–42.

Gillam, R., Cowan, N., & Marler, J. (1998). Information processing by school-age children with specific language impairment: Evidence from a modality effect paradigm. *Journal of Speech, Language, and Hearing Research, 41*, 913–926.

Gillam, R., Hoffman, L., Marler, J., & Wynn-Dancy, M. (2002). Sensitivity to increased task demands: Contributions from data-driven and conceptually driven processing deficits. *Topics in Language Disorders, 22*(3), 30–49.

Gillam, R., Peña, E., & Miller, L. (1999). Dynamic assessment of narrative and expository discourse. *Topics in Language Disorders, 20*(1), 33–47.

Gillberg, C. (1991). Outcome in autism and autistic-like conditions. *Journal of the American Academy of Child and Adolescent Psychiatry, 30*, 375–382.

Gillon, G., & Young, A. (2002). The phonological awareness skills of children who are blind. *Journal of Visual Impairment and Blindness, 96*, 38–49.

Giorcelli, L. (1991). *Programming communication for students with severe intellectual disability.* Parramatta, Australia: NSW Department of School Education.

Girolametto, L. (1988). Improving the social-conversational skills of developmentally delayed children: An intervention study. *Journal of Speech and Hearing Disorders, 53*, 156–167.

Girolametto, L. (1997). Development of a parent report measure for profiling the conversational skills of preschool children. *American Journal of Speech-Language Pathology, 6*(4), 25–33.

Girolametto, L., Pearce, P., & Weitzman, E. (1996). Interactive focused stimulation for toddlers with expressive vocabulary delays. *Journal of Speech and Hearing Research, 39,* 1274–1283.

Girolametto, L., & Weitzman, E. (2002). Responsiveness of child care providers in interactions with toddlers and preschoolers. *Language, Speech, and Hearing Services in Schools, 33,* 268–281.

Girolametto, L., Weitzman, E., & Greenberg, J. (2000). *Teacher Interaction and Language Rating Scale.* Toronto, Canada: The Hanen Centre.

Girolametto, L., Weitzman, E., van Lieshout, R., & Duff, D. (2000). Directiveness in teachers' language input to toddlers and preschoolers in day care. *Journal of Speech, Language, and Hearing Research, 43,* 1101–1114.

Girolametto, L., Weitzman, E., Wiigs, M., & Pearce, P. (1999). The relationship between maternal language measures and language development in toddlers with expresssive vocabulary delays. *American Journal of Speech-Language Pathology, 8,* 364–374.

Girolametto, L., Wiigs, M., Smyth, R., Weitzman, E., & Pearce, P. (2001). Children with a history of expressive vocabulary delay: Outcomes at 5 years of age. *American Journal of Speech-Language Pathology, 10,* 358–369.

Gisel, E. G., Birnbaum, R., & Schwartz, S. (1998). Feeding impairments in children: Diagnosis and effective intervention. *International Journal of Orofacial Myology, 24,* 27–33.

Givens, G., & Seidemann, M. (1977). Middle ear measurements in a difficult to test mentally retarded population. *Mental Retardation, 15,* 40–42.

Glass, A. L., & Perna, J. (1986). The role of syntax in reading disability. *Journal of Learning Disabilities, 19,* 354–359.

Glenn, C., & Stein, N. (1980). *Syntactic structures and real world themes in stories generated by children.* Urbana: University of Illinois Center for the Study of Reading.

Goldfarb, W., Braunstein, P., & Lorge, I. (1956). A study of speech patterns in a group of schizophrenic children. *American Journal of Orthopsychiatry, 26,* 544–555.

Goldstein, B. (2001). Transcription of Spanish and Spanish-influenced English. *Communication Disorders Quarterly, 23*(1), 54–60.

Goldstein, B., & Iglesias, A. (2001). The effect of dialect on phonological analysis: Evidence from Spanish-speaking children. *American Journal of Speech-Language Pathology, 10,* 394–406.

Goldstein, H., English, K., Shafer, K., & Kaczmarek, L. (1997). Interaction among preschoolers with and without disabilities: Effects of across-the-day peer intervention. *Journal of Speech, Language, and Hearing Research, 40,* 33–48.

Goldstein, H., & Ferrell, D. R. (1987). Augmenting communicative interaction between handicapped and nonhandicapped preschool children. *Journal of Speech and Hearing Disorders, 52,* 200–211.

Goldstein, H., & Mousetis, L. (1989). Generalized language learning by children with severe mental retardation:

Effects of peers' expressive modeling. *Journal of Applied Behavior Analysis, 22,* 245–259.

Golinkoff, R., Mervis, C. B., & Hirsh-Pasek, K. (1994). Early object labels: The case for a developmental lexical principles framework. *Journal of Child Language, 21,* 125–155.

Gonzalez-Lopez, A., & Kamps, D. M. (1997). Social skills training to increase social interactions between children with autism and their typical peers. *Focus on Autism and Other Developmental Disabilities, 12*(1), 2–14.

Goodluck, H. (1986). Children's knowledge of prepositional phrase structure: An experimental test. *Journal of Psycholinguistic Research, 15,* 177–188.

Goodyer, I. (2000). Language difficulties and psychopathology. In D. V. M. Bishop & L. Leonard (Eds.), *Speech and language impairment in children: Causes, characteristics, intervention and outcome* (pp. 227–244). East Sussex, UK: Psychology Press.

Goossens, C., & Crain, S. (1986). *Guidelines for selecting an initial core vocabulary for early intervention.* Wauconda, IL: Don Johnston.

Goossens, C., Crain, S., & Elder, P. S. (1992). *Engineering the preschool environment for interactive, symbolic communication.* Birmingham, AL: Southeast Augmentative Communication Conference Publications.

Gopnik, A. (1981). The development of non-nominal expressions: Why the first words are not about things. In D. Ingram & P. Dale (Eds.), *Child language: An international perspective.* Baltimore, MD: University Park Press.

Gopnik, M. (1990). Feature-blind grammar and dysphasia. *Nature, 344,* 715.

Gottardo, A. (2002). The relationship between language and reading skills in bilingual Spanish-English speakers. *Topics in Language Disorders, 22*(5), 46–70.

Graham, J. T., & Graham, L. W. (1971). Language behavior of the mentally retarded: Syntactic characteristics. *American Journal of Mental Deficiency, 75,* 623–629.

Graham, S., & Harris, K. (1999). Assessment and intervention in overcoming writing difficulties: An illustration from the self-regulated strategy development model. *Language, Speech, and Hearing Services in Schools, 30,* 255–264.

Grandin, T. (1995). *Thinking in pictures and other reports from my life with autism.* New York: Doubleday.

Granlund, M. (1991). Staff in-service training on intervention with persons with impairments. *European Journal of Special Needs Education, 6*(3), 165–175.

Granlund, M., Björck-Åkesson, E., Brodin, J., & Olsson, C. (1995). Communication intervention for persons with profound disabilities: A Swedish perspective. *Augmentative and Alternative Communication, 11*(1), 49–59.

Granlund, M., Björck-Åkesson, E., Olsson, C., & Rydeman, B. (2001). Working with families to introduce augmentative and alternative communication systems. In H. Cockerill

& L. Carroll-Few (Eds.), *Communication without speech: Practical communication for children* (pp. 88–102). Cambridge, UK: Mac Keith Press.

Gravel, J., & Wallace, I. (1992). Listening and language at 4 years of age. *Journal of Speech and Hearing Research, 35,* 588–595.

Gray, D., Achilles, J., Keller, T., Tate, D., Haggard, L., Rolfs, R., Cazier, C., Workman, J., & McMahon, W. (2002). Utah Youth Suicide Study. *Journal of the American Academy of Child and Adolescent Psychiatry, 41,* 427–434.

Gray, S. (2003a). Diagnostic accuracy and test-retest reliability of nonword repetition and digit span tasks administered to preschool children with specific language impairment. *Journal of Communication Disorders, 36,* 129–151.

Gray, S. (2003b). Word-learning by preschoolers with specific language impairment: What predicts success? *Journal of Speech, Language, and Hearing Research, 46,* 56–67.

Gray, S., Plante, E., Vance, R., & Henrichsen, M. (1999). The diagnostic accuracy of four vocabulary tests administered to preschool-age children. *Language, Speech, and Hearing Services in Schools, 30,* 196–206.

Greenfield, P., & Smith, J. (1976). *The structure of communication in early language development.* New York: Academic Press.

Greenfield, P., & Zukow, P. (1978). Why do children say what they say when they say it? An experimental approach to the psychogenesis of presupposition. In K. Nelson (Ed.), *Children's language* (Vol. 1). New York: Gardner Press.

Grejda, G. F., & Hannafin, M. J. (1992). Effects of word processing on sixth graders' holistic writing and revisions. *Journal of Education Research, 85,* 144–149.

Grela, B. G. (2003). Do children with Down syndrome have difficulty with argument structure? *Journal of Communication Disorders, 36,* 263–279.

Griffin, C. C., & Tulbert, B. L. (1995). The effect of graphic organizers on students' comprehension and recall of expository text: A review of the research and implications for practice. *Reading and Writing Quarterly, 11*(1), 73–89.

Grossman, H. J. (Ed.). (1983). *Classification in mental retardation.* Washington, DC: American Association on Mental Deficiency.

Grosz, D., Zimmerman, J., & Asnis, G. (1995). Suicidal behavior in adolescents: A review of risk and protective factors. In J. Zimmerman & G. Asnis (Eds.), *Treatment approaches with suicidal adolescents* (pp. 17–43). Oxford, UK: Wiley.

Grove, N., & Walker, M. (1990). The Makaton Vocabulary: Using manual signs and graphic symbols to develop interpersonal communication. *Augmentative & Alternative Communication, 6,* 15–18.

Grunwell, P., & Russell, J. (1987). Vocalisations before and after cleft palate surgery: A pilot study. *British Journal of Disorders of Communication, 22,* 1–17.

Gualtieri, L., Koriath, U., Van Bourgondien, M., & Saleeby, N. (1983). Language disorders in children referred for psychiatric services. *Journal of the American Academy of Child Psychiatry, 22,* 165–171.

Guilford, A., Scheuerle, J., & Shonburn, S. (1981). Aspects of language development in the gifted. *Gifted Child Quarterly, 25,* 159–163.

Gummersall, D., & Strong, C. (1999). Assessment of complex sentence production in a narrative context. *Language, Speech, and Hearing Services in Schools, 30,* 152–164.

Gunnell, D., Lopatatzidis, A., Dorling, D., Wehner, H., Southall, H., & Frankel, S. (1999). Suicide and unemployment in young people: Analysis of trends in England and Wales, 1921–1995. *British Journal of Psychiatry, 175*(9), 263–270.

Guralnick, M. J., & Paul-Brown, D. (1986). Communicative interactions of mildly delayed and normally developing preschool children: Effects of listener's developmental level. *Journal of Speech and Hearing Research, 29,* 2–10.

Gutiérrez-Clellen, V. (1999). Language choice in intervention with bilingual children. *American Journal of Speech-Language Pathology, 8,* 291–302.

Gutiérrez-Clellen, V., & Peña, E. (2001). Dynamic assessment of diverse children: A tutorial. *Language, Speech, and Hearing Services in Schools, 32,* 212–224.

Gutiérrez-Clellen, V., Restrepo, M., Bedore, L., Peña, E., & Anderson, R. (2000). Language sample analysis in Spanish-speaking children: Methodological considerations. *Language, Speech, and Hearing Services in Schools, 31,* 88–98.

Hadley, P. (1998). Language sampling protocols for eliciting text-level discourse. *Language, Speech, and Hearing Services in Schools, 29,* 132–147.

Hadley, P. (1999). Validating a rate-based measure of early grammatical abilities: Unique syntactic types. *American Journal of Speech-Language Pathology, 8,* 261–272.

Hadley, P., & Rice, M. (1991). Conversational responsiveness of speech- and language-impaired preschoolers. *Journal of Speech and Hearing Research, 34,* 1308–1317.

Hadley, P., & Schuele, C. M. (1998). Facilitating peer interaction: Socially relevant objectives for preschool language intervention. *American Journal of Speech-Language Pathology, 7*(4), 25–36.

Hadley, P., Simmerman, A., Long, M., & Luna, M. (2000). Facilitating language development for inner-city children: Experimental evaluation of a collaborative, classroom-based intervention. *Language, Speech, and Hearing Services in Schools, 31,* 280–295.

Haggard, M., Birkin, J., & Pringle, D. (1994). Consequences of otitis media for speech and language. In B. McCormick (Ed.), *Pediatric Audiology.* London, UK: Whurr.

Hale-Benson, J. (1986). *Black children: Their roots, culture, and learning styles* (2nd ed.). Baltimore, MD: Johns Hopkins University Press.

Haley, S. M., Cioffi, M. I., Lewin, J. E., & Baryza, M. J. (1990). Motor dysfunction in children and adolescents after traumatic brain injury. *Journal of Head Trauma Rehabilitation, 5,* 77–90.

Hall, E. (1959). *The silent language.* New York: Fawcett.

Hall, P., & Tomblin, J. B. (1978). A follow-up study of children with articulation and language disorders. *Journal of Speech and Hearing Disorders, 43,* 227–241.

Halliday, M. (1974). A sociosemiotic perspective on language development. *Bulletin of the School of Oriental and African Studies, 37,* Part 1.

Halliday, M. (1975). *Learning how to mean: Explorations in the development of language.* London, UK: Edward Arnold.

Hammill, D. (1990). On defining learning disabilities: An emerging consensus. *Journal of Learning Disabilities, 23,* 74–84.

Hammill, D. (1998). *Detroit Test of Learning Aptitude—4.* Austin, TX: Pro-Ed.

Hammill, D., Brown, V., Larsen, S., & Wiederholt, J. L. (1994). *Test of Adolescent and Adult Language—3.* Austin, TX: Pro-Ed.

Hammill, D., & Bryant, B. (1991). *Detroit Tests of Learning Aptitude—Adult.* Austin, TX: Pro-Ed.

Hammill, D., & Larsen, S. (1974). The effectiveness of psycholinguistic training. *Exceptional Children, 40,* 5–14.

Hammill, D., Mather, N., & Roberts, R. (2001). *Illinois Test of Psycholinguistic Abilities—3.* Austin, TX: Pro-Ed.

Hammill, D., & Newcomer, P. (1997). *Test of Language Development: Intermediate—3.* Austin, TX: Pro-Ed.

Hammill, D., Pearson, N., & Wiederholt, J. L. (1996). *Comprehensive Test of Nonverbal Intelligence.* Austin, TX: Pro-Ed.

Hannah, E. (1977). *Applied linguistic analysis II.* Pacific Palisades, CA: SenCom Associates.

Hanzlik, J. R., & Stevenson, M. B. (1986). Interaction of mothers with their infants who are mentally retarded, retarded with cerebral palsy, or nonretarded. *American Journal of Mental Deficiency, 90,* 513–520.

Hargrove, P. (1997). Prosodic aspects of language impairment in children. *Topics in Language Disorders, 17*(4), 76–83.

Harris, G. (1985). Considerations in assessing English language performance of Native American children. *Topics in Language Disorders, 5*(4), 42–52.

Harris, M. (1992). *Language experience and early language development.* Hove, UK: Lawrence Erlbaum.

Harris, S. L., Handleman, J. S., Gordon, R., Kristoff, B., & Fuentes, F. (1991). Changes in cognitive and language functioning of preschool children with autism. *Journal of Autism and Developmental Disorders, 21,* 281–290.

Harris, S. L., Handleman, J. S., Kristoff, B., Bass, L., & Gordon, R. (1990). Changes in language development among autistic and peer children in segregated and integrated preschool settings. *Journal of Autism and Developmental Disorders, 20,* 23–31.

Hart, B., & Risley, T. (1995). *Meaningful differences in the everyday experience of young American children.* Baltimore, MD: Paul H. Brookes.

Hartas, D., & Donahue, M. (1997). Conversational and social problem-solving skills in adolescents with learning disabilities. *Learning Disabilities Research and Practice, 12,* 213–220.

Harter, S., Whitesell, N. R., & Junkin, L. J. (1998). Similarities and differences in domain-specific and global self-evaluations of learning-disabled, behaviorally disordered, and normally achieving adolescents. *American Educational Research Journal, 35*(4), 653–680.

Hasle, H., Clemmensen, I. H., & Mikkelsen, M. (2000). Risks of leukaemia and solid tumours in individuals with Down's syndrome. *Lancet, 355,* 165–169.

Hass, W., & Wepman, J. (1974). Dimensions of individual difference in the spoken syntax of school children. *Journal of Speech and Hearing Research, 17,* 455–469.

Hawley, C. A., Ward, A. B., Magnay, A. R., & Long, J. (2003). Parental stress and burden following traumatic brain injury amongst children and adolescents. *Brain Injury, 1,* 1–23.

Hayakawa, S. (1964). *Language in thought and action* (2nd ed.). New York: Harcourt, Brace & World.

Haynes, W., Haak, N., Moran, M., Rice, R., & Johnson, V. (1995, December). The Preschool Language Assessment Instrument (PLAI): Performance differences in rural southern African American and White Headstart children. Paper presented at the Annual Convention of the American Speech-Language-Hearing Association, Orlando, FL.

Hazen, N., & Black, B. (1989). Preschool peer communication skills: The role of social status and interaction context. *Child Development, 60,* 867–876.

Hécaen, H. (1976). Acquired aphasia in children and the ontogenesis of hemispheric functional specialization. *Brain and Language, 3,* 114–134.

Hedrick, D., Prather, E., & Tobin, A. (1975). *Sequenced inventory of communication development.* Seattle: University of Washington.

Hegde, M. (1980). An experimental-clinical analysis of grammatical and behavioral distinctions between verbal auxiliary and copula. *Journal of Speech and Hearing Research, 23,* 864–877.

Hegde, M., Noll, M., & Pecora, R. (1979). A study of some factors affecting generalization of language training. *Journal of Speech and Hearing Disorders, 44,* 301–320.

Heibeck, T., & Markman, E. (1987). Word learning in children: An examination of fast mapping. *Child Development, 58,* 1021–1034.

Hemmeter, M. L. (2000). Classroom-based interventions: Evaluating the past and looking toward the future. *Topics in Early Childhood Special Education, 20*(1), 56–61.

Henderson, C. (2001). *College freshmen with disabilities: A biennial statistical profile.* Washington, DC: American Council on Education.

Henry, F., Reed, V. A., & McAllister, L. (1995). Adolescents' perceptions of the relative importance of selected communication in their positive peer relationships. *Language, Speech, and Hearing Services in Schools, 26,* 263–272.

Hernandez, R. (1994). Reducing bias in the assessment of culturally and linguistically diverse populations. *Journal of Educational Issues of Language Minority Students, 14,* 269–300.

Hester, E. (1996). Narratives of young African American children. In A. Kamhi, K. Pollock, & J. Harris (Eds.), *Communication development and disorders in African American children: Research, assessment, and intervention* (pp. 227–245). Baltimore, MD: Paul H. Brookes.

Hill, S., & Haynes, W. (1992). Language performance in low-achieving elementary school students. *Language, Speech, and Hearing Services in Schools, 23,* 169–175.

Hillis, A. E., & Bahr, D. C. (2001). Neurological and anatomical bases. In D. C. Bahr (Ed.), *Oral motor assessment and treatment: Ages and stages* (pp. 1–41). Boston: Allyn & Bacon.

Hirshoren, A., & Ambrose, W. (1976). The Wepman Auditory Discrimination Test and Southern Piedmont children. *Language, Speech, and Hearing Services in Schools, 7,* 86–90.

Hirst, E., & Brittion, L. (1998). Specialised service to children with specific language impairment in mainstream schools. *International Journal of Language and Communication Disorders, 33,* 593–598.

Hobson, R. P. (1993). *Autism and the development of mind.* Mahwah, NJ: Lawrence Erlbaum.

Hodapp, R. M., Evans, D. W., & Ward, B. A. (1989). Communicative interaction between teachers and children with severe handicaps. *Mental Retardation, 27,* 388–395.

Hoff-Ginsberg, E., & Naigles, L. (1999, July). Fast mapping is only the beginning: Complete word learning requires multiple exposures. Paper presented at the VIIth International Congress for the Study of Child Language, San Sebastian, Spain.

Holland, A. (1975). Language therapy for children: Some thoughts on context. *Journal of Speech and Hearing Disorders, 40,* 514–523.

Holm, V., & Kunze, L. (1969). Effects of chronic otitis media on language and speech development. *Paediatrics, 43,* 833.

Holmes, D. L. (1998). *Autism through the lifespan: The Eden model.* Bethesda, MD: Woodbine House.

Hood, L. (1998). Auditory neuropathy: What it is and what we can do about it. *Hearing Journal, 51*(8), 10–18.

Horner, R. H., & Budd, C. M. (1985, March). Acquisition of manual sign use: Collateral reduction of maladaptive behavior, and factors limiting generalization. *Education and Training of the Mentally Retarded, 39*–47.

Horstmeier, D., & MacDonald, J. (1978). *The Environmental Language Intervention Program.* Columbus, OH: Merrill.

Hotz, G., Helm-Estabrooks, N., & Nelson, N. W. (2001). Development of the Pediatric Test of Traumatic Brain Injury. *Journal of Head Trauma Rehabilitation, 16*(5), 426–440.

Howard, J. B. (1994). Addressing needs through strengths: Five instructional practices for use with gifted/learning disabled students. *Journal of Secondary Gifted Education, 5*(3), 23–34.

Howe, M. J. A. (1990). *The origins of exceptional abilities.* Cambridge, MA: Basil Blackwell.

Howe, M. J. A., Davidson, J. W., & Sloboda, J. A. (1998). Innate talents: Reality or myth? *Behavioral and Brain Sciences, 21,* 399–442.

Howie, V. (1975). Natural history of otitis media. *Annals of Otolaryngology, Rhinology, and Laryngology, 19*(Suppl.), 67–72.

Howlin, P., Wing, L., & Gould, J. (1995). The recognition of autism in children with Down syndrome—Implications for intervention and some speculations about pathology. *Developmental Medicine and Child Neurology, 37,* 404–414.

Huang, R., Hopkins, J., & Nippold, M. (1997). Satisfaction with standardized language testing: A survey of speech-language pathologists. *Language, Speech, and Hearing Services in Schools, 28,* 12–29.

Hubbell, R. (1981). *Children's language disorders: An intergrated approach.* Englewood Cliffs, NJ: Prentice-Hall.

Hughes, D. (1989). Generalization from language therapy to classroom academics. *Seminars in Speech and Language, 10,* 218–229.

Hughes, D. (1998). Effects of preparation time for two quantitative measures of narrative production. *Perceptual and Motor Skills, 87*(1), 343–352.

Hughes, D., McGillivray, L., & Schmidek, M. (1997). *Guide to narrative language.* Eau Claire, WI: Thinking Publications.

Hulit, L. M., & Howard, M. R. (2002). *Born to talk: An introduction to speech and language development* (3rd ed.). Boston: Allyn & Bacon.

Hulme, C., & MacKenzie, S. (1992). *Working memory and severe learning difficulties.* London, UK: Erlbaum.

Hummel, L., & Prizant, B. (1993). Language and social skills in the school-age population: A socioemotional perspective for understanding social difficulties of school-age children with language disorders. *Language, Speech, and Hearing Services in Schools, 24,* 216–224.

Hunt, K. (1965). *Grammatical structures written at three grade levels.* Urbana, IL: National Council of Teachers of English.

Hunt, P., Alwell, M., & Goetz, L. (1988). Acquisition of conversation skills and the reduction of inappropriate social behaviors. *Journal of the Association for Persons with Severe Handicaps, 13*(1), 20–27.

Hunt, P., Alwell, M., & Goetz, L. (1991). Interactions with peers through conversation turn taking with a communication book adaptation. *Augmentative and Alternative Communication, 7*(2), 117–126.

Hunt, P., Soto, G., Maier, E., Müller, E., & Goetz, L. (2002). Collaborative teaming to support students with augmentative and alternative communication needs in general classrooms. *Augmentative & Alternative Communication, 18,* 20–35.

Hutchinson, T. (1996). What to look for in the technical manual: Twenty questions for users. *Language, Speech, and Hearing Services in Schools, 27,* 109–121.

Hutson-Nechkash, P. (1990). *Storybuilding: A guide to structuring oral narratives.* Eau Claire, WI: Thinking Publications.

Huttenlocher, J., Haight, W., Bryk, A., Seltzer, M., & Lyons, T. (1991). Early vocabulary growth: Relation to language input and gender. *Developmental Psychology, 27,* 236–248.

Hux, K., Morris-Friehe, M., & Sanger, D. (1993). Language sampling practices: A survey of nine states. *Language, Speech, and Hearing Services in Schools, 24,* 84–91.

Hux, K., Walker, M., & Sanger, D. D. (1996). Traumatic brain injury: Knowledge and self-perceptions of school speech-language pathologists. *Language, Speech, and Hearing Services in Schools, 27,* 171–184.

Hwa-Froelich, D., Hodson, B., & Edwards, H. (2002). Characteristics of Vietnamese Phonology. *American Journal of Speech-Language Pathology, 11,* 264–273.

Hyter, Y. (1998). *Ties that bind: The sounds of African American English.* Multicultural Electronic Journal of Communication Disorders. Retrieved December 2, 2002, from www.asha.ucf.edu/hyter.html

Hyter, Y., Rogers-Adkinson, D., Self, T., Simmons, B., & Jantz, J. (2001). Pragmatic language intervention for children with language and emotional/behavioral disorders. *Communication Disorders Quarterly, 23,* 4–16.

Iacono, T. A. (1992). Individual language learning styles and augmentative and alternative communication. *Augmentative and Alternative Communication, 8*(1), 33–40.

Iacono, T. A., Chan, J. B., & Waring, R. E. (1998). Efficacy of a parent implemented early language intervention based on collaborative consultation. *International Journal of Language and Communication Disorders, 33,* 281–303.

Iacono, T. A., & Duncum, J. E. (1995). Comparison of sign alone and in combination with an electronic communication device in early language intervention: Case study. *Augmentative and Alternative Communication, 11*(4), 249–259.

Iacono, T., Mirenda, P., & Beukelman, D. (1993). Comparison of unimodal and multimodal AAC techniques for children with intellectual disabilities. *Augmentative and Alternative Communication, 9*(2), 83–94.

Iacono, T. A., & Parsons, C. L. (1987). Stepping beyond the teaching manuals into signing in the "real world." *Australian Journal of Human Communication Disorders, 15*(2), 101–116.

Iglesias, A., & Anderson, N. (1993). Dialectal variations. In N. W. Bernthal (Ed.), *Articulation and phonological disorders* (3rd ed.). Englewood Cliffs, NJ: Prentice Hall.

Immunization Safety Review Committee—Institute of Medicine. (2001). *Immunization safety review: Measles-mumps-rubella vaccine and autism.* Washington, DC: National Academy Press. Retrieved July 2002, from http://books.nap.edu/html/mmr/report.pdf

Ingram, D. (1989a). *First language acquisition: Method, description, and explanation.* Cambridge, UK: Cambridge University Press.

Ingram, D. (1989b). *Phonological disability in children* (2nd ed.). London, UK: Cole & Whurr.

Irlen, H. (2002). *Reading by the colors: Overcoming dyslexia and other reading disabilities through the Irlen method.* New York: Berkley Publishing Group.

Iwan, S., & Siegel, G. (1982). The effects of feedback on referential communication of preschool children. *Journal of Speech and Hearing Research, 25,* 224–229.

Jackson, N. E. (1988). Precocious reading ability: What does it mean? *Gifted Child Quarterly, 32,* 200–204.

Jackson, N. E., & Kearney, J. M. (1995). Achievement of precocious readers in middle childhood and young adulthood. In N. Colangelo & S. Assouline (Eds.), *Talent Development III* (pp. 203–218). Scottsdale, AZ: Gifted Psychology Press.

Jackson, T., & Plante, E. (1996). Gyral morphology in the posterior sylvian region in families affected by developmental language disorders. *Neuropsychology Review, 6*(2), 81–94.

Jackson-Maldonado, D., Bates, E., & Thal, D. (1992). *Fundación MacArthur: Inventario del desarrollo de habilidades comunicativas.* San Diego, CA: San Diego State University.

Jacoby, G., Levin, L., Lee, L., Creaghead, N., & Kummer, A. (2002). The number of individual treatment units necessary to facilitate functional communication improvements in the speech and language of young children. *American Journal of Speech-Language Pathology, 11,* 370–380.

Jan, J. E., Groenveld, M., Sykanda, A. M., & Hoyt, C. S. (1987). Behavioural characteristics of children with permanent cortical visual impairment. *Developmental Medicine and Child Neurology, 29,* 571–576.

Janicki, M. P., & Dalton, A. J. (2000). Prevalence of dementia and impact on intellectual disability services. *Mental Retardation, 38*(3), 276–288.

Jarrold, C., Baddeley, A. D., & Hewes, A. K. (1999). Genetically dissociated components of working memory: Evidence from Down's and William's syndrome. *Neuropsychologia, 37,* 637–651.

Javorsky, J. (1996). An examination of youth with attention deficit/hyperactivity disorder and language learning disabilities: A clinical study. *Journal of Learning Disabilities, 29*(3), 247–259.

JCIHS. (1995). Joint Committee on Infant Screening 1994 position paper. *Paediatrics, 95,* 152–156.

JCIHS. (2000). Joint Committee of Infant Hearing Screening: Year 2000 position statement. Principles and guidelines for early hearing detection and intervention programs. *Audiology Today,* Special Issue, August, 6–27.

Jenkins, C. (1993). Expressive language delay in children with Down's syndrome: A specific cause for concern. *Down Syndrome: Research and Practice, 1,* 10–14.

Jensen, J. (1973). Do gifted children speak an intellectual dialect? *Exceptional Children, 39,* 337–338.

Jerger, J. (1998). Controversial issues in central auditory processing disorders. *Seminars in Hearing, 19,* 393–397.

Jerger, J., & Musiek, F. (2000). Report on the Consensus Conference on the Diagnosis of Auditory Processing Disorders in School-Aged Children. *Journal of the Academy of Audiology, 11*(9), 467–474.

Jerger, S., & Jerger, J. (1983). Evaluation of diagnostic audiometric tests. *Audiology, 22*(2), 144–161.

Jerome, A., Fujiki, M., Brinton, B., & James, S. (2002). Self-esteem in children with specific language impairment. *Journal of Speech, Language, and Hearing Research, 45,* 700–714.

Johnson, C. (1995). Expanding norms for narration. *Language, Speech, and Hearing Services in Schools, 26,* 326–341.

Johnson, C., & Anglin, J. (1995). Qualitative developments in the content and form of children's definitions. *Journal of Speech and Hearing Research, 38,* 612–629.

Johnson, C., Beitchman, J., Young, A., Escobar, M., Atkinson, L., Wilson, B., et al. (1999). Fourteen-year follow up of children with and without speech/language impairments: Speech/language stability and outcomes. *Journal of Speech, Language, and Hearing Research, 42,* 744–760.

Johnson, M. H., Siddons, F., Frith, U., & Morton, J. (1992). Can autism be predicted on the basis of infant screening tests? *Developmental Medicine and Child Neurology, 34,* 316–320.

Johnson, R., Liddell, S., & Erting, C. (1989). *Unlocking the curriculum: Principle for achieving access in deaf education (Working Paper 89-3).* Washington, DC: Gallaudet University Press, Gallaudet Research Institute.

Johnson, S. S., & Reichle, J. (1993). Designing and implementing interventions to decrease challenging behavior.

Language, Speech, and Hearing Services in Schools, 24, 225–235.

John-Steiner, V., & Panofsky, C. (1992). Narrative competence: Cross-cultural comparisons. *Journal of Narrative and Life History, 2,* 219–233.

Johnston, J. (1994). Cognitive abilities of children with language impairment. In R. Watkins & M. Rice (Eds.), *Specific language impairments in children* (pp. 107–121). Baltimore, MD: Paul H. Brookes.

Johnston, J. (2001). An alternate MLU calculation: Magnitude and variability. *Journal of Speech, Language, and Hearing Research, 44,* 156–164.

Johnston, J., & Wong, M.-Y. A. (2002). Cultural differences in beliefs and practices concerning talk to children. *Journal of Speech, Language, and Hearing Research, 45,* 916–926.

Johnston, W., & Packer, A. (1987). *Workforce 2000: Work and workers for the 21st century.* Indianapolis, IN: Hudson Institute.

Jones, O. H. M. (1977). Mother–child communication with prelinguistic Down's syndrome and normal infants. In H. R. Schaffer (Ed.), *Studies in mother–infant interaction.* London, UK: Academic Press.

Jones, R., Lennings, C., Ward, P., Neville, M., Howard, J., & Mackdacy, E. (1999). Descriptions of youth who self harm: The Mackay-Mooranbah Youth Suicide Prevention Project. *Journal of Applied Health Behavior, 1*(2), 23–30.

Joos, M. (1976). The style of the five clocks. In N. Johnson (Ed.), *Current topics in language: Introductory readings.* Cambridge, MA: Winthrop.

Jordan, F., & Ashton, R. (1996). Language performance of severely closed head injured children. *Brain Injury, 10*(2), 91–97.

Jordan, F., Cremona-Meteyard, S., & King, A. (1996). High-level linguistic disturbances subsequent to childhood closed head injury. *Brain Injury, 10*(10), 729–738.

Jordan, F., & Murdoch, B. (1994). Severe closed-head injury in childhood: Linguistic outcomes into adulthood. *Brain Injury, 8*(6), 501–508.

Jordan, F., Murdoch, B., Buttsworth, D., & Hudson-Tennent, L. (1995). Speech and language performance of brain-injured children. *Aphasiology, 9*(1), 23–32.

Jordan, F., Murdoch, B., Hudson-Tennent, L., & Boon, D. (1996). Naming performance of brain-injured children. *Aphasiology, 10*(8), 755–766.

Juan-Garau, M., & Perez-Vidal, C. (2001). Mixing and pragmatic parental strategies in early bilingual acquisition. *Journal of Child Language, 28*(1), 59–86.

Just, M., & Carpenter, P. (1992). A capacity theory of comprehension: Individual differences in working memory. *Psychological Review, 99,* 122–149.

Justice, L., & Ezell, H. (2000). Enhancing children's print and word awareness through home-based parent intervention. *American Journal of Speech-Language Pathology, 9*, 257–269.

Justice, L., & Ezell, H. (2002). Use of storybook reading to increase print awareness in at-risk children. *American Journal of Speech-Language Pathology, 11*, 17–29.

Justice, L., Invernizzi, M., & Meier, J. (2002). Designing and implementing an early literacy screeing protocol: Suggestions for the speech-language pathologist. *Language, Speech, and Hearing Services in Schools, 33*, 84–101.

Justice, L., Weber, S., Ezell, H., & Bakeman, R. (2002). A sequential analysis of children's responsiveness to parental print references during shared book-reading interactions. *American Journal of Speech-Language Pathology, 11*, 30–40.

Kahn, J. (1984). Cognitive training and initial use of referential speech. *Topics in Language Disorders, 5*, 14–23.

Kail, R. (1992). General slowing of information-processing by persons with mental retardation. *American Journal of Mental Retardation, 97*(3), 333–341.

Kail, R., Hale, C., Leonard, L., & Nippold, M. (1984). Lexical storage and retrieval in language-impaired children. *Applied Psycholinguistics, 5*, 37–49.

Kail, R., & Leonard, L. (1986). *Word-finding abilities in language-impaired children.* Rockville, MD: American Speech-Language-Hearing Association.

Kamhi, A., & Catts, H. (1986). Toward an understanding of developmental language and reading disorders. *Journal of Speech and Hearing Disorders, 51*, 337–347.

Kamhi, A., & Catts, H. (1991). *Reading disabilities: A developmental language perspective.* Boston: Allyn & Bacon.

Kamhi, A., Catts, H., & Mauer, D. (1990). Explaining speech production deficits in poor readers. *Journal of Learning Disabilities, 23*, 632–636.

Kamhi, A., & Johnston, J. R. (1982). Towards an understanding of retarded children's linguistic deficiencies. *Journal of Speech and Hearing Research, 25*, 435–445.

Kamhi, A., & Koenig, L. (1985). Metalinguistic awareness in normal and language-disordered children. *Language, Speech, and Hearing Services in Schools, 16*, 199–210.

Kangas, K. A., & Lloyd, L. (1988). Early cognitive skills as prerequisites to augmentative and alternative communication use: What are we waiting for? *Augmentative and Alternative Communication, 4*(4), 211–221.

Kanner, L. (1943). Autistic disturbances of affective contact. *Nervous Child, 2*, 217–250.

Kapell, D., Nightingale, B., Rodriquez, A., Lee, J. H., Zigman, W. B., & Schupf, N. (1998). Prevalence of chronic medical conditions in adults with MR: Comparison with the general population. *Mental Retardation, 36*, 269–279.

Kaplan, J., & Kies, D. (1994). Strategies to increase critical thinking in the undergraduate classroom. *College Student Journal, 28*, 24–31.

Karr, S. (1999). Action: School services. *Language, Speech, and Hearing Services in Schools, 30*, 212–216.

Kasari, C., Freeman, S. F. N., & Paparella, T. (2001). Early intervention in autism: Joint attention and symbolic play. In L. M. Glidden (Ed.), *International review of research in mental retardation: Autism* (Vol. 23, pp. 207–232). San Diego, CA: Academic Press.

Kasari, C., & Hodapp, R. M. (1996). Is Down syndrome different? Evidence from social and family studies. *Down Syndrome Quarterly, 1*(4), 1–8.

Katz, R. (1996). Object-naming errors and reading ability. *Annals of Dyslexia, 46*, 189–208.

Katz, W. F., Curtiss, S., & Tallal, P. (1992). Rapid automatized naming and gesture by normal and language-impaired children. *Brain and Language, 43*(4), 623–641.

Kauffman, J. (2001). *Characteristics of emotional and behavioral disorders of children and youth* (7th ed.). Columbus, OH: Merrill.

Kaufman, A., & Kaufman, N. (1983). *Kaufman Assessment Battery for Children (K-ABC).* Circle Pines, MN: American Guidance Service.

Kavale, K. A., & Forness, S. (1985). *The science of learning disabilities.* Boston: College-Hill Press.

Kay-Raining Bird, E., & Chapman, R. (1994). Sequential recall in individuals with Down syndrome. *Journal of Speech and Hearing Research, 37*, 1369–1380.

Kay-Raining Bird, E., Cleave, P. L., & McConnell, L. (2000). Reading and phonological awareness in children with Down syndrome: A longitudinal study. *American Journal of Speech-Language Pathology, 9*, 319–330.

Kay-Raining Bird, E., & Vetter, D. (1994). Storytelling in Chippewa-Cree children. *Journal of Speech and Hearing Research, 37*, 1354–1368.

Keen, D., Woodyatt, G., & Sigafoos, J. (2002). Verifying teacher perceptions of the potential communicative acts of children with autism. *Communication Disorders Quarterly, 23*, 133–142.

Keenan, E. (1975). Evolving discourse—The next step. *Papers and Reports on Child Language Development, 10*, 80–87.

Keith, R. (1986). *SCAN: A Screening Test for Auditory Processing Disorders.* San Diego, CA: The Psychological Corporation.

Keith, R. (1994a). *Auditory Continuous Performance Test.* San Antonio, TX: Psychological Corporation.

Keith, R. (1994b). *SCAN—A: A test for auditory processing disorders in adolescents and adults.* San Antonio, TX: Psychological Corporation.

Keith, R. (1999). Clinical issues in central auditory processing disorders. *Language, Speech, and Hearing Services in the Schools, 30*(4), 339–344.

Keith, R. (2000). *Test for Auditory Processing Problems in Children—Revised.* San Antonio, TX: Psychological Corporation.

Kekelis, L. S., & Prinz, P. M. (1996). Blind and sighted children with their mothers: The development of discourse skills. *Journal of Visual Impairment and Blindness, 90,* 423–436.

Kelly, D. (1998). A clinical synthesis of the "late talker" literature: Implications for service delivery. *Language, Speech, and Hearing Services in Schools, 29,* 76–84.

Kelly, D., & Rice, M. (1994). Preferences for verb interpretation in children with specific language impairment. *Journal of Speech and Hearing Research, 37,* 182–192.

Kemp, K., & Klee, T. (1997). Clinical speech and language sampling practices: Results of a survey of speech-language pathologists in the United States. *Child Language Teaching and Therapy, 13,* 161–176.

Kennedy, E. J., & Flynn, M. C. (2003). Training phonological awareness skills in children with Down syndrome. *Research in Developmental Disabilities, 24,* 44–57.

Kent, R. D. (1999). Motor control: Neurophysiology and functional development. In A. J. Caruso & E. A. Strand (Eds.), *Clinical management of motor speech disorders in children* (pp. 29–71). New York: Thieme Medical Publishers.

Kent, R. D., Osberger, M. J., Netsell, R., & Hustedde, C. G. (1987). Phonetic development in identical twins differing in auditory function. *Journal of Speech and Hearing Disorders, 52*(1), 64–75.

Kerbel, D., & Grunwell, P. (1997). Idioms in the classroom: An investigation of language unit and mainstream teachers' use of idioms. *Child Language Teaching and Therapy, 13,* 113–123.

Kessel, F. (1970). The role of syntax in children's comprehension from ages six to twelve. *Monographs of the Society for Research in Child Development, 35,* 1–95.

Kiernan, B., & Snow, D. (1999). Bound-morpheme generalization by children with SLI: Is there a functional relationship with accuracy of response to training. *Journal of Speech, Language, and Hearing Research, 42,* 649–662.

Kiese-Himmel, C. (2002). Unilateral sensorineural hearing impairment in childhood: Analysis of 31 consecutive cases. *International Journal of Audiology, 41,* 57–63.

Kim, Y., & Lombardino, L. (1991). The efficacy of script contexts in language comprehension intervention with children who have mental retardation. *Journal of Speech and Hearing Research, 34,* 845–857.

Kindler, A. (2002). *Survey of the states' limited English proficient students and available educational programs and services, 2000–2001 summary report.* Washington, DC: National Clearinghouse for English Language Acquisition & Language Instruction Educational Programs.

King, R., Schwab-Stone, M., Flisher, A., Greenwald, S., Kramer, R., Goodman, S., et al. (2001). Psychosocial and risk behavior correlates of youth suicide attempts and suicidal ideation. *Journal of the American Academy of Child and Adolescent Psychiatry, 40,* 837–846.

Kirchner, C., & Diament, S. (1999). Usable data report: Estimates of the number of visually impaired students, their

teachers, and orientation and mobility specialists: Part I. *Journal of Visual Impairment and Blindness, 93*(9), 600–606.

Kirk, J., & Reid, G. (2001). An examination of the relationship between dyslexia and offending in young people and the implications for the training system. *Dyslexia, 7,* 77–84.

Kirk, S., McCarthy, J., & Kirk, W. (1968). *The Illinois Test of Psycholinguistic Abilities* (Revised ed.). Urbana: University of Illinois Press.

Kitson, N., & Fry, R. (1990). Prelingual deafness and psychiatry. *British Journal of Hospital Medicine, 44,* 353–356.

Kitzinger, M. (1984). The role of repeated and echoed utterances in communication with a blind child. *British Journal of Disorders of Communication, 19,* 135–146.

Klecan-Aker, J., & Hedrick, D. (1985). A study of the syntactic language skills of normal school-age children. *Language, Speech, and Hearing Services in Schools., 16,* 187–198.

Klee, T. (1985). Clinical language sampling: Analysing the analyses. *Child Language Teaching and Therapy, 1,* 182–198.

Klee, T., Carson, D., Gavin, W., Hall, L., Kent, A., & Reece, S. (1998). Concurrent and predictive validity of an early language screening program. *Journal of Speech, Language, and Hearing Research, 41,* 627–641.

Klee, T., & Fitzgerald, M. (1985). The relation between grammatical development and mean length of utterance in morphemes. *Journal of Child Language, 12,* 251–269.

Klee, T., Pearce, K., & Carson, D. (2000). Improving the positive predictive value of screening for developmental language disorder. *Journal of Speech, Language, and Hearing Research, 43,* 821–833.

Klee, T., Schaffer, M., May, S., Membrino, I., & Mougey, K. (1989). A comparison of the age–MLU relation in normal and specifically language-impaired preschool children. *Journal of Speech and Hearing Disorders, 54,* 226–233.

Klin, A. (1991). Young autistic children's listening preferences in regard to speech: A possible characterization of the symptom of social withdrawal. *Journal of Autism and Developmental Disorders, 21,* 29–42.

Klink, M., Gerstman, L., Raphael, L., Schlanger, B., & Newsome, L. (1986). Phonological process usage by young EMR children and nonretarded preschool children. *American Journal of Mental Deficiency, 91,* 190–195.

Knight-Arest, I. (1984). Communicative effectiveness of learning disabled and normally achieving 10- to 13-year-old boys. *Learning Disability Quarterly, 7,* 237–245.

Koegel, L. (2000). Interventions to facilitate communication in autism. *Journal of Autism and Developmental Disorders, 30*(5), 384–391.

Koegel, L., Koegel, R., Frea, W., & Green-Hopkins, I. (2003). Priming as a method of coordinating educational services for students with autism. *Language, Speech, and Hearing Services in Schools, 34,* 228–235.

Koegel, R., O'Dell, M. C., & Koegel, L. (1987). A natural language teaching paradigm for nonverbal autistic children. *Journal of Autism and Developmental Disorders, 17,* 187–200.

Koeppe, R. (1996). Language differentiation in bilingual children: The development of grammatical and pragmatic competence. *Linguistics, 34*(5), 927–954.

Kohler, F. W., & Strain, P. S. (1999). Maximizing peer-mediated resources in integrated preschool classrooms. *Topics in Early Childhood Special Education, 19*(2), 92–102.

Kohnert, K., Bates, E., & Hernandez, A. (1999). Balancing bilinguals: Lexical-semantic production and cognitive processing in children learning Spanish and English. *Journal of Speech, Language, and Hearing Research, 42,* 1400–1413.

Konstantareas, M. M., & Homatidis, S. (1987). Brief report: Ear infections in autistic and normal children. *Journal of Autism and Developmental Disorders, 17,* 585–593.

Koppenhaver, D., Coleman, P., Kalman, P., & Yoder, D. (1992). The implications of emergent literacy research for children with developmental disabilities. *American Journal of Speech-Language Pathology, 1,* 38–44.

Koppenhaver, D., Pierce, P., Steelman, J., & Yoder, D. (1995). Contexts of early literacy intervention for children with developmental disabilities. In M. Fey, J. Windsor, & S. Warren (Eds.), *Language intervention: Preschool through elementary years* (pp. 241–274). Baltimore, MD: Paul H. Brookes.

Kramer, C., James, S., & Saxman, J. (1979). A comparison of language samples elicited at home and in the clinic. *Journal of Speech and Hearing Disorders, 44,* 321–330.

Kreschek, J., & Nicolosi, L. (1973). A comparison of black and white children's scores on the Peabody Picture Vocabulary Test. *Language, Speech, and Hearing Services in Schools, 4,* 37–40.

Kuhl, P. (1990). Auditory perception and the ontogeny and phylogeny of human speech. *Seminars in Speech and Language, 11,* 77–91.

Kuhl, P., & Meltzoff, A. (1988). Speech as an intermodal object of perception. In A. Yonas (Ed.), *Minnesota symposia in child psychology: The development of perception* (pp. 235–266). Hillsdale, NJ: Lawrence Erlbaum.

Kumin, L. (2001). *Classroom language skills for children with Down syndrome: A guide for parents and teachers.* Bethesda, MD: Woodbine House.

Ladefoged, P. (2001). *A course in phonetics* (4th ed.). Orlando, FL: Harcourt College Publishers.

Lahey, M. (1988). *Language disorders and language development.* Columbus, OH: Macmillan.

Lahey, M. (1990). Who shall be called language disordered? Some reflections and one perspective. *Journal of Speech and Hearing Disorders, 55,* 612–620.

Lahey, M. (1994). Grammatical morpheme acquisition: Do norms exist? [Letter to the editor]. *Journal of Speech and Hearing Research, 37,* 1192–1194.

Lahey, M., & Bloom, L. (1994). Variability and language learning disabilities. In G. Wallach & K. Butler (Eds.), *Language-learning disabilities in school-age children and adolescents: Some principles and applications* (pp. 354–372). Boston: Allyn & Bacon.

Lahey, M., & Edwards, J. (1995). Specific language impairment: Preliminary investigation of factors associated with family history and with patterns of language performance. *Journal of Speech and Hearing Research, 38,* 643–657.

Lahey, M., Liebergott, J., Chesnick, M., Menyuk, P., & Adams, J. (1992). Variability in children's use of grammatical morphemes. *Applied Psycholinguistics, 13,* 373–398.

Lamberts, R., & Weener, P. (1976). M. R. children's competence in processing negation. *American Journal of Mental Deficiency, 81,* 181–186.

Landa, R., Folstein, S. E., & Isaacs, C. (1991). Spontaneous narrative-discourse performance of parents of autistic individuals. *Journal of Speech and Hearing Research, 34,* 1339–1345.

Landau, B., & Gleitman, L. (1985). *Language and experience: Evidence from the blind child.* Cambridge, MA: Harvard University Press.

Landry, S. H., & Loveland, K. A. (1989). The effect of social context on the functional communication skills of autistic children. *Journal of Autism and Developmental Disorders, 19,* 283–299.

Langacker, R. (1968). *Language and its structure: Some fundamental linguistic concepts.* New York: Harcourt, Brace & World.

Langlois, J. (Ed.). (2000). *Traumatic brain injury in the United States: Assessing outcomes in children.* Atlanta, GA: Centers for Disease Control and Prevention.

Lapadat, J. C. (1991). Pragmatic language skills of students with language and/or learning disabilities: A quantitative synthesis. *Journal of Learning Disabilities, 24,* 147–158.

Larson, V. Lord, & McKinley, N. (1985). General intervention principles with language impaired adolescents. *Topics in Language Disorders, 5,* 70–77.

Larson, V. Lord, & McKinley, N. (1987). *Communication assessment and intervention strategies for adolescents.* Eau Claire, WI: Thinking Publications.

Larson, V. Lord, & McKinley, N. (1988). Language disorders in the adolescent: Intervention. In D. Yoder & R. Kent (Eds.), *Decision making in speech-language pathology.* Burlington, Ontario: B.C. Decker.

Larson, V. Lord, & McKinley, N. (1995). *Language disorders in older students: Preadolescents and adolescents.* Eau Claire, WI: Thinking Publications.

Larson, V. Lord, & McKinley, N. (1998). Characteristics of adolescents' conversations: A longitudinal study. *Clinical Linguistics and Phonetics, 12,* 183–203.

Larson, V. Lord, & McKinley, N. (2003). *Communication solutions for older students.* Eau Claire, WI: Thinking Publications.

Lazar, R., Warr-Leeper, G., Nicholson, C., & Johnson, S. (1989). Elementary school teachers' use of multiple meaning expressions. *Language, Speech, and Hearing Services in Schools, 20,* 420–430.

Leadholm, B., & Miller, J. (1992). *Language sample analysis: The Wisconsin guide.* Madison: Wisconsin Department of Public Instruction.

Leap, W. (1993). *American Indian English.* Salt Lake City: University of Utah Press.

Lee, A., Hobson, R. P., & Chiat, S. (1994). I, you, me and autism: An experimental study. *Journal of Autism and Developmental Disorders, 24,* 155–176.

Lee, L. L. (1974). *Developmental sentence analysis.* Evanston, IL: Northwestern University Press.

Lee, L. L., Koenigsknecht, R., & Mulhern, S. (1975). Interactive language development teaching. Evanston, IL: Northwestern University Press.

Lee, R. F., & Kamhi, A. (1990). Metaphoric competence in children with learning disabilities. *Journal of Learning Disabilities, 23,* 476–482.

Leifer, J. S., & Lewis, M. (1984). Acquisition of conversational response skills by young Down syndrome and nonretarded young children. *American Journal of Mental Deficiency, 88,* 610–618.

Lenneberg, E. (1967). *Biological foundations of language.* New York: Wiley.

Lenz, B. K., Bulgren, J., & Kissam, B. (1995). *Pedagogies for academic diversity in secondary schools: Smarter planning.* Lawrence: University of Kansas—Center for Research on Learning.

Leonard, L. (1979). Language impairment in children. *Merrill Palmer Quarterly, 25*(3), 205–232.

Leonard, L. (1981). Facilitating linguistic skills in children with specific language impairment. *Applied Psycholinguistics, 2,* 89–118.

Leonard, L. (1982). Early language development and language disorders. In G. Shames & E. Wiig (Eds.), *Human communication disorders: An introduction.* Columbus, OH: Merrill/Macmillan.

Leonard, L. (1983). Defining the boundaries of language disorders in children. In J. Miller, D. Yoder, & R. Schiefelbusch (Eds.), *Contemporary issues in language intervention.* Rockville, MD: American Speech-Language-Hearing Association.

Leonard, L. (1984). Normal language acquisition: Some recent findings and clinical implications. In A. Holland (Ed.), *Language disorders in children.* San Diego, CA: College-Hill Press.

Leonard, L. (1987). Is specific language impairment a useful construct? In S. Rosenberg (Ed.), *Advances in applied psycholinguistics: Disorders of first-language development* (Vol. 1, pp. 1–39). New York: Cambridge University Press.

Leonard, L. (1991). Specific language impairment as a clinical category. *Language, Speech, and Hearing Services in Schools, 22,* 66–68.

Leonard, L. (1998). *Children with specific language impairment.* Cambridge, MA: MIT Press.

Leonard, L., Bolders, J., & Miller, J. (1976). An examination of the semantic relations reflected in the language usage of normal and language-disordered children. *Journal of Speech and Hearing Research, 19,* 371–392.

Leonard, L., Bortolini, U., Caselli, M., McGregor, K., & Sabbadini, L. (1992). Morphological deficits in children with specific language impairment: The status of features in the underlying grammar. *Language Acquisition, 2,* 151–179.

Leonard, L., Camarata, S., Rowan, L., & Chapman, K. (1982). The communicative functions of lexical usage by language-impaired children. *Applied Psycholinguistics, 3,* 109–126.

Leonard, L., Deevy, P., Miller, C., Rauf, L., Charest, M., & Kurtz, R. (2003). Surface forms and grammatical functions: Past tense and passive particple use by children with specific language impairment. *Journal of Speech, Language, and Hearing Research, 46,* 43–55.

Leonard, L., Eyer, J., Bedore, L., & Grela, B. (1997). Three accounts of the grammatical morpheme difficulties of English-speaking children with specific language impairment. *Journal of Speech, Language, and Hearing Research, 40,* 741–753.

Leonard, L., McGregor, K., & Allen, G. (1992). Grammatical morphology and speech perception in children with specific language impairment. *Journal of Speech and Hearing Research, 35,* 1076–1085.

Leonard, L., Miller, C., Deevy, P., Rauf, L., Gerber, E., & Charest, M. (2002). Production operations and the use of nonfinite verbs by children with specific language impairment. *Journal of Speech, Language, and Hearing Research, 45,* 744–758.

Leonard, L., Miller, C., & Gerber, E. (1999). Grammatical morphology and the lexicon in children with specific language impairment. *Journal of Speech, Language, and Hearing Research, 42,* 678–689.

Leonard, L., Miller, C., Grela, B., Holland, A., Gerber, E., & Petucci, M. (2000). Production operations contribute to the grammatical morpheme limitations of children with specific language impairment. *Journal of Memory and Language, 43,* 362–378.

Leonard, L., Nippold, M., Kail, R., & Hale, C. (1983). Picture naming in language-impaired children. *Journal of Speech and Hearing Research, 26,* 609–615.

Leonard, L., Prutting, C., Perozzi, J., & Berkley, R. (1978). Nonstandard approaches to the assessment of language behaviors. *Asha, 20,* 371–379.

Leonard, L., Schwartz, R., Chapman, K., Rowan, L., Prelock, P., Terrell, B., et al. (1982). Early lexical acquisition in children with specific language impairment. *Journal of Speech and Hearing Research, 25,* 554–564.

Leonard, L., Schwartz, R., Morris, B., & Chapman, K. (1981). Factors influencing early lexical acquisition: Lexical orientation and phonological composition. *Child Development, 52,* 882–887.

Lerner, J. (2000). *Learning disabilities: Theories, diagnosis, and teaching strategies* (8th ed.). Boston: Houghton Mifflin.

Lewis, B., & Thompson, L. (1992). A study of developmental speech and language disorders in twins. *Journal of Speech and Hearing Research, 35,* 1086–1094.

Lewis, G., & Sloggett, A. (1998). Suicide, deprivation, and unemployment. *British Medical Journal, 317,* 1283–1286.

Lieberman, R., Heffron, A., West, S., Hutchinson, E., & Swem, T. (1987). A comparison of four adolescent language tests. *Language, Speech, and Hearing Services in Schools, 18,* 250–266.

Lieberman, R., & Michael, A. (1986). Content relevance and content coverage in tests of grammatical ability. *Journal of Speech and Language Disorders, 51,* 71–81.

Light, J. (1997). "Let's go star fishing": Reflections on the contexts of language learning for children who use aided AAC. *Augmentative and Alternative Communication, 13*(3), 158–171.

Light, J., Collier, B., & Parnes, P. (1985a). Communicative interaction between young nonspeaking physically disabled children and their primary caregivers: Part 1—discourse patterns. *Augmentative and Alternative Communication, 1*(2), 74–83.

Light, J., Collier, B., & Parnes, P. (1985b). Communicative interaction between young nonspeaking physically disabled children and their primary caregivers: Part II—communicative function. *Augmentative and Alternative Communication, 1*(3), 98–107.

Light, J., Collier, B., & Parnes, P. (1985c). Communicative interaction between young nonspeaking physically disabled children and their primary caregivers: Part III—modes of communication. *Augmentative and Alternative Communication, 1*(4), 125–133.

Light, J., Datillo, J., English, J., Gutierrez, L., & Hartz, J. (1992). Instructing facilitators to support the communication of people who use augmentative communication systems. *Journal of Speech and Hearing Research, 35,* 865–875.

Light, J., Roberts, B., Dimarco, R., & Greiner, N. (1998). Augmentative and alternative communication to support receptive and expressive communication for people with autism. *Journal of Communication Disorders, 31,* 153–180.

Liles, B. (1985). Cohesion in the narratives of normal and language-disordered children. *Journal of Speech and Hearing Disorders, 28,* 123–133.

Lilly, M. (1979). *Children with exceptional needs: A survey of special education.* New York: Holt, Rinehart & Winston.

Limber, J. (1973). The genesis of complex sentences. In T. Moore (Ed.), *Cognitive development and the acquisition of language.* New York: Academic Press.

Linares-Orama, N., & Sanders, L. (1977). Evaluation of syntax in three-year-old Spanish-speaking Puerto Rican children. *Journal of Speech and Hearing Research, 20,* 350–357.

Lincoln, A., Courchesne, E., Harms, L., & Allen, M. (1995). Sensory modulation of auditory stimuli in children with autism and receptive developmental language disorder: Event-related brain potential evidence. *Journal of Autism and Developmental Disorders, 25,* 521–539.

Lindamood, C., & Lindamood, P. (1979). *Lindamood Auditory Conceptualization Test—Revised.* Austin, TX: Pro-Ed.

Livingstone, M. S., Rosen, G. D., Drislane, F. W., & Galaburda, A. M. (1991). Physiological and anatomical evidence for a magnocellular defect in developmental dyslexia. *Proceedings of the National Academy of Sciences, 88,* 7943–7947.

Lloyd, J. W., Hallahan, D. P., Kauffman, J. M., & Keller, C. E. (1998). Academic problems. In R. J. Morris & T. R. Kratochwill (Eds.), *The practice of child therapy* (pp. 167–198). Boston: Allyn & Bacon.

Lloyd, L., & Fulton, R. (1972). Audiology's contribution to communications programming with the retarded. In J. McLean, D. Yoder, & R. Schiefelbusch (Eds.), *Language intervention with the retarded.* Baltimore, MD: University Park Press.

Loban, W. (1976). *Language development: Kindergarten through grade twelve.* Urbana, IL: National Council of Teachers of English.

Loeb, D., Kinsler, K., & Bookbinder, L. (2000, November). Current language sampling practices in preschools. Paper presented at the American Speech-Language-Hearing Association, Washington, DC.

Loeb, D., & Leonard, L. (1991). Subject case marking and verb morphology in normally developing and specifically language-impaired children. *Journal of Speech and Hearing Research, 34,* 340–346.

Loeb, D., Pye, C., Redmond, S., & Richardson, L. (1996). Eliciting verbs from children with specific language impairment. *American Journal of Speech-Language Pathology, 5,* 17–30.

Long, E. (1998). Native American children's performance on the Preschool Language Scale—3. *Journal of Children's Communication Development, 19*(2), 43–47.

Long, E., & Christensen, J. (1998). Indirect language assessment tool for English-speaking Cherokee Indian children. *Journal of American Indian Education, 38*(1), 1–14.

Long, S. (1999a). About time: A comparison of computerized and manual procedures for grammatical and phonological analysis. *Clinical Linguistics and Phonetics, 15,* 399–426.

Long, S. (1999b). Technology applications in the assessment of children's language. *Seminars in Speech and Hearing, 20,* 117–132.

Long, S., & Channell, R. (2001). Accuracy of four language analysis procedures performed authomatically. *American Journal of Speech-Language Pathology, 10,* 180–188.

Long, S., Fey, M., & Channell, R. (2000). Computerized profiling (CP) (Version 9.2.7) [MS-DOS computer software]. Cleveland, OH: Department of Communication Sciences, Case Western Reserve University.

Long, S., Olswang, L., Brian, J., & Dale, P. (1997). Productivity of emerging word combinations in toddlers with specific expressive language impairment. *American Journal of Speech-Language Pathology, 6,* 34–47.

Longhurst, T. M. (1972). Assessing and increasing descriptive communication skills in retarded children. *Mental Retardation, 19,* 42–45.

Longhurst, T. M. (1974). Communication in retarded adolescents: Sex and intelligence level. *American Journal of Mental Deficiency, 78,* 607–618.

Longhurst, T. M., & Berry, G. W. (1975). Communication in retarded adolescents: Response to listener feedback. *American Journal of Mental Deficiency, 80,* 158–164.

Lonigan, C., Bloomfield, B., Anthony, J., Bacon, K., Phillips, B., & Samwel, C. (1999). Relations among emergent literacy skills, behavior problems, and social competence in preschool children from low- and middle-income households. *Topics in Early Childhood Special Education, 19,* 40–53.

Lord, C. (1997). Diagnostic instruments in autism spectrum disorders. In D. J. Cohen & F. R. Volkmar (Eds.), *Handbook of Autism and Pervasive Developmental Disorders* (2nd ed., pp. 460–483). New York: Wiley.

Lord, C., Rutter, M., DiLavore, P. C., & Risi, S. (1999). *Autism diagnostic observation schedule.* Los Angeles: Western Psychological Services.

Louis, B., & Lewis, M. (1992). Parental beliefs about giftedness in young children and their relation to actual ability level. *Gifted Child Quarterly, 36,* 27–31.

Lovaas, O. I. (1977). *The autistic child: Language development through behavior modification.* New York: Irvington.

Lovaas, O. I., Schaeffer, B., & Simmons, J. Q. (1965). Building social behavior in autistic children by use of electric shock. *Journal of Experimental Research in Personality, 1,* 99–109.

Lovell, K., & Bradbury, B. (1967). The learning of English morphology in educationally subnormal special school children. *American Journal of Mental Deficiency, 71,* 609–615.

Lucas, E. (1980). *Semantic and pragmatic language disorders: Assessment and remediation.* Rockville, MD: Aspen.

Ludlow, J. R., & Allen, L. M. (1979). The effect of early intervention and pre-school stimulus on the development of the Down's syndrome child. *Journal of Mental Deficiency Research, 23,* 29–44.

Lund, N., & Duchan, J. (1993). *Assessing children's language in naturalistic contexts* (3rd ed.). Englewood Cliffs, NJ: Prentice-Hall.

Lunday, A. (1996). A collaborative communication skills program for Job Corps centers. *Topics in Language Disorders, 16,* 23–36.

Luria, A. (1961). *The role of speech in the regulation of normal and abnormal processes in the child.* Baltimore, MD: Penguin.

Luria, A. (1963). *The mentally retarded child.* Oxford, UK: Pergamon Press.

Luria, A., & Yudovich, F. (1971). *Speech and the development of mental processes in the child.* Baltimore, MD: Penguin.

Lutzker, J., & Sherman, J. A. (1974). Producing generative sentence usage by imitation and reinforcement procedures. *Journal of Applied Behavior Analysis, 7,* 447–460.

Lynch, M. P., & Eilers, R. E. (1991). Perspectives on early language from typical development and Down syndrome. *International Review of Research in Mental Retardation, 17,* 55–89.

Lynch, M. P., Oller, D. K., Steffens, M. L., Levine, S. L., Basinger, D. L., & Umbel, V. M. (1995). Development of speech-like vocalizations in infants with Down syndrome. *American Journal of Mental Retardation, 100,* 68–86.

Lyon, G. R., Fletcher, J. M., Shaywitz, S. E., Shaywitz, B. A., Torgesen, J. K., Wood, F. B., et al. (2001). Rethinking learning disabilities. In C. E. Finn, J. Rotherham, & J. C. R. Hokanson (Eds.), *Rethinking special education for a new century* (pp. 259–288). Washington, DC: Thomas B. Fordham Foundation.

Lyon, G. R., & Risucci, D. (1988). Classification of learning disabilities. In K. A. Kavale (Ed.), *Learning disabilities: State of the art and practice* (pp. 44–70). Boston: College-Hill Press.

MacArthur, C. A., & Graham, S. (1987). Learning disabled students' composing under three methods of text production: Handwriting, word processing, and dictation. *Journal of Special Education, 21,* 22–42.

MacDonald, J., Blott, J., Gordon, K., Spiegel, B., & Hartmann, M. (1974). An experimental parent-assisted program for preschool language-delayed children. *Journal of Speech and Hearing Disorders, 39,* 395–415.

MacDonald, J., & Horstmeier, D. S. (1978). *Environmental Language Intervention Program (ELIP)*. San Antonio, TX: Psychological Corporation.

MacDuff, G., Krantz, P., & McClannahan, I. (1993). Teaching children with autism to use photographic activity schedules: Maintenance and generalization of complex response chains. *Journal of Applied Behavior Analysis, 26,* 89–98.

Mack, A., & Warr-Leeper, G. (1992). Language abilities in boys with chronic behavior disorders. *Language, Speech, and Hearing Services in Schools, 23,* 214–223.

Mackie, K., & Dermody, P. (1986). Use of a monosyllabic adaptive speech test (MAST) with young children. *Journal of Speech and Hearing Research, 29*(2), 275–281.

MacLachlan, B., & Chapman, R. (1988). Communication breakdowns in normal and language learning-disabled children's conversation and narration. *Journal of Speech and Hearing Disorders, 53,* 2–9.

MacMillan, D. L., & Siperstein, G. N. (2001). Learning disabilities as operationally defined by schools. Paper presented at the Learning Disabilities Summit: Building a Foundation for the Future, Washington, DC.

MacWhinney, B. (1996). The CHILDES system. *American Journal of Speech-Language Pathology, 5*(1), 5–14.

MacWhinney, B. (2000). *The CHILDES project: Tools for analyzing talk* (3rd ed.). Mahwah, NJ: Lawrence Erlbaum.

Madding, C. (2002). Socialization practices of Latinos. In A. E. Brice (Ed.), *The Hispanic child: Speech, language, culture and education* (pp. 68–84). Boston: Allyn & Bacon.

Mahoney, G., Glover, A., & Finger, I. (1981). Relationship between language and sensorimotor development of Down syndrome and nonretarded children. *American Journal of Mental Deficiency, 86,* 21–27.

Mahoney, G., & Seely, P. (1977). The role of the social agent in language acquisition. In H. Ellis (Ed.), *International review of research in mental retardation* (Vol. 8). New York: Academic Press.

Maino, D. M., Rado, M., & Pizzi, W. J. (1996). Ocular anomalies of individuals with mental illness and dual diagnosis. *Journal of the American Optometric Association, 67*(12), 740–748.

Malone, L. D., & Mastropieri, M. A. (1992). Reading comprehension instruction: Summarization and self-monitoring training for students with learning disabilities. *Exceptional Children, 58,* 270–279.

Malvy, J., Roux, S., Zakian, A., Debuly, S., Sauvage, D., & Barthelemy, C. (1999). A brief clinical scale for the early evaluation of imitation disorders in autism. *Autism, 3*(4), 357–369.

Mann, V. A., Cowin, E., & Schoenheimer, J. (1989). Phonological processing, language comprehension, and reading ability. *Journal of Learning Disabilities, 22,* 76–89.

Mantovani, J. F., & Landau, W. M. (1980). Acquired aphasia with convulsive disorder: Course and prognosis. *Neurology, 30,* 524–529.

Marcell, M. M. (1995). Relationships between hearing and auditory cognition in Down's syndrome youth. *Down Syndrome: Research and Practice, 3,* 75–91.

March of Dimes Birth Defects Foundation. (2002). *March of Dimes: Health library: Infant health statistics.* Retrieved July 2002, from www.modimes.org/HealthLibrary/334_606.htm.

Marchant, J. M. (1992). Deaf-blind handicapping conditions. In P. J. McLaughlin & P. Wehman (Eds.), *Developmental disabilities: A handbook for best practices.* Boston: Andover Medical.

Marchman, V., Wulfeck, B., & Ellis Weismer, S. (1999). Morphological productivity in children with normal language and SLI: A study of the English past tense. *Journal of Speech, Language, and Hearing Research, 42,* 206–219.

Marcon, R. (1998, March). Impact of language deficits on maladaptive behavior of inner-city early adolescents: A longitudinal analysis. Paper presented at the Biennial Conference on Human Development, Mobile, AL.

Marcus, R. (1996). The friendships of delinquents. *Adolescence, 31,* 145–159.

Margalit, M., & Levin-Alyagon, M. (1994). Learning disability sub-typing, loneliness, and classroom adjustment. *Learning Disability Quarterly, 17,* 297–310.

Markman, E. (1989). *Categorization and naming in children.* Cambridge, MA: MIT Press.

Markman, E., & Wachtel, G. (1988). Children's use of mutual exclusivity to constrain the meaning of words. *Cognitive Psychology, 20,* 121–157.

Marland, S. (1972). *Education of the gifted and talented: Report to the Congress of the United States by the U.S. Commissioner of Education.* Washington, DC: U.S. Office of Education.

Mars, A. E., Mauk, J. E., & Dowrick, P. (1998). Symptoms of pervasive developmental disorders as observed in prediagnostic home videos of infants and toddlers. *Journal of Pediatrics, 132,* 500–504.

Marshall, N., Hegrenes, J., & Goldstein, S. (1973). Verbal interactions: Mothers and their retarded children vs mothers and their non-retarded children. *American Journal of Mental Deficiency, 77,* 415–419.

Marshall, R. M., & Hynd, G. W. (1997). Academic underachievement in ADD subtypes. *Journal of Learning Disabilities, 30*(6), 635–643.

Martin, B. A. (1997). Primary care of adults with mental retardation living in the community. *American Family Physician, 56,* 485–494.

Martin Luther King Jr. Elementary School children v. Ann Arbor School District Board. (1977). 473 Federal Supplement 1371c ED. Michigan.

Martins, I. P., & Ferro, J. M. (1992). Recovery of acquired aphasia in children. *Aphasiology, 6*(4), 431–438.

Martins, I. P., Ferro, J. M., & Trindade, A. (1987). Acquired crossed aphasia in a child. *Developmental Medicine and Child Neurology, 29,* 96–100.

Marton, K., & Schwartz, R. (2003). Working memory capacity and language processes in children with specific language impairment. *Journal of Speech, Language, and Hearing Research, 46,* 1138–1153.

Marvin, C. (1994). Cartalk! Conversational topics of preschool children en route home from preschool. *Language, Speech, and Hearing Services in Schools, 25,* 146–155.

Marvin, C., Beukelman, D., & Bilyeu, D. (1994). Vocabulary-use patterns in preschool children: Effects of context and time sampling. *Augmentative and Alternative Communication, 10*(4), 224–236.

Marvin, C., & Privratsky, A. (1999). After-school talk: The effects of materials sent home from preschool. *American Journal of Speech-Language Pathology, 8,* 231–240.

Massa, J., & Eggert, L. (2001). Activity involvement among suicidal and nonsuicidal high-risk and typical adolescents. *Suicide and Life-Threatening Behavior, 31*(3), 265–281.

Masters, L., & March, G. (1978). Middle ear pathology as a factor in learning disabilities. *Journal of Learning Disabilities, 11,* 103–106.

Masterson, J. (1997). Interrelationships in children's language production. *Topics in Language Disorders, 17*(4), 11–22.

Masterson, J., & Crede, L. A. (1999). Learning to spell: Implications for assessment and intervention. *Language, Speech, and Hearing Services in Schools, 30,* 243–254.

Masterson, J., & Kamhi, A. (1991). The effects of sampling conditions on sentence production in normal, reading-disabled, and language-learning-disabled children. *Journal of Speech and Hearing Research, 34,* 549–558.

Masterson, J., & Kamhi, A. (1992). Linguistic trade-offs in school-age children with and without language disorders. *Journal of Speech and Hearing Research, 35,* 1064–1075.

Mathinos, D. A. (1991). Conversational engagement of children with learning disabilities. *Journal of Learning Disabilities, 24,* 439–446.

Mattis, S., French, J., & Rapin, I. (1975). Dyslexia in children and young adults: Three independent neuropsychological syndromes. *Developmental Medicine and Child Neurology, 17,* 150–163.

Mauk, G., White, K. R., & Mortensen, L. B. (1991). The effectiveness of hearing screening programs based on high risk characteristics in early identification of hearing impairment. *Ear and Hearing, 12,* 312–319.

Maurer, H., & Sherrod, K. B. (1987). Context of directives given to young children with Down syndrome and non-retarded children: Development over two years. *American Journal of Mental Deficiency, 91,* 579–590.

Mayberry, R. I., & Eichen, E. B. (1991). The long lasting advantage of learning sign language in childhood: Another look at the critical period for language acquisition. *Journal of Memory and Language, 30,* 486–512.

Mayes, S. D., Calhoun, S. L., & Crites, D. L. (2001). "Does DSM-IV Asperger's disorder exist?" *Journal of Abnormal Child Psychology, 29,* 263–271.

McCaffrey, H. (1999). Multichannel cochlear implantation and the organisation of the early speech. *Volta Review, 101*(1), 5–29.

McCarthren, R., Warren, S., & Yoder, P. (1996). Prelinguistic predictors of later language development. In K. Cole, P. Dale, & D. Thal (Eds.), *Assessment of communication and language* (pp. 57–75). Baltimore, MD: Paul H. Brookes.

McCauley, R. (1996). Familiar strangers: Criterion-referenced measures in communication disorders. *Language, Speech, and Hearing Services in Schools, 27,* 122–131.

McCauley, R., & Demetras, M. (1990). Identification of language impairment in the selection of specifically language-impaired subjects. *Journal of Speech and Hearing Disorders, 55,* 468–475.

McCauley, R., & Swisher, L. (1984). Use and misuse of norm-referenced tests in clinical assessment: A hypothetical case. *Journal of Speech and Hearing Disorders, 49,* 338–348.

McCluskey, K. W., & Walker, K. D. (1986). *The doubtful gift.* Kingston, Ontario: Ronald P. Frye.

McCormick, L. (1997). Language intervention and support. In L. McCormick, D. Loeb, & R. Schiefelbusch (Eds.), *Supporting children with communication difficulties in inclusive settings: School-based language intervention* (pp. 257–306). Boston: Allyn & Bacon.

McCune, L., Kearney, B., & Checkoff, M. (1989). Forms and functions of communication by children with Down syndrome and nonretarded children with their mothers. In S. von Tetzchner, L. S. Siegel, & L. Smith (Eds.), *The social and cognitive aspects of normal and atypical language development* (pp. 113–127). New York: Springer-Verlag.

McDonald, S. (1993). Pragmatic language skills after closed head injury: Ability to meet the informational needs of the listener. *Brain and Language, 44*(1), 28–46.

McDonald, S., & Turkstra, L. (1998). Adolescents with traumatic brain injury: Assessing pragmatic language function. *Clinical Linguistics and Phonetics, 12*(3), 237–248.

McFadden, T. (1998). The immediate effects of pictographic representation on children's narratives. *Child Language Teaching and Therapy, 14,* 51–67.

McFadden, T., & Gillam, R. (1996). An examination of the qualitiy of narratives produced by children with language disorders. *Language, Speech, and Hearing Services in Schools, 27,* 48–56.

McFarland, D. J., & Cacace, A. T. (1997). Modality specificity of auditory and visual pattern recognition: Implications for assessment of central auditory processing disorders. *Audiology, 36*(5), 249–260.

McGee, G. C., Almeida, M. C., & Sulzer-Azaroff, B. (1992). Promoting reciprocal interactions via peer incidental teaching. *Journal of Applied Behavior Analysis, 25,* 117–126.

McGivern, A. B., Rieff, M. L., & Vender, B. F. (1978). *Language stories: Teaching language to developmentally disabled children.* New York: John Day.

McGregor, K. (1997a). Prosodic influences on children's grammatical morphology. *Topics in Language Disorders, 4,* 63–75.

McGregor, K. (1997b). The nature of word-finding errors of preschoolers with and without word-finding deficits. *Journal of Speech, Language, and Hearing Research, 40,* 1232–1244.

McGregor, K., Friedman, R., Reilly, R., & Newman, R. (2002). Semantic representation and naming in young children. *Journal of Speech, Language, and Hearing Research, 45,* 332–346.

McGregor, K., & Leonard, L. (1989). Facilitating word-finding skills of language-impaired children. *Journal of Speech and Hearing Disorders, 54,* 141–147.

McGregor, K., Newman, R., Reilly, R., & Capone, N. (2002). Semantic representation and naming in children with specific language impairment. *Journal of Speech, Language, and Hearing Research, 45,* 998–1014.

McGregor, K., & Windsor, J. (1996). Effects of priming on the naming accuracy of preschoolers with word-finding deficits. *Journal of Speech and Hearing Research, 39,* 1048–1058.

McKinley, N., & Larson, V. Lord. (1989). Students who can't communicate: Speech-language service at the secondary level. *Curriculum Report, 19*(2), 1–8.

McLaren, J., & Bryson, S. E. (1987). Review of recent epidemiological studies of mental retardation: Prevalence, associated disorders, and etiology. *American Journal of Mental Retardation, 92,* 243–254.

McLaughlin, S. (1998). *Introduction to language development.* San Diego, CA: Singular.

McLean, J. (1992). Facilitated communication: Some thoughts on Biklen's and Calculator's interaction. *American Journal of Speech-Language Pathology, 1,* 25–27.

McLean, J., McLean, L., Brady, N. C., & Etter, R. (1991). Communication profiles of two types of gesture using nonverbal persons with severe to profound mental retardation. *Journal of Speech and Hearing Research, 34,* 294–308.

McLean, J., & Snyder-McLean, L. (1999). *How children learn language.* San Diego, CA: Singular.

McLean, L., Brady, N. C., McLean, J., & Behrens, G. A. (1999). Communication forms and functions of children and adults with severe mental retardation in community and institutional settings. *Journal of Speech, Language, and Hearing Research, 42,* 231–240.

McLean, L., & Cripe, J. (1997). The effectiveness of early intervention for children with communication disorders. In M. Guralnick (Ed.), *The effectiveness of early intervention* (pp. 349–428). Baltimore, MD: Paul H. Brookes.

McLeavey, B. C., Toomey, J. F., & Dempsey, P. J. R. (1982). Nonretarded and mentally retarded children's control over syntactic structures. *American Journal of Mental Deficiency, 86,* 485–494.

McLeod, S., van Doorn, J., & Reed, V. A. (2001a). Consonant cluster development in two-year-olds: General trends and individual differences. *Journal of Speech, Language, and Hearing Research, 44,* 1144–1171.

McLeod, S., van Doorn, J., & Reed, V. A. (2001b). Normal acquisition of consonant clusters. *American Journal of Speech-Language Pathology, 10,* 99–110.

McNaughton, D. (1991). Augmentative and alternative communication intervention for a child with acquired aphasia and convulsive disorder: A case study. *Journal of Speech-Language Pathology and Audiology, 15,* 35–41.

McNulty, M. (2003). Dyslexia and the life course. *Journal of Learning Disabilities, 36,* 363–381.

McWilliams, B., Morris, H., & Shelton, R. (1990). *Cleft palate speech.* Philadelphia: B. C. Decker.

Mehl, A. L., & Thomson, V. (1998). Newborn hearing screening: The great omission. *Paediatrics, 101,* 1–6.

Meltzer, L., Roditi, B., & Fenton, T. (1986). Cognitive and learning profiles of delinquent and learning disabled adolescents. *Adolescence, 21,* 581–591.

Mendaglio, S. (1993). Counseling gifted learning disabled: Individual and group counseling techniques. In L. K. Silverman (Ed.), *Counseling the gifted and talented* (pp. 131–149). Denver, CO: Love.

Menn, L., & Stoel-Gammon, C. (2001). Phonological development: Learning sounds and sound patterns. In J. Berko-Gleason (Ed.), *The development of language* (5th ed., pp. 70–124). Boston: Allyn & Bacon.

Menyuk, P. (1969). *Sentences children use.* Cambridge, MA: MIT Press.

Menyuk, P., Chesnick, M., Leibergott, J., Korngold, B., D'Agostino, R., & Belanger, A. (1991). Predicting reading problems in at-risk children. *Journal of Speech and Hearing Research, 34,* 893–903.

Menyuk, P., Liebergott, J., Schultz, M., Chesnick, M., & Ferrier, L. (1991). Patterns of early lexical and cognitive development in premature and full-term infants. *Journal of Speech and Hearing Research, 34,* 88–94.

Mercer, C. D., Jordan, L., Allsopp, D. H., & Mercer, A. R. (1996). Learning disabilities definitions and criteria used by state education departments. *Learning Disabilities Quarterly, 19,* 217–232.

Merchen, M. A. (1984). Technology and people. *Communication Outlook, 6*(2), 12–13.

Merchen, M. A. (1990). Some reasons for being passive from a personal perspective. *Communication Outlook, 12*(1), 10–11.

Merrell, A., & Plante, E. (1997). Norm-referenced test interpretation in the diagnostic process. *Language, Speech, and Hearing Services in Schools, 28,* 50–58.

Merrill, E. C., & Mar, H. H. (1987). Differences between mentally retarded and nonretarded persons' efficiency of auditory sentence processing. *American Journal of Mental Deficiency, 91,* 406–414.

Mervis, C., Yeargin-Allsopp, M., Winter, S., & Boyle, C. (2000). Aetiology of childhood vision impairment, metropolitan Atlanta, 1991–93. *Paediatric and Perinatal Epidemiology, 14,* 70–77.

Mervis, C. B. (1990). Early conceptual development of children with Down syndrome. In D. Cicchetti & M. Beeghly (Eds.), *Children with Down Syndrome: A developmental perspective.* Cambridge, UK: Cambridge University Press.

Mervis, C. B., & Bertrand, J. (1994). Acquisition of the novel name-nameless category (N_3C) principle. *Child Development, 65,* 1646–1662.

Merzenich, M., Jenkins, W., Johnston, P., Schreiner, C., Miller, S., & Tallal, P. (1996). Temporal processing deficits of language-learning impaired children ameliorated by training. *Science, 271,* 77–81.

Meyer, M. S., Wood, F. B., Hart, L. A., & Felton, R. H. (1998). Selective predictive value of rapid automatized naming in poor readers. *Journal of Learning Disabilities, 31,* 107–117.

Miles, S., & Chapman, R. S. (2002). Narrative content as described by individuals with Down syndrome and typically developing children. *Journal of Speech, Language, and Hearing Research, 45,* 175–189.

Miller, C., Kail, R., Leonard, L., & Tomblin, J. B. (2001). Speech of processing in children with specific language impairment. *Journal of Speech, Language, and Hearing Research, 44,* 416–433.

Miller, C., & Leonard, L. (1998). Deficits in finite verb morphology: Some assumptions in recent accounts of specific language impairment. *Journal of Speech, Language, and Hearing Research, 41,* 701–707.

Miller, G., & Gildea, P. (1987). How children learn words. *Scientific American, 257,* 94–99.

Miller, J. (1981). *Assessing language production in children: Experimental procedures.* Boston: Allyn & Bacon.

Miller, J. (1983). Identifying children with language disorders and describing their language performance. In J. Miller, D. Yoder, & R. Schiefelbusch (Eds.), *Comtemporary issues in language intervention* (pp. 61–74). Rockville, MD: American Speech-Language-Hearing Association.

Miller, J. (1984). Mental retardation. In W. H. Perkins (Ed.), *Language handicaps in children.* New York: Thieme-Stratton.

Miller, J. (1988). The developmental asynchrony of language development in children with Down syndrome. In L. Nadel (Ed.), *The psychobiology of Down syndrome* (pp. 168–198). Cambridge, MA: MIT Press.

Miller, J. (1992). Lexical development in young children with Down syndrome. In R. S. Chapman (Ed.), *Processes in language acquisition and disorder.* St. Louis, MO: Mosby Year Book.

Miller, J. (1996). Progress in assessing, describing, and defining child language disorder. In K. Cole, P. Dale, & D. Thal (Eds.), *Assessment of communication and language* (pp. 309–324). Baltimore, MD: Paul H. Brookes.

Miller, J., Budde, M., Bashir, A., & LaFollette, L. (1987). Lexical productivity in children with Down syndrome. Paper presented at the American Speech-Language-Hearing Association Annual Convention, New Orleans, LA.

Miller, J., Campbell, T., Chapman, R., & Ellis Weismer, S. (1984). Language behavior in acquired childhood aphasia. In A. L. Holland (Ed.), *Language disorders in children: Recent advances.* San Diego, CA: College-Hill.

Miller, J., & Chapman, R. (1984). Disorders of communication: Investigating the development of language of mentally retarded children. *American Journal of Mental Deficiency, 88,* 536–545.

Miller, J., & Chapman, R. (2000). Systematic Analysis of Language Transcripts (SALT) (Version 6.1) [Windows computer software]. Madison: Language Analysis Laboratory, Waisman Center on Mental Retardation and Human Development, University of Wisconsin—Madison.

Miller, J., & Paul, R. (1995). *The clinical assessment of language comprehension.* Baltimore, MD: Paul H. Brookes.

Miller, J., & Weinert, R. (1998). *Spontaneous spoken language. Syntax and discourse.* Oxford, UK: Clarendon Press.

Mills, C. J., & Durden, W. G. (1992). Cooperative learning and ability grouping: An issue of choice. *Gifted Child Quarterly, 36,* 11–16.

Mills, D. L., Coffey-Corina, S. A., & Neville, H. J. (1993). Language acquisition and cerebral specialization in 20-month-old infants. *Journal of Cognitive Neuroscience, 5*(3), 317–334.

Mindell, P., & Stracher, D. (1980). Assessing reading and writing of the gifted: The warp and woof of the language program. *Gifted Child Quarterly, 24,* 72–80.

MindWeavers. (1996). *MindWeavers history.* Retrieved February 2004, from www.mindweavers.co.uk/HTML/news. html#history.

Minino, A. M., & Smith, B. L. (2001). Deaths: Preliminary data for 2000. *National Vital Statistics Reports, 49*(12), 1–40.

Minner, S. (1990). Teacher evaluations of case descriptions of LD gifted children. *Gifted Child Quarterly, 34,* 37–45.

Miranda, A. E., McCabe, A., & Bliss, L. S. (1998). Jumping around and leaving things out: A profile of the narrative abilities of children with specific language impairment. *Applied Psycholinguistics, 19,* 647–667.

Mirenda, P. (1997). Supporting individuals with challenging behavior through functional communication training and AAC: Research review. *Augmentative and Alternative Communication, 13,* 207–225.

Mirenda, P. (2001). Autism, augmentative communication and assistive technology: What do we really know? *Focus on Autism and Other Developmental Disabilities, 16,* 141–159.

Mirenda, P. (2003). Toward functional augmentative and alternative communication for students with autism: Manual signs, graphic symbols, and voice output communication aids. *Language, Speech, and Hearing Services in Schools, 34,* 203–216.

Mirenda, P., & Erickson, K. (2000). Augmentative communication and literacy. In B. M. Prizant (Ed.), *Autism spectrum disorder: A transactional approach* (pp. 333–369). Baltimore, MD: Paul H. Brookes.

Mirenda, P., & Locke, P. A. (1989). A comparison of symbol transparency in nonspeaking persons with intellectual disabilities. *Journal of Speech and Hearing Disorders, 54,* 131–140.

Mirenda, P., & Mathy-Laikko, P. (1989). Augmentative and alternative communication applications for persons with severe congenital communication disorders: An introduction. *Augmentative and Alternative Communication, 5,* 3–13.

Mirenda, P., & Schuler, A. L. (1988). Augmenting communication for people with autism: Issues and strategies. *Topics in Language Disorders, 9*(1), 24–42.

Mitchell, P. R. (1997). Prelinguistic vocal development: A clinical primer. *Contemporary Issues in Communication Science and Disorders, 24,* 87–93.

Mody, M., Studdert-Kennedy, M., & Brady, S. (1997). Speech perception deficits in poor readers: Auditory processing or phonological coding? *Journal of Experimental Child Psychology, 64*(2), 199–231.

Moeller, M., & Luetke-Stahlman, B. (1990). Parent's use of SEE-II: A descriptive analysis. *Journal of Speech and Hearing Disorders, 55,* 327–338.

Moerk, E. (1976). Processes of language teaching and training in the interactions of mother–child dyads. *Child Development, 47,* 1064–1078.

Montague, M., Maddux, C. D., & Dereshiwsky, M. I. (1990). Story grammar and comprehension and production of narrative prose by students with learning disabilities. *Journal of Learning Disabilities, 23,* 190–197.

Montgomery, J. (2000). Verbal working memory and sentence comprehension in children with specific language impairment. *Journal of Speech, Language, and Hearing Research, 43,* 293–308.

Montgomery, J. (2002a). Information processing and language comprehension in children with specific langauge impairment. *Topics in Language Disorders, 22*(3), 62–84.

Montgomery, J. (2002b). Understanding the language difficulties of children with specific language impairments: Does verbal working memory matter? *American Journal of Speech-Language Pathology, 11,* 77–91.

Montgomery, J., & Leonard, L. (1998). Real-time inflectional processing by children with specific language impairment: Effects of phonetic substance. *Journal of Speech, Language, and Hearing Research, 41,* 1432–1443.

Moore, L., Clibbens, J., & Dennis, I. (1998). Reference and representation in children with Down syndrome. *Down Syndrome: Research and Practice, 5,* 63–70.

Moore, V., & McConachie, H. (1994). Communication between blind and severely visually impaired children and their parents. *British Journal of Developmental Psychology, 12,* 491–502.

Moran, M. (1975). *Verb inflections of normal and learning disabled children.* Lawrence: University of Kansas.

Mordecai, D., & Palin, M. (1982). Lingquest 1 & 2 [Computer software]. Napa, CA: Lingquest Software.

Morehead, D., & Ingram, D. (1973). The development of base syntax in normal and linguistically deviant children. *Journal of Speech and Hearing Research, 16,* 330–352.

Morgan, D., & Guilford, A. (1984). *Adolescent Language Screening Test.* Austin, TX: Pro-Ed.

Morris, S. E., & Klein, K. D. (1987). *Pre-feeding skills: A comprehensive resource for therapists.* Tucson, AZ: Therapy Skill Builders.

Morrow, D. R., Mirenda, P., Beukelman, D., & Yorkston, K. M. (1993). Vocabulary selection for augmentative communication systems: A comparison of three techniques. *American Journal of Speech-Language Pathology, 2*(2), 19–30.

Morse, J. L. (1988). Assessment procedures for people with mental retardation: The dilemma and suggested adaptive procedures. In S. N. Calculator & J. L. Bedrosian (Eds.), *Communication assessment and intervention for adults with mental retardation* (pp. 109–138). London, UK: Taylor & Francis.

Mundy, P., Kasari, C., Sigman, M., & Ruskin, E. (1995). Nonverbal communication and early language acquisition in children with Down syndrome and in normally developing children. *Journal of Speech and Hearing Research, 38,* 157–167.

Mundy, P., & Markus, J. (1997). On the nature of communication and language impairment in autism. *Mental Retardation and Developmental Disabilities Research Reviews, 3*(4), 343–349.

Mundy, P., Sigman, M. D., & Kasari, C. (1990). A longitudinal study of joint attention and language development in autistic children. *Journal of Autism and Developmental Disorders, 20,* 115–128.

Murphy, C. C., Boyle, C., Schendel, D., Decoufle, P., & Yeargin-Allsopp, M. (1998). Epidemiology of mental retardation in children. *Mental Retardation and Developmental Disabilities Research Reviews, 4*(1), 6–13.

Murphy, V., & Hicks-Stewart, K. (1991). Learning disabilities and attention deficit-hyperactivity disorder: An interactional perspective. *Journal of Learning Disabilities, 24,* 386–388.

Murray, L., & Andrews, L. (2001). *Your social baby: Understanding babies' communication from birth.* Melbourne, Australia: Australian Council for Education Research.

Muscular Dystrophy Campaign. (2002). *Duchenne MD.* Retrieved 12/02/02, from the World Wide Web: www.muscular-dystrophy.org/information/KeyFacts/duchenne.html

Musiek, F. E. (1999). Central auditory tests. *Scandinavian Audiology, 28*(Suppl. 51), 33–46.

Musselwhite, C. R., & St. Louis, K. W. (1988). *Communication programming for persons with severe handicaps: vocal and augmentative strategies* (2nd ed.). Boston: College-Hill Press.

Muter, V. (1998). Phonological awareness: Its nature and its influence over early literacy development. In C. Hulme & R. M. Joshi (Eds.), *Reading and spelling: Development and disorders* (pp. 113–126). Mahwah, NJ: Lawrence Erlbaum.

Myklebust, H. (1954). *Auditory disorders in children. A manual for differential diagnosis.* New York: Grunne & Stratton.

Naisbitt, J. (1988). Back to basics: U.S. businesses tackle remedial education. *John Naisbitt's Trend Letters, 7*(15), 8.

Namazi, M., & Johnston, J. (1996, June). The relationship between grammatical morphology and semantic complexity in the utterances of language-impaired children. Paper presented at the Symposium on Research in Child Language Disorders, Madison, WI.

Nation, K., & Hulme, C. (1997). Phonemic segmentation, not onset-rime segmentation, predicts early reading and spelling skills. *Reading Research Quarterly, 32,* 154–167.

National Center for Children in Poverty. (2002). *Low-income children in the United States: A brief demographic profile.* Retrieved July 2002, from http://cpmcnet.columbia.edu/dept/nccp/YCPfact302.pdf.

National Institute of Child Health and Human Development. (2001). *Autism facts—Autism research at the NICHD.* Washington, DC: National Institutes of Health.

National Joint Committee for the Communication Needs for Persons with Severe Disabilities. (2002). Supporting documentation for the position statement of access to communication and supports. *Communication Disorders Quarterly, 23,* 145–153.

National Joint Committee on Learning Disabilities. (1989). Issues in learning disabilities: Assessment and diagnosis. *Asha, 31,* 111–112.

National Joint Committee on Learning Disabilities. (1991a). Learning disabilities: Issues on definition. *Asha, 33* (Suppl. 5), 18–20.

National Joint Committee on Learning Disabilities. (1991b). Providing appropriate education for students with learning disabilities in regular education classrooms. *Asha, 33*(Suppl. 5), 15–17.

National Joint Committee on Learning Disabilities. (1998). Operationalizing the NJCLD definition of learning disabilities for ongoing assessment in schools. *Learning Disabilities Quarterly, 21,* 186–193.

Needleman, H. (1977). Effects of hearing loss from early recurrent otitis media on speech and language development. In B. Jaffe (Ed.), *Hearing loss in children.* Baltimore, MD: University Park Press.

Nelson, K., Camarata, S., Welsh, J., Butkovsky, L., & Camarata, M. (1996). Effects of imitative and conversational recasting treatment on the acquisition of grammar in children with specific language impairment and younger normal children. *Journal of Speech and Hearing Research, 39,* 850–859.

Nelson, K., Carskaddon, G., & Bonvillian, J. (1973). Syntax acquistion: Impact of experimental variation in adult verbal interaction with the child. *Journal of Child Language, 44,* 497–504.

Nelson, K., Welsh, J., Camarata, S., Butkovsky, L., & Camarata, M. (1995). Available input for language-impaired children and younger children of matched language levels. *First Language, 43,* 1–18.

Nelson, N. (1998). *Childhood language disorders in context: Infancy through adolescence* (2nd ed.). Boston: Allyn & Bacon.

Nelson, N., & Hyter, Y. (1990). Black English sentence scoring: Development and use as a tool for non-biased assessment. Paper presented at the Annual Convention of the American Speech-Language-Hearing Association, Seattle, WA.

Nettelbladt, U., & Hansson, K. (1999). Mazes in Swedish preschool children with specific language impairment. *Clinical Linguistics and Phonetics, 13,* 483–497.

Neville, H., Coffey, S., Holcomb, P., & Tallal, P. (1993). The neurobiology of sensory and language processing in language-impaired children. *Journal of Cognitive Neuroscience, 5,* 235–253.

Nevins, H., & Chute, P. (1996). *Children with cochlear implants in educational settings.* London, UK: Singular.

Newcomer, P., & Hammill, D. (1977). Test of language development. Austin, TX: Pro-Ed.

Newfield, M., & Schlanger, B. (1968). The acquisition of English morphology by normal and educable mentally retarded children. *Journal of Speech and Hearing Research, 11,* 82–95.

New Zealand Guidelines Group. (1998). *Traumatic brain injury rehabilitation guidelines.* Retrieved December 2, 2002, from www.nzgg.org.nz/library/gl_complete/tbi/TBI_guideline.pdf

Nicholas, J., & Geers, A. (2003). Personal, social, and family adjustment in school-aged children with cochlear implant. *Ear and Hearing, 24*(1 Suppl.), 69S–81S.

Nichols, L. M. (1996). Pencil and paper versus word processing: A comparative study of creative writing in the elementary school. *Journal of Research on Computing in Education, 29,* 159–166.

Nicoladis, E., & Secco, G. (2000). The role of a child's productive vocabulary in the language choice of a bilingual family. *First Language, 20*(58), 3–28.

Nietupski, J., Scheutz, G., & Ockwood, L. (1980). The delivery of communication therapy services to severely handicapped students: A plan for change. *Journal of the Association for the Severely Handicapped, 5,* 13–23.

Nippold, M. (Ed.). (1988). *Later language development: Ages nine through nineteen.* Boston: Little, Brown.

Nippold, M. (1991). Evaluating and enhancing idiom comprehension in language-disordered students. *Language, Speech, and Hearing Services in Schools, 22,* 100–106.

Nippold, M. (1993). Developmental markers in adolescent language: Syntax, semantics, and pragmatics. *Language, Speech, and Hearing Services in Schools, 24,* 21–28.

Nippold, M. (1994a). Persuasive talk in social contexts: Development, assessment, and intervention. *Topics in Language Disorders, 14*(3), 1–12.

Nippold, M. (1994b). Third-order verbal analogical reasoning: A developmental study of children and adolescents. *Contemporary Educational Psychology, 19,* 101–107.

Nippold, M. (1995). School-age children and adolescents: Norms for word definition. *Language, Speech, and Hearing Services in Schools, 26,* 320–325.

Nippold, M. (1998). *Later language development: The school-age and adolescent years.* Austin, TX: Pro-Ed.

Nippold, M. (1999). Word definition in adolescents as a function of reading proficiency: A research note. *Child Language Teaching and Therapy, 15,* 171–176.

Nippold, M. (2000). Language development during the adolescents years: Aspects of pragmatics, syntax, and semantics. *Topics in Language Disorders, 20*(2), 15–28.

Nippold, M. (2002). Lexical learning in school-age children, adolescents, and adults: A process where language and literacy converge. *Journal of Child Language, 29*(2), 474–478.

Nippold, M., Allen, M., & Kirsch, D. (2001). Proverb comprehension as a function of reading proficiency in preadolescents. *Language, Speech, and Hearing Services in Schools, 32,* 90–100.

Nippold, M., Cuyler, J., & Braunbeck-Price, R. (1988). Explanation of ambiguous advertisements: A developmental study with children and adolescents. *Journal of Speech and Hearing Research, 31,* 466–474.

Nippold, M., Hegel, S., Sohlberg, M., & Schwarz, I. (1999). Defining abstract entities: Development in the preadolescents, adolescents, and young adults. *Journal of Speech, Language, and Hearing Research, 42,* 473–481.

Nippold, M., Hegel, S., Uhden, L., & Bustamante, S. (1998). Development of proverb comprehension in adolescents: Implications for instruction. *Journal of Children's Communication Development, 19,* 49–55.

Nippold, M., Leonard, L., & Anastopoulos, A. (1982). Development in the use and understanding of polite forms in children. *Journal of Speech and Hearing Research, 25,* 193–202.

Nippold, M., Leonard, L., & Kail, R. (1984). Syntactic and conceptual factors in children's understanding of metaphors. *Journal of Speech and Hearing Research, 27,* 197–205.

Nippold, M., & Martin, S. (1989). Idiom interpretation in isolation versus context: A developmental study with adolescents. *Journal of Speech and Hearing Research, 32,* 59–66.

Nippold, M., Moran, C., & Schwarz, I. (2001). Idiom understanding in preadolescents: Synergy in action. *American Journal of Speech-Language Pathology, 10,* 169–179.

Nippold, M., & Rudzinski, M. (1993). Familiarity and transparency in idiom explanation: A developmental study with children and adolescents. *Journal of Speech and Hearing Research, 36,* 728–737.

Nippold, M., & Schwarz, I. (1996). Children with slow expressive language development: What is the forecast for school achievement? *American Journal of Speech-Language Pathology, 5*(2), 22–25.

Nippold, M., Schwarz, I., & Undlin, R. (1992). Use and understanding of adverbial conjuncts: A developmental study of adolescents and young adults. *Journal of Speech and Hearing Research, 35,* 108–118.

Nippold, M., & Taylor, C. (1995). Idiom understanding in youth: Further examination of familiarity and transparency. *Journal of Speech and Hearing Research, 38,* 426–433.

Nippold, M., & Taylor, C. (2002). Judgments of idiom familiarity and transparency: A comparison of children and adolescents. *Journal of Speech, Language, and Hearing Research, 45,* 384–391.

Nippold, M., Taylor, C., & Baker, J. (1996). Idiom understanding in Australian youth: A cross-cultural comparison. *Journal of Speech and Hearing Research, 39,* 442–447.

Nippold, M., Uhden, L., & Schwarz, I. (1997). Proverb explanation through the lifespan: A developmental study of adolescents and adults. *Journal of Speech, Language, and Hearing Research, 40,* 245–253.

Nolan, M., McCartney, E., McArthur, K., & Rowson, V. (1980). A study of the hearing and receptive vocabulary of the trainees of an adult training centre. *Journal of Mental Deficiency Research, 24,* 271–286.

Nopoulos, P., Berg, S., Canady, J., Richman, L., Van Demark, D., & Andreasen, N. (2000). Abnormal brain morphology in patients with isolated cleft lip, cleft palate, or both: A preliminary analysis. *Cleft Palate-Craniofacial Journal, 37,* 441–446.

Norris, J. (1995). Expanding language norms for school-age children and adolescents: Is it pragmatic? *Language, Speech, and Hearing Services in Schools, 26,* 342–352.

Northern, J., & Downs, M. (2002). *Hearing in Children* (5th ed.). Philadelphia: Lippincott, Williams & Wilkins.

Northern, J., & Hayes, D. (1994). Universal screening for infant hearing impairment: Necessary, beneficial and justifiable. *Audiology Today, 6*(2), 10–13.

O'Carroll, P., Crosby, A., Mercy, J., Lee, R., & Simon, T. (2001). Interviewing suicide "decedents": A fourth strategy for risk factor assessment. *Suicide and Life-Threatening Behavior, 32*(Suppl.), 3–6.

Odom, S. L., & Watts, E. (1991). Reducing teacher prompts in peer-mediated interventions for young children with autism. *Journal of Special Education, 25,* 26–33.

Oetting, J., & Horohov, J. (1997). Past-tense marking by children with and without specific language impairment. *Journal of Speech, Language, and Hearing Research, 40,* 62–74.

O'Gara, M. M., & Logemann, J. A. (1988). Phonetic analyses of the speech development of babies with cleft palate. *Cleft Palate Journal, 25,* 122–134.

Ogletree, B. T., & Hahn, W. E. (2001). Augmentative and alternative communication for persons with autism: History, issues and unanswered questions. *Focus on Autism and Other Developmental Disabilities, 16,* 138–142.

Olenchak, F. R. (1994). Talent development. *Journal of Secondary Gifted Education, 5*(3), 40–52.

Oliver, B., & Buckley, S. (1994). The language development of children with Down's syndrome: First words to two-word phrases. *Down Syndrome: Research and Practice, 2,* 71–75.

Oller, D. K. (1980). The emergence of the sounds of speech in infancy. In G. Yeni-Komshian, J. A. Kavanagh, & C. Ferguson (Eds.), *Child Phonology* (Vol. 1). New York: Academic Press.

Oller, D. K., & Eilers, R. (1988). The role of audition in infant babbling. *Child Development, 59,* 441–449.

Oller, D. K., Eilers, R. E., Neal, A. R., & Schwartz, H. K. (1999). Precursors to speech in infancy: The prediction of speech and language disorders. *Journal of Communication Disorders, 32,* 223–245.

Oller, D. K., Levine, S., Cobo-Lewis, A., Eilers, R., & Pearson, B. (1998). Vocal precursors to linguistic communication: How babbling is connected to meaningful speech. In R. Paul (Ed.), *Exploring the speech-language connection* (pp. 1–23). Baltimore, MD: Paul H. Brookes.

Olswang, L., & Bain, B. (1991a). Intervention issues for toddlers with specific language impairments. *Topics in Language Disorders, 11,* 69–86.

Olswang, L., & Bain, B. (1991b). When to recommend intervention. *Language, Speech, and Hearing Services in Schools, 22,* 255–263.

Olswang, L., & Bain, B. (1996). Assessment information for predicting upcoming change in language production. *Journal of Speech and Hearing Research, 39,* 414–423.

Olswang, L., & Carpenter, R. (1978). Elicitor effects on the language obtained from young language-impaired children. *Journal of Speech and Hearing Disorders, 43,* 76–88.

Olswang, L., Johnson, G., & Crooke, P. (1992, November). Single to multi-words: A journey with SLI children. Paper presented at the Annual Convention of the American Speech-Language-Hearing Association, San Antonio, TX.

Olswang, L., Long, S., & Fletcher, P. (1997). Verbs in the emergence of word combinations in young children with specific expressive language impairment. *European Journal of Disorders of Communication, 32,* 15–33.

Olswang, L., Rodriguez, B., & Timler, G. (1998). Recommending intervention for toddlers with specific language learning difficulties: We may not have all the answers, but we know a lot. *American Journal of Speech-Language Pathology, 7*(1), 23–32.

Oram, J., Fine, J., Okamoto, C., & Tannock, R. (1999). Assessing the language of children with attention deficit hyperactivity disorder. *American Journal of Speech-Language Pathology, 8,* 72–80.

Osberger, M. J., Chute, P., Pope, M., Kessler, D. K., Carotta, C., Firstz, J., et al. (1991). Speech perception abilities of children with cochlear implants, tactile aids or hearing aids. *American Journal of Otology, 12*(Suppl.), 80–88.

Osberger, M. J., & McGarr, N. S. (1982). Speech production characteristics of the hearing impaired. In N. Lass (Ed.), *Speech and language: advances in research and practice* (Vol. 8). New York: Academic Press.

Osberger, M. J., Robbins, A. M., Berry, S., Todd, S. L., Hesketh, L., & Sedey, A. (1991). Analysis of the spontaneous speech samples of children with cochlear implants or tactile aids. *American Journal of Otology, 12*(Suppl.), 151–164.

Osberger, M. J., Robbins, A. M., Todd, S. L., & Riley, A. I. (1996). Cochlear implants and tactile aids for children with profound hearing impairment. In F. Bess, J. Gravel, & A. Tharpe (Eds.), *Amplification for children with auditory deficits* (pp. 283–308). Nashville, TN: Bill Wilkerson Press.

Oshima-Takane, Y., & Benaroya, S. (1989). An alternative view of pronominal errors in autistic children. *Journal of Autism and Developmental Disorders, 19,* 73–85.

Osterling, J., & Dawson, G. (1994). Early recognition of children with autism: A study of first birthday home videotapes. *Journal of Autism and Developmental Disorders, 24,* 247–257.

Outhred, L. (1989). Word processing: Its impact on children's writing. *Journal of Learning Disabilities, 22,* 262–264.

Owen, A., & Leonard, L. (2002). Lexical diversity in the spontaneous speech of children with specific langauge impairment: Application of D. *Journal of Speech, Language, and Hearing Research, 45,* 927–937.

Owens, R. (1999). *Language disorders: A functional approach to assessment and intervention* (3rd ed.). Boston: Allyn & Bacon.

Owens, R. (2001). *Language development: An Introduction* (5th ed.). Boston: Allyn & Bacon.

Owens, R., & MacDonald, J. (1982). Communicative uses of the early speech of nondelayed and Down syndrome children. *American Journal of Mental Deficiency, 86,* 503–510.

Owings, N. O., & McManus, M. D. (1980). An analysis of communication functions in the speech of a deinstitutionalized adult mentally retarded client. *Mental Retardation, 18,* 309–314.

Oyler, R. F., Oyler, A. L., & Matkin, N. D. (1987). Warning: A unilateral hearing loss may be detrimental to a child's academic career. *Hearing Journal, 40*(9), 18–22.

Oyler, R. F., Oyler, A. L., & Matkin, N. D. (1988). Unilateral hearing loss: Demographics and educational impact. *Language, Speech, and Hearing Services in Schools, 19,* 201–209.

Ozonoff, S., Pennington, B. F., & Rogers, S. J. (1991). Executive function deficits in high-functioning autistic individuals: Relationship to theory of mind. *Journal of Child Psychology and Psychiatry, 32,* 1081–1105.

Pajewski, A., & Enriquez, L. (1996). *Teaching from a Hispanic perspective: A handbook for non-Hispanic adult educators.* Retrieved December 2, 2002, from http://literacynet.org/lp/hperspectives

Pan, B., & Berko-Gleason, J. (2001). Semantic development: Learning the meanings of words. In J. Berko-Gleason (Ed.), *The development of language* (5th ed., pp. 125–161). Boston: Allyn & Bacon.

Paradise, J. L., Elster, B., & Lingshi, T. (1994). Evidence in infants with cleft lip and palate that breast milk protects against otitis media. *Pediatrics, 94*(6), 853–860.

Parke, K., Shallcross, R., & Anderson, R. (1980). Differences in coverbal behavior between blind and sighted persons during dyadic communication. *Journal of Visual Impairment and Blindness, 74,* 142–146.

Parker, R., Tindal, G., & Hasbrouck, J. (1991). Countable indices of writing quality: Their suitability for screening-eligibility decisions. *Exceptionality, 2,* 1–17.

Parsons, C. L., Iacono, T. A., & Rozner, L. (1987). Effect of tongue reduction on articulation in children with Down syndrome. *American Journal of Mental Deficiency, 91,* 328–332.

Paul, P. V. (1998). *Literacy and deafness.* Boston: Allyn & Bacon.

Paul, R. (1981). Analyzing complex sentence development. In J. Miller (Ed.), *Assessing language production in children.* Baltimore, MD: University Park Press.

Paul, R. (1991). Profiles of toddlers with slow expressive language development. *Topics in Language Disorders, 11*(4), 1–13.

Paul, R. (1993). Outcomes of early expresssive language delay. *Journal of Childhood Communication Disorders, 15,* 7–14.

Paul, R. (1996). Clinical implications of the natural history of slow expressive language development. *American Journal of Speech-Language Pathology, 5*(2), 5–21.

Paul, R. (1997a). Introduction: Special section on language development in children who use AAC. *Augmentative and Alternative Communication, 13,* 139–140.

Paul, R. (1997b). Understanding language delay: A response to van Kleeck, Gillam, and Davis. *American Journal of Speech-Language Pathology, 6*(2), 40–49.

Paul, R. (2000). Predicting outcomes of early expressive language delay: Ethical implications. In D. V. M. Bishop & L. Leonard (Eds.), *Speech and language impairments in children: Causes, characteristics, intervention and outcomes* (pp. 195–209). East Sussex, UK: Psychology Press.

Paul, R. (2001). *Language disorders from infancy through adolescence: Assessment and intervention* (2nd ed.). St. Louis, MO: Mosby.

Paul, R., & Cohen, D. J. (1984). Responses to contingent queries in adults with mental retardation and pervasive developmental disorders. *Applied Psycholinguistics, 5,* 349–357.

Paul, R., Hernandez, R., Taylor, L., & Johnson, K. (1996). Narrative development in late talkers: Early school age. *Journal of Speech and Hearing Research, 39,* 1295–1303.

Paul, R., & Jennings, P. (1992). Phonological behavior in toddlers with slow expressive language development. *Journal of Speech and Hearing Research, 35,* 99–107.

Paul, R., Looney, S., & Dahm, P. (1991). Communication and socialization skills at ages 2 and 3 in "late-talking" young children. *Journal of Speech and Hearing Research, 34,* 858–865.

Paul, R., Murray, C., Clancy, K., & Andrews, D. (1997). Reading and metaphonological outcomes in late talkers. *Journal of Speech, Language, and Hearing Research, 40,* 1037–1047.

Paul, R., & Smith, R. (1993). Narrative skills in 4-year-olds with normal, impaired, and late-developing language. *Journal of Speech and Hearing Research, 36,* 592–598.

Peacock, T., & Day, D. (1999). *Teaching American Indian and Alaska Native languages in the schools: What has been learned.* Retrieved July 2002, from www.ed.gov/databases/ERIC_Digests/ed438155.html.

Pearce, P. S., & Darwish, H. (1984). Correlation between EEG and auditory perceptual measures in auditory agnosia. *Brain and Language, 22,* 41–48.

Pearl, R., Donahue, M., & Bryan, T. H. (1985). The development of tact: Children's strategies for delivering bad news. *Journal of Applied Developmental Psychology, 6,* 141–149.

Pearl, R., Farmer, T. W., Van Acker, R., Rodkin, P., Bost, K. K., Coe, M., et al. (1998). The social integration of students with mild disabilities in general education classrooms: Peer group membership and peer-assessed social behavior. *Elementary School Journal, 99,* 167–185.

Peck, C. A. (1985). Increasing opportunities for social control by children with autism and severe handicaps: Effects on student behavior and perceived classroom climate. *Journal of the Association for Persons with Severe Handicaps, 10*(4), 183–193.

Pehrsson, R. S., & Denner, P. R. (1988). Semantic organizers: Implications for reading and writing. *Topics in Language Disorders, 8,* 24–37.

Pehrsson, R. S., & Denner, P. R. (1989). *Semantic organizers: A study strategy for special needs learners.* Rockville, MD: Aspen.

Peña, E. (1996). Dynamic assessment: The model and its language applications. In K. Cole, P. Dale, & D. Thal (Eds.), *Assessment of communicaiton and language* (pp. 281–307). Baltimore, MD: Paul H. Brookes.

Peña, E., Bedore, L., & Rappazzo, C. (2003). Comparison of Spanish, English, and bilingual children's performance across semantic tasks. *Language, Speech, and Hearing Services in Schools, 34,* 5–16.

Peña, E., Bedore, L., & Zlatic-Giunta, R. (2002). Category-generation performances of bilingual children: The influence of condition, category, and language. *Journal of Speech, Language, and Hearing Research, 45,* 938–947.

Peña, E., Iglesias, A., & Lidz, C. (2001). Reducing test bias through dynamic assessment of children's word learning ability. *American Journal of Speech-Language Pathology, 10,* 138–154.

Perera, K. (1984). *Children's writing and reading: Analysing classroom language.* London, UK: Basil Blackwell.

Perez-Pereira, M., & Conti-Ramsden, G. (1999). *Language development and social interaction in blind children.* Hove, East Sussex, UK: Psychology Press.

Peterson, S. E. (1993). A comparison of student revisions when composing with pen and paper versus word-processing. *Computers in the Schools, 9,* 55–69.

Pharoah, P. O., Cooke, T., Johnson, M. A., King, R., & Mutch, L. (1998). Epidemiology of cerebral palsy in England and Scotland, 1984–9. *Archives of Disease in Childhood: Fetal and Neonatal Edition, 79*(1), F21–F25.

Phelps-Terasaki, D., & Phelps-Gunn, T. (1992). *Test of Pragmatic Language.* Austin, TX: Pro-Ed.

Phillips, J. (1973). Syntax and vocabulary of mothers' speech to young children: Age and sex comparisons. *Child Development, 44,* 182–185.

Piaget, J. (1954). *The origins of intelligence.* New York: Basic Books.

Pine, J. (1999, July). Tense optionality and children's use of verb morphology: Testing the optional infinitive hypothesis. Paper presented at the International Association for the Study of Child Language, San Sebastian, Spain.

Piven, J., Chase, G. A., Landa, R., Wzorek, M., Gayle, J., Cloud, D., et al. (1991). Psychiatric disorders in the parents of autistic individuals. *Journal of the American Academy of Child and Adolescent Psychiatry, 30,* 471–478.

Piven, J., Gayle, J., Landa, R., Wzorek, M., & Folstein, S. E. (1991). The prevalence of Fragile X in a sample of autistic individuals diagnosed using a standardized interview. *Journal of the American Academy of Child and Adolescent Psychiatry, 30,* 825–830.

Plante, E. (1996a). Observing and interpreting behaviors: An introduction to the clinical forum. *Language, Speech, and Hearing Services in Schools, 27,* 99–101.

Plante, E. (1996b). Phenotypic variability in brain-behavior studies of specific language impairment. In M. Rice (Ed.), *Toward a genetics of language* (pp. 317–335). Hillsdale, NJ: Lawrence Erlbaum.

Plante, E. (1998). Criteria for SLI: The Stark and Tallal legacy and beyond. *Journal of Speech, Language, and Hearing Research, 41,* 951–957.

Plante, E., Boliek, C., Binkiewicz, A., & Erly, W. (1996). Elevated androgen, brain development, and language/learning disabilities in children with congenital adrenal hyperplasia. *Developmental Medicine and Child Neurology, 38,* 432–437.

Plante, E., Shenkman, K., & Clark, M. (1996). Classification of adults for family studies of developmental language disorders. *Journal of Speech and Hearing Research, 39,* 661–667.

Plante, E., Swisher, L., Vance, R., & Rapcsak, S. (1991). MRI findings in boys with specific language impairment. *Brain and Language, 41,* 52–66.

Plante, E., & Vance, R. (1994). Selection of preschool language tests: A data-based approach. *Language, Speech, and Hearing Services in Schools, 25,* 15–24.

Platt, J., & Coggins, T. (1990). Comprehension of social-action games in prelinguistic children: Levels of participation and effects of adult structure. *Journal of Speech and Hearing Disorders, 55,* 315–326.

Plomin, R., & Dale, P. (2000). Genetics and early language development: A UK study of twins. In D. V. M. Bishop & L. Leonard (Eds.), *Speech and language impairments in children: Causes, characteristics, intervention and outcomes* (pp. 35–51). East Sussex, UK: Psychology Press.

Plomin, R., DeFries, J., McClearn, G., & McGuffin, P. (2001). *Behavioral genetics* (4th ed.). New York: Worth.

Plomin, R., Fulker, D., Corley, R., & DeFries, J. (1997). Nature, nurture and cognitive development from 1 to 16 years: A parent-offspring adoption study. *Psychological Science, 8,* 442–447.

Pollio, M., & Pollio, H. (1979). A test of metaphoric comprehension: Preliminary data. *Journal of Child Language, 6,* 111–120.

Pollock, K. (2001). *Phonological features of African American vernacular English.* Retrieved December 2, 2002, from www.ausp.memphis.edu/phonology/features.htm

Poole, E. (1934). Genetic development of articulation of consonant sounds in speech. *Elementary English Review, 11,* 159–161.

Porch, B. E. (1979). *Porch Index of Communicative Ability in Children.* Palo Alto, CA: Consulting Psychologists Press.

Power, R., Taylor, C., & Nippold, M. (2001). Comprehending literally-true versus literally-false proverbs. *Child Language Teaching and Therapy, 17,* 1–18.

Powls, A., Botting, N., Cooke, R. W., Stephenson, G., & Marlow, N. (1997). Visual impairment in very low birthweight children. *Archives of Disease in Childhood, 76*(2), F82–F87.

Prather, E., Breecher, S., Stafford, M., & Wallace, E. (1980). *Screening Test of Adolescent Language.* Seattle: University of Washington Press.

Prather, E., Brenner, A., & Hughes, K. (1981). A mini-screening language test for adolescents. *Language, Speech, and Hearing Services in Schools, 12,* 67–73.

Preece, D. (2002). Consultation with children with autistic spectrum disorders about their experience of short-term residential care. *British Journal of Learning Disabilities 30*(3), 97–104.

President's Commission on Excellence in Special Education. (2002). *A new era: Revitalizing special education for children and their families.* Retrieved December 20, 2002, from www.ed.gov/inits/commissionsboards/whspecialeducation/reports.html

Price, E. (1976). How 37 gifted children learned to read. *Reading Teacher, 30,* 44–48.

Prinz, P., & Ferrier, L. (1983). "Can you give me that one?": The comprehension, production and judgment of directives in language-impaired children. *Journal of Speech and Hearing Disorders, 48,* 44–54.

Prizant, B., Audet, L., Burke, G., Hummel, L., Maher, S., & Theadore, G. (1990). Communication disorders and emotional and behavioral disorders in children and adolescents. *Journal of Speech and Hearing Disorders, 55,* 179–192.

Prizant, B., Schuler, A. L., Wetherby, A. M., & Rydell, P. J. (1997). Enhancing language and communication development: Language approaches. In D. J. Cohen & F. R. Volkmar (Eds.), *Handbook of Autism and Pervasive Developmental Disorders* (2nd ed., pp. 572–605). New York: Wiley.

Prizant, B., & Wetherby, A. M. (1998). Understanding the continuum of discrete-trial traditional behavioral to social-pragmatic developmental approaches in communication enhancement for young children with autism/PDD. *Seminars in Speech and Language, 19,* 329–353.

Proctor, A. (1989). Stages of normal noncry vocal development in infants: A protocol for assessment. *Topics in Language Disorders, 10*(1), 26–42.

Proctor-Williams, K., Fey, M., & Loeb, D. (2001). Parental recasts and production of copulas and articles by children with specific language impairment and typical language. *American Journal of Speech-Language Pathology, 10,* 155–168.

Pruess, J. B., Vadasy, P. F., & Fewell, R. R. (1987). Language development in children with Down syndrome: An overview of recent research. *Education and Training of the Mentally Retarded, 22,* 44–55.

Prutting, C. (1979). Process: The action of moving forward progressively from one point to another on the way to completion. *Journal of Speech and Hearing Disorders, 44,* 3–30.

Prutting, C. (1982). Pragmatics as social competence. *Journal of Speech and Hearing Disorders, 47,* 123–134.

Pueschel, S. M. (1990). Clinical aspects of Down syndrome from infancy to adulthood. *American Journal of Medical Genetics, 7,* 52–56.

Pueschel, S. M. (1992). Phenotypic characteristics. In S. M. Pueschel & J. K. Pueschel (Eds.), *Biomedical concerns in persons with Down syndrome* (pp. 1–12). Baltimore, MD: Paul H. Brookes.

Pueschel, S. M. (1998). Should children with Down syndrome be screened for atlantoaxial instability? *Archives of Pediatric and Adolescent Medicine, 152,* 123–125.

Pueschel, S. M., & Gieswein, S. (1993). Ocular disorders in children with Down syndrome. *Down Syndrome: Research and Practice, 1,* 129–132.

Pye, C. (1987). Pye Analysis of Language (PAL) [DOS computer software]. Lawrence: University of Kansas.

Qi, C. H., Kaiser, A. P., Milan, S. E., Yzquierdo, Z., & Hancock, T. B. (2003). The performance of low-income, African American children on the Preschool Language Scale—3. *Journal of Speech, Language, and Hearing Research, 46,* 576–590.

Quiroga, T., Lemos-Britton, Z., Mostafapour, E., Abbott, R., & Berninger, V. (2002). Phonological awareness and beginning reading in Spanish-speaking ESL first graders: Research into practice. *Journal of School Psychology, 40*(1), 85–111.

Raffaelli, M., & Duckett, E. (1989). "We were just talking . . . ": Conversations in early adolescence. *Journal of Youth and Adolescence, 18,* 567–582.

Rapin, I. (1996). Developmental language disorders: A clinical update. *Journal of Child Psychology and Psychiatry, 37,* 643–656.

Rapin, I., & Allen, D. (1987). Developmental dysphasia and autism in preschool children: Characteristics and subtypes. In J. Martin, P. Fletcher, P. Grunwell, & D. Hall (Eds.), *Proceedings of the First International Symposium on Specific Speech and Language Disorders in Children* (pp. 20–35). London, UK: AFASIC.

Rattigan, K., Reed, V. A., & Lee, K. (2002). An investigation into the phonological processing and literacy skills of children using cochlear implants. Paper presented at the A. G. Bell Association for the Deaf and Hard of Hearing, St. Louis, MO.

Rauch, A. (Ed.). (1994). *Behaviour management: An approach for the 90s.* Newcastle, Australia: ASSID Publications.

Raven, C. (1998). *Raven's Progressive Matrices.* San Antonio, TX: Psychological Corporation.

Raybarman, C. (2002). Landau-Kleffner syndrome: A case report. *Neurology India, 50,* 212–213.

Redmond, S. (2003). Children's productions of the affix *-ed* in past tense and past participle contexts. *Journal of Speech, Language, and Hearing Research, 46,* 1095–1109.

Redmond, S., & Rice, M. (1998). The socioemotional behaviors of children with SLI: Social adaptation or social deviance? *Journal of Speech, Language, and Hearing Research, 41,* 688–700.

Redmond, S., & Rice, M. (2001). Detection of irregular verb violations by children with and without SLI. *Journal of Speech, Language, and Hearing Research, 44,* 655–669.

Reed, V. A. (1990, March). Differences in the language skills of 8- and 14-year-old children. Paper presented at the Annual Conference of the Australian Association of Speech and Hearing, Sydney.

Reed, V. A. (1991). What Crocodile Dundee never told us. *American Journal of Speech-Language Pathology, 1*(1), 11–12.

Reed, V. A. (1992). Associations between phonology and other language components in children's communicative performance. *Australian Journal of Human Communication Disorders, 20,* 75–87.

Reed, V. A., Bradfield, M., & McAllister, L. (1998). The relative importance of selected communication skills for successful adolescent peer interactions: Speech pathologists' opinions. *Clinical Linguistics and Phonetics, 12,* 205–220.

Reed, V. A., & Evernden, A. (2001, November). Verb morphology of older children with reading difficulties. Paper presented at the Annual Convention of the American Speech-Language-Hearing Association, New Orleans, LA.

Reed, V. A., Griffith, F. A., & Rasmussen, A. (1998). Morphosyntactic structures in the spoken language of older children and adolescents. *Clinical Linguistics and Phonetics, 12,* 163–181.

Reed, V., MacMillan, V., & McLeod, S. (2001). Elucidating the effects of different definitions of "utterance" on selected syntactic measures of older children's language samples. *Asia Pacific Journal of Speech, Language, and Hearing, 6,* 39–45.

Reed, V. A., McLeod, K., & McAllister, L. (1999). Importance of selected communication skills for talking with peers and teachers: Adolescents' opinions. *Language, Speech, and Hearing Services in Schools, 30,* 32–49.

Reed, V. A., & Miles, M. (1989). *Adolescent language disorders: A video inservice for educators.* Eau Claire, WI: Thinking Publications.

Reed, V. A., & Spicer, L. (2003). The relative importance of selected communication skills for adolescents' interactions with their teachers: High school teachers' opinions. *Language, Speech, and Hearing Services in Schools, 34,* 343–357.

Rees, N. S. (1973). Auditory processing factors in language disorders: The view from Procrustes' bed. *Journal of Speech and Hearing Disorders, 38*(3), 304–315.

Rees, N. S. (1982). Saying more than we know: Is auditory processing disorder a meaningful concept. In R. Keith (Ed.), *Central Auditory and Language Disorders in Children.* San Diego, CA: College-Hill Press.

Reich, P. A. (Ed.). (1986). *Langauge development.* Englewood Cliffs, NJ: Prentice-Hall.

Reichle, J., Williams, W., & Ryan, S. (1981). Selecting signs for the formulation of an augmentative communicative modality. *Journal of the Association for the Severely Handicapped, 6,* 48–56.

Reid, R. (1996). Research in self-monitoring with students with learning disabilities: The present, the prospects, the pitfalls. *Journal of Learning Disabilities, 29,* 317–331.

Reilly, P., & Simpson, D. (1988). Assessing the conscious level in infants and young children: A paediatric version of the Glasgow Coma Scale. *Child's Nervous System, 4,* 30–33.

Rescorla, L. (1989). The Language Development Survey: A screening tool for delayed language in toddlers. *Journal of Speech and Hearing Disorders, 54,* 587–599.

Rescorla, L. (1991). Identifying expressive language delay at age two. *Topics in Language Disorders, 11,* 14–20.

Rescorla, L. (1993). Outcome of toddlers with specific expressive delay at ages 3, 4, 5, 6, 7, & 8. Paper presented at the Biennial Meeting of the Society for Research in Child Development, New Orleans, LA.

Rescorla, L. (2002). Language and reading outcomes to age 9 in late-talking toddlers. *Journal of Speech, Language, and Hearing Research, 45,* 360–371.

Rescorla, L., & Achenbach, T. (2002). Use of the Language Development Survey (LDS) in a national probability sample of children 18 to 35 months old. *Journal of Speech, Language, and Hearing Research, 45,* 733–743.

Rescorla, L., Alley, A., & Christine, J. (2001). Word frequencies in toddlers' lexicons. *Journal of Speech, Language, and Hearing Research, 44,* 598–609.

Rescorla, L., Dahlsgaard, K., & Roberts, J. (2000). Late-talking toddlers: MLU and IPSyn outcomes at 3;0 and 4;0. *Journal of Child Language, 27,* 643–664.

Rescorla, L., & Goossens, M. (1992). Symbolic play development in toddlers with expressive specific language impairment. *Journal of Speech and Hearing Research, 35,* 1290–1302.

Rescorla, L., Hadicke-Wiley, M., & Escarce, E. (1993). Epidemiological investigation of expressive language delay at age two. *First Language, 13,* 5–22.

Rescorla, L., & Lee, E. (2001). Language impairment in young children. In T. Layton, E. Crais, & L. Watson (Eds.), *Handbook of early language impairment in children: Nature* (pp. 11–55). Albany, NY: Delmar.

Rescorla, L., & Ratner, N. (1996). Phonetic profiles of toddlers with specific expressive language impairments (SLI-E). *Journal of Speech and Hearing Research, 39,* 153–165.

Restrepo, M. (1998). Identifiers of Spanish-speaking children with specific language impairment. *Journal of Speech, Language, and Hearing Research, 41,* 1398–1411.

Restrepo, M., & Silverman, S. (2001). Validity of the Spanish Preschool Language Scale—3 for use with bilingual children. *American Journal of Speech-Language Pathology, 10,* 392–393.

Retherford, K. (2000). *Guide to analysis of language transcripts* (3rd ed.). Eau Claire, WI: Thinking Publications.

Rettig, M. (1994). The play of young children with visual impairments: Characteristics and interventions. *Journal of Visual Impairments and Blindness, 88,* 410–420.

Reynolds, C., & Bigler, E. (1994). *Test of Memory and Learning.* Austin, TX: Pro-Ed.

Riccio, C. A., & Jemison, S. J. (1998). ADHD and emergent literacy: Influences of language factors. *Reading and Writing Quarterly, 14*(1), 43–59.

Rice, M. (1983). Contemporary accounts of the cognition/language relationship: Implications for speech-language clinicians. *Journal of Speech and Hearing Disorders, 38,* 347–359.

Rice, M. (1990). Preschoolers' QUIL: Quick incidental learning of words. In G. Conti-Ramsden & C. Snow (Eds.), *Children's language* (Vol. 7, pp. 171–195). Hillsdale, NJ: Lawrence Erlbaum.

Rice, M. (Ed.). (1996). *Toward a genetics of language.* Hillsdale, NJ: Lawrence Erlbaum.

Rice, M. (2000). Grammatical symptoms of specific language impairment. In D. V. M. Bishop & L. Leonard (Eds.), *Speech and language impairment in children: Causes,* *characteristics, intervention and outcome* (pp. 17–34). East Sussex, UK: Psychology Press.

Rice, M., & Bode, J. (1993). GAPs in the verb lexicons of children with specific language impairment. *First Language, 13,* 113–131.

Rice, M., Buhr, J., & Nemeth, M. (1990). Fast mapping word-learning abilities of language-delayed preschoolers. *Journal of Speech and Hearing Disorders, 55,* 33–42.

Rice, M., Buhr, J., & Oetting, J. (1992). Specific-language-impaired children's quick incidental learning of words: The effect of a pause. *Journal of Speech and Hearing Research, 35,* 1040–1048.

Rice, M., & Hadley, P. (1995). Language outcomes of the language-focused curriculum. In M. Rice & K. Wilcox (Eds.), *Building a language-focused curriculum for the preschool classroom: A foundation for lifelong communication* (Vol. I, pp. 155–169). Baltimore, MD: Paul H. Brookes.

Rice, M., Huston, A., Truglio, R., & Wright, J. (1990). Words from "Sesame Street": Learning vocabulary while viewing. *Developmental Psychology, 26,* 421–428.

Rice, M., Oetting, J., Marquis, J., Bode, J., & Pae, S. (1994). Frequency of input effects on word comprehension of children with specific language impairment. *Journal of Speech and Hearing Research, 37,* 106–122.

Rice, M., Sell, M., & Hadley, P. (1990). The Social Interactive Coding System (SICS): An on-line, clinically relevant descriptive tool. *Language, Speech, and Hearing Services in Schools, 21,* 2–14.

Rice, M., Sell, M., & Hadley, P. (1991). Social interactions of speech- and language-impaired children. *Journal of Speech and Hearing Research, 34,* 1299–1307.

Rice, M., Spitz, R., & O'Brien, M. (1999). Semantic and morphosyntactic language outcomes in biologically at-risk children. *Journal of Neurolinguistics, 12,* 213–234.

Rice, M., & Watkins, R. (1996). "Show me X": New views on an old assessment technique. In K. Cole, P. Dale, & D. Thal (Eds.), *Assessment of communication and language* (pp. 183–206). Baltimore, MD: Paul H. Brookes.

Rice, M., & Wexler, K. (1996). Toward tense as a clinical marker of specific language impairment in English-speaking children. *Journal of Speech and Hearing Research, 39,* 1239–1257.

Rice, M., & Wexler, K. (2001). *Rice/Wexler Test of Early Grammatical Impairment.* San Antonio, TX: Psychological Corporation.

Rice, M., Wexler, K., & Cleave, P. (1995). Specific language impairment as a period of extended optional infinitive. *Journal of Speech and Hearing Research, 38,* 850–863.

Rice, M., Wexler, K., & Hershberger, S. (1998). Tense over time: The longitudinal course of tense acquisition in children with specific language impairment. *Journal of Speech, Language, and Hearing Research, 41,* 1412–1431.

Rice, M., Wexler, K., Marquis, J., & Hershberger, S. (2000). Acquisition of irregular past tense by children with specific language impairment. *Journal of Speech, Language, and Hearing Research, 43,* 1126–1145.

Rice, M., & Wilcox, K. (Eds.). (1995). *Building a language-focused curriculum for the preschool classroom: A foundation for lifelong communication* (Vol. I). Baltimore, MD: Paul H. Brookes.

Rice, M., & Woodsmall, L. (1988). Lessons from television: Children's word learning when viewing. *Child Development, 59,* 420–429.

Richard, G., & Hanner, A. (1995). *Language Processing Test—Revised.* East Moline, IL: LinguiSystems.

Richman, L., & Eliason, M. (1993). Disorders of communication, developmental language disorders and cleft palate. In C. E. Walker & M. Roberts (Eds.), *Handbook of child clinical psychology—Revised* (pp. 537–552). New York: Wiley.

Richman, L., Eliason, M., & Lindgren, S. (1988). Reading disability in children with clefts. *Cleft Palate Journal, 25,* 21–25.

Rickford, J. (1998). The creole origins of African American vernacular English: Evidence from copula absence. In S. S. Mufwene, J. R. Rickford, G. Bailey, & J. Baugh (Eds.), *African-American English: Structure, History, and Usage* (pp. 154–200). London, UK: Routledge.

Rickford, J., & Rickford, A. (1995). Dialect readers revisited. *Linguistics and Education, 7*(2), 107–128.

Ridgeway, S. (1998). A deaf personality? In S. Gregory, P. Knight, W. McCracken, S. Powers, & L. Watson (Eds.), *Issues in deaf education.* London, UK: David Fulson.

Rimmer, J. H., Braddock, D., & Fujiura, G. (1993). Prevalence of obesity in adults with MR: Implications for health promotion and disease prevention. *Mental Retardation, 31,* 105–110.

Ripich, D. N., & Griffith, P. L. (1988). Narrative abilities of children with learning disabilities and nondisabled children: Story structure, cohesion, and propositions. *Journal of Learning Disabilities, 21,* 165–173.

Robert, E., Kallen, B., & Harris, J. (1996). The epidemiology of orofacial clefts. 1. Some general epidemiological characteristics. *Journal of Craniofacial Genetics and Developmental Biology, 16*(4), 234–241.

Roberts, J. M. A. (1989). Echolalia and comprehension in autistic children. *Journal of Autism and Developmental Disorders, 19,* 271–281.

Roberts, J. E., Rabinowitch, S., Bryant, D., Burchinal, M., Koch, M., & Ramey, C. (1989). Language skills of children with different preschool experiences. *Journal of Speech and Hearing Research, 32,* 773–786.

Robertson, S. B., & Ellis Weismer, S. (1997). The influence of peer models on the play scripts of children with specific language impairment. *Journal of Speech, Language, and Hearing Research, 40,* 49–61.

Robertson, S. B., & Ellis Weismer, S. (1999). Effects of treatment on linguistic and social skills in toddlers with delayed language development. *Journal of Speech, Language, and Hearing Research, 42,* 1234–1248.

Robinson, G. L., Foreman, P. J., & Dear, K. B. G. (1996). The familial incidence of symptoms of scotopic sensitivity/Irlen syndrome. *Perceptual and Motor Skills, 79,* 467–483.

Robinson-Zañartu, C. (1996). Serving Native American children and families: Considering cultural variables. *Language, Speech, and Hearing Services in Schools, 27,* 373–384.

Rock, S. L., Head, D. N., Bradley, R. H., Whiteside, L., & Brisby, J. (1994). Use of the HOME Inventory with families of young visually impaired children. *Journal of Visual Impairment and Blindness, 88,* 140–151.

Rogers, K., & Silverman, L. (1997). *A study of 241 profoundly gifted children.* Retrieved July 2002, from www.gifteddevelopment.com/Articles/Astudyof241 ExtraordGC.htm.

Roid, G. H., & Miller, L. J. (1997). *Leiter International Performance Scale* (Revised ed.). Wood Dale, IL: Stoelting.

Rom, A., & Bliss, L. (1981). A comparison of verbal communicative skills of language impaired and normal speaking children. *Journal of Communication Disorders, 14,* 133–140.

Romski, M. A., & Sevcik, R. A. (1996). *Breaking the speech barrier: Language development through augmented means.* Baltimore, MD: Paul H. Brookes.

Romski, M. A., Sevcik, R. A., & Adamson, L. B. (1997). Framework for studying how children with developmental disabilities develop language through augmented means. *Augmentative and Alternative Communication, 13,* 172–178.

Romski, M. A., Sevcik, R. A., & Forrest, S. (2000). Assistive technology and augmentative and alternative communication in early childhood programs. In M. J. Guralnick (Ed.), *Early childhood inclusion* (pp. 465–479). Baltimore, MD: Paul H. Brookes.

Rondal, J. A. (1988). Down's syndrome. In D. V. M. Bishop & K. Mogford (Eds.), *Language development in exceptional circumstances.* New York: Churchill Livingstone.

Rosenberg, S. (1982). The language of the mentally retarded: Development, processes, and intervention. In S. Rosenberg (Ed.), *Handbook of applied psycholinguistics: Major thrusts of research and theory* (pp. 329–392). Hillsdale, NJ: Lawrence Erlbaum.

Rosenberg, S., & Abbeduto, L. (1993). *Language and communication in mental retardation. Development, processes, and intervention.* Hillsdale, NJ: Lawrence Erlbaum.

Rosenhall, U., Nordin, V., Sandstroem, M., Ahlsen, G., & Gillberg, C. (1999). Autism and hearing loss. *Journal of Autism and Developmental Disorders, 29*(5), 349–357.

Ross, P. O. (1993). *National excellence: A case for developing America's talent.* Washington, DC: Office of Educational Research and Improvement, U.S. Department of Education.

Rossetti, L. (1995). *The Rossetti Infant-Toddler Language Scale: A measure of communication and intervention.* East Moline, IL: LinguiSystems.

Roth, F. (1987). Temporal characteristics of maternal verbal styles. In K. Nelson & A. van Kleeck (Eds.), *Children's language* (Vol. 6). Hillsdale, NJ: Lawrence Erlbaum.

Roth, F., & Spekman, N. (1984a). Assessing the pragmatic abilities of children: Part 1. Organizational framework and assessment parameters. *Journal of Speech and Hearing Disorders, 49,* 2–11.

Roth, F., & Spekman, N. (1984b). Assessing the pragmatic abilities of children: Part 2. Guidelines, considerations, and specific evaluation procedures. *Journal of Speech and Hearing Disorders, 49,* 12–17.

Roth, F., & Spekman, N. (1986). Narrative discourse: Spontaneously generated stories of learning-disabled and normally achieving students. *Journal of Speech and Hearing Disorders, 51,* 8–23.

Roth, F., & Spekman, N. (1989). The oral syntactic proficiency of learning disabled students: A spontaneous story sampling analysis. *Journal of Speech and Hearing Research, 32,* 67–77.

Rowan, L., Leonard, L., Chapman, K., & Weiss, A. (1983). Performative and presuppositional skills in language-disordered and normal children. *Journal of Speech and Hearing Research, 26,* 97–106.

Rowland, C., & Schweigert, P. (1989). Tangible symbols: Symbolic communication for individuals with multisensory impairments. *Augmentative and Alternative Communication, 5*(3), 226–234.

Rowland, C., & Schweigert, P. (1990). *Tangible symbols: Symbolic communication for individuals with multisensory impairments.* Tucson, AZ: Communication Skill Builders.

Rubin, S. S., Rimmer, J. H., Chicoine, B., Braddock, D., & McGuire, D. E. (1998). Overweight prevalence in persons with Down syndrome. *Mental Retardation, 36,* 175–181.

Rubinstein, J. (2002). Pediatric cochlear implantation: Prosthetic hearing and language development. *Lancet, 360,* 483–487.

Rueda, R., & Chan, K. (1980). Referential communication skill levels of moderately mentally retarded adolescents. *American Journal of Mental Deficiency, 85,* 45–52.

Rueda, R., & Perozzi, J. (1977). A comparison of two Spanish tests of receptive language. *Journal of Speech and Hearing Disorders, 42,* 210–215.

Rukeyser, L. (1988, August 30). U.S. firms make it their business to help ease the dropout dilemma. *Minneapolis Star Tribune,* p. 2D.

Runco, M. A. (1997). Is every child gifted? *Roeper Review, 19*(4), 220–224.

Rutter, M. (1978). Diagnosis and definition of childhood autism. *Journal of Autism and Childhood Schizophrenia, 8,* 139–161.

Rutter, M., Bailey, A., Simonoff, E., & Pickles, A. (1997). Genetic influences and autism. In D. J. Cohen & F. R. Volkmar (Eds.), *Handbook of Autism and Pervasive Developmental Disorders* (2nd ed., pp. 370–387). New York: Wiley.

Rutter, T., & Buckley, S. (1994). The acquisition of grammatical morphemes in children with Down's syndrome. *Down Syndrome: Research and Practice, 4,* 76–82.

Rutter, M., & Schopler, E. (1987). Autism and pervasive developmental disorders: Concepts and diagnostic issues. *Journal of Autism and Developmental Disorders, 17,* 159–186.

Rydell, P. J., & Mirenda, P. (1994). Effects of high and low constraint utterances on the production of immediate and delayed echolalia in young children with autism. *Journal of Autism and Developmental Disorders, 24,* 719–735.

Sabers, D. (1996). By their tests we will know them. *Language, Speech, and Hearing Services in Schools, 27,* 102–108.

Saenz, R. B. (1999). Primary care of infants and young children with Down's syndrome. *American Family Physician, 59,* 381–390.

Sainsbury, S. (1986). *Deaf worlds: A study of integration, segregation and disability.* London, UK: Hutchison.

Salas-Provance, M., Erickson, J., & Reed, J. (2002). Disabilities as viewed by four generations of one Hispanic family. *American Journal of Speech-Language Pathology, 11,* 151–162.

Sanger, D. (1999). The communication skills of female juvenile delinqents: A selected review. *Journal of Correctional Education, 50,* 90–94.

Sanger, D., Creswell, J., Dworak, J., & Schultz, L. (2000). Cultural analysis of communication behaviors among juveniles in a correctional facility. *Journal of Communication Disorders, 33,* 31–57.

Sanger, D., Hux, K., & Belau, D. (1997). Language skills of female juvenile delinquents. *American Journal of Speech-Language Pathology, 6,* 70–76.

Sanger, D., Hux, K., & Ritzman, M. (1999). Female juvenile delinquents' pragmatic awareness of conversational interactions. *Journal of Communication Disorders, 32,* 281–295.

Sanger, D., Moore-Brown, B., & Alt, E. (2000). Advancing the discussion on communication and violence. *Communication Disorders Quarterly, 22,* 43–48.

Sanger, D., Moore-Brown, B., Magnuson, G., & Svoboda, N. (2001). Prevalence of language problems among adolescent delinquents: A closer look. *Communication Disorders Quarterly, 23,* 17–26.

San Miguel, S. K., Forness, S. R., & Kavale, K. A. (1996). Social skills deficits in learning disabilities: The psychiatric comorbidity hypothesis. *Learning Disability Quarterly, 19,* 252–261.

Sardegna, J., & Otis, T. P. (1991). *The encyclopedia of blindness and vision impairment.* New York: Facts on File.

Sarno, M. T. (1998). Recovery and rehabilitation in aphasia. In M. T. Sarno (Ed.), *Acquired aphasia* (3rd ed., pp. 595–631). San Diego, CA: Academic Press.

Sattler, J. (2001). *Assessment of children: cognitive applications* (4th ed.). San Diego, CA: J. Sattler.

Satz, P., & Bullard-Bates, C. (1981). Acquired aphasia in children. In M. T. Sarno (Ed.), *Acquired aphasia* (2nd ed.). New York: Academic Press.

Satz, P., & Morris, R. (1981). Learning disability subtypes: A review. In F. J. Priozzolo & M. C. Wittrock (Eds.), *Neuropsychological and cognitive processes in reading* (pp. 104–141). New York: Academic Press.

Savage, R. C. (1991). Identification, classification, and placement issues for students with traumatic brain injuries. *Journal of Head Trauma Rehabilitation, 6,* 1–9.

Savage, R. C., & Wolcott, G. (1994). *Educational dimensions of acquired brain injury.* Austin, TX: Pro-Ed.

Saville-Troike, M. (1988). Private speech: Evidence for second language learning strategies during the "silent" period. *Journal of Child Language, 15,* 567–590.

Sax, M. (1972). A longitudinal study of articulation change. *Language, Speech, and Hearing Services in Schools, 3,* 41–48.

Saywitz, K., & Cherry-Wilkinson, L. (1982). Age-related differences in metalinguistic awareness. In S. Kuczaj (Ed.), *Language development: Vol 2. Language, thought and culture.* Hillsdale, NJ: Lawrence Erlbaum.

Scarborough, H. (1990). Index of Productive Syntax (IPSyn). *Applied Psycholinguistics, 11,* 1–22.

Scarborough, H. (1998). Early identification of children at risk for reading disabilities. In B. Shapiro, P. Accardo, & A. Capute (Eds.), *Specific reading disabilities: A view of the spectrum* (pp. 75–119). Timonium, MD: York Press.

Scarborough, H., & Dobrich, W. (1990). Development of children with early language delay. *Journal of Speech and Hearing Research, 33,* 70–83.

Scarborough, H., Wyckoff, J., & Davidson, R. (1986). A reconsideration of the relation between age and mean utterance length. *Journal of Speech and Hearing Research, 29,* 394–399.

Schachar, R. J., Tannock, R., & Logan, G. (1993). Inhibitory control, impulsiveness, and attention deficit hyperactivity disorder. *Clinical Psychology Review, 13,* 721–739.

Scherer, N., & D'Antonio, L. (1997). Language and play development in toddlers with cleft lip and/or palate. *American Journal of Speech-Language Pathology, 6*(4), 48–54.

Scherer, N., D'Antonio, L., & Kalbfleisch, J. (1999). Early speech and language development in children with velocardiofacial syndrome. *American Journal of Medical Genetics, 88,* 714–723.

Schiff, M., Kaufman, A., & Kaufman, N. (1981). Scatter analysis of WISC-R profiles for learning disabled children with superior intelligence. *Journal of Learning Disabilities, 14,* 400–404.

Schiff, N. (1979). *The development of form and meaning in the language of hearing children of deaf parents.* New York: Columbia University.

Schlosser, R. W., & Blischak, D. (2001). Is there a role for speech output in intervention for person's with autism? A review. *Focus on Autism and Other Developmental Disabilities, 16,* 170–186.

Schmidt, J., Deshler, D., Schumaker, J., & Alley, G. (1989). Effects of generalization instruction on the written language performance of adolescents with learning disabilities in the mainstream classroom. *Journal of Reading, Writing, and Learning Disabilities, 4,* 291–311.

Schneider, P., & Watkins, R. (1996). Applying Vygotskian developmental theory to language intervention. *Language, Speech, and Hearing Services in Schools, 27,* 157–170.

Schober-Peterson, D., & Johnson, C. (1989). Conversational topics of 4-year-olds. *Journal of Speech and Hearing Research, 32,* 857–870.

Schopler, E., Reichler, R. J., & Renner, B. R. (1988). *Childhood Autism Rating Scale.* Los Angeles: Western Psychological Services.

Schumaker, J., & Sherman, J. A. (1970). Training generative verb usage by imitation and reinforcement procedures. *Journal of Applied Behavior Analysis, 3,* 273–287.

Schwartz, R., & Leonard, L. (1982). Do children pick and choose? An examination of phonological selection and avoidance in early lexical acquisition. *Journal of Child Language, 9,* 319–336.

Schwartz, R., Leonard, L., Folger, M., & Wilcox, M. (1980). Early phonological behavior in normal-speaking and language disordered children: Evidence for a synergistic view of linguistic disorders. *Journal of Speech and Hearing Disorders, 45,* 357–377.

Schwartzman, A., & Ledingham, J. (1992). Early disruptive behavior, poor school achievement, delinquent behavior, and delinquent personality: Longitudinal analyses. *Journal of Consulting and Clinical Psychology, 60,* 64–72.

Scientific Learning Corporation. (1997). *Fast ForWord training program for children. Procedure manual for professionals.* Berkeley, CA: Author.

Scott, C. M. (1984). Adverbial connectivity in conversations of children 6 to 12. *Journal of Child Language, 11,* 423–452.

Scott, C. M. (1988). Producing complex sentences. *Topics in Language Disorders, 8,* 44–62.

Scott, C. M. (1991). Problem writers: Nature, assessment, and intervention. In A. G. Kamhi & H. W. Catts (Eds.), *Reading disabilities: A developmental language perspective* (pp. 303–344). Boston: Allyn & Bacon.

Scott, C. M., & Rush, D. (1985). Teaching adverbial connectivity: Implications from current research. *Child Language Teaching and Therapy, 1,* 264–280.

Scott, C. M., & Stokes, S. (1995). Measures of syntax in school-age children and adolescents. *Language, Speech, and Hearing Services in Schools, 26,* 309–319.

Scott, C. M., & Windsor, J. (2000). General language performance measures in spoken and written narrative and expository discourse of school-age children with language learning disabilities. *Journal of Speech, Language, and Hearing Research, 43,* 324–339.

Secord, W., & Wiig, E. (1993). Interpreting figurative language expressions. *Folia Phoniatrica, 45*(1), 1–9.

Seidenberg, P. L., & Bernstein, D. K. (1986). The comprehension of similes and metaphors by learning-disabled and nonlearning-disabled children. *Language, Speech, and Hearing Services in Schools, 17,* 219–229.

Semel, E., Wiig, E., & Secord, W. (1996a). *CELF—3 Observational rating scales.* San Antonio, TX: Psychological Corporation.

Semel, E., Wiig, E., & Secord, W. (1996b). *Clinical Evaluation of Language Fundamentals screening test (CELF)—3.* San Antonio, TX: Psychological Corporation.

Semel, E., Wiig, E., & Secord, W. (2003). *Clinical Evaluation of Language Fundamentals (CELF)—4.* San Antonio, TX: Psychological Corporation.

Serry, T., & Blamey, P. (1999). A 4-year investigation into phonetic inventory development in young cochlear implant users. *Journal of Speech, Language, and Hearing Research, 42,* 141–154.

Sevcik, R. A., Romski, M. A., & Adamson, L. B. (1999). Measuring AAC interventions for individuals with severe developmental disabilities. *Augmentative and Alternative Communication, 15,* 38–45.

Seyfried, D. N., & Kricos, P. B. (1996). Language and speech of the deaf and hard of hearing. In R. L. Schow & M. A. Nerbonne (Eds.), *Introduction to audiological rehabilitation* (3rd ed., pp. 168–228). Boston: Allyn & Bacon.

Seymour, H., Bland-Stewart, L., & Green, L. (1998). Difference versus deficit in child African American English. *Language, Speech, and Hearing Services in Schools, 29*(2), 96–108.

Seymour, H., Roeper, T., & de Villiers, J. (2003). *Diagnostic Evaluation of Language Variance (DELV)—Criterion Referenced.* San Antonio, TX: Psychological Corporation.

Seymour, H., & Seymour, C. (1981). Black English and Standard American English contrasts in consonantal development of four- and five-year-old children. *Journal of Speech and Hearing Disorders, 46,* 274–280.

Shane, H. C., & Bashir, A. S. (1980). Election criteria for adoption of an augmentative communication system: Preliminary considerations. *Journal of Speech and Hearing Disorders, 45,* 408–444.

Shapiro, E. S., DuPaul, G. J., & Bradley-Klug, K. L. (1998). Self-management as a strategy to improve classroom behavior of adolescents with ADHD. *Journal of Learning Disabilities, 31,* 545–555.

Shapiro, E. S., & Lentz, F. E., Jr. (1991). Vocational-technical programs: Follow-up of students with learning disabilities. *Exceptional Children, 58,* 47–59.

Shatz, M., Bernstein, D., & Shulman, M. (1980). The responses of language-disordered children to indirect directives in varying contexts. *Applied Psycholinguistics, 1,* 295–306.

Shatz, M., & Gelman, R. (1973). The development of communication skills: Modifications in the speech of young children as a function of listener. *Monographs of the Society for Research in Child Development, 38,* 1–37.

Shatz, M., & Gelman, R., & O'Reilly, A. (1990). Conversational or communicative skill? A reassessment of two-year-olds' behavior in miscommunication episodes. *Journal of Child Language, 17,* 131–146.

Shavelle, R. M., Strauss, D. J., & Pickett, J. (2001). Causes of death in autism. *Journal of Autism and Developmental Disorders, 31,* 569–576.

Shaywitz, B. A., Fletcher, J. M., & Shaywitz, S. E. (1995). Defining and classifying learning disabilities and attention-deficit/hyperactivity disorder. *Journal of Child Neurology, 10*(1), S50–S57.

Shields, J. D., Green, R.-J., Cooper, B. A. B., & Ditton, P. (1995). The impact of adults' communication clarity versus communication deviance on adolescents with learning disabilities. *Journal of Learning Disabilities, 28*(6), 382–384.

Shipley, K., & McAfee, J. (1998). *Assessment in speech-language pathology: A resource manual* (2nd ed.). San Diego, CA: Singular.

Shore, B. M., & Delacourt, M. A. (1997). Effective curricular and program practices in gifted education and the interface with general education. *Journal for the Education of the Gifted, 20*(2), 138–154.

Short, A. B., & Schopler, E. (1988). Factors relating to age of onset in autism. *Journal of Autism and Developmental Disorders, 18,* 207–216.

Shoumaker, R. D., Bennett, D. R., Bray, P. F., & Curless, R. G. (1974). Clinical and EEG manifestations of an unusual aphasia syndrome in children. *Neurology, 24,* 10–16.

Shreibman, L., Kaneko, W., & Koegel, R. L. (1991). Positive affect of parents of autistic children: A comparison across two teaching techniques. *Behavior Therapy, 22,* 479–490.

Shriberg, L., Gruber, F., & Kwiatkowski, J. (1994). Developmental phonological disorders III: Long-term speech-sound normalization. *Journal of Speech and Hearing Research, 37,* 1151–1177.

Shriberg, L., & Kwiatkowski, J. (1988). A follow-up study of children with phonologic disorders of unknown origin. *Journal of Speech and Hearing Disorders, 53,* 144–155.

Shriberg, L., & Kwiatkowski, J. (1994). Developmental phonological disorders I: A clinical profile. *Journal of Speech and Hearing Research, 37,* 1100–1126.

Shriberg, L., & McSweeny, J. (2002). Classification and misclassification of childhood apraxia of speech. Paper presented at the Ninth Meeting of The International Clinical Phonetics and Linguistics Association, Hong Kong.

Shriberg, L., Paul, R., McSweeny, J. L., Klin, A., & Cohen, D. J. (2001). Speech and prosody characteristics of adolescents and adults with high-functioning autism and Asperger syndrome. *Journal of Speech, Language, and Hearing Research, 44,* 1097–1115.

Shulz, T., & Horibe, F. (1974). Development of the appreciation of verbal jokes. *Developmental Psychology, 10,* 13–20.

Shulz, T., & Pilon, R. (1973). Development of the ability to detect linguistic ambiguity. *Child Development, 44,* 728–733.

Siegel, B., Vukicevic, J., Elliott, G. R., & Kraemer, H. C. (1989). The use of signal detection theory to assess DSM-III-R criteria for autistic disorder. *Journal of the American Academy of Child and Adolescent Psychiatry, 28,* 542–548.

Siegel, E. B., & Cress, C. (2002). Overview of the emergence of early AAC behaviors: Progression from communicative to symbolic skills. In J. Reichle, D. Beukelman, & J. Light (Eds.), *Exemplary practices for beginning AAC users and their partners* (pp. 25–58). Baltimore, MD: Paul H. Brookes.

Siegel-Causey, E., & Guess, D. (1989). *Enhancing nonsymbolic communication interactions among learners with severe disabilities.* Baltimore, MD: Paul H. Brookes.

Sieratzki, J. S., Calvert, G. A., Brammer, M., David, A., & Woll, B. (2001). Accessibility of spoken, written, and sign language in Landau-Kleffner syndrome: A linguistic and functional MRI study. *Epileptic Disorders, 3*(2), 79–89.

Sigafoos, J., & Dempsey, R. (1992). Assessing choice making among children with multiple disabilities. *Journal of Applied Behavior Analysis, 25,* 747–755.

Sigafoos, J., Didden, R., & O'Reilly, M. (2003). Effects of speech output on maintenance of requesting and frequency of vocalizations in three children with developmental disabilities. *Augmentative and Alternative Communication, 19,* 37–47.

Sigafoos, J., & Iacono, T. (1993). Selecting augmentative communication devices for persons with severe disabil-

ities: Some factors for educational teams to consider. *Australia and New Zealand Journal of Developmental Disabilities, 16*(3), 133–146.

Sigafoos, J., Kerr, M., Roberts, D., & Couzens, D. (1994). Increasing opportunities for requesting in classrooms serving children with developmental disabilities. *Journal of Autism and Developmental Disabilities, 24,* 631–645.

Sigafoos, J., Roberts, D., Kerr, M., Couzens, D., & Baglioni, A. (1994). Opportunities for communication in classrooms serving children with developmental disabilities. *Journal of Autism and Developmental Disabilities, 24,* 259–279.

Sigafoos, J., & Tucker, M. (2000). Brief assessment and treatment of multiple challenging behaviors. *Behavioral Intervention, 15,* 53–70.

Silliman, E. R., Diehl, S. F., Bahr, R. H., Hnath-Chisolm, T., Zenlo, C. B., & Friedman, S. A. (2003). A new look at performance on theory-of-mind tasks by adolescents with autism spectrum disorder. *Language, Speech, and Hearing Services in Schools, 34,* 236–252.

Silverman, L. K., Chitwood, D. G., & Waters, J. L. (1986). Young gifted children: Can parents identify giftedness? *Topics in Early Childhood Special Education, 6*(1), 23–38.

Simkin, Z., & Conti-Ramsden, G. (2001). Non-word repetition and grammatical morphology: normative data for children in their final year of primary school. *International Journal of Language and Communication Disorders, 36,* 395–404.

Simon, C. (1987). *Classroom communication screening procedure for early adolescents.* Tempe, AZ: Communi-Cog.

Simon, C. (1998). When big kids don't learn: Contextual modifications and intervention strategies for age 8–18 at-risk students. *Clinical Linguistics and Phonetics, 12,* 249–280.

Simon, C., & Holway, C. (1991). Presentation of communication evaluation information. In C. Simon (Ed.), *Communication skills and classroom success: Assessment and therapy methodologies for language and learning disabled students* (pp. 151–197). Eau Claire, WI: Thinking Publications.

Simon, N. (1975). Echolalic speech in childhood autism. *Archives of General Psychiatry, 32,* 1439–1446.

Simpson, D. A., Cockington, R. A., Hanieh, A., Raftos, J., & Reilly, P. L. (1991). Head injuries in infants and young children: The value of the Paediatric Coma Scale. Review of literature and report on a study. *Child's Nervous System, 7,* 183–190.

Singer, B., & Bashir, A. (1999). What are executive functions and self-regulation and what do they have to do with language-learning disorders? *Language, Speech, and Hearing Services in Schools, 30,* 265–273.

Sinson, J., & Wetherick, N. (1982). Mutual gaze in preschool Down's and normal children. *Journal of Mental Deficiency Research, 26,* 123–129.

Skarakis, E., & Greenfield, P. (1982). The role of new and old information in the verbal expression of language-disordered children. *Journal of Speech and Hearing Research, 25,* 462–467.

Skarakis-Doyle, E., MacLellan, N., & Mullin, K. (1990). Nonverbal indicants of comprehension monitoring in language-disordered children. *Journal of Speech and Hearing Disorders, 55,* 461–467.

Skarakis-Doyle, E., & Woodall, S. (1988). The effects of modeling upon the verbal elaboration of a language disordered child's pretend play. *Human Communication, 12,* 29–35.

Skidmore, M. D., Rivers, A., & Hack, M. (1990). Increased risk of cerebral palsy among very low-birthweight infants with chronic lung disease. *Developmental Medicine and Child Neurology, 32,* 325–332.

Skinner, B. (1957). *Verbal behavior.* Englewood Cliffs, NJ: Prentice-Hall.

Slobin, D. (1973). Cognitive prerequisites for the development of grammar. In C. Ferguson & D. Slobin (Eds.), *Studies of child language development.* New York: Holt, Rinehart & Winston.

Smeets, P., & Streifel, S. (1976). Training the generative usage of article-noun responses in severely retarded males. *Journal of Mental Deficiency Research, 20,* 121–127.

Smit, A. (1993a). Phonologic error distributions in the Iowa-Nebraska articulation norms project: Consonant singletons. *Journal of Speech and Hearing Research, 36,* 533–547.

Smit, A. (1993b). Phonologic error distributions in the Iowa-Nebraska Articulation Norms Project: Word-initial consonant clusters. *Journal of Speech and Hearing Research, 36,* 931–947.

Smit, A., Hand, L., Freilinger, J., Bernthal, J., & Bird, A. (1990). The Iowa Articulation Norms Project and its Nebraska replication. *Journal of Speech and Hearing Disorders, 55,* 779–798.

Smith, A., McCauley, R., & Guitar, B. (2000). Development of the "Teacher Assessment of Student Communicative Competence (TASCC)" for grades 1 through 5. *Communication Disorders Quarterly, 22,* 3–11.

Smith, B. L., & Oller, D. K. (1981). A comparative study of premeaningful vocalizations produced by normally developing and Down's syndrome infants. *Journal of Speech and Hearing Disorders, 46,* 46–51.

Smith, B. L., & Stoel-Gammon, C. (1983). A longitudinal study of the development of stop consonant production in normal and Down's syndrome children. *Journal of Speech and Hearing Disorders, 48,* 114–118.

Smith, B. L., & Stoel-Gammon, C. (1996). A quantitative analysis of the reduplicated and variegated babbling in vocalizations by Down syndrome infants. *Clinical Linguistics and Phonetics, 10,* 119–130.

Smith, C. (1975). Residual hearing and the speech production of deaf children. *Journal of Speech and Hearing Research, 18,* 795–811.

Smith, L. (1989). Case studies of maternal speech to prelinguistic children in the format of object transfer. In S. von Tetzchner, L. S. Siegel, & L. Smith (Eds.), *The social and cognitive aspects of normal and atypical language development* (pp. 69–93). New York: Springer-Verlag.

Smith, L., & von Tetzchner, S. (1986). Communicative, sensorimotor, and language skills of young children with Down syndrome. *American Journal of Mental Deficiency, 91,* 57–66.

Smitherman, G. (2000). *Words and phrases from the Hood to the Amen Corner* (Revised ed.). Boston: Houghton Mifflin.

Smoski, W. J., Brunt, M. A., & Tannahill, J. C. (1992). Listening characteristics of children with central auditory processing disorders. *Language, Speech, and Hearing Services in Schools, 23,* 145–152.

Snow, C. (1972). Mothers' speech to children learning language. *Child Development, 43,* 549–565.

Snow, C. (1977). The development of conversation between mothers and babies. *Journal of Child Language, 4,* 1–22.

Snow, C., Burns, M., & Griffin, P. (Eds.). (1998). *Preventing reading difficulties in young children.* Washington, DC: National Academy Press.

Snow, P. (2000). Language disabilities: Comorbid developmental disorders and risk for drug abuse in adolescence. *Brain Impairment, 1,* 165–176.

Snowling, M., Adams, J., Bishop, D. V. M., & Stothard, S. (2001). Educational attainments of school leavers with a preschool history of speech-language impairments. *International Journal of Language and Communication Disorders, 36*(2), 173–183.

Snowling, M., Adams, J., Bowyer-Crane, C., & Tobin, V. (2000). Levels of literacy among juvenile offenders: The incidence of specific reading difficulties. *Criminal Behaviour and Mental Health, 10*(4), 229–241.

Snowling, M., Bishop, D. V. M., & Stothard, S. (2000). Is preschool language impairment a risk for dyslexia in adolescence? *Journal of Child Psychology and Psychiatry, 41,* 587–600.

Snyder, L. (1975). Pragmatics in language-deficient children: Their prelinguistic and early verbal performatives and presuppositions. Unpublished doctoral dissertation, University of Colorado, Boulder.

Snyder, L. (1978). Communicative and cognitive abilities and disabilities in the sensorimotor period. *Merrill-Palmer Quarterly, 24,* 161–180.

Snyder, L. (1984). Developmental language disorders: Elementary school age. In A. Holland (Ed.), *Language disorders in children.* San Diego, CA: College-Hill Press.

Snyder, L., & Downey, D. (1991). The language-reading relationship in normal and reading-disabled children. *Journal of Speech and Hearing Research, 34,* 129–140.

Solomon, M. (1972). Stem endings and the acquisition of inflections. *Language Learning, 22,* 43–50.

Solter, A. J. (2001). *The aware baby.* Goleta, CA: Shining Star Press.

Soprano, A. M., Garcia, E. F., Caraballo, R., & Fejerman, N. (1994). Acquired epileptic aphasia: Neuropsychologic follow-up of 12 patients. *Pediatric Neurology, 11*(3), 230–235.

Sparrow, S., Balla, D., & Ciccetti, D. (1984). *Vineland Adaptive Behavior Scales.* Circle Pines, MN: American Guidance Service.

Sparrow, S., Marans, W., Klin, A., Carter, A., Volkmar, F. R., & Cohen, D. J. (1997). Developmentally based assessments. In D. J. Cohen & F. R. Volkmar (Eds.), *Handbook of autism and pervasive developmental disorders* (2nd ed., pp. 411–447). New York: Wiley.

Spector, C. (1990). Linguistic humor comprehension of normal and language-impaired adolescents. *Journal of Speech and Hearing Disorders, 55,* 533–541.

Spector, C. (1996). Children's comprehension of idioms in the context of humor. *Language, Speech, and Hearing Services in Schools, 27,* 307–313.

Speltz, M. L., Endriga, M. C., Hill, S., Maris, C. L., Jones, K., & Omnell, M. L. (2000). Brief report: Cognitive and psychomotor development of infants with orofacial clefts. *Journal of Pediatric Psychology, 25*(3), 185–190.

Spragale, D., & Micucci, D. (1990). Signs of the week: A functional approach to manual sign training. *Augmentative and Alternative Communication, 6*(1), 29–37.

St. Charles, J., & Costantino, M. (2000). *Reading and the Native American learner. Research report.* Olympia, WA: Office of Superintendent of Public Instruction, Office of Indian Education.

Stahmer, A. C. (1999). Using pivotal response training to facilitate appropriate play in children with autistic spectrum disorders. *Child Language Teaching and Therapy, 15*(1), 29–40.

Stainton, T., & Besser, H. (1998). The positive impact of children with an intellectual disability on the family. *Journal of Intellectual and Developmental Disability, 23*(1), 57–70.

Stanford, L. D., & Hynd, G. W. (1994). Congruence of behavioral symptomology in children with ADD/H, ADD/WO, and learning disabilities. *Journal of Learning Disabilities, 27*(4), 243–254.

Stanovich, K. (1986). Matthew effects in reading: Some consequences of individual differences in the acquisition of literacy. *Reading Research Quarterly, 21,* 360–364.

Stanovich, K., & Siegel, L. (1994). Phenotypic performance profile of children with reading disabilities: A regression-based test of the phonological-core-variable-difference model. *Journal of Educational Psychology, 86,* 24–53.

Stansbury, K., & Zimmermann, L. (1999). Relations among child language skills, maternal socializations of emotion regulation, and child behavior problems. *Child Psychiatry and Human Development, 30,* 121–142.

Stark, R. (1980). Stages of speech development in the first year. In G. Yeni-Komshian, J. A. Kavanagh, & C. Ferguson (Eds.), *Child Phonology* (Vol. 1). New York: Academic Press.

Steffens, M. L., Oller, D. K., Lynch, M., & Urbano, R. C. (1992). Vocal development in infants with Down syndrome and infants who are developing normally. *American Journal of Mental Retardation, 97,* 235–246.

Stein, N., & Glenn, C. (1979). An analysis of story comprehension in elementary school children. In R. Freedle (Ed.), *New directions in discourse processing* (Vol. 2, pp. 53–120). Norwood, NJ: Ablex.

Stephens, M. (1976). Elicited imitation of selected features of two American English dialects in Head Start children. *Journal of Speech and Hearing Research, 19,* 493–508.

Stephens, M., & Montgomery, A. (1985). A critique of recent relevant standardized tests. *Topics in Language Disorders, 5,* 21–45.

Stockman, I. (1996a). Phonological development and disorders in African American children. In A. Kamhi, K. Pollock, & J. Harris (Eds.), *Communication development and disorders in African American children: Research, assessment and intervention* (pp. 117–153). Baltimore, MD: Paul H. Brookes.

Stockman, I. (1996b). The promises and pitfalls of language sample analysis as an assessment tool for linguistic minority children. *Language, Speech, and Hearing Services in Schools, 27,* 355–366.

Stoel-Gammon, C. (1980). Phonological analysis of four Down's syndrome children. *Applied Psycholinguistics, 1,* 31–48.

Stoel-Gammon, C. (1981). Speech development of infants and children with Down syndrome. In J. Darby, Jr. (Ed.), *Speech evaluation in medicine* (pp. 341–360). New York: Grune & Stratton.

Stoel-Gammon, C. (1987). The phonological skills of two-year-olds. *Language, Speech, and Hearing Services in Schools, 18,* 323–329.

Stoel-Gammon, C. (1988). Prelinguistic vocalizations of hearing-impaired and normally hearing subjects: A comparison of consonantal inventories. *Journal of Speech and Hearing Disorders, 53*(3), 302–315.

Stoel-Gammon, C. (1990). Down syndrome. *Asha, 32*(9), 42–44.

Stoel-Gammon, C. (1991). Normal and disordered phonology in two-year-olds. *Topics in Language Disorders, 11,* 21–32.

Stoel-Gammon, C. (2001). Down syndrome phonology: Developmental patterns and intervention strategies. *Down Syndrome: Research and Practice, 7*(3), 93–100.

Stoel-Gammon, C., & Dunn, C. (1985). *Normal and disordered phonology in children.* Austin, TX: Pro-Ed.

Stoel-Gammon, C., & Kehoe, M. (1994). Hearing impairment in infants and toddlers. In J. Bernthal & N. Bankson (Eds.), *Child phonology: Characteristics, assessment and intervention in special populations* (pp. 163–181). New York: Thieme.

Stone, W. L., & Caro-Martinez, L. M. (1990). Naturalistic observations of spontaneous communication in autistic children. *Journal of Autism and Developmental Disorders, 20,* 437–453.

Stoneman, Z., Brody, G., & Abbott, D. (1983). In-home observations of young Down syndrome children with their mothers and fathers. *American Journal of Mental Deficiency, 87,* 591–600.

Stores, R. (1993). Sleep problems in children with Down's syndrome: A summary report. *Down Syndrome: Research and Practice, 1,* 72–74.

Storkel, H. (2003). Learning new words II: Phonotactic probability in verb learning. *Journal of Speech, Language, and Hearing Research, 46,* 1312–1323.

Stothard, S., Snowling, M., Bishop, D. V. M., Chipchase, B., & Kaplan, C. (1998). Language-impaired preschoolers: A follow-up into adolescence. *Journal of Speech, Language, and Hearing Research, 41,* 407–418.

Strauss, A. A., & Kephart, N. C. (1955). *Psychopathology and education of the brain-injured child, Vol. II. Progress in theory and clinic.* New York: Grune & Stratton.

Strauss, A. A., & Lehtinen, L. E. (1947). *Psychopathology and education of the brain-injured child.* New York: Grune & Stratton.

Strong, C. (1998). *Strong Narrative Assessment Procedure.* Eau Claire, WI: Thinking Publications.

Sullivan, P. (1978). A comparison of administration modifications on the WISC-R perfomance scale with different categories of deaf children. Unpublished doctoral dissertation, University of Iowa, Iowa City.

Sutton-Smith, B. (1986). The development of fictional narrative performances. *Topics in Language Disorders, 7,* 1–10.

Svensson, I., Lundberg, I., & Jacobson, C. (2001). The prevalence of reading and spelling difficulties among inmates of institutions for compulsory care of juvenile delinquents. *Dyslexia, 7,* 62–76.

Swan, D., & Goswami, U. (1997). Picture-naming deficits in developmental dyslexia: The phonological representations hypothesis. *Brain and Language, 56,* 334–353.

Swanson, L., & Leonard, L. (1994). Duration of function-word vowels in mothers' speech to young children. *Journal of Speech and Hearing Research, 37,* 1394–1405.

Swenson, N. (2000). Comparing traditional and collaborative settings for language intervention. *Communication Disorders Quarterly, 22,* 12–18.

Swift, E., & Rosin, P. (1990). A remediation sequence to improve speech intelligibility for students with Down syndrome. *Language, Speech, and Hearing Services in Schools, 21,* 140–146.

Swisher, K. (1991). *American Indian/Alaskan Native learning styles: Research and practice.* Retrieved July 2002, from www.ed.gov/databases/ERIC_Digests/ed335175.html.

Swisher, L. (1985). Language disorders in children. In J. K. Darby (Ed.), *Speech and language evaluation in neurology: Childhood disorders.* Orlando, FL: Grune & Stratton.

Swisher, L., Restrepo, M., Plante, E., & Lowell, S. (1995). Effect of implicit and explicit "rule" presentation on bound-morpheme generalization in specific language impairment. *Journal of Speech and Hearing Research, 38,* 168–173.

Swisher, L., & Snow, D. (1994). Learning and generalization components of morphological acquisition by children with specific language impairment: Is there a functional relation? *Journal of Speech and Hearing Research, 37,* 1406–1413.

Tager-Flusberg, H. (1981). On the nature of linguistic functioning in early infantile autism. *Journal of Autism and Developmental Disorders, 11,* 45–56.

Tager-Flusberg, H. (1992). Autistic children's talk about psychological states: Deficits in the early acquisition of a theory of mind. *Child Development, 63,* 161–172.

Tager-Flusberg, H. (2001). Putting words together: Morphology and syntax in the preschool years. In J. Berko-Gleason (Ed.), *The development of language* (5th ed., pp. 162–212). Boston: Allyn & Bacon.

Tager-Flusberg, H., & Calkins, S. (1990). Does imitation facilitate the acquisition of grammar? Evidence from a study of autistic, Down's syndrome and normal children. *Journal of Child Language, 17,* 591–606.

Tallal, P. (1975). Perceptual and linguistic factors in the language impairment of developmental dysphasics: An experimental investigation with the Token Test. *Cortex, 11*(3), 196–205.

Tallal, P. (1976). Rapid auditory processing in normal and disordered language development. *Journal of Speech and Hearing Research, 19,* 561–571.

Tallal, P. (1980). Language and reading: Some perceptual prerequisites. *Bulletin of the Orton Society, 30,* 170–178.

Tallal, P., Miller, S., Bedi, G., Byma, G., Wang, X., Nagarajan, S., Schreiner, C., Jenkins, W., & Merzenich, M. (1996). Language comprehension in language-learning impaired children improved with acoustically modified speech. *Science, 271*(5245), 81–84.

Tallal, P., & Piercy, M. (1973a). Defects of nonverbal auditory perception in children with developmental dysphasia. *Nature, 241,* 468–499.

Tallal, P., & Piercy, M. (1973b). Developmental aphasia: Impaired rate of non-verbal processing as a function of sensory modality. *Neuropsychologia, 11*(4), 389–398.

Tallal, P., & Piercy, M. (1974). Developmental aphasia: Rate of auditory processing and selective impairment of consonant perception. *Neuropsychologia, 12*(1), 83–93.

Tallal, P., & Piercy, M. (1975). Developmental aphasia: The perception of brief vowels and extended stop consonants. *Neuropsychologia, 13*(1), 69–74.

Tallal, P., Ross, R., & Curtiss, S. (1989). Familial aggregation in specific language impairment. *Journal of Speech and Hearing Disorders, 54,* 167–173.

Tallal, P., Stark, R. E., & Curtis, B. (1976). The relation between speech perception impairment and speech production impairment in children with developmental dysphasia. *Brain and Language, 3,* 305–317.

Tallal, P., Townsend, J., Curtiss, S., & Wulfeck, B. (1991). Phenotypic profiles of language-impaired children based on genetic/family history. *Brain and Language, 41,* 81–95.

Tannock, R. (1988). Mothers' directiveness in their interactions with their children with and without Down syndrome. *American Journal of Mental Retardation, 93,* 154–165.

Tate, R., & Douglas, J. (2002). Editorial: Evidence-based clinical practice in rehabilitation. *Brain Impairment, 3,* ii–iv.

Taylor, B. A., & Harris, S. L. (1995). Teaching children with autism to seek information: Acquisition of novel information and generalization of responding. *Journal of Applied Behavior Analysis, 28,* 3–14.

Taylor, H. G., Yeates, K. O., Wade, S. L., Drotar, D., Stancin, T., & Minich, N. (2002). A prospective study of short- and long-term outcomes after traumatic brain injury in children: Behavior and achievement. *Neuropsychology, 16*(1), 15–27.

Taylor, M., Bennie, S., & Buckley, S. (1996). Classroom behaviour, language competence, and the acceptance of children with Down syndrome by their mainstream peers. *Down Syndrome: Research and Practice, 4,* 100–109.

Taylor, O. (1987). Clinical practice as a social occasion. In V. R. Deal (Ed.), *Communication disorders in multicultural populations.* Rockville, MD: American Speech-Language-Hearing Association.

Taylor, O. (1990). *Cross-cultural communication: An essential dimension of effective education.* Retrieved December 2, 2002, from www.nwrel.org/cnorse/booklets/ccc

Taylor, R. L., & Kaufmann, S. (1991). Trends in classification usage in the mental retardation literature. *Mental Retardation, 29,* 367–371.

Teasdale, G., & Jennett, B. (1974). Assessment of coma and impaired consciousness: A practical scale. *Lancet, 2,* 81–84.

Tempest, P. (1998). Local Navajo norms for the Wechsler Intelligence Scale for Children—Third Edition. *Journal of American Indian Education, 37*(3), 18–30.

Templin, M. (1957). *Certain language skills in children: Their development and interrelationships.* Minneapolis: University of Minnesota Press.

Terman, L., & Merrill, M. (1973). *Stanford-Binet Intelligence Scale.* Boston: Houghton Mifflin.

Teuber, J. F., & Furlong, M. F. (1985). The concurrent validity of the Expressive One-Word Picture Vocabulary Test for Mexican-American children. *Psychology in the Schools, 22,* 269–273.

Tew, B. (1991). The effects of spina bifida upon learning and behaviour. In C. M. Bannister & B. Tew (Eds.), *Current concepts in spina bifida and hydrocephalus.* Cambridge, UK: Mac Keith Press.

Thal, D., Jackson-Maldonado, D., & Acosta, D. (2000). Validity of a parent report measure of vocabulary and grammar for Spanish-speaking toddlers. *Journal of Speech-Language-Hearing Research, 5,* 1087–1100.

Thal, D., & Katich, J. (1996). Predicaments in early identification of specific language impairment: Does the early bird always catch the worm? In K. Cole, P. Dale, & D. Thal (Eds.), *Assessment of communication and language* (pp. 1–28). Baltimore, MD: Paul H. Brookes.

Thal, D., Oroz, M., Evans, D., Katich, J., & Leasure, K. (1995, June). From first words to grammar in late-talking toddlers. Paper presented at the Symposium on Research in Child Language Disorders, Madison, WI.

Thal, D., & Tobias, S. (1988). Language and gesture in late talkers. *Journal of Speech and Hearing Research, 34,* 115–123.

Thal, D., & Tobias, S. (1992). Communicative gestures in children with delayed onset of oral expressive vocabulary. *Journal of Speech and Hearing Research, 35,* 1281–1289.

Thal, D., & Tobias, S. (1994). Relationships between language and gesture in normally developing and late-talking toddlers. *Journal of Speech and Hearing Research, 37,* 157–170.

Thal, D., Tobias, S., & Morrison, D. (1991). Language and gesture in late talkers: A 1-year follow-up. *Journal of Speech and Hearing Research, 34,* 604–612.

Tharp, R., & Yamauchi, L. (1994). *Effective instructional conversation in Native American classrooms (Educational Practice Report No. 10).* Santa Cruz, CA, and Washington, DC: National Center for Research on Cultural Diversity and Second Language Learning.

Thompson, L., & Dodd, B. J. (2001). The nature of speech disorder in children with Down syndrome. *International Journal of Intellectual Disability, 45,* 8–16.

Thordardottir, E. T., & Ellis Weismer, S. (2002). Content mazes and filled pauses in narrative language samples of children with specific language impairment. *Brain and Cognition, 48*(2–3), 587–592.

Thorndike, R. L., Hagen, E. P., & Sattler, J. M. (1996). *The Stanford Binet Intelligence Scale* (4th ed.). Itasca, IL: Riverside.

Thorum, A. (1986). *Fullerton Language Test for Adolescents* (2nd ed.). Austin, TX: Pro-Ed.

Thurston, K. (1998). Mitigating barriers to Navajo students' success in English courses. *Teaching English in the Two-Year College, 26*(1), 29–38.

Tobey, E., Geers, A., & Brenner, C. (1994). Speech production results: Speech feature acquisition. *Volta Review, 96,* 109–129.

Tobin, K. (1986). Effects of teacher wait time on discourse characteristics in mathematics and language arts classes. *American Educational Research Journal, 23,* 191–200.

Tobin, K. (1987). The role of wait time in higher cognitive level learning. *Review of Educational Research, 57,* 69–95.

Tomblin, J. B. (1983). An examination of the concept of disorder in the study of language variation. *Proceedings of the Fourth Wisconsin Symposium on Research in Child Language Disorders.* Madison: University of Wisconsin Press.

Tomblin, J. B., Abbas, P., Records, N., & Brenneman, L. (1995). Auditory evoked responses to frequency-modulated tones in children with specific language impairment. *Journal of Speech and Hearing Research, 38,* 387–393.

Tomblin, J. B., & Buckwalter, P. (1998). Heritability of poor language achievement among twins. *Journal of Speech, Language, and Hearing Research, 41,* 188–199.

Tomblin, J. B., Freese, P., & Records, N. (1992). Diagnosing specific language impairment in adults for the purpose of pedigree analysis. *Journal of Speech and Hearing Research, 35,* 832–843.

Tomblin, J. B., Hardy, J., & Hein, H. (1991). Predicting poor-communication status in preschool children using risk factors present at birth. *Journal of Speech and Hearing Research, 34,* 1096–1105.

Tomblin, J. B., Records, N., Buckwalter, P., Zhang, X., Smith, E., & O'Brien, M. (1997). Prevalence of specific language impairment in kindergarten children. *Journal of Speech, Language, and Hearing Research, 40,* 1245–1260.

Tomblin, J. B., Records, N., & Zhang, X. (1996). A system for the diagnosis of specific language impairment in kindergarten children. *Journal of Speech and Hearing Research, 39,* 1284–1294.

Tomblin, J. B., Smith, E., & Zhang, X. (1997). Epidemiology of specific language impairment: Prenatal and perinatal risk factors. *Journal of Communication Disorders, 30,* 325–344.

Tomblin, J. B., Spencer, L., Flock, S., Tyler, R., & Gantz, B. (1999). A comparison of language achievement in children with cochlear implants and children using hearing aids. *Journal of Speech, Language, and Hearing Research, 42*(2), 497–511.

Tomblin, J. B., Zhang, X., Buckwalter, P., & O'Brien, M. (2003). The stability of primary language disorder: Four years after kindergarten diagnosis. *Journal of Speech, Language, and Hearing Research, 46,* 1283–1296.

Tonge, B. J. (2002). Autism, autistic spectrum and the need for better definition. *Medical Journal of Australia, 176*(9), 412–413.

Tooher, R. (2002). Making their way in the world: An investigation into the outcomes of cochlear implantation for adolescents using a biopsychosocial approach. Unpublished doctoral dissertation, University of Sydney, Sydney, Australia.

Tooher, R., Hogan, A., & Reed, V. A. (2002a, March). Quality of life and psychosocial outcomes of paediatric cochlear implantation in adolescents. Paper presented at the XXVI International Congress of Audiology, Melbourne, Australia.

Tooher, R., Hogan, A., & Reed, V. A. (2002b, September). "The Hearing's not enough, its just enough to get by . . . " What is life like for young people who use cochlear implants to hear? Paper presented at the 7th International Cochlear Implant Conference, Manchester, UK.

Toppelberg, C., Medrano, L., Pena Morgens, L., & Nieto-Castanon, A. (2002). Bilingual children referred for psychiatric services: Associations of language disorders, language skills, and psychopathology. *Journal of the American Academy of Child and Adolescent Psychiatry, 41*(6), 712–722.

Toppelberg, C., Snow, C., & Tager-Flusberg, H. (1999). Severe developmental disorders and bilingualism. *Journal of the American Academy of Child and Adolescent Psychiatry, 38,* 1197–1199.

Toronto, A. (1976). Developmental assessment of Spanish grammar. *Journal of Speech and Hearing Disorders, 41,* 150–171.

Tough, J. (1977). *The development of meaning.* New York: Halsted Press.

Townsend, J., Courchesne, E., & Egaas, B. (1996). Slowed orienting of covert visual-spatial attention in autism: Specific deficits associated with cerebellar and parietal abnormality. *Development and Psychopathology, 8,* 563–584.

Trauner, D., Wulfeck, B., Tallal, P., & Hesselink, J. (1995). *Neurologic and MRI profiles of language impaired children: Technical Report CND-9513.* San Diego: Center for Research in Language, University of California.

Treiman, R. (1997). Spelling in normal children and dyslexics. In B. Blachman (Ed.), *Foundations of reading acquisition and dyslexia* (pp. 191–218). Mahwah, NJ: Lawrence Erlbaum.

Treiman, R., Tincoff, R., Rodriguez, K., Mouzaki, A., & Francis, D. J. (1998). The foundations of literacy: Learning the sounds of letters. *Child Development, 69,* 1524–1540.

Treuting, J. J., & Hinshaw, S. P. (2001). Depression and self-esteem in boys with attention-deficit/hyperactivity disorder: Associations with comorbid aggression and explanatory attributional mechanisms. *Journal of Abnormal Child Psychology, 29,* 23–39.

Troster, H., Hecker, W., & Brambring, M. (1993). Early motor development in blind infants. *Journal of Applied Developmental Psychology, 14,* 83–106.

Tucker, B. F., & Colson, S. E. (1992). Traumatic brain injury: An overview of school re-entry. *Intervention in School and Clinic, 27*(4), 198–206.

Tucker, M., Sigafoos, J., & Bushell, H. (1998a). Analysis of conditions associated with low rates of challenging behavior in two adolescents with multiple disabilities. *Behavior Change, 15,* 126–139.

Tucker, M., Sigafoos, J., & Bushell, H. (1998b). Use of noncontingent reinforcement in the treatment of challenging behavior. *Behavior Modification, 22,* 529–547.

Turkstra, L. (1999). Language testing in adolescents with brain injury: A consideration of the CELF-3. *Language, Speech, and Hearing Services in Schools, 30,* 132–140.

Turkstra, L., & Holland, A. L. (1998). Assessment of syntax after adolescent brain injury: Effects of memory on test performance. *Journal of Speech, Language, and Hearing Research, 41*(1), 137–149.

Turkstra, L., McDonald, S., & Kaufmann, P. (1996). Assessment of pragmatic communication skills in adolescents after traumatic brain injury. *Brain Injury, 10*(5), 329–345.

Turner, R. C., Robinette, M. S., & Bauch, C. D. (1999). Clinical decisions. In F. Musiek & W. F. Rintelmann (Eds.), *Contemporary perspective in hearing assessment* (pp. 437–463). Boston: Allyn & Bacon.

Turnure, J. E. (1991). Long-term memory and mental retardation. *International Review of Research in Mental Retardation, 17,* 193–217.

Tyack, D., & Venable, G. (1999). *Language sampling, analysis and training: A handbook* (3rd ed.). Austin, TX: Pro-Ed.

Tye-Murray, N. (1998). *Foundations of aural rehabilitation: Children, adults, and their family members.* San Diego, CA: Singular.

Tye-Murray, N., & Kirk, K. I. (1993). Vowel and diphthong production by young users of cochlear implants and the relationship between the phonetic level evaluation and spontaneous speech. *Journal of Speech and Hearing Research, 36*(3), 488–502.

Uberti, H., Scruugs, T., & Mastropieri, M. (2003). Keywords make the difference! Mnemonic instruction in inclusive classrooms. *Teaching Exceptional Children, 35*(3), 46–61.

Ukrainetz, T., Harpell, S., Walsh, C., & Coyle, C. (2000). A preliminary investigation of dynamic assessment with Native American kindergartners. *Language, Speech, and Hearing Services in Schools, 31,* 142–154.

Ullman, M., & Gopnik, M. (1994). Past tense production: Regular, irregular and nonsense verbs. *McGill Working Papers in Linguistics, 10,* 81–118.

United Cerebral Palsy. (2002). *Cerebral palsy—Facts & figures.* Retrieved December 2, 2002, from www.ucpa.org/ucp_generaldoc.cfm/1/9/37/37–37/447

U.S. Bureau of the Census. (2000). *Statistical abstract of the United States* (115th ed.). Washington, DC: U.S. Department of Commerce.

U.S. Bureau of the Census. (2001). *The Hispanic population.* Washington,DC: U.S. Department of Commerce.

U.S.Department of Education. (1999). *Twenty-first annual report to congress on the implementation of The Individuals with Disabilities Education Act.* Washington, DC: Author.

U.S. Department of Education. (2000). *Twenty-second annual report to congress on the implementation of The Individuals with Disabilities Education Act.* Washington, DC: Author.

U.S. Department of Education. (2001a). *Digest of education statistics:* Washington, DC: Author.

U.S. Department of Education. (2001b). *Twenty-third annual report to Congress on the implementation of The Individuals with Disabilities Education Act (IDEA).* Washington, DC: Author.

Urwin, C. (1984). Language for absent things: Learning from visually handicapped children. *Topics in Language Disorders, 4,* 24–37.

van de Sandt-Koenderman, W. M. E., Smit, I. A. C., van Dongen, H. R., & van Hest, J. B. C. (1984). A case of acquired aphasia and convulsive disorder: Some linguistic aspects of recovery and breakdown. *Brain and Language, 21,* 174–183.

van Dongen, H. R., Paquier, P. F., Creten, W. L., van Borsel, J., & Catsman-Berrevoets, C. E. (2001). Clinical evaluation of conversational speech fluency in the acute phase of acquired childhood aphasia: Does a fluency/nonfluency dichotomy exist? *Journal of Child Neurology, 16*(5), 345–351.

van Kleeck, A. (1994a). Metalinguistic development. In G. P. Wallach & K. G. Butler (Eds.), *Language learning disabilities in school-age children and adolescents: Some principles and applications* (2nd ed., pp. 53–98). Boston: Allyn & Bacon.

van Kleeck, A. (1994b). Potential cultural bias in training parents as conversational partners with their children who have delays in language development. *American Journal of Speech-Language Pathology, 3,* 67.

van Kleeck, A. (1998). Preliteracy domains and stages: Laying the foundations for beginning reading. *Journal of Children's Communication Development, 20,* 33–51.

van Kleeck, A., Gillam, R., & Davis, B. (1997). When is "watch and see" warranted? A response to Paul's 1996 article, "Clinical implications of the natural history of slow expressive language development." *American Journal of Speech-Language Pathology, 6*(2), 34–39.

van Kleeck, A., Gillam, R., Hamilton, L., & McGrath, C. (1997). The relationship between middle-class parents' book-sharing discussion and their preschoolers' abstract language development. *Journal of Speech, Language, and Hearing Research, 40,* 1261–1271.

van Kleeck, A., & Richardson, A. (1988). Language delay in the child. In N. J. Lass, L. V. McReynolds, J. L. Northern, & D. E. Yoder (Eds.), *Handbook of speech-language pathology and audiology.* Philadelphia: B. C. Decker.

VanMeter, L., Fein, D., Morris, R., Waterhouse, L., & Allen, D. (1997). Delay versus deviance in autistic social behavior. *Journal of Autism and Developmental Disorders, 27*(5), 557–569.

VanTassel-Baska, J. (1992). Educational decision making on acceleration and grouping. *Gifted Child Quarterly, 36,* 68–72.

VanTassel-Baska, J. (1998). *Excellence in educating gifted and talented learners.* Denver, CO: Love.

Vaughn, S., Elbaum, B., & Boardman, A. G. (2001). The social functioning of students with learning disabilities: Implications for inclusion. *Exceptionality, 9*(1–2), 47–65.

Vaughn-Cooke, F. (1983). Improving language assessment in minority children. *Asha, 25,* 29–34.

Ventry, I. (1983). Research design issues in studies of the effects of middle ear effusion. *Pediatrics, 71,* 644.

Vicker, B. (1996). *Using tangible symbols for communication purposes: An optional step in building the two-way communication process.* Bloomington: Indiana University, Indiana Resource Center for Autism.

Vicker, B., & Monahan, M. (1988). The diagnosis of autism by state agencies. *Journal of Autism and Developmental Disorders, 18,* 231–240.

Viding, E., Price, T., Spinath, F., Bishop, D. V. M., Dale, P., & Plomin, R. (2003). Genetic and environmental mediation of the relationship between language and nonverbal impairment in 4-year-old twins. *Journal of Speech, Language, and Hearing Research, 46,* 1271–1282.

Vihman, M. M. (1996). *Phonological development: The origins of language in the child.* Cambridge, MA: Blackwell.

Vogel, S. A. (1990). Gender differences in intelligence, language, visual-motor abilities, and academic achievement in students with learning disabilities: A review of the literature. *Journal of Learning Disabilities, 23,* 44–52.

Volden, J., & Lord, C. (1991). Neologisms and idiosyncratic language in autistic speakers. *Journal of Autism and Developmental Disorders, 21,* 109–130.

Volkmar, F. R., & Nelson, D. S. (1990). Seizure disorders in autism. *Journal of the American Academy of Child and Adolescent Psychiatry, 29,* 127–129.

Volterra, V., & Taeschner, R. (1978). The acquisition and development of language by bilingual children. *Journal of Child Language, 5,* 311–326.

von Tetzchner, S. (1999). Introduction to language development. In F. T. Loncke, J. Clibbens, H. H. Arvidson, & L. L. Lloyd (Eds.), *Augmentative and alternative communication: New directions in research and practice* (pp. 3–7). London, UK: Whurr.

von Tetzchner, S., & Martinsen, H. (2000). *Introduction to augmentative and alternative communication* (2nd ed.). London, UK: Whurr.

Vygotsky, L. (1962). *Thought and language.* Cambridge, MA: MIT Press.

Vygotsky, L. (1978). *Mind in society: The development of higher psychological processes.* Cambridge, MA: Harvard University Press.

Wacker, P., Berg, W. K., & Harding, J. W. (2002). Replacing socially unacceptable behavior with acceptable communication responses. In J. Reichle, D. Beukelman, & J. Light (Eds.), *Exemplary practices for beginning AAC users and their partners* (pp. 97–123). Baltimore, MD: Paul H. Brookes.

Wagner, R., Torgesen, J., & Rashotte, C. (1999). *Comprehensive Test of Phonological Processing.* Austin, TX: Pro-Ed.

Waldron, K. A., Saphire, D. G., & Rosenblum, S. A. (1987). Learning disabilities and giftedness: Identification based on self-concept, behavior, and academic patterns. *Journal of Learning Disabilities, 29,* 422–427.

Walker, M. (1976). *Language programmes for use with the Revised Makaton Vocabulary.* Surrey, UK: M. Walker.

Walker, M. (Ed.). (1985). *Symbols for Makaton.* Camberley, UK: Makaton Vocabulary Development Project.

Walker, M., & Cooney, A. (1984). *Line drawings to use with the Revised Makaton Vocabulary (Australian Version).* Newcastle, UK: Makaton Vocabulary Development Project.

Wallace, G., & Hammill, D. (2002). *Comprehensive Receptive and Expressive Vocabulary—2.* Austin, TX: Pro-Ed.

Waltzman, S., Cohen, N., Gomolin, R., Green, J., Shapiro, W., Brackett, D., et al. (1997). Perception and production results in children implanted between 2 and 5 years of age. *Advances in Oto-Rhino-Laryngology, 52,* 177–180.

Warden, D. (1976). The influence of context on children's use of identifying expressions and references. *British Journal of Psychology, 67,* 101–112.

Warren, S. F., & Bambara, L. M. (1989). An experimental analysis of milieu language intervention: Teaching the action-object form. *Journal of Speech and Hearing Disorders, 54,* 448–461.

Warren, S. F., & Kaiser, A. P. (1986). Incidental language teaching: A critical review. *Journal of Speech and Hearing Disorders, 51,* 291–299.

Watamori, T. S., Sasanuma, S., & Ueda, S. (1990). Recovery and plasticity in child-onset aphasics: Ultimate outcome at adulthood. *Aphasiology, 4,* 9–30.

Watkins, R., Kelly, D., Harbers, H., & Hollis, W. (1995). Measuring children's lexical diversity: Differentiating typical and impaired learners. *Journal of Speech and Hearing Research, 38,* 1349–1355.

Watkins, R., & Rice, M. (1991). Verb particle and preposition acquisition in language-impaired preschoolers. *Journal of Speech and Hearing Research, 34,* 1130–1141.

Watkins, R., Rice, M., & Moltz, C. (1993). Verb use by language-impaired and normally developing children. *First Language, 13,* 133–143.

Watkinson, J. T., & Lee, S. W. (1992). Curriculum-based measures of written expression for learning-disabled and nondisabled students. *Psychology in the Schools, 29,* 184–191.

Watson, L. R. (2001). Issues in early comprehension development of children with autism. In E. Schopler & N. Yirmiya (Eds.), *The research basis for autism intervention* (pp. 135–150). New York: Kluwer Academic/Plenum.

Webb, J. T. (1993). Nurturing social-emotional development of gifted children. In K. A. Heller, F. J. Monks, & A. H. Passow (Eds.), *International handbook for research on giftedness and talent* (pp. 525–538). Oxford, UK: Pergamon Press.

Wechsler, D. (1991). *Wechsler Intelligence Scale for Children—III.* San Antonio, TX: Psychological Corporation.

Wechsler, D. (2002). *Wechsler Preschool and Primary Scale of Intelligence—III.* San Antonio, TX: Psychological Corporation.

Wegner, J., & Rice, M. (1988, November). The acquisition of verb-particle constructions: How do children figure them out? Paper presented at the Annual Convention of the American Speech-Language-Hearing Association, Boston.

Wehrebian, A. (1970). Measures of vocabulary and grammatical skills for children up to age six. *Developmental Psychology, 2,* 439–446.

Weiner, P. (1974). A language-delayed child at adolescence. *Journal of Speech and Hearing Disorders, 39,* 202–212.

Weisenberger, J. (1976). A choice of words: Two-year-old speech from a situational point of view. *Journal of Child Language, 3,* 272–281.

Weiss, A., & Nakamura, M. (1992). Children with normal language skills in preschool classrooms for children with language impairments: Differences in modeling styles. *Language, Speech, and Hearing Services in Schools, 23,* 64–70.

Wells, G. (1985). *Language development in the pre-school years.* New York: Cambridge University Press.

Wepman, J. (1958). *Wepman Auditory Discrimination Test.* Chicago: Language Research Association.

West, D., & Bloomberg, K. (1997). *Picture it project: Assessment tools.* Melbourne, Australia: SCIOP.

Westby, C. (1991). Assessing and remediating comprehension problems. In A. Kamhi & H. Catts (Eds.), *Reading disabilities: A developmental language perspective* (pp. 199–260). Boston: Allyn & Bacon.

Westby, C. (1998). Communicative refinement in school age and adolescence. In W. Hayes & B. Shulman (Eds.), *Communication development: Foundations, processes, and clinical applications* (pp. 311–360). Baltimore, MD: Williams & Wilkins.

Westby, C., & Atencio, D. (2002). Computers, culture, and learning. *Topics in Language Disorders, 22*(4), 70–87.

Westby, C., & Roman, R. (1995). Finding the balance: Learning to live in two worlds. *Topics in Language Disorders, 15*(4), 68–88.

Westby, C., Stevens Dominguez, M., & Oetter, P. (1996). A performance/competence model of observational assessment. *Language, Speech, and Hearing Services in Schools, 27,* 144–156.

Wetherby, A. M. (1989). Language intervention for autistic children: A look at where we have come in the past 25 years. *Journal of Speech, Language Pathology, and Audiology, 13,* 15–28.

Wetherby, A. M., & Prizant, B. (1992). Profiling young children's communicative competence. In J. Reichle (Ed.), *Causes and effects in communication and language intervention* (pp. 217–253). Baltimore, MD: Paul H. Brookes.

Wetherby, A. M., & Prizant, B. (1993). *Communication and symbolic behavior scales.* Chicago: Riverside.

Wetherby, A. M., & Rodriguez, G. (1992). Measurement of communicative intentions in normally developing children during structured and unstructured contexts. *Journal of Speech and Hearing Research, 35,* 130–138.

Wetherby, A. M., Warren, S. F., & Reichle, J. (Eds.). (1998). *Transitions in prelinguistic communication.* Baltimore, MD: Paul H. Brookes.

Wexler, K., Schütze, C., & Rice, M. (1998). Subject case in children with SLI and unaffected controls: Evidence for the Agr/Tns omission model. *Language Acquisition, 7,* 317–344.

Wheldall, K. (1976). Receptive language development in the mentally handicapped. In P. Berry (Ed.), *Language and communication in the mentally handicapped.* Baltimore, MD: University Park Press.

White, H., & Sreenivasan, V. (1987). Epilepsy-aphasia syndrome in children: An unusual presentation to psychiatry. *Canadian Journal of Psychiatry, 32,* 599–601.

White, S., & White, R. (1987). The effects of hearing status of the family and age of intervention on reception and expressive oral language skills in hearing impaired infants. In H. Levitt, N. S. McGarr, & D. Geffner (Eds.), *Development of language and communication skills in hearing impaired children.* Washington, DC: Asha.

Whitehurst, G., & Fischel, J. (1994). Early developmental language delay: What, if anything should the clinician do about it? *Journal of Child Psychology and Psychiatry, 35,* 613–648.

Whitehurst, G., Fischel, J., Arnold, D., & Lonigan, C. (1992). Evaluating outcomes with children with expressive language delay. In W. Warren & J. Reichle (Eds.), *Causes and effects in communication and language intervention* (pp. 277–314). Baltimore, MD: Paul H. Brookes.

Whitehurst, G., Fischel, J., Lonigan, C., Valdez-Menchaca, M., Arnold, D., & Smith, M. (1991). Treatment of early expressive language delay: If, when, and how. *Topics in Language Disorders, 11,* 55–68.

Whitehurst, G., & Lonigan, C. (1998). Child development and emergent literacy. *Child Development, 69,* 848–872.

Whitehurst, G., Smith, M., Fischel, J., Arnold, D., & Lonigan, C. (1991). The continuity of babble and speech in children with specific expressive language delay. *Journal of Speech and Hearing Research, 34,* 1121–1129.

Whitmire, K. (2000). Adolescence as a developmental phase: A tutorial. *Topics in Language Disorders, 20*(2), 1–14.

Wiegner, S., & Donders, J. (2000). Predictors of parental distress after congenital disabilities. *Journal of Developmental and Behavioral Pediatrics, 21,* 271–277.

Wiener, F., Lewnau, L., & Erway, E. (1983). Measuring language competency in speakers of Black American English. *Journal of Speech and Hearing Disorders, 48,* 76–84.

Wiener, J., Harris, P. J., & Shirer, C. (1990). Achievement and social-behavioral correlates of peer status in LD children. *Learning Disabilities Quarterly, 13,* 114–127.

Wiig, E. (1982a). Identifying language disorders in adolescents. Paper presented at the Gunderson Clinic, La Crosse, WI.

Wiig, E. (1982b). *Let's talk inventory for adolescents.* San Antonio, TX: Psychological Corporation.

Wiig, E. (1986). Language disabilities in school-age children and youth. In G. Shames & E. Wiig (Eds.), *Human communication disorders: An introduction* (2nd ed., pp. 331–379). Columbus, OH: Merrill/Macmillan.

Wiig, E. (1989). *Steps to language competence: Developing metalinguistic strategies.* San Antonio, TX: Psychological Corporation.

Wiig, E. (1990a). Linguistic transitions and learning disabilities: A strategic learning perspective. *Learning Disability Quarterly, 13,* 128–140.

Wiig, E. (1990b). *Wiig Criterion-Referenced Inventory of Language.* San Antonio, TX: Psychological Corporation.

Wiig, E. (1995). Assessment of adolescent language. *Seminars in Speech and Language, 16*(1), 14–30.

Wiig, E., Gilbert, M., & Christian, S. (1978). Developmental sequences in the perception and interpretation of lexical and syntactic ambiguities. *Perceptual and Motor Skills, 44,* 959–969.

Wiig, E., & Secord, W. (1989). *Test of Language Competence—Expanded Edition.* San Antonio, TX: Psychological Corporation.

Wiig, E., & Secord, W. (1992). *Test of Word Knowledge.* San Antonio, TX: Psychological Corporation.

Wiig, E., & Semel, E. (1974). Logio-grammatical sentence comprehension by learning disabled adolescents. *Perceptual and Motor Skills, 38,* 1331–1334.

Wiig, E., & Semel, E. (1984). *Language assessment and intervention for the learning disabled* (2nd ed.). New York: Merrill/Macmillan.

Wiig, E., Semel, E., & Crouse, M. (1973). The use of morphology by high-risk and learning disabled children. *Journal of Learning Disabilities, 6,* 457–465.

Wiig, E., Zureich, P., & Chan, H.-N. H. (2000). A clinical rationale for assessing rapid automatized naming in children with language disorders. *Journal of Learning Disabilities, 33*(4), 359–374.

Wilcox, K., & Aasby, S. (1988). The performance of monolingual and bilingual Mexican children on the TACL. *Language, Speech, and Hearing Services in Schools, 19,* 34–40.

Wilcox, M. J. (1984). Developmental language disorders: Preschoolers. In A. Holland (Ed.), *Language disorders in children.* San Diego, CA: College-Hill Press.

Wilcox, M. J. (1989). Delivering communication-based services to infants, toddlers, and their families: Approaches and models. *Topics in Language Disorders, 10*(1), 68–79.

Willadsen, E., & Enemark, H. (2000). A comparative study of prespeech vocalizations in two groups of toddlers with cleft palate and a noncleft group. *Cleft Palate-Craniofacial Journal, 37*(2), 172–178.

Willcutt, E. G., & Pennington, B. F. (2000). Comorbidity of reading disability and attention-deficit/hyperactivity disorder: Differences by gender and subtype. *Journal of Learning Disabilities, 33,* 179–191.

Willeford, J. (1977). Assessing central auditory behaviour in children: A test battery approach. In R. W. Keith (Ed.), *Central auditory dysfunction.* New York: Grune & Stratton.

Williams, C., & Tillman, M. (1968). Word associations for selected form classes of children varying in age and intelligence. Paper presented at the Annual Meeting of the American Educational Research Association, Chicago.

Williams, D. (1996). *Autism: An inside out approach.* London, UK: Jessica Kingsley.

Williams, G., Donley, C. R., & Keller, J. W. (2000). Teaching children with autism to ask questions about hidden objects. *Journal of Applied Behavior Analysis, 33*(4), 627–630.

Williams, M. B. (2000). Just an independent guy who leads a busy life. In M. Fried-Oken & H. Bersani (Eds.), *Speaking up and spelling it out* (pp. 231–235). Baltimore, MD: Paul H. Brookes.

Williams, P. D., Williams, A. R., Graff, J. C., Hanson, S., Stanton, A., Hafeman, C., et al. (2002). Interrelationships among variables affecting well siblings and mothers in families of children with a chronic illness or disability. *Journal of Behavioral Medicine, 25*(5), 411–424.

Williams, S., & McGee, R. (1994). Reading attainment and juvenile delinquency. *Journal of Child Psychology and Psychiatry and Allied Disciplines, 35,* 441–459.

Windfuhr, K., Faragher, B., & Conti-Ramsden, G. (2002). Lexical learning skills in young children with specific language impairment. *International Journal of Language and Communication Disorders, 37,* 415–432.

Windsor, J., & Fristoe, M. (1989). Key word signing: Listeners' classification of signed and spoken narratives. *Journal of Speech and Hearing Disorders, 54,* 374–382.

Windsor, J., Milbrath, R., Carney, E., & Rakowski, S. (2001). General slowing in language impairment: Methodological considerations in testing the hypothesis. *Journal of Speech, Language, and Hearing Research, 44,* 446–461.

Winebrenner, S. (2003). Teaching strategies for twice-exceptional students. *Intervention in School and Clinic, 38,* 131–137.

Wing, L. (1981). Language, social, and cognitive impairments in autism and severe mental retardation. *Journal of Autism and Developmental Disorders, 11,* 31–44.

Wing, L. (1997). Syndromes of autism and atypical development. In D. J. Cohen & F. R. Volkmar (Eds.), *Handbook of autism and pervasive developmental disorders* (2nd ed., pp. 148–170). New York: Wiley.

Winne, P. H., Woodlands, M. J., & Wong, B. Y. L. (1982). Comparability of self-concept among learning disabled, normal, and gifted students. *Journal of Learning Disabilities, 15,* 470–475.

Winner, E., Rosenstiel, A., & Gardner, H. (1976). The development of metaphoric understanding. *Developmental Psychology, 12,* 289–297.

Wishart, J. (1993). Learning the hard way: Avoidance strategies in young children with Down's syndrome. *Down Syndrome: Research and Practice, 1,* 47–55.

Wolf, M., Bowers, P. G., & Biddle, K. (2000). Naming-speed processes, timing, and reading: A conceptual review. *Journal of Learning Disabilities, 33,* 387–407.

Wolfram, W., & Schilling-Estes, N. (1998). *American English: Dialects and variation.* Oxford, UK: Blackwell.

Wolk, L., & Giesen, J. (2000). A phonological investigation of four siblings with childhood autism. *Journal of Communication Disorders, 33,* 371–389.

Wood, L. A., Lasker, J., Siegel-Causey, E., Beukelman, D., & Ball, L. (1998). Input framework for augmentative and alternative communication. *Augmentative and Alternative Communication, 14*(4), 261–276.

Woodcock, R. (1991). *Woodcock Language Proficiency Battery—Revised.* Chicago: Riverside.

Woods, J. J., & Wetherby, A. M. (2003). Early identification of and intervention for infants and toddlers who are at risk for autism spectrum disorder. *Language, Speech, and Hearing Services in Schools, 34,* 180–193.

Work, R. (1991). Children of poverty: What is their future? *Asha, 33,* 61.

Work, R., Cline, J., Ehren, B., Keiser, D., & Wujek, C. (1993). Adolescent language programs. *Language, Speech, and Hearing Services in Schools, 24,* 43–53.

World Health Organization. (1993). *International code of diseases* (10th ed.). New York: World Health Organization.

Wright, H. H., & Newhoff, M. (2001). Narration abilities of children with language-learning disabilities in response to oral and written stimuli. *American Journal of Speech-Language Pathology, 10,* 308–319.

Wright, M., Purcell, A., & Reed, V. A. (2001a, March). Cochlear implants for babies: Expectations and outcomes. Paper presented at the 8th Symposium on Cochlear Implants in Children, Los Angeles.

Wright, M., Purcell, A., & Reed, V. A. (2001b, June). Communicative intents in infants pre- and post-cochlear implantation: Preliminary results. Paper presented at the 22nd Annual Symposium on Research in Child Language Disorders, Madison, WI.

Wright, M., Purcell, A., & Reed, V. A. (2002). Cochlear implants and infants: Expectations and outcomes. *Annals of Otology, Rhinology and Laryngology, 111*(5, Part 2, Suppl. 189), 131–137.

Yates, C. M., Berninger, V. W., & Abbott, R. D. (1995). Specific writing difficulties in intellectually gifted children. *Journal for the Education of the Gifted, 18*(2), 131–155.

Yirmiya, N., Erel, O., Shaked, M., & Solomonika, D. (1998). Is the deficit in theory of mind abilities unique to autism?: Meta analyses comparing theory of mind abilities of individuals with autism, individuals with mental retardation, and normally developing individuals. *Psychological Bulletin, 124,* 283–308.

Yirmiya, N., Sigman, M. D., Kasari, C., & Mundy, P. (1992). Empathy and cognition in high-functioning children with autism. *Child Development, 63,* 150–160.

Ylvisaker, M. (1989). Cognitive and psychosocial outcome following head injury in children. In T. M. Cole (Ed.), *Mild to moderate head injury.* London, UK: Blackwell.

Ylvisaker, M., & Gioia, G. A. (1998). Cognitive assessment. In M. Ylvisaker (Ed.), *Traumatic brain injury rehabilitation: Children and adolescents* (2nd ed., pp. 159–179). Boston: Butterworth-Heinemann.

Ylvisaker, M., Hartwick, P., & Stevens, M. (1991). School reentry following head injury: Managing the transition from hospital to school. *Journal of Head Trauma Rehabilitation, 6,* 10–22.

Ylvisaker, M., & Holland, A. L. (1984). Head injury. In W. H. Perkins (Ed.), *Language handicaps in children.* New York: Thieme-Stratton.

Ylvisaker, M., & Szekeres, S. F. (1989). Metacognitive and executive impairments in head-injured children and adults. *Topics in Language Disorders, 9,* 34–49.

Yoder, P., Kaiser, A., & Alpert, C. (1991). An exploratory study of the interaction between language teaching methods and child characteristics. *Journal of Speech and Hearing Research, 34,* 155–167.

Yont, K. (1998). The source of conversational breakdowns in typically developing preschoolers. Unpublished manuscript. University Park, PA: The Pennsylvania State University.

Yont, K., & Hewitt, L. (1999, November). Nature of conversational breakdowns in children with specific language impairment. Paper presented at the Annual Convention of the American Speech-Language-Hearing Association, San Francisco.

Yont, K., Hewitt, L., & Miccio, A. (2000). A coding system for describing conversational breakdowns in preschool children. *American Journal of Speech-Language Pathology, 9,* 300–309.

Yorkston, K. M., Jaffe, K. M., Liao, S., & Polissar, N. L. (1999). Recovery of written language production in children with traumatic brain injury: Outcomes at one year. *Aphasiology, 13,* 691–700.

Yoshinaga, H. (2000). Development of audition and speech: Implications for early intervention with infants who are deaf or hard of hearing. *Volta Review, 100,* 213–234.

Yoshinaga, H., & Downey, D. M. (1996). Development of school aged deaf, hard of hearing and normally hearing students' written language. *Volta Review, 98,* 3–7.

Yoshinaga-Itano, C. (1998). Development of audition and speech: Implications for early intervention with infants who are deaf or hard of hearing. *Volta Review, 100*(5), 212–234.

Yoshinaga-Itano, C., Stredler-Brown, A., & Jancosek, E. (1992). From phone to phoneme: What can we understand from babble. *Volta Review, 94*(3), 283–313.

Young, E., & Perachio, J. (1993). *The Patterned Elicitation Syntax Test with Morphological Analysis.* Tuscon, AZ: Communication Skill Builders.

Zachman, L., Huisingh, R., Barrett, M., Orman, J., & Blagden, C. (1989). *The Word Test—Adolescent.* Moline, IL: LinguiSystems.

Zhang, X., & Tomblin, J. B. (2000). The association of intervention receipt with speech-language profiles and social-demographic variables. *American Journal of Speech-Language Pathology, 9,* 345–357.

Zigler, E., & Balla, D. (1982). Introduction: The developmental approach to mental retardation. In E. Zigler & D. Balla (Eds.), *Mental retardation: The developmental-difference controversy* (pp. 3–8). Hillsdale, NJ: Lawrence Erlbaum.

Zigler, E., & Hodapp, R. M. (1986). *Understanding mental retardation.* New York: Cambridge University Press.

Zigler, E., & Hodapp, R. M. (1991). Behavioral functioning in individuals with mental retardation. *Annual Review of Psychology, 42,* 29–50.

Zimmerman, I., Steiner, V., & Pond, R. (1992). *Preschool Language Scale—3.* San Antonio, TX: Psychological Corporation.

Zimmerman, I., Steiner, V., & Pond, R. (1993). *Preschool Language Scale—3: Spanish edition.* San Antonio, TX: Psychological Corporation.

Zimmerman, I., Steiner, V., & Pond, R. (2002). *Preschool Language Scale—4.* San Antonio, TX: Psychological Corporation.

Zintz, M. (1970). *The reading process.* Dubuque, IA: William C. Brown.

NAME INDEX

SUBJECT INDEX